SIXTH EDITION

INNOVATIVE TEACHING STRATEGIES

IN NURSING

and Related Health Professions

Edited by

Martha J. Bradshaw, PhD, RN
Consultant
Professional Writing
Nursing Education
Dallas, Texas

Arlene J. Lowenstein, PhD, RN
Professor and Director
Health Professions Education Doctorate Program
Simmons College
Boston, Massachusetts

JONES & BARTLETT
LEARNING

World Headquarters
Jones & Bartlett Learning
5 Wall Street
Burlington, MA 01803
978-443-5000
info@jblearning.com
www.jblearning.com

Jones & Bartlett Learning books and products are available through most bookstores and online booksellers. To contact Jones & Bartlett Learning directly, call 800-832-0034, fax 978-443-8000, or visit our website, www.jblearning.com.

Production Credits

Executive Publisher: William Brottmiller
Senior Editor: Amanda Harvey
Associate Managing Editor: Sara Bempkins
Production Editor: Keith Henry
Senior Marketing Manager: Jennifer Stiles
V.P., Manufacturing and Inventory Control:
    Therese Connell
Composition: Laserwords Private Limited, Chennai, India
Cover Design: Kristin E. Parker
Cover Image: © Elenamiv/ShutterStock, Inc.
Printing and Binding: Edwards Brothers Malloy
Cover Printing: Edwards Brothers Malloy

Library of Congress Cataloging-in-Publication Data
Innovative teaching strategies in nursing and related health professions / [edited by] Martha J. Bradshaw and Arlene J. Lowenstein.—6th edition.
        p. ; cm.
    Preceded by Innovative teaching strategies in nursing and related health professions / edited by Martha J. Bradshaw, Arlene J. Lowenstein. 5th edition. 2011.
    Includes bibliographical references and index.
    ISBN 978-1-284-03099-0 (pbk.)
    I. Bradshaw, Martha J., editor of compilation. II. Lowenstein, Arlene J., editor of compilation.
    [DNLM: 1. Education, Nursing—methods. 2. Teaching—methods.   WY 18]
    RT71
    610.73071—dc23
                                                                                    2013020663
6048

Printed in the United States of America
17 16 15 14   10 9 8 7 6 5 4 3

Dedication

To teachers—past, present, and future.
May you continue to inspire, uplift, and transform.

And to students—past, present, and future.
May you always be enriched by good teaching.

Contents

■ Section VI: Evaluation   489

Preface

This edition of *Innovative Teaching Strategies in Nursing and Related Health Professions* continues the theme of interdisciplinary collaboration in health professions education. The need to capitalize on the contributions of numerous healthcare professionals is increasingly more important in light of the current, complex healthcare system. Education has a knowledge base that crosses over disciplinary lines and is one we need to understand in order to be effective in our work.

This text incorporates educational principles and techniques to encourage and advance learning for students in all higher education settings, at the graduate and the undergraduate levels. Learning is the focus, and educators can choose strategies that best address the learning needs of students in their professions. The diversity of learners has increased at all levels of higher education, such as cultural and ethnic diversity, generational differences, and lifestyle diversity, including the impact of the need to continue education despite the stresses of financial issues or special needs. Strategies for recognizing and working with a diverse student population are considered in this book. Learning about diversity is also presented in the use of study abroad programs.

As technology continues to rapidly grow and evolve, it is not possible to present all methods and versions that are available, but new and different ways to utilize technology to enhance learning are presented. What needs to be remembered by educators is that technology is a means, not an end, to enhance teaching effectiveness. It is the individual teacher who makes decisions based upon best education principles, about which strategy or form of technology to use in order to meet learning goals of both educators and students. The educational setting may also determine which technologies are available to use, but faculty may be able to encourage the purchase and development of technologies in their settings when they are aware of how they can be used to increase learning. Some students grasp the use of technology quickly and can benefit from the incorporation of technology in their learning, but other students are not as comfortable and may need additional faculty and support to promote a positive outcome. The chapters in this book address working with mixed media, simulations, distance and blended learning, and social media, among others.

Learning assessment and evaluation are important concepts for educators to be aware of and work with. Chapters in this book provide information and strategies to use in relation to assessing student learning in both theory and clinical practice and to programmatic evaluation, but also to finding and evaluating resources for use in planning and teaching.

It is our intent that this book will be a useful resource for educators in all health professions to become aware of and utilize strategies that encourage students to enhance and deepen their learning.

Martha J. Bradshaw
Arlene J. Lowenstein

Contributors

Stephanie S. Allen, RN, MSN, CNS
Clinical Nurse Specialist
Children's Medical Center Dallas
Dallas, Texas

Catherine Bailey, PhD, RN, CNE
College of Nursing
Texas Woman's University
Dallas, Texas

Martha J. Bradshaw, PhD, RN
Consultant
Professional Writing
Nursing Education
Dallas, Texas

LaDonna L. Christian, MSN, APRN-BC
Associate Professor of Practice and Nursing
Director of the Dotson Bridge and Mentoring Program
Simmons College
Boston, Massachusetts

Liliana Coman, BHSc(PT), MSc, MD
Assistant Professor
McMaster University, School of Rehabilitation Science
Hamilton, Ontario, Canada

Sharon M. Cosper, MHS, OTR/L
Georgia Regents University
SAHS, Department of Occupational Therapy
Augusta, Georgia

Mariana D'Amico, EdD, OTR/L, BCP
Associate Professor
College of Allied Health Sciences, Georgia Regents University
Augusta, Georgia

Brian M. French, RN, MS, BC
The Institute for Patient Care
Massachusetts General Hospital
Boston, Massachusetts

Shanti Freundlich, BA, MSLIS
Research Science, Liaison Librarian
Simmons College
Boston, Massachusetts

Miriam Greenspan, RN, MS
Brigham and Women's Hospital
Boston, Massachusetts

Maureen Harris, PT, DPT
Simmons College
Boston, Massachusetts

Lynn Jaffe, ScD, OTR/L
Georgia Regents University
SAHS, Department of Occupational Therapy
Augusta, Georgia

Judy Johnson-Russell, EdD, RN
Clinical Educator, Medical Education Technologies, Inc.
Professor Emerita, Texas Woman's University, Dallas
Sarasota, Florida

Ellen M. Landis, PhD, ADTR
Adjunct Faculty, Lesley University
Division of Expressive Therapies
Clinical Director, Sharevision, Inc.
Family Counseling and Consulting Group
Amherst, Massachusetts

Kimberly Leighton, PhD, RN
Associate Director, Simulation Center of Excellence, DeVry University
Downers Grove, Illinois

Arlene J. Lowenstein, PhD, RN
Professor and Director, Health Professions Education Doctoral Program
Simmons College
Professor Emerita
MGH Institute of Health Professions
Boston, Massachusetts

Jennifer E. Mackey, MA, CCC-SLP
MGH Institute of Health Professions
Department of Communication Sciences and Disorders
Boston, Massachusetts

Hendrika Maltby, PhD, RN, FACN
College of Nursing and Health Sciences
University of Vermont
Burlington, Vermont

Gail Matthews-DeNatale, PhD
Associate Dean, Graduate and Professional Programs
Emmanuel College
Formerly Interim Director
Academic Technology
Simmons College
Boston, Massachusetts

Lesley Maxwell
MGH Institute of Health Professions
Department of Communication Sciences and Disorders
Boston, Massachusetts

Marjorie Nicholas, PhD, CCC-SLP
Associate Chair, MGH Institute of Health Professions
Department of Communication Sciences and Disorders
School of Health and Rehabilitation Sciences
Boston, Massachusetts

Gregory G. Passmore, PhD, CNMT
Professor
Georgia Regents University
Augusta, Georgia

Shawna Patrick, RN, MS
Nurses for Nursing
Snowmass, Colorado

Lynda M. Pesta, RN, MSN
Louise Herrington School of Nursing
Baylor University
Dallas, Texas

Llewellyn S. Prater, RN, MSN, PhD
Louise Herrington School of Nursing
Baylor University
Dallas, Texas

Jeanine Salfi, PhD, RN
McMaster University
School of Nursing
Faculty of Health Sciences
Hamilton, Ontario, Canada

Patricia Solomon, PhD, PT
McMaster University
Faculty of Health Sciences
School of Rehabilitation Science
Hamilton, Ontario, Canada

Deborah Tapler, PhD, RN, CNE
College of Nursing
Texas Woman's University
Dallas, Texas

Karen H. Teeley, MS, RN, AHC-BC, CNE
Simmons College
Boston, Massachusetts

Cheryl A. Tucker, MSN, RN, CNE
Senior Lecturer & Undergraduate Theory Coordinator
Louise Herrington School of Nursing
Baylor University
Dallas, Texas

Julie Vosit-Steller, DNP, FNP-BC, AOCN
Simmons College
School of Nursing and Health Sciences
Boston, Massachusetts

Astrid Wilson, DSN, RN
Professor
WellStar School of Nursing
Kennesaw State University
Kennesaw, Georgia

Barbara C. Woodring, EdD, RN, CPN
Dean and Professor, Retired
Georgia State University
Byrdine F. Lewis School of Nursing
Atlanta, Georgia

Richard C. Woodring, BA, MDiv, DMin
Georgia Regents University
Division of Continuing Education
Augusta, Georgia

SECTION I

Introduction

Creating an effective learning environment is not an easy task in today's world, and it is even more complex in education programs for the health professions. Students entering the fields of health care are extremely diverse. Traditional undergraduates, entering college directly from high school, interact with a vast variety of nontraditional students returning to school after experiences in the workplace and/or having completed previous college degrees. There is a wide range of ages and experience within the student body. Educators are challenged to recognize different learning needs and respect and utilize the knowledge and experiences that students bring to the learning settings. The teaching strategies and examples throughout this text may be adapted for use in a variety of situations, at undergraduate and graduate levels, taking into account the diversity of learning needs.

The chapters in Section I provide a foundation for understanding, selecting, and adapting specific teaching strategies to the educator's setting and student body. The contributors provide a theory base for learning and critical thinking and bring in various dimensions of effective learning that include creativity, humor, and exploration of diverse viewpoints and ways of processing information.

CHAPTER 1

Effective Learning: What Teachers Need to Know

■ MARTHA J. BRADSHAW ■

"Knowing is a process, not a product."

— *Jerome Bruner (1966)*

What brings about effective learning in nursing students? Is it insight on the part of the student? A powerful clinical experience? Perhaps it is the dynamic, creative manner in which the nurse educator presents information or structures the learning experience. Effective learning likely is the culmination of all of these factors, in addition to others. In this chapter, dimensions of effective learning will be explored as a foundation for use of the innovative teaching strategies presented in subsequent chapters. The monumental growth in the use of technology has definitely changed the teaching–learning environment. Learners also have changed regarding how they access and use information and their expectations regarding feedback. The field of health professions education is experiencing a difference in learners, yet how individuals learn is essentially unchanged.

■ Theories of Learning

We approach learning individually, based largely on cognitive style (awareness of and taking in of relevant information) and preferred approaches to learning, or learning style. Some students are aware of their style and preference, some gain insight into these patterns as they become more sophisticated learners, and some students never have been guided to determine how they learn best.

Theoretical underpinnings classify learning as behavioristic or cognitive. Behavioristic learning was the earliest pattern identified through research. Psychologists such as Skinner and Thorndike described learning as a change in behavior and used stimulus response actions as an example. Subsequent theorists have described more complex forms of behaviorist learning. Bandura's (1977) theory of social learning describes human learning as coming from others through observation, imitation, and reinforcement. We learn from society, and we learn to be social. This type of learning is evident when we describe the need to socialize students to the profession of nursing.

Robert Gagne (1968) formulated suggestions for sequencing of instruction, conditions by which learning takes place, and outcomes of learning, or categories in which human learning occurs. These learning categories are based on a hierarchical arrangement of learning theories, moving from simple to complex learning, and include intellectual and motor skills, verbal information, cognitive strategies, and attitudes. For example, within the category of intellectual skills are the following stages:

- *Discrimination learning*: Distinguishing differences, so as to respond appropriately
- *Concept learning*: Detecting similarities, so as to understand common characteristics
- *Rule learning*: Combination of two or more concepts, as a basis for action in new situations

Gagne's ideas seem to combine behaviorism and cognitive theories. Use of behaviorism in nursing education was especially popular in the 1970s and early 1980s through the use of concrete, measurable, specific behavioral objectives. Even though nursing education has moved away from the concrete methods of learning and evaluation, use of the hierarchical arrangement is seen in curriculum development and learning outcomes.

Cognitive theories address the perceptual aspect of learning. Cognitive learning results in the development of perceptions and insight—also called gestalt—that bring about a change in thought patterns (causing one to think, "Aha") and related actions. Jerome Bruner (1966) described cognitive learning as processes of conceptualization and categorization. He contended that intellectual development includes awareness of one's own thinking, the ability to recognize and deal with several alternatives and sequences, and the ability to prioritize. Bruner also saw the benefit of discovery learning to bring about insights. Ausubel's (1968) assimilation theory focuses on meaningful learning, in which the individual develops a more complex cognitive structure by associating new meanings with old ones that already exist within the learner's frame of reference. Ausubel's theory relies heavily on the acquisition of previous knowledge. These principles are useful for introducing the new student to the healthcare environment by relating information to what the student knows about health and illness. The same principles are fundamental to curriculum development based upon transition from simple to complex situations. Having a good grasp of what is known is extremely helpful as learners move into new or unknown patient situations. This can be seen in the chapters on problem-based learning, clinical reasoning, and concept mapping, Gardner's theory of multiple intelligences recognizes cognition as more than knowledge acquisition. Based on his definition of intelligence as "the ability to solve problems or fashion products that are valued in more than one setting" (Gardner & Hatch, 1990, p. 5), Gardner has described the following seven forms of intelligence:

1. *Linguistic:* Related to written and spoken words and language, and use and meaning of language(s)
2. *Musical/rhythmic:* Based on sensitivity to rhythm and beat, recognition of tonal patterns and pitch, and appreciation of musical expression
3. *Logical/mathematical:* Related to inductive and deductive reasoning, abstractions, and discernment of numerical patterns
4. *Visual/spatial:* Ability to visualize an object or to create internal (mental) images, and thus able to transform or re-create the image
5. *Bodily kinesthetic.* The taking in and processing of knowledge through use of bodily sensations; learning is accomplished through physical movement or use of body language
6. *Interpersonal:* Emphasizes communication and interpersonal relationships, recognition of mood, temperament, and other behaviors
7. *Intrapersonal:* Related to inner thought processes, such as reflection and metacognition; includes spiritual awareness and self-knowledge (Gardner & Hatch, 1990)

Some educational programs use assessment tools based upon the work of Gardner and Hatch or similar assessments to guide incoming students on their approaches to learning and to better direct study skills. Faculty can benefit from this information as well and will find that student performance, as a group, is enhanced when a variety of teaching strategies are used. As an example, Slater, Lujan, and DiCarlo (2007) found that among first-year medical students, the females were more diverse in their sensory modalities and thus preferred multiple forms of information presentation.

Cognitive theories that address learning stages appropriate for college students include Perry's (1970) model of intellectual and ethical development. This model recognizes the following four nonstatic stages in which students progress: (1) dualism (black versus white), (2) multiplicity (diversity and tolerance), (3) relativism (decision made by reasoned support), and (4) commitment to relativism (recognition of value set for decision making). Perry's ideas can serve to explain how critical thinking is developed over time.

A related behavior pattern that can be associated with success in professional education is categorized as Executive functions (Lesaca, 2001). Executive functions are mental activities that are related to internal self-control and ability to employ goal-directed behavior. These functions then lead the individual to problem-solving ability and flexibility. Consequently, use of Executive functions promote better study skills and the ability to apply content knowledge to purposeful, professional actions.

■ Approaches to Learning

Emerging from learning theories are descriptions of preferred styles or approaches to learning. Categorized as cognitive styles and learning styles, these approaches to learning are the ways that individuals acquire knowledge, which are concerned more with form or process than content (Miller & Babcock, 1996). Cognitive style deals with information process, the natural, unconscious internal process concerned with thinking and memory. It is the stable and enduring manner in which individuals organize and handle information. The most common example of cognitive style is Witkin and colleagues' field dependent–field independent style (Witkin, Moore, Goodenough, & Cox, 1977). The field dependent–field independent style describes one's field of perception, or how one takes in information or data. Whereas one style generally predominates, people possess the capacity for both styles. Field-dependent individuals are global, are open to external sources of information, are influenced by their surroundings, and therefore see the situation as a whole, rather than identifying and focusing on the separate aspects of it. Field-dependent people tend to be social, people oriented, and sensitive to social cues. Learners in which the field-dependent style predominates may be externally motivated and therefore take a spectator or passive role in the learning process, preferring to be taught rather than to actively participate. Field-independent individuals are less sensitive to the social environment than field-dependent individuals, and thus take on a more analytical approach to information. By identifying aspects of the situation separately, they are able to restructure information and to develop their own system of classification. Field-independent learners enjoy concepts, challenges, and hypotheses and are task oriented (Miller & Babcock, 1996).

An aspect of learning style related to student behavior is response style. Kagan (1965) pioneered work, with school-age children, on the concepts of reflection and impulsiveness. These dimensions of cognitive response style describe personal tendencies regarding possibilities to solutions and choice selection. Individuals who have the impulsivity tendency prefer the quick, obvious answer, especially in highly uncertain problems, thus selecting the nearly correct answer as first choice. Reflective individuals identify and carefully consider alternatives before making a decision or choice. The implications for education in the health professions are apparent and will be discussed further. One problem that emerges with individuals who have a strong tendency in one of these dimensions is that the impulsive individual acts too quickly, based on an instant decision. Conversely, the reflective individual may be immobilized in decision making, which has outcomes implications.

Reflection, as associated with learning, was described as early as 1916 by John Dewey as being a process of inquiry (Miller & Babcock, 1996). To reflect on a situation, experience, or collection of information is to absorb, consider, weigh, speculate, contemplate, and deliberate. Such reflection serves either as a basis for reasoned action or to gain understanding or attach meaning to an experience. The most notable descriptions of reflection, especially as related to nursing, have been presented by Schön (1983). In his work, Schön related reflection to problem solving. He pointed out that traditional means of teaching and learning result in structured problem solving where the ends are clear and fixed. In the reality of health care, such ends are not always so concrete.

Schön also believed that professionals in practice demonstrate a unique proficiency of thinking, and he has described the following three aspects of this thinking: (1) knowing-in-action (use of a personally constructed knowledge base), (2) reflection-in-action (conscious thinking about what one is doing, awareness of use of knowledge), and (3) reflection-on-action (a retrospective look at thoughts and actions, to conduct self-evaluation and make decisions for future events). Reflection results in synthesis. This outcome is evident when the individual carries over thoughts, feelings, and conclusions to other situations. Teaching includes reflection-in-action, in which the teacher spontaneously adapts to learner reactions. Thus, reflection is the foundation for growth through experience. Reflection, as a form of thinking and learning, can be cultivated. Educators improve their teaching when they reflect upon episodes of teaching that were successful as well as those that were failures (Pinsky, Monson, & Irby, 1998).

One of the best-known descriptions of learning styles is Kolb's, which emerged from Dewey's seminal theory on experiential learning (Kolb, 1984). Dewey pioneered educational thinking regarding the relationship between learning and experience. The relationship between the learning environment and personal factors such as motivation and goals can lead the learner through a stream of experiences that, once connected, bring about meaningful learning (Kelly & Young, 1996). Using these ideas, Kolb went on to describe learning as occurring in the following stages: concrete experiences, observation and reflection on the experience, conceptualization and generalization, then theoretical testing in new and more complex situations. Learning is cyclical, with new learning coming from new experiences. Consequently, learning occurs in a comprehensive means, beginning with performance (concrete experience) and ending with educational growth. Kolb further explained that individuals go about this learning along the following two basic dimensions: grasping experiences (prehension), with abstract–concrete poles, and transforming, with action–reflection poles (Kelly & Young, 1996). Applying his experiential learning theory to his dimensions, Kolb identified these four basic learning styles:

1. *Convergers:* Prefer abstract conceptualization and active experimentation. These individuals are detached and work better with objects than people. They are problem solvers and apply ideas in a practical manner.
2. *Divergers:* Prefer concrete experience and reflective observation. Individuals with this tendency are good at generating ideas and displaying emotionalism and interest in others. Divergers are imaginative and can see the big picture.
3. *Assimilators:* Prefer abstract conceptualization and reflective observation. Assimilators easily bring together diverse items into an integrated entity,

sometimes overlooking practical aspects or input from others. Theoreticians likely are assimilators.

4. *Accommodators:* Prefer concrete experience and active experimentation. These individuals, while intuitive, are risk takers and engage in trial-and-error problem solving. Accommodators are willing to carry out plans, and they like and adapt to new circumstances (Miller & Babcock, 1996).

Gregorc's (1979) categorization of learning styles is similar to Kolb's, except that Gregorc believes that an individual's style is static, even in light of the changing educational setting. Thus, even through maturity and further learning, an individual still approaches learning in the same way. Gregorc uses the learning style categories of concrete sequential, concrete random, abstract sequential, and abstract random. In his research, Gregorc determined that individuals have preferences in one or two categories. In studying both first-year and fourth-year baccalaureate nursing students, Wells and Higgs (1990) discovered that these students have preferences in the concrete sequential and abstract random categories (total 81% of first-year students, 74% of fourth-year students).

■ Use of Learning Styles and Preferences

Theoretical foundations regarding learning and descriptive studies of cognitive and learning styles provide insight and understanding of self. It would be difficult to address research on all modes of learning in this one chapter. A summary application of information from the vast field of knowledge about learning theory and cognitive and learning styles has been developed by Svinicki (1994) as six operating principles, which are:

1. If information is to be learned, it must first be recognized.
2. During learning, learners act on information in ways that make it more meaningful.
3. Learners store information in long-term memory in an organized fashion related to their existing understanding of the world.
4. Learners continually check understanding, which results in refinement and revision of what is retained.
5. Transfer to new contexts is not automatic but results from exposure to multiple applications.
6. Learning is facilitated when learners are aware of their learning strategies and monitor their use (Svinicki, 1994, p. 275).

To understand one's own learning styles helps to understand one's own thinking, to be aware of a fit between style and strategies for learning, and thus to select the most effective and efficient means to go about learning. Some students are aware of how they learn best and gravitate toward that strategy. Instructors see this process in students who choose to sit in the front row of the class, take many notes, and feel involved with the topic, or students who prefer online learning, choose to not come to class but instead read course material, watch Internet clips or videos, and acquire information as it pertains to a clinical assignment. Some students adhere to tradition-bound forms of learning, such as lecture and reading, yet do not maximize their learning. This result explains why these students benefit more from direct clinical experiences. Many students find learning to be more powerful when they experience something new or significant in a clinical environment, then explore information and reflect on the experience. Learning experiences can be adapted to the environment and are influenced by the environment in which they occur. Awareness and comprehension of one's style of learning enables one to tailor the learning environment for optimal outcomes. A simple test that will guide the student in discovering his or her learning style(s) is presented in the teaching example at the end of this chapter.

Feedback from an observer, such as the instructor, can heighten awareness of personal styles. The knowledgeable educator also can guide the student in enhancing predominant styles or in beginning to cultivate additional dimensions of thinking and responding. For example, a student who is predominantly impulsive in decision making should be guided to explore outcomes of decisions and encouraged to increase reflection time as appropriate. Conversely, the student who is highly reflective may need to explore reasons that bring about hesitancy or prolonged deliberation and the outcomes of such behaviors.

■ Effective Teaching for Effective Learning

A knowledgeable and insightful educator is the key to effective learning in many situations. Consequently, the educator should call upon a knowledge base in learning and teaching as well as an extensive repertoire of useful strategies to reach learning goals. Faculty in health professions education are challenged to be directive in their teaching, addressing measurable learning outcomes that are directly linked to professional standards. This is juxtaposed with the importance of freeing the student from linear thinking and encouraging broader approaches to learning that are accomplished through dialogue, expression, and attribution of meaning. Instructors must determine best use of time, both for themselves and for students. So, difficult decisions must be made regarding what to leave in and what to omit from teaching episodes. In the health professions, faculty have to choose between teaching for practical judgment or for disciplinary knowledge. Specialized knowledge from within the discipline can clarify issues involved in practical situations, but it cannot determine judgment or a course of action (Sullivan & Rosin, 2008). This is where the role of the instructor, as a seasoned practitioner, is indispensible.

In their research to discover attributes of successful teachers at the rank of full professor, Rossetti and Fox (2009) developed these four categories for teaching success:

1. *Presence of the teacher:* Being there or available for the students, becoming acquainted with students, and cultivating mutual respect and trust

2. *Promotion of learning:* Interest in students' learning and finding meaning in their education
3. *Teachers as learners:* Staying current in the discipline and teaching strategies, and continually updating and refreshing courses
4. *Enthusiasm:* Conveying an interest in the subject and passion for the work

Regardless of setting, whether it be a traditional classroom, clinical care, synchronous or asynchronous electronic instruction, these principles of teaching success are applicable.

As students advance in their education, their established, comfortable ways of knowing, thinking, and reflection are challenged. This is especially true in the health professions, where students explore value systems that differ from their own and identify ethical dilemmas in practice or circumstances in which there is more than one right answer or no clear choice. In situations in which the research evidence diverges from existing paradigms that are known to students, and thus cause conflict in thinking, the instructor should be prepared to adapt and modify teaching to address this conflict (Fryer, 2008). Therefore, the instructor needs to be patently aware of his or her own teaching styles and how to amend his or her style for the circumstances.

Regarding the teaching strategies presented in this text, each strategy will have different effects on the attainment of learning outcomes in each student, based on the attributes and use of the strategy, in addition to learning and cognitive styles and learning preferences. Here are some broad suggestions for applying information about learning in teaching situations. The specific strategies addressed in subsequent chapters provide detailed information that enable faculty to use each method in an optimal way.

Underlying assumptions regarding the nature of professional education are derived in part from principles on adult learning, as formulated by Knowles (1978). Key principles include assuming responsibility for one's own learning and recognition of meaning or usefulness of information to be learned. Students in health professions are career oriented and need to see practical value in their educational endeavors. As consumers, adult students need to believe that they are receiving the maximum benefit from learning experiences. Furthermore, taking charge of one's own learning is empowering. Students who gain a sense of self-responsibility can feel empowered in other areas of their lives, such as professional practice. Faculty, in turn, have the responsibility to cultivate empowerment and to affect learning outcomes.

The teaching–learning experience, whether it is in a classroom environment or online, should be fresh and challenging each time the class convenes. Faculty should endeavor to provide variety in the manner in which they teach, rather than the same, predictable, albeit comfortable method of telling, rather than teaching. As providers of information, instructors need to remember that learning is best brought about by a combination of motivation and stimulation. The effective instructor should be the facilitator of learning in the students. In professional education, motivation is gained when the relationship to the well-being of the client is pointed out. The value of faculty experience is evident when the nurse-teacher shares from his or her own professional experiences and uses these anecdotes as examples for client outcomes. Nursing students and faculty agree that nontraditional strategies such as collaborative or cooperative learning, active involvement, and participation in the learning experience are desirable for effective learning. Students in professional education programs do respond positively to opportunities to choose or structure some of their learning experiences (Melrose, 2004). This approach should be used frequently by the teacher, to not only promote active learning but also to instill in students a sense of empowerment, which is an important attribute for the clinical setting. Technology-based learning activities direct the student to engage in independent learning, research, and use visual cues, such as video, to enhance comprehension.

As can be seen from the information on learning styles, students are more likely to remember information with which they can agree or relate and if they can attach meaning to the item or information. Disagreement or disharmony should be explored in an objective fashion. Viewpoints can then be strengthened or altered. Questioning and discussion should be based on the diversity that exists among the students. An instructor who is able to establish a sense of trust and confidence with the students can promote the expression of different perspectives likely to be found in the group. Professional educators should support students who are at various levels of cognitive growth, looking upon students from a criterion framework, rather than a normative one. Faculty should show that various viewpoints are welcome, legitimate, and worthy of discussion.

Effective educators guide students to see how their thought processes occur. They ask, "What do you know about ____?" or "How did you arrive at that answer/conclusion?" Teachers cultivate further development in the individual learners by demonstrating how to critique a theory, develop a rationale, or work through the steps of problem solving. These strategies will facilitate growth in students who are in an early cognitive stage such as dualism or will challenge more advanced students to a commitment to realism (Perry, 1970).

Delivery of information should be based on instructional theory in addition to content expertise. Using Ausubel's (1968) principles of advanced organizer, the teacher can develop inductive discovery by which students can build on previously acquired, simplistic knowledge to develop new or broader concepts. Effective learning experiences that emerge from identified styles should be developed and used in both class and clinical settings. Information from Kolb's four dimensions serves as an excellent example. Students who are convergers readily become bored with straight lecture, especially with topics that are abstract in nature. These individuals work better by themselves, so they are less likely to participate well in group projects. Learners with the diverger style learn from case studies and will actively participate in discussion, but they may have difficulty detaching personal values from the issue. These students often are visionary group leaders. Individuals with the assimilator style manipulate ideas well, so they will participate well in discussion or write comprehensive papers; however, these students may be less practical and have difficulty with some of the realism of clinical practice. Accommodators usually enjoy case studies, new or unusual teaching strategies, skills labs, and tinkering with new equipment. These learners will be most responsive to a challenging, complex client. With the multitude of learning opportunities available through electronic resources and patient simulation, teachers can readily craft a learning experience that meets most learning styles and preferences.

Skiba, Connors, and Jeffries (2009) cite nursing education as the field considered by many to be pioneers in the use of educational technology. Nursing, along with the other health professions, must face the challenges of incorporating core competencies, use of emerging technologies, and practice in informatics-intensive healthcare environments. However, one-way learning, such as web-based instruction, will not fully replace the competency-based instruction and verification that is needed in the applied disciplines of health care (Knapp, 2004).

In the clinical setting, the instructor may wish to provide introductory motivation through discovery learning. One way to accomplish this goal is to have each student observe or follow an individual in the clinical setting to gain exposure to the myriad tasks and responsibilities of a professional healthcare provider. Whereas students may have some rudimentary ideas of what healthcare providers do, they discover the depth and demands required in day-to-day work by observing actual practice. This strategy should broaden their perspectives and set the stage for meaningful learning, which includes increased retention of material and greater inquiry.

As students develop clinical written summaries about their clients, instructors should be flexible with the type of written work submitted. Traditionally, nursing students develop some form of a care plan based on the nursing process. The structured, linear method has taken criticism as the only way to look at clients. As a concrete, methodical strategy, the nursing process care plan is effective for students who are field independent and who can readily discern the data and related information needed for each step.

Additional methods of client summary or analysis should be introduced, and students should be encouraged to try each method. In doing so, students may broaden their ways of seeing clients and nursing problems, thus setting the stage for increased insight, analysis, and confidence. For example, use of the concept map is a way in which a student can envision the client or care situation in a holistic manner. Concept maps provide a fluidity that enhances the ability to determine relationships and make connections. Therefore, this strategy likely will be used positively by students who demonstrate Gardner's categories of visual/spatial or interpersonal intelligence. Learners who are field dependent also should do well with the concept map strategy because of their tendency to see the situation as a whole. Concept mapping should be effective for learners with all of Kolb's styles but for different reasons and with different outcomes.

Guided reflection, especially reflection-on-action, helps the student bring closure to the clinical experience, as well as conduct self-evaluation and gain from the experience. Journal writing is one of the most effective means by which the student can capture thoughts and responses and preserve these ideas in writing for subsequent consideration. This strategy is particularly useful as a means by which students can identify and modify impulsive-reflective tendencies. Journal writing will have the best results with divergers and assimilators, and some students may benefit from open discussion about the experiences entered into their journals. Again, feedback from the faculty is crucial and should be as thoughtful as the entries provided by the student. Faculty reading journals should guide the students in growth of insight and patterns of reflection.

Effective teachers in the health professions are those who possess content expertise, create an active learning environment, and use carefully selected teaching strategies (Wolf, Bender, Beitz, Wieland, & Vito, 2004). One of the greatest challenges for faculty is in developing the blend of strategies to bring about effective learning in all students. Part of the challenge is the fit between the faculty's styles and learning preferences and that of each of the learners. Faculty especially should be on guard against favoritism to students who possess the same attributes as the instructor. Conversely, the congruency between styles of the teacher and of the student may enhance a relationship that is especially meaningful and may evolve into professional mentoring.

■ Future Considerations

From this chapter, many ideas that are worthy of more detailed scrutiny emerge. The majority of research on cognitive styles, learning style, and learning preferences was conducted in the 1970s and 1980s. This was before the widespread accepted use of electronic technology. Use of technology in teaching and learning may be influenced by learning preferences, such as in visual and kinesthetic learners. Have some students learned to modify their preferences to become more comfortable with technology? Online education is widely accepted, and the role of the instructor is changing. The extent to which learners continue to value the presence of the instructor for spontaneous teaching is worthy of investigation. Currently, there is a shift in education toward student-centered, active learning for the development of critical thinking, coupled with generations of students who are used to immediate feedback and a variety of stimulation. Educators must determine if selected strategies are useful for genuine learning or, if not used properly, merely providing entertainment.

■ Conclusion

Effective learning is more than merely the results of good teaching. It is enhanced by a learning environment that includes active interactions among faculty, students, and student peers. Effective learning is achieved through the use of creative strategies designed not to entertain but to inform and stimulate. The best ways faculty can bring about effective learning are by recognizing students as individuals, with unique, personal ways of knowing and learning, by creating learning situations that recognize diversity, and by providing empowering experiences in which students are challenged to think.

TEACHING EXAMPLE:

How Do I Learn Best?

This instrument typically takes 4–6 minutes to complete and can be self-scored. The style categories are visual, aural, read/write, and kinesthetic, which correspond with categories found in Gardner's multiple forms of intelligence. Students are directed to answer the brief questions, then are shown the learning modalities that best fit predominant styles.

HOW DO I LEARN BEST?

This test is to find out something about your preferred learning method. Research on left brain/right brain differences and on learning and personality differences suggests that each person has preferred ways to receive and communicate information.

Choose the answer that best explains your preference and put the key letter in the box. If a single answer does not match your perception, please enter two or more choices in the box. Leave blank any question that does not apply. Once you have completed the test, find the totals for each of the letters (*V, A, R, K*) that correspond with a learning preference. Then look at the table of learning modalities (**Table 1-1**) to see which strategies best support your learning preference.

Table 1-1   Learning Modalities

	In Class	*When Studying*	*For Exams*
Visual	Underline Use different colors Use symbols, charts, arrangements on a page	Recall visual aspects of presentation Reconstruct images in different ways Redraw pages from memory Replace words with symbols and initials	Recall the pictures on the pages Draw, use diagrams where appropriate Practice turning visuals back into words

	In Class	*When Studying*	*For Exams*
Aural	Attend lectures and listen Discuss topics with students Use a tape recorder Discuss overheads, pictures, and other visual aids Leave space in notes for later recall	May take poor notes because of preference for voices Expand notes by talking out ideas Explain new ideas to another student Read assignments out loud	Speak the answers/ tutorials Practice writing answers to an old exam Read questions to yourself or have someone read them to you
Reading/writing	Use lists, headings Write out lists and definitions Use handouts and textbooks	Write out the words Reread notes silently Rewrite ideas in other words Use lecture notes/ read	Practice with multiple-choice questions Write paragraphs, beginnings, endings Organize diagrams into statements
Kinesthetic: use all of the senses	May take notes poorly because topics do not seem relevant Go to lab, take field trips Use trial-and-error method Listen to real-life examples	Put examples in note summaries Talk about notes, especially with another kinesthetic person Use pictures and photos to illustrate	Write practice answers Role-play the exam situation in one's head

1. Suppose you are about to give directions to a person. She is staying in a hotel in town and wants to visit your house. She has a rental car. Would you:
   V) draw a map on paper?
   R) write down the directions (without a map)?
   A) tell her the directions by phone?
   K) collect her from the hotel in your car?

(continued)

2. Suppose you are staying in a hotel and have a rental car. You would like to visit a friend whose address/location you do not know. Would you like him to:
   V) draw you a map on paper?
   R) write down the directions (without a map)?
   A) tell you the directions by phone?
   K) collect you from the hotel in his car?

3. Imagine that you have just received a copy of your itinerary for a world trip. This is of interest to a friend. Would you:
   A) call her immediately and tell her about it?
   R) send her a copy of the printed itinerary?
   V) show her the itinerary on a map of the world?

4. Suppose you are going to cook a dessert as a special treat for your family. Do you:
   K) cook something familiar without need for instructions?
   V) thumb through the cookbook looking for ideas from the pictures?
   R) refer to a specific cookbook where there is a good recipe?
   A) ask for advice from others?

5. Suppose a group of tourists has been assigned to you to find out about national parks. Would you:
   K) drive them to a national park?
   R) give them a book on national parks?
   V) show them slides and photographs?
   A) give them a talk on national parks?

6. Imagine that you are about to purchase a new stereo. Other than price, what would most influence your decision?
   A) A friend talking about it.
   K) Listening to it.
   R) Reading the details about it.
   V) Its distinctive, upscale appearance.

7. Recall a time in your life when you learned how to do something like playing a new board game. Try to avoid choosing a very physical skill, such as riding a bike. How did you learn best? By:
   V) visual clues—pictures, diagrams, charts?
   A) listening to somebody explaining it?
   R) written instructions?
   K) doing it?

8. Which of these games do you prefer?
   V) Pictionary
   R) Scrabble
   K) Charades

9. Suppose you are about to learn to use a new program on a computer. Would you:
   K) ask a friend to show you?
   R) read the manual that comes with the program?
   A) telephone a friend and ask questions about it?

10. Imagine that you are not sure whether a word should be spelled *d-e-p-e-n-d-e-n-t* or *d-e-p-e-n-d-a-n-t*. Do you:
    R) look it up in the dictionary?
    V) see the word in your mind and choose the best way it looks?
    A) sound it out in your mind?
    K) write both versions down?

11. Apart from price, what would most influence your decision to buy a particular book?
    K) Using a friend's copy.
    R) Skimming parts of it.
    A) A friend talking about it.
    V) It looks OK.

12. Suppose a new movie has arrived in town. What would most influence your decision to go or not go?
    A) Friends talked about it.
    R) You read a review about it.
    V) You saw a preview of it.

13. Do you prefer a lecturer/teacher who likes to use:
    R) handouts and/or a textbook?
    V) flow diagrams, charts, and slides?
    K) field trips, labs, and practical sessions?
    A) discussion and guest speakers?

Source: Gardner & Hatch, 1990.

REFERENCES

Ausubel, D. P. (1968). *Educational psychology: A cognitive view.* New York, NY: Holt, Rinehart and Winston.

Bandura, A. (1977). *Social learning theory.* Morristown, NJ: General Learning Press.

Bruner, J. (1966). *Toward a theory of instruction.* New York, NY: W. W. Norton & Co.

Fryer, G. (2008). Teaching critical thinking in osteopathy: Integrating craft knowledge and evidence-informed approaches. *International Journal of Osteopathic Medicine, 11*(2), 56–61.

Gagne, R. M. (1968). Learning hierarchies. *Educational Psychologist, 6,* 1–9.

Gardner, H., & Hatch, T. (1990). *Multiple intelligences go to school: Educational implications of the theory of multiple intelligences* (Technical Report No. 4). New York, NY: Center for Technology in Education.

Gregorc, A. F. (1979). Learning/teaching styles: Their nature and effects. In National Association of Secondary School Principals (Eds). *Student learning styles* (pp. 19–26). Reston, VA: National Association of Secondary School Principals.

Kagan, J. (1965). Reflection-impulsivity and reading ability in primary grade children. *Child Development, 36,* 609–628.

Kelly, E., & Young, A. (1996). Models of nursing education for the 21st century. In K. Stevens (Ed.), *Review of research in nursing education* (vol. vii, pp. 1–39). New York, NY: National League for Nursing.

Knapp, B. (2004). Competency: An essential component of caring in nursing. *Nursing Administration Quarterly, 28,* 285–287.

Knowles, M. A. (1978). *The adult learner: A neglected species* (2nd ed.). Houston, TX: Gulf Publishing.

Kolb, D. A. (1984). *Experiential learning theory.* Englewood Cliffs, NJ: Prentice-Hall.

Lesaca, T. (2001). Executive functions in parents with ADHD. *Psychiatric Times, 18*(11), 4.

Melrose, S. (2004). What works? A personal account of clinical teaching strategies in nursing. *Education for Health, 17,* 236–239.

Miller, M. A., & Babcock, D. E. (1996). *Critical thinking applied to nursing.* St. Louis, MO: Mosby.

Perry, W. G. (1970). *Forms of intellectual and ethical development in the college years: A scheme.* New York, NY: Holt, Rinehart and Winston.

Pinsky, L. E., Monson, D., & Irby, D. M. (1998). How excellent teachers are made: Reflecting on success to improve teaching. *Advances in Health Sciences Education, 3,* 207–215.

Rossetti, J., & Fox, P. G. (2009). Factors related to successful teaching by outstanding professors: An interpretive study. *Journal of Nursing Education, 48*(1), 11–16.

Schön, D. A. (1983). *The reflective practitioner: How professionals think in action.* New York, NY: Basic Books.

Skiba, D. J., Connors, H. R., & Jeffries, P. R. (2008). Information technologies and the transformation of nursing education. *Nursing Outlook, 56*(5), 225–230.

Slater, J. A., Lujan, H. L., & DiCarlo, S. E. (2007). Does gender influence learning style preferences of first-year medical students? *Advances in Physiology Education, 31,* 336–342.

Sullivan, W. M., & Rosin, M. S. (2008). A life on the mind for practice: Bridging liberal and professional education. *Change, 40*(2), 44–47.

Svinicki, M. D. (1994). Practical implications of cognitive theories. In K. A. Feldman & M. B. Paulsen (Eds.), *Teaching and learning in the college classroom* (pp. 274–281). Needham Heights, MA: Ginn Press.

Wells, D., & Higgs, Z. R. (1990). Learning and learning preferences of first and fourth semester baccalaureate degree nursing students. *Journal of Nursing Education, 29,* 385–390.

Witkin, H. A., Moore, C. A., Goodenough, D. R., & Cox, P. W. (1977). Field-dependent and field-independent cognitive styles and their implications. *Review of Educational Research, 47,* 1–64.

Wolf, Z. R., Bender, P. J., Beitz, J. M., Wieland, D. M., & Vito, K. O. (2004). Strengths and weaknesses of faculty teaching performance reported by undergraduate and graduate nursing students: A descriptive study. *Journal of Professional Nursing, 20,* 118–128.

CHAPTER 2

Culture and Diversity in the Classroom

■ ARLENE J. LOWENSTEIN AND LADONNA L. CHRISTIAN ■

Today's classrooms are very different from those in the past. Immigration, both forced and voluntary, has shaped the face of the United States. Each new wave of immigrants adds to the mosaic that is the United States. A mosaic is made up of many pieces, each different in size and shape; some may be brightly colored and others pale, transparent, or with no color added. Each piece does not mean much by itself, but when put together, the pieces change, forming new designs and an overall effect very different from the mosaic's component pieces. The strength of that mosaic is the ability to capitalize on new and different ideas. Its weakness is the clash between cultures that feeds prejudice and discriminatory behaviors. Health professions educators and leaders have recognized this change, and cultural competence of practitioners is now being stressed in both education and service. By using the strengths and originality of diverse students, the final classroom product can be much stronger than the product of an assimilated, cookie cutter one.

A new emphasis on civil rights, feminism, sexuality, and morality issues in the late 1960s and 1970s brought about drastic changes in what had been considered accepted societal behavior. Those changes shaped the move toward increased diversity of both patients and student body in our world today and provided new and different opportunities and challenges from those of the past. Change continues as you read this, and classrooms in the future may look very different. Educators need to be flexible, aware of trends and patterns, and able to respond to continuing challenges. This chapter presents a brief glimpse at some of the diversity issues in the past and present day, and it discusses some of the issues and strategies involved in working with a diverse classroom population.

■ The Past

In the 1950s, healthcare professional education was almost nonexistent for African Americans (Blacks), other *multicultural students*, and persons with disabilities. Men went into medicine, while women became nurses. Other health professions may have had some of each gender, but women were often in the majority (Moffat, 2003). Educational facilities were often segregated culturally and religiously, not only in the South, which had a history of legal segregation at that time, but in the North as well (Carnegie, 1991, 2005). Catholic and Jewish hospitals often had their own schools of nursing, and there were religious and ethnic student quotas in many colleges and universities. This meant that most classes were homogenized, with a large majority of Caucasian (White) and Protestant students in all but the religion-sponsored or minority-established programs, and those were few and far between. Very few Hispanic, Asian, Islamic, or Muslim students were admitted to the schools. For multicultural students who were admitted, retention rates were often low (Carnegie, 1991).

Nursing education was founded in hospital diploma programs using the apprentice system of education. From the early days in the late 1800s through the 1950s, there were very few graduate nurses in hospitals. Most graduate nurses moved into private duty after graduation, with some going into public health and a few staying on primarily in managerial or teaching positions. Student nurses were the major providers of care for hospital patients. Very ill patients on the hospital wards were most often assigned a private-duty nurse to care for them, usually paid for by the patients and their families, although hospitals absorbed the cost in some instances.

In 1946, shortly after World War II, the Hill-Burton Act was passed in Congress and signed into law. It provided funds to hospitals for renovation, expansion, capital projects, and new hospital buildings. As hospitals expanded, more nurses and other healthcare professionals were needed. Another trend was the development of intensive care units in the mid-1950s, and skilled nurses were needed for those areas as well. The nursing students and nurses in the labor pool during those years were still primarily Caucasian and Protestant with few minorities.

During that time, although it seems hard to believe in today's world, very few nursing schools admitted married students. Female students were dismissed from the program if they chose to get married, if the secret marriages that occurred were found out by school authorities, and even if they were almost ready to graduate. In the few schools where married students were permitted, pregnant women were excluded, and pregnancy out of wedlock was an unforgivable sin for health professions education.

Nursing was viewed as a women's profession, and few men were permitted in. Those men who were nurses had severe restrictions in clinical experiences such as obstetrics and gynecology, but they could be welcomed in psychiatric facilities because it was thought that they were stronger and could work better with distraught and violent patients. It was generally considered that students with disabilities would not be able to participate in providing all aspects of care, so they were not admitted to programs. There were no allowances made. In Augusta, Georgia, from the early 1900s through the early 1960s, University Hospital had two schools of nursing, the Lamar school for Blacks and the Barrett school for Whites (Lowenstein, 1990, 1994). The two schools joined together in 1965, after the passage of civil rights legislation. The Barrett school accepted more nursing students and had a higher graduation rate than the Lamar school. One year, three Asian students applied and were admitted to the Barrett school, but only one graduated. In Augusta, as in most of the South, and often in the North (although no one talked about that), Black students were assigned to the units with Black patients, and White students with Whites. Supervisors, administrators, and teachers were almost always White.

The late 1960s and early 1970s brought a revolutionary change, which has continued expanding since that time. The civil rights movement sparked a feminist movement, and those movements opened previously closed doors in education. Women had more opportunities to be admitted to healthcare professions that were previously male dominated. A few men were admitted into programs that had only women students, although the numbers were still small and discrimination prevalent, especially due to the belief that male nurses were homosexual. The sexual revolution of those years also brought a change in thinking about sexual orientation, although many attitudes of the past persist today, and discrimination still occurs. In nursing, the rules against marriage were dropped, and women could attend school while pregnant. Although the changes have been gradual, the face of the classroom is continuing its transformation.

During this period of time, the community college movement began, which provided more access to multicultural students, to those who could not afford private college tuition, and to students who needed educational facilities closer to their homes. This was a boon to older women, including women of color, and those with families who could attend less expensive schools that were closer to home. Part-time attendance was possible in some programs, and nursing students no longer needed to live at the hospitals. Graduates of associate degree programs in nursing were eligible for licensure as registered nurses and took less time to graduate than the typical 3-year diploma program students. Many hospital diploma schools began to close, although that was a prolonged fight. During those years, nursing leaders recognized the discrimination against women in college and university admissions. They were pleased that nursing education had moved out of the hospital program, but they were not satisfied. In an effort to raise the status of women in the profession, they began a move toward baccalaureate education for all nurses by 1984, which also helped the demise of hospital programs. However, for many reasons, the baccalaureate goal was not achieved.

The physical therapy profession and its professional organization, the American Physical Therapy Association (APTA), were begun by women, but men were recognized in the profession by the 1920s. However, even with the feminist movements of the 1960s and 1970s, it took until the early 1990s for the APTA to feel it important enough to address women's issues and the inequities in the profession as it pertained to the disparities in the professional and economic status of women. The board of directors appointed the first Committee on Women in Physical Therapy, and in 1994 the Office of Women's Issues was created at APTA headquarters in Alexandria, Virginia. The Office of Minority Affairs also became an integral part of the APTA headquarters at this time, as the profession tried to recruit more minorities (Moffat, 2003). Those years also saw the beginning of affirmative action, and an increased number of multicultural students began to be admitted to colleges, although the numbers were still small. The end of the Vietnam War began an Asian migration to the United States, and we have seen other migrations since that time, creating increased Latino/Hispanic, Muslim, Indian, and Russian-Jewish populations in the United States, among others. Those migrations have meant more diverse students accepted into health professions programs. In 1990, the Americans with Disabilities Act (ADA) was passed by Congress and signed into law. It required educators to think differently about what could be done to provide access and retention for disabled persons who would be able to work in some, if not all, aspects of their chosen health profession and thereby provide a valuable service for the profession and its patients.

■ The Present

So where has this history led us in the classroom in today's world? The health professions classroom is more diverse than ever before. However, diversity no longer means ethnic background alone. The age range may be wide and gender ratios may have changed, although nursing still has a minority of male students. In medicine it worked the other way around, and more women have gone into that field than ever before. There is diversity in sexual orientation, though discrimination on this basis still exists.

There are diverse social and family issues in the classroom. Many divorced and single parents have gone back to school, but often have great responsibility in raising their children alone, which may interfere with the amount of time that can be allotted to school work (Grosz, 2005; Ogunsiji & Wilkes, 2005). In some places, disadvantaged students have come into the health professions classrooms as new economic relief programs are put into place (Wessling, 2000). Students, especially older ones, may have caretaker responsibilities for their parents or other relatives including children with disabilities. Those in the "sandwich generation" may have caretaker responsibilities for both their parents and their children.

We also have wealthy students, for whom textbook purchases and other expenses are not a problem, and need-based scholarship students and other students who may have real concerns about the financial issues that can impact on their doing well and completing their program. Tuition increases and the spectre of repayment of student loans may create additional stress. Financially secure students do not always have it easy just because they have the financial means, because they may have other family and social problems that affect them and their classroom abilities.

The number of disabled students, with both physical and learning disabilities, has increased. Due to technological advances and better awareness, educational institutions are now able to provide more accommodations for students with disabilities. These may include policy modifications, equipment, and physical changes to increase handicap access. Students with disabilities often have concerns about how they are being perceived by others and worry that other students and faculty are expecting them to fail. Research has shown that creative problem solving and faculty support can be developed for students with disabilities, and health professions education programs can be enriched by their presence (Carroll, 2004).

Colleges and universities are being encouraged to promote diversity in both hiring faculty and in student recruitment and admissions, although success rates are still low (Silver, 2002; Barbee & Gibson 2001). Even though affirmative action has been under fire, it is recognized that there is still a need to make higher education more accessible for both minorities and students with disabilities. Although diversity in admissions and hiring may be strongly encouraged, retaining diverse students and faculty is often difficult. However, Splenser and his colleagues (Splenser, Canlas, Sanders, & Melzer, 2003), in a study of physical therapy educational programs, found that when schools provided special retention efforts, they were effective in increasing the numbers of graduating multicultural students. They also found a positive correlation between increased applications from diverse students and the presence of multicultural faculty in a program.

Other researchers have found that many multicultural students experience significant culture shock when entering the collegiate world, which may be very different from their previous life experiences. In schools or programs with low numbers of diverse students and faculty, the recruited multicultural students often feel excluded in an educational system in which their values, knowledge, and practices are largely ignored. Because Blacks are frequently in the minority in such a classroom, feelings of isolation, alienation, and loneliness, as well as perceived racism, can cause academic difficulties. Inadequate academic preparation for the rigor of college, family conflicts, and lack of financial resources can contribute to that failure. In many cases, support services are offered by institutions but might not be used (Kosowski, Grams, Taylor, & Wilson, 2001). Bain (2004) reported that negative stereotypes are often internalized by multicultural students. The resulting educational disparities are evident in learning outcomes. That can apply to disabled persons as well (Bain, 2004). These feelings can be compounded by impersonal, and sometimes hostile, treatment from faculty, who are still predominately White. **Multicultural faculty** also face these feelings, and, in turn, this often leads to students dropping out of school and faculty leaving educational positions (Evans, 2004; Kosowski et al., 2001; Vasquez, 1990).

There are many causes for the lack of success of multicultural students in the classroom. Kirkland (1998) found a difference in psychological stress between Black and White nursing students. Blacks often felt more stress and perceived their environment differently. Because of the history of discrimination and their previous experiences with discrimination, Blacks may perceive discrimination, even though White students, employers, or other employees in a healthcare setting do not feel that discrimination exists (Lowenstein & Glanville, 1995). Kosowski and colleagues (2001) noted that the failure rate for Black students can be higher than that for their White counterparts. These issues are not limited to Blacks but often affect other multicultural students, as well as White students from poorer economic strata. Evans (2004) found Hispanic/Latino and Native American nursing students struggled with similar feelings. Those in the study described the impact of perceived lack of options for multicultural students. Even before they entered the program, it was difficult for them to imagine themselves being successful in a healthcare profession. Language issues can be difficult to overcome. Lack of family support due to financial or cultural expectations and ignorance of academic demands was also identified as a barrier to success for some students, especially those who were the first in their families to attend college. Students who successfully confronted those barriers were helped by faculty who recognized these stressors, worked to respect students' intense obligation to family and community, and provided long-term, personal encouragement to continue in the program (Evans, 2004).

■ The Importance of Culture in Education

Language, ethnicity, religion, class, lifestyle, gender, and power shape culture. A person's cultural relevance is confirmed through values, beliefs, and traditions. Other cultural influences include ways of thinking and being. These characteristics are shared and identifiable in groups of people with a common geography, history, and communication system (Sieffert, 2006).

One of the main challenges of education is creating a learning environment that preserves cultural integrity for all students while enhancing their educational achievement (Phuntsog, 1999). Many educational institutions attempt to acknowledge cultures by offering a course in multicultural education, which is expected to address a breadth and depth of cultural diversity. Educators are expected to overcome years of deep-rooted societal beliefs that question or challenge cultural hegemony and adopt transformational curricula of social justice. However, there is a need for educators to recognize that culture is central to who we are. Attempts to dismiss it or mandate complete acculturation may have injurious effects on the ability of multicultural students to experience positive learning outcomes. Successful student-centered learning requires that educators are prepared to adapt their curricula based on the cultural needs of the community in which they serve (Phuntsog, 1999). Teachers who have been successful with diverse students have set up situations where positive expectations are verbalized and integrated into the classroom. Letting multicultural students know that there is respect for their abilities has been shown to lead to improvement in pass rates (Bain, 2004).

Researchers have confirmed the benefits of creating a learning environment that is relevant to, and reflective of, student realities, customs, and beliefs.

Encouraging cultural and ethnic identity in the classroom diminishes negative experiences, increases self-confidence and self-esteem, and promotes resiliency in multicultural students (Kana'iaupuni, Ledward, & Jensen, 2009). Culturally inclusive pedagogical approaches are associated with the survival of ethnicity, tradition, and language. Culture is also vital to the functioning of social and family networks and support systems that may contribute to the sustainability of diverse ethnic groups in the classroom (Kana'iaupuni et al., 2009). However, a focus on individual groups and classrooms can obscure the role and responsibility of broader society in addressing educational inequity (Nasir & Hand, 2006). Hancock (2004) described the convergence of numerous aspects of social identity and memberships in marginalized multicultural communities as intersectionality. These inequities create a multiplicity of barriers and add important implications to our consideration of cultural differences in education (Hancock, 2004). Think about the term *minority*. This term is often used to describe multicultural and diverse students. What does that label mean to students? The connotation is that they are out of the mainstream, not as good as the majority students, and often expected to fail. Bain noted that even students who had a strong self-image could fall into the trap of feeling that they needed to prove themselves, leading to increased anxiety, stress, and eventually failure (Bain, 2004).

■ Culture and Educational Theories

The definition of *culture* depends on whether the author's viewpoint is sociological or anthropological. In the sociological view, education socializes people into society's mainstream. Thus education focuses on forming an organized social structure by bringing people together from multifarious backgrounds and Americanizing them (Sieffert, 2006). Early researchers in sociological education sought to explain racial deficits in learning and achievements as both biological and cultural. In the 1970s, educational sociologists began to argue that multicultural children were not deficient in their cognitive and social orientations, but rather were different than mainstream society in their learning styles. Sociologists then began to develop new conceptual models to better understand cultural differences and to explore ways to design pedagogical approaches and classroom environments to support culturally diverse children (Nasir & Hand, 2006).

Educational anthropologists define culture as a complex whole including knowledge, beliefs, morals, customs, and a social heritage that are transmitted and shared from one generation to another. The anthropological approach to education reduces ethnocentrism by instilling an appreciation for other cultures and contributes to the understanding of other human beings (Nasir & Hand, 2006). The anthropologist theory of education takes into consideration the many aspects of culture and is concerned with cultural transmission. Cultural transmission involves both enculturation and acculturation or the movement of cultural beliefs across traditional educational lines (Sieffert, 2006). There are three major influences of the anthropological view that contribute to our understanding of how culturally diverse students learn. First, there is the belief is that culturally diverse students are no less capable than members of the majority population, but their variances in learning are attributed to language, culture, life experiences, and learning styles. Second, educational anthropology looks beyond exam scores and takes into account the entire schooling experience. Third, educational anthropologists view education as a process in which all participants contribute in shaping the outcomes (Jacob & Jordan, 1996, pp. 15–23).

Many theorists have attempted to rationalize the apertures in student performance. Most have focused on home, environment, communication styles, language, and cultural mismatch as the major problems with culture and learning (Jacob & Jordan, 1996). Oppositional theorists have cited societal inequities and experiences with discrimination as participatory causes explaining why students of minority cultures have difficulty learning (Kana'iaupuni et al., 2009). Although both sociological and anthropological education theories have their advantages, current researchers have demonstrated that understanding the culture of the population that we serve in our classroom makes a positive difference in learning outcomes. Anthropologists highlight the roles of communication styles, social interaction, and cultural norms with a focus on ethnographic process–based descriptions of teaching and learning. The fundamental idea of educational anthropology is that learning occurs as teachers negotiate complex social interactions that are often formed by a set of cultural differences in customs and resolutions (Nasir & Hand, 2006).

■ Pedagogy and Cultural Influences

All educational systems and institutions of learning are ingrained in a particular cultural worldview. The issue of culture has had a strong influence on pedagogy, and learning has not improved to date. Education is affected by culture, and the role of culture is germane to instructional design. Culture affects not only what students learn, but also how they learn. Cultural values and beliefs provide a basis for how a person interacts when learning and how a person perceives learning. Thus, culture and learning are intertwined and intricate. Pedagogy does not begin and end in the classroom. It should also reflect the practices of the community that it serves, locally, nationally, and internationally (Dale, 2009, pp. 27–37). Pedagogical strategies that include multicultural education, cultural competence, and cultural inclusivity must have an increased representation in curricula (Nasir & Hand, 2006). Because learning theories are not necessarily inclusive or compatible, educators must borrow from many different approaches (Vincent & Ross, 2001). Approaches to learning should be modified to include learning styles from different cultural backgrounds, because cultural diversity contributes to innovation and creativity within an educational environment (Sieffert, 2006).

■ Learning Styles and Cultural Implications

In most traditional classrooms, the pedagogical process functions according to mainstream assumptions about culture, which empowers some voices more than others. Some Asian Americans come from cultures where eye contact and active participation are not normal experiences and may be uncomfortable with them (Suinn, 2006). They also tend to remain silent out of consideration for others and do not interrupt class members. This can manifest as minimal participation in class discussion, and they may sit back and not offer comments in class, even when they have a good understanding of the material and would have information that would be helpful to the class or need clarification and additional help with a concept (Fiume, 2005). Hawaiians and Native Americans are accustomed to helping one another instead of working at their desks independently. Both cultures feel strongly about this way of learning and collaboration is the norm. Participants may not want to stand out from the group because individual praise is discouraged. They believe that it spotlights a person and is culturally incongruous, whereas group praise is anthropologically acceptable (Swisher, 1991; Vogt, Jordan, & Tharp, 1987). Other researchers have indicated that students of African descent and Latinos are also more group oriented, cooperative, and less competitive than those of European descent. Traditionally, most educators see unassigned group work as cheating and not collaborating or modeling (Griggs & Dunn, 1996). The cultural values of European Americans thrive on collaboration and discussion and getting their opinions heard. Class discussion is more acceptable because it is what they are used to and offers an opportunity to show off their knowledge base. They also tend to be more individualistic and often competitive (Fiume, 2005). Of course, students raised in the American culture can also be shy or nonparticipating, especially in large classes, and small-group discussions can be helpful for them as well. In higher education, the phenomenon of group assessment, collaboration, and cooperative learning is becoming a positive trend.

Although we are making improvements toward developing new innovative pedagogical assessment tools, group collaboration on exams is still viewed negatively and forbidden in many classrooms. Additionally, Pewewardy (2002) stated that many culturally diverse students are field dependent, where European-descent students are field independent. Field dependency or global processing is a learning style in which students are unable to perceive themselves as separate from their environment. These students are holistic learners, right-brain dominant, highly relational, visual/spatial, intuitive, integrative, and contextual. The field-dependent learner establishes meaning only in relation to the whole and prefers a loosely structured learning environment that includes group work and collaboration (Graybill, 1997). Field-independent learners tend to be linear or hierarchical, analytical, logical, and temporal. These learners often prefer classroom activity that requires competition and individual gain as well as impersonal work. Field-independent learners are able divide and subdivide the whole into minute pieces. When classroom information is presented in an analytical and sequential manner, this places field-dependent learners at a disadvantage (Graybill, 1997).

■ Learning Styles and Pedagogical Strategies

Researchers have suggested that no single instructional method will be effective in a culturally diverse classroom. Therefore, more attention must be given to helping educators develop a repertoire of instructional and assessment methods that include cultural differences and address various learning styles (Hurtado, 1996). Classroom teaching practices grounded in anthropological and constructivist education theory may be able to meet the challenges presented by culturally diverse classrooms. One of the primary beliefs of constructivist pedagogy is that knowledge comes about through the efforts of people interacting with each other and crossing various diverse social borders (Fuime, 2005). Phuntsog (1999) also acknowledged the need for culturally responsive teaching, which may require teachers to change the structure of classroom interactions and activities to be able to meet the needs of students with different learning styles. Understanding the learning styles of our culturally diverse students can benefit not only educators but also their students. When students understand how they learn, this empowers them to better manage their learning. Educators benefit by developing curricula to include various classroom assessment tools that disseminate the information across the spectrum of learning styles (Vincent & Ross, 2001).

Teaching methods should be determined by distinct learning objectives adapted for variables such as goals to be attained and the learning styles of individual students. Some of the more well-known learning styles presented in the literature include Howard Gardner's seven distinct learning intelligences, Anthony Gregorc's learning styles models, Alice Kolb's four learning modes, Myers and Briggs's learning types preferences, and Carol Kanar's visual, auditory, and kinesthetic learning styles that are related to physiological factors. Although most educators agree that different learning styles do exist and have a substantial effect on the learning process, this wealth of available information can sometimes be confusing because there is no real consensus on acceptable criteria for practice (Vincent & Ross, 2001).

The diversity of cultures and learning styles in their classroom inspired Green and Stortz (2006) to search for a common culture that was accessible to everyone regardless of their race, ethnicity, or culture. Their first goal was to understand the learning styles of their students. They were able to accomplish this by asking students about their own preferred modes of learning and their prior experiences. Second, they wanted to help the students better understand their own learning styles. Third, they wanted the students to learn to appreciate the diversity in the classroom and see it as a resource and not an obstacle. According to Fuime (2005), active discussion is one instructional method that unites the many social borders that come together in culturally diverse classrooms. Other pedagogical practices that enhance learning include small-group work, debates around specific topics, case studies, dialogue, role-play/simulation, and opportunities for open responses and language immersion (Fuime, 2005; Klein, 2008). It is important for the students' voices to be heard by relating their personal experiences to scholarship and by promoting these experiences as an essential pedagogical tool. When students feel comfortable contributing to discussion in the classroom, they are not only empowered, but also function as agents in construction of their own knowledge (Fuime, 2005). Classroom social interactions, including cooperative learning, that cross age, gender, and cultural barriers can help students make connections with other cultures and develop a community of learners. Student-taught classrooms require that each person act as an expert in an assigned subject. The students are then required to work collaboratively and teach one another. The use of this pedagogical tool will promote higher success for the entire class, rather than certain individuals (Ladson-Billings, 2008). Immediate assessment tools, called feedback loops, using free writing or specific questions, can help to evaluate whether the students are learning. The goal of culturally inclusive pedagogy is to combine cognitive and experiential learning strategies that will allow exploration of individual learning styles and facilitate learning. Discovering their learning style will allow students to apply those strategies to actual interpersonal and cross-cultural situations with an emphasis on personal growth and development (Reggy-Mamo, 2008). As educators, our role is to facilitate learning by setting a positive climate for learning. A better knowledge and understanding of learning styles allows the educator to teach in a multifarious fashion that both reaches the greatest number of students and challenges all students to grow as learners (Gilakjani, 2011).

■ Working with a Diverse Student Body

Diversity can have a positive impact on teaching and learning. When encouraged by faculty, recognition and understanding of differences and an introduction to other cultures can broaden viewpoints and stimulate discussion and ideas (Villaruel, Canales, & Torres, 2001). However, it is important to point out that although this chapter covers some cultural traits, there is a wide range in cultural responses and traits within a single culture. Members of a racial or cultural group may or may not adhere to some of the traditions of their background culture and ethnic group, and they may not even identify as a member of that group. Gutierrez and Rogoff warned that relating learning styles to certain cultures may negate a person's individuality and result in stereotyping and defined limitations on how members of a certain culture can learn (Scott, 2010). Although it is important to understand the learning styles of individuals in different cultures, overgeneralizing can also be harmful (Morgan, 2009). Faculty members must remember that people are individuals who react differently and must be treated individually. Students who are members of a cultural group cannot be expected to be a spokesperson for their group. There are too many variations within the groups themselves, and what is appropriate for one sect within a group may not be acceptable to another sect in that group.

Discrimination is always a difficult issue, and faculty, staff, administrators, and patients are not immune from it. We all have our likes, dislikes, and moral beliefs. Because of their previous experiences, many multicultural students will see discrimination where others do not. That needs to be respected and cannot be brushed off, but sometimes it also needs to be faced, corrected, or worked with. The major thrust here needs to be concentration on providing appropriate learning opportunities and meeting learning objectives. Seeking ways to help students learn about each other can be a positive force in changing discriminatory attitudes. Many myths of prejudice and discrimination can be dismantled and dismissed when students who have led sheltered lives begin to know those who are different from them and understand that although there are cultural differences, there are also many similarities.

However, conflict between cultural groups does occur in the classroom. There can be other sources for conflict that have nothing to do with ethnicity, as well as conflicts that are ethnicity and values led. In some instances, mediation may be helpful to define limits and focus the groups back onto the learning tasks at hand. Separation may work for other groups, but that is usually a temporary situation until the strong feelings subside. Encouraging groups to learn about each other is a strategy that can be used to defuse potential conflict, but this strategy needs to be carefully managed, and the instructor needs to observe group dynamics and be on the alert for peer-influenced negative ideas and peer pressure to adopt those ideas.

Baumgartner and Johnson-Bailey (2008) note that traditionally we, as teachers, work to avoid emotions in working with diversity, with negative emotions to be avoided and emotions to be kept under control. Baumgartner and Johnson-Bailey stress that while it is important to not get mired down in emotions when discussing challenging issues, there is also an opportunity for a good teaching moment to explore.

> Positive emotions can enhance the learning process. Moreover, emotions are always to be acknowledged, not judged. We contend that emotions that are on display are a sign that students care and are engaged. When a student expresses a strong emotion, it is a good time to take an intellectual breather, not a break or a recess, and say, "Do you mind if we explore that?" "I missed that side of it," or "How about we step back from this emotional terrain and deconstruct this premise." Take advantage of the energy that learners bring to your classroom even when it means departing from the syllabus. These rare challenging teachable moments should be embraced as opportunities to knock down walls. (Baumgartner & Johnson-Bailey, 2008, p. 52)

Developing a welcoming and supportive environment is essential, not only for multicultural students, but also for the other groups mentioned as part of the diverse classroom, including single parents, disabled students, and those with age and gender disparities. Faculty availability and interest are critical elements in developing a positive environment. Instructors need to be aware of potential issues, know their students, and demonstrate interest in them and their success in the program. The importance of cultural and linguistic role models (e.g., community health professionals of color and/or those from minority-based professional organizations, including those who speak a similar language) cannot be overemphasized because it has a universal effect on overcoming obstacles and achieving academic success for students of color and English-as-a-second-language (ESL) students (Heller & Lichtenberg, 2003; Yoder, 1996). Mentoring has shown success, whether it comes from outside the school or from an advanced student of one's own ethnic or cultural origin, especially when there are no faculty members of color. Those same principles apply to gender-based multicultural students, who may also feel isolated or unwelcome in the profession.

When learning difficulties appear in any group of students, it is important to look for behavioral patterns that may be impacting on their success or other stresses or anxieties that seem present. Some students need to be encouraged to be tested for learning disabilities. A diagnosis of a learning disorder, confirmed by testing, allows the student access to the resources required under ADA regulations. Faculty need to learn about student support services in their college. They need to know to whom and how to make referrals for students in areas such as financial aid, study skills, test-taking skills and tutorial assistance, mental and physical health services, and social services. It is extremely important that students are supported and encouraged to take advantage of those services.

Age Range

Older students will have a sense of history during their lifetime that is very different from the 18-year-olds, and they have learned how to deal with many situations that 18-year-olds haven't yet faced, which can be valuable when there are opportunities for sharing. However, depending on their success or frustration levels in working with those situations, older students can also hold a cynical or ingrained view that comes through and needs to be worked with and mediated at times. Older students may not value the young lifestyle and find younger students immature. Building on some of the strengths of the younger groups growing up in the technology age can be helpful to older students who are not comfortable with the technology.

Young students can be bored by the older students' experiences, tired of listening to them, or not relate those experiences to their own, or they can be interested and learn from them. Younger students may relate to older students as parental figures— which can be good or bad—viewing them as caring or the extreme of dictatorial or authoritarian, which is often based in their experiences with older adults.

The most important task is getting students in different age groups to respect and learn from each other. Small-group work can create diverse working groups. Monitoring group work is important to identify conflict areas. However, when students in different age levels get to know each other better and have success in working together toward a common goal of meeting learning objectives, negative perceptions can change, and the students can be a positive support for each other.

Communication

Communication can be problematic between minority cultural and ethnic groups and the majority group. The learning goals and objectives need to be clearly understood by both students and the teacher in a diverse classroom. Communication is often an issue and at the same time is the key to understanding and acceptance of those goals. A diverse group of students may have their own individual goals and objectives based on their interests and learning experiences, and may or may not be willing to share them with the instructor. An instructor needs to be open to listen to and encourage ideas that can be different than the ones he or she planned for the class, and allow for appropriate analytic, creative, and practical knowledge to be utilized. It may be easier for ESL students to read English than it is to understand English conversation, so written instructions or handouts may be helpful and allow students more time to clarify concepts. Instructors need to speak slowly and clearly in classroom presentations, and conversational pauses may need to be longer so that students can be encouraged to speak up, but also allow them to catch up with what is being said and with note taking.

Students and faculty may have a difference in perception, especially if English is not the primary language. Ideas may not translate well. One of the authors had the experience of presenting a lecture in Taiwan and worked with a Taiwanese nurse who spoke English well and was responsible for translating comments to the audience into their native language. The author and translator met and went over the lecture notes. While the translator wrote her translations, things seemed to be going very well, until she asked the author, "What is custodial care?" The author immediately realized that she had assumed the translator understood everything that was being discussed, but that was not necessarily the case. The pair went over the speech again until the author was comfortable that the translator understood concepts and would be able to translate them appropriately.

American ideals and values may be different from what some students are used to. One of the most important aspects in working with all students, but especially with multicultural and ESL students, is what the authors call "know your PVCs." This is not the cardiac term most of us are familiar with, but instead stands for *perception, validation,* and *clarification.* Each person perceives an event differently. An inquiry to see if there are any questions or areas they do not understand needs to have more depth than just asking if the students understand and expecting and getting a *yes* answer. Students need to be encouraged to articulate what they think was said, and that is where the differences show up. Formal classroom assessment techniques can also be helpful in identifying problem areas (Angelo & Cross, 1994).

When an instructor feels a student lacks understanding of the materials, it is important to question that *perception* with the student, *validate* that what was meant to be communicated is in reality what the student understood to be communicated, and, when there is a difference, *clarify.* Students who are not proficient in English may smile and seem to understand, but often they do not, and they may not want to ask in front of the whole class for clarification or statements to be repeated. It is important for faculty to be aware of this possibility, and follow-through outside of the classroom environment may be necessary.

Accommodation

The passage of the Americans with Disabilities Act in 1990 has made a major difference in today's classroom. Instructors need to adjust to accommodations that may be necessary. Think about the following: If a health professional is injured or comes down with a debilitating illness or is wheelchair bound, can accommodations be made so he or she can continue working? In most cases employees can and will be accommodated in various jobs within the profession, even those employees who become deaf or legally blind. These jobs may not be those involving the usual clinical care, but they are still jobs that need a health professional to perform and are essential for quality care. Think about jobs that a disabled person could perform in your specialty—those that may be possible, despite the fact that some jobs will not be performed at all or as completely. Assistive devices can often be used to allow the employee to perform safely and appropriately in limited activities if he or she has the appropriate clinical knowledge required for the specific position. This being the case, why does the door to the profession need to be closed and applicants with disabilities turned away? Think about ways in which a disabled student could be prepared to work in those jobs within the profession, and the types of clinical experiences that a disabled student can carry out that will provide appropriate experiences for a future job. The technology field is rapidly expanding, and assistive devices are improving and becoming more cost-effective and more available.

Faculty must become well aware of the disability regulations and student support services that colleges have set up because of those regulations. Faculties need to develop awareness of the barriers and regulations that are present for disabled students and need to be addressed, and where resources can be found to help both faculty members and students. One issue that needs to be worked out in a positive manner is making sure these accommodations are fair to the nondisabled students. What does *fair* mean? Disabilities—in particular, learning disabilities or certain physical disabilities such as back problems—may not be visible to others. Rules of privacy may not allow a faculty member to discuss a disabled student's condition, but they can encourage the student to discuss this issue with others and provide support as necessary.

For many years, teachers were authoritarians in the classrooms, with rigid standards and rules and regulations. Things are different today. Student demonstrations in the late 1960s and early 1970s began a students' rights movement that altered college cultures. But some questions need to be asked. How much compromise is possible, and how do we work within regulated issues? A very positive part of students' rights has been that faculties have had to look at what they were doing and assess whether they were working by ritual or providing real learning opportunities. Such faculties have learned to work successfully with students who, in the past, would not have had the opportunities available to them today.

Making accommodations is also an important concept to those with heavy personal responsibilities. Older students may be faced with family issues, such as caring for children and/or elderly parents. They and single parents may have responsibilities that interfere with their ability to meet deadlines or come to class. Rigid attendance policies are often more ritualistic than real. The focus needs to be on what is necessary for the learning experience. Sitting in a class does not guarantee that a student is attentive and learning. Teachers are well aware that students daydream, have conversations with their classmates, and even fall asleep, and that they will forget a good portion of what was presented, even though we as teachers believe that every word we say is valuable. It may be more important for a student to attend a small seminar-type class because the learning is more dependent on participation in discussion than it is for sitting in a large lecture session. The important determining issue is what the goals and objectives are for the course, and whether there are other ways to meet them without perfect attendance. That may sound heretical, but there are other ways for conscientious and motivated students to meet learning objectives and set priorities. The use of the Internet, library services, and out-of-class assignments can afford some flexibility if needed. Attendance at clinical experiences may be more problematic because of the need for scheduling and faculty availability, but there are ways to design a program with a student that may afford some flexibility for specific instances. Again, it is important to keep the learning goal of the experience or class in mind and consider creative and flexible ways to work with students to plan for what they feel they can accomplish.

Financially challenged students may not be able to participate in some activities because they may need to work in addition to their school responsibilities. They may have difficulty in buying books and special or technological equipment or participating in outside learning opportunities, such as conferences or lectures that have a fee attached. These students may not be able to spend hours in the library because of their work and family schedules, and finding study time may be difficult. Anxiety and worry over finances can impact their learning experience.

There is no easy solution to these issues, but again, student services can often be an ally. Student lives outside the classroom need to be respected, but the responsibility for learning is theirs, not yours. Students and faculty can work together to assess what is needed to achieve the objectives of the learning experiences and to facilitate their learning. Are there alternative ways of achieving those objectives that don't meet up with the "Is it fair to others?" question? It is important for instructors to meet with student services to find out just what they do and how they do it. Student services can help students set up workable schedules, tutorial services, and study and testing guidance. They can also counsel students on student life issues and refer students to outside resources when needed. Faculty should also be familiar with financial aid issues and regulations, which can be quite complicated because of differences in governmental and private sources, and with outside services for referrals when appropriate.

Academic Issues

Students with academic problems need to be identified early and encouraged to discuss the issue with faculty without the spectre of punishment or embarrassment. It is important to discover patterns of negative behavior, discuss them directly with the students involved, and develop a plan that the students and faculty agree to and believe can be implemented and carried out. Unfortunately, not all students can be helped, and some will drop out or fail out, but others will be successful and benefit from the encouragement.

Students with learning disabilities and ESL students may have problems with timed tests. ESL students may need more time to read and digest test questions because they may be translating the questions into their primary language, and some words and phrases do not translate well. Students with learning disabilities are supported in the need for additional time by the ADA regulations, but that is not true for ESL students. To evaluate and accurately grade the level of knowledge, faculty can provide opportunities for various types of testing other than timed tests—take home tests being one example. There may be a limit to this, however, when students need to improve in timed testing because they will be subjected to that in the licensure testing. Again, students with a learning disability can have additional time because the regulations support them, but ESL can be a cause for failure in timed tests, and those students may need practice and/or tutorial assistance to become more proficient in testing so as to pass a licensing exam and enter the profession.

■ Conclusion

Although working with diverse students can be challenging, it can also be stimulating and exciting. As healthcare professionals, we and our students are in a clinical environment, and ideally learning about new cultures and disabilities will be translated into increased cultural competence when working with patients.

Remember that the responsibility for learning lies with the learner, but feelings of anxiety and isolation can cause stress that impacts the learning process and may affect graduation rates and successful entrance into the profession. Family responsibilities can also interfere with a student's ability to carry out the required work. Faculty members need to learn to develop sensitivity and awareness of issues that impact the learning process and work with students to meet the learning goals. They need to develop their knowledge of services and resources that can be utilized by students. A culturally inclusive pedagogy that also incorporates learning styles allows the teacher to reach the greatest number of students. Flexibility, patience, and creativity are needed to develop a supportive environment that enhances learning. A major role of faculty is offering support, guidance, and referrals as appropriate and developing a community of students who view diversity as a strength that provides an opportunity to learn from each other as well as from their teachers. It is painful but necessary to understand that this will not work for all students, but it will be appreciated by and benefit many students. Our reward for the efforts expended is that we can rightly celebrate and be proud of the successful students whom we have helped enter the profession and who are now providing a valuable service to their patients, communities, and profession.

REFERENCES

Angelo, T. A., & Cross, K. P. (1994). *Classroom assessment techniques: A handbook for college teachers* (2nd ed.). San Francisco, CA: Jossey-Bass.

Bain, K. (2004). *What the best college teachers do.* Cambridge, MA: Harvard University Press.

Barbee, E., & Gibson, S. (2001). Our dismal progress: The recruitment of non-Whites into nursing [Electronic version]. *Journal of Nursing Education, 40,* 243–244.

Baumgartner, L. M., & Johnson-Bailey, J. (2008). Fostering awareness of diversity and multiculturalism in adult and higher education. *New Directions for Adult & Continuing Education, 120,* 45–53.

Carnegie, M. E. (1991). *The path we tread: Blacks in nursing 1834–1990.* New York, NY: National League for Nursing.

Carnegie, M. E. (2005). Educational preparation of Black nurses: A historical perspective. *ABNF Journal, 16*(1), 6–7.

Carroll, S. M. (2004). Inclusion of people with physical disabilities in nursing education. *Journal of Nursing Education, 43*(5), 207–212.

Dale, R. (2009). *Education theories, cultures, and learning: A critical perspective* (pp. 27–37). New York, NY: Routledge, Taylor & Francis Group.

Evans, B. C. (2004). Application of the caring curriculum to education of Hispanic/Latino and American Indian nursing students. *Journal of Nursing Education, 43*(5), 219–228.

Gilakjani, A.P. (2011). Visual, auditory, kinesthetic learning styles and their impact on English language teaching. *Journal of Studies in Education, 2*(1), 104–112.

Graybill, S. W. (1997). Questions of race and culture: How they relate to the classroom for African American students. *Clearing House, 70*(6), 311–318.

Green, B., & Stortz, M. (2006). The syllabus as passport into a common culture of teaching and learning: Developing and assessing strategies for dealing with diversity. *Teaching Theology & Religion, 9*(4), 221–228.

Griggs, D., & Dunn, R. (1996). Hispanic-American students and learning style. *ERIC Digest.* Retrieved from ERIC database. (ED393607)

Grosz, R. (2005). The forgotten (?) minority. *Internet Journal of Allied Health Sciences and Practice, 3*(3). Retrieved from http://ijahsp.nova.edu/articles/vol3num3/grosz_commentary.htm

Hancock, D. (2004). Cooperative learning and peer orientation effects on motivation and achievement. *The Journal of Educational Research, 97*(3), 159–166.

Heller, B. R., & Lichtenberg, L. P. (2003). Addressing the shortage: Strategies for building the nursing workforce. *Nursing Leadership Forum, 8*(1), 34–39.

Hurtado, S. (1996). How diversity affects teaching and learning. *Educational Record, 77*(4), 27–29. Retrieved from http://www.diversityweb.org/research_and_trends/research_evaluation_impact/benefits_of_diversity/sylvia_hurtado.cfm

Jacob, E., & Jordan, C. (1996). *Minority education: Anthropological perspectives.* Norwood, NJ: Ablex Publishing.

Kana'iaupuni, S., Ledward, B., & Jensen, U. (2009). Culture based education and its relationship to student outcomes. *Kamehameha Schools Research and Evaluation.* Retrieved from http://www.ksbe.edu/spi/PDFS/CBE_relationship_to_student_outcomes.pdf

Kirkland, M. L. S. (1998). Stressors and coping strategies among successful female African American baccalaureate nursing students. *Journal of Nursing Education, 37*(1), 5–13.

Klein, A. M. (2008). Sensitivity to the learning needs of newcomers in foreign language settings. *Multicultural Education, 16*(2), 41–44. ERIC document (EJ832227). Retrieved from http://www .teqjournal.org/sample_issue/article_6.htm

Kosowski, M. M., Grams, K. M., Taylor, G. J., & Wilson, C. B. (2001). They took the time … they started to care: Stories of African-American nursing students in intercultural caring groups. *Advances in Nursing Science, 23*(3), 11–27.

Ladson-Billings, G. (2008). Toward a theory of culturally relevant pedagogy. *American Educational Research Journal, 32*(3), 465–491.

Lowenstein, A. (1990, March 28–April 1). Racial segregation and nursing education in Georgia: The Lamar experience. *Proceedings of the National Association for Equal Opportunity in Higher Education's (NAFEO's) 15th National Conference on Blacks in Higher Education.* Washington, DC.

Lowenstein, A. (1994, September). *Racial segregation and nursing education in Georgia: The Lamar experience.* Paper presented at the annual convention of the Transcultural Nursing Society. Atlanta, GA.

Lowenstein, A. J., & Glanville, C. (1995). Cultural diversity and conflict in the health care workplace. *Nursing Economics, 13*(4), 203–209, 247.

Moffat, M. (2003). The history of physical therapy practice in the United States. *Journal of Physical Therapy Education, 17*(3), 15–25.

Morgan, H. (2009). What every teacher needs to know to teach Native American students. *Multicultural Education, 16*(4), 10–12.

Nasir, S. N., & Hand, V. M. (2006). Exploring sociocultural perspectives on race, culture, and learning. *Review of Educational Research, 76*(4), 449–475.

Ogunsiji, O., & Wilkes, L. (2005). Managing family life while studying: Single mothers' lived experience of being students in a nursing program. *Contemporary Nurse, 18*(1–2), 108–123.

Phuntsog, N. (1999). The magic of culturally responsive pedagogy: In search of the genie's lamp in multicultural education. *Teacher Education Quarterly, 26*(3). Retrieved from http://www.teqjournal .org/sample_issue/article_6.htm

Reggy-Mamo, M. (2008). An experiential approach to intercultural education. *Christian Higher Education, 7*(2), 110–122.

Scott, C. (2010). The enduring appeal of learning styles. *Australian Journal of Education, 54*(1), 5–17.

Sieffert, S. (2006). *Placing culture at the forefront.* Saskatoon, Canada: University of Saskachewan. Retrieved from http://www.usask.ca/education/coursework/802papers/seiffert/index.htm

Silver, J. H., Sr. (2002). Diversity issues. In R. Diamond (Ed.), *Field guide to academic leadership* (pp. 357–372). San Francisco, CA: Jossey-Bass.

Splenser, P. E., Canlas, H. L., Sanders, B., & Melzer, B. (2003). Minority recruitment and retention strategies in physical therapist education programs. *Journal of Physical Therapy Education, 17*(1), 18–26.

Suinn, R. M. (2006). Teaching culturally diverse students. In W. J. McKeachie & M. Svinicki (Eds.), *McKeachie's teaching tips* (12th ed., pp. 152–171). Boston, MA: Houghton Mifflin.

Swisher, K. (1991). American Indian/Native American learning styles: Research and practice. *ERIC Digest.* Retrieved from ERIC database. (ED335175)

Vasquez, J. (1990). Instructional responsibilities of college faculty to minority students. *Journal of Negro Education, 59,* 599–610.

Villaruel, A. M., Canales, M., & Torres, S. (2001). Educational mobility of Hispanic nurses. *Journal of Nursing Education, 40*(6), 245–251.

Vincent, A., & Ross, D. (2001). Learning styles awareness: A basis for developing teaching and learning strategies. *Journal of Research on Technology in Education, 33*(5), 1–10.

Vogt, L. A., Jordan, C., & Tharp, R. G. (1987). Explaining school failure, producing school success: Two cases. *Anthropology and Education Quarterly, 18*(4) 276–286.

Wessling, S. (2000, Fall). Coming home: Two unique programs are giving homeless and disadvantaged persons an opportunity to start again as nursing professionals. *Minority Nurse,* 32–35.

Yoder, M. (1996). Instructional responses to ethnically diverse nursing students. *Journal of Nursing Education, 35,* 315–321.

RECOMMENDED READING

Barbee, E., & Gibson, S. (2001). Our dismal progress: The recruitment of non-Whites into nursing [Electronic version]. *Journal of Nursing Education, 40,* 243–244.

Byrne, M. (2001). Uncovering racial bias in nursing fundamentals textbooks. *Nursing and Health Care Perspectives, 22,* 299–303.

Dickerson, S., & Neary, M. (1999). Faculty experiences teaching Native Americans in a university setting. *Journal of Transcultural Nursing, 10*(1), 56–64.

Edward, J. (2000). Teaching strategies for foreign nurses. *Journal for Nurses in Staff Development, 16*(4), 171–173.

Evans, B. C. (2004). Application of the caring curriculum to education of Hispanic/Latino and American Indian nursing students. *Journal of Nursing Education, 43*(5), 219–228.

Griffiths, M., & Tagliareni, E. (1999). Challenging traditional assumptions about minority students in nursing education. *Nursing & Health Care Perspectives, 20,* 290–295.

Grosz, R. (2005, July). The forgotten (?) minority. [Commentary]. *Internet Journal of Allied Health Sciences and Practice, 3*(3). Retrieved from http://ijahsp.nova.edu/articles/vol3num3/grosz_commentary.htm

Gurin, P., Dey, E. L., Hurtado, S., & Gurin, G. (2002). Diversity and higher education: Theory and impact on educational outcomes. *Harvard Educational Review, 72*(3), 330–366.

Kosowski, M. M., Grams, K. M., Taylor, G. J., & Wilson, C. B. (2001). They took the time—they started to care: Stories of African-American nursing students in intercultural caring groups. *Advances in Nursing Science, 23*(3), 11–27.

Maruyama, G., Moreno, J. F., Gudeman, R. H., & Marin, P. (2000). *Does diversity make a difference? Three research studies on diversity in college classrooms.* Washington, DC: American Association of University Professors. Retrieved from ERIC database. (ED444409)

Maville, J., & Huerta, C. (1997). Stress and social support among Hispanic student nurses: Implications for academic achievement. *Journal of Cultural Diversity, 4*(1), 18–25.

Miller, J. E., & Hollenshead, C. (2005). Gender, family, and flexibility—why they're important in the academic workplace. *Change, 37*(6), 58–62.

Splenser, P. E., Canlas, H. L., Sanders, B., & Melzer, B. (2003). Minority recruitment and retention strategies in physical therapist education programs. *Journal of Physical Therapy Education, 17*(1), 18–26.

Taylor, V., & Rust, G. (1999). The needs of students from diverse cultures. *Academic Medicine, 74,* 302–304.

Vasquez, J. (1990). Instructional responsibilities of college faculty to minority students. *Journal of Negro Education, 59,* 599–610.

Weaver, H. (2001). Indigenous nurses and professional education: Friends or foe? *Journal of Nursing Education, 40*(6), 252–258.

Yoder, M. (1996). Instructional responses to ethnically diverse nursing students. *Journal of Nursing Education, 35*(7), 315–321.

Yurkovich, E. (2001). Working with American Indians toward educational success. *Journal of Nursing Education, 40*(6), 259–269.

ELECTRONIC RESOURCES

Griggs, D., & Dunn, R. (1996). Hispanic-American students and learning style. *ERIC Digest.* Retrieved from ERIC database. (ED393607)

Kana'iaupuni, S., Ledward, B., & Jensen, U. (2009). Culture based education and its relationship to student outcomes. *Kamehameha Schools Research and Evaluation.* Available at www.ksbe.edu/spi

Sieffert, S. (2006). *Placing culture at the forefront.* Saskatoon, Canada: University of Saskachewan. Retrieved from http://www.usask.ca/education/coursework/802papers/seiffert/index.htm

Swisher, K. (1991). American Indian/Native American learning styles: Research and practice. *ERIC Digest.* Retrieved from ERIC database. (ED335175)

U.S. Department of Justice. *ADA regulations and technical assistance materials.* Retrieved from http://www.usdoj.gov/crt/ada/publicat.htm

CHAPTER 3

Strategies for Innovation

■ Arlene J. Lowenstein ■

The scope of change in health care has been enormous, and the rate at which change occurs continues to accelerate. Today's technology and therapeutics were inconceivable even a few decades ago. Over time, the growth of the health professions has been influenced by those new technologies and therapeutics, but there are many other influencing factors and forces, including, but not limited to:

- The appearance of new diseases, such as swine flu (H1N1), HIV/AIDS, and Lyme disease and the rapid growth of new treatments, medications, and noninvasive surgeries.
- War and its consequences, which brought new techniques to care for burns and radiation, growth of the use of penicillin and other antibiotics, treatments for posttraumatic stress syndrome, growth of nursing, and rehabilitation services in the military and veterans' systems.
- Sociocultural issues, including the civil rights movement, the feminist movement, the consumer revolution of the late 1960s and 1970s, and changing immigration and demographic patterns, which brought dramatic changes in maternity care ranging from shortened length of stay to sibling visitation, increased focus on care of the elderly, and end-of-life care. Diversity has increased in healthcare education and practice, and more emphasis has been placed on culturally competent care.
- Religious issues, which brought ethical components of care and the development of parish nursing.
- Changing economics as evidenced by the recent recession and political/legal issues, which brought us Medicare, Medicaid, managed care, legalized abortion, and the current debate over healthcare reform, even though a bill was passed in Congress and signed by President Obama.

■ Changes in education that brought nursing into academic settings and gave rise to nursing science and nursing research, thereby changing practice and creating new roles, such as advanced practice nursing and the newest credential, the doctor of nursing practice (DNP). Physical therapy embraced the doctor of physical therapy (DPT) as an entry-level degree, and other health professions have developed and evolved as well.

These forces are not isolated but are part of the total environment in which we live and work. They are ever changing and interacting, challenging health professions educators to keep on top of the trends, technologies, and resources, while enabling self-directed student learning. Graduates who are self-directed learners understand and are responsive to healthcare system changes when they are in practice and out of the school setting, where there are no faculty members with whom to consult.

Healthcare educators straddle the fields of healthcare practice and education. They need to be knowledgeable about changes in practice and technology in both fields. What healthcare practitioners learn, as well as how they are taught, must keep pace with the changing milieu. The field of education has also changed over the years through many of the same forces that affected health care. Technology and therapeutics in health care can be compared to a new understanding of learning theories and teaching methods in education. The student entering a healthcare profession from high school today is most likely much more comfortable with the use of computers than the RN returning to school or an older student who has chosen a health profession as a second career. Online courses are now in the mainstream.

Health professions classrooms are also more culturally diverse than ever before. More men are entering the nursing profession, and more women are going to medical schools. Younger students may have had very different cultural experiences in their secondary schools than did older students. Older students may be dealing with the added stress of parenthood and job responsibilities. Different cultures and experiences may produce different expectations of teaching and learning. Respecting learning-need differences and establishing an innovative climate in the classroom can help to prepare students for the changes they will face in practice. An educational climate that values different viewpoints and experiences among students encourages those students to create their own innovations. Those innovations will serve them in good stead by enhancing positive interactions with the wide variety of persons for whom they will be caring and with whom they will be working.

Omachonu and Einspruch (2010) saw four areas of potential innovation in health care: product innovation; process innovation (which includes healthcare practices), marketing innovation, and organizational innovation. There are many new opportunities for innovation. Sources of information have multiplied. The Internet has laid at our doors the possibility of learning over long distances. The barrier of geography has been breached. Even nurses in rural communities have access to continued learning by highly qualified nurse educators. Innovative computer-based materials can provide technical training within the classroom—audio and video combining to offer a breadth of exposure previously available only through many hours at the bedside. Instant messaging is available, and we can listen to lectures over podcasts and locate reference material instantly through our very own personal digital assistants (PDAs). We can have two-way access between health settings and homes with the use of Skype, a software application that provides the ability to make voice calls, complete with pictures, over the Internet, and telemedicine, so a person many miles away can join you in your living room or in a health facility. The use of simulators has increased. This capability is becoming much more important as productivity pressures make clinical sites for student experience harder and harder to find.

How do we teach more and more information to our students without overwhelming them? And how do we maintain the underlying paradigm of care and compassion? How do we maintain the threads of patient-centered, holistic, and compassionate care within the complex scientific information our students must master? In this text, we hope to provide health professions educators with ideas and examples that have been used to allow students to master the facts and theory as well as the perspective of a caring professional. Implementing and adapting these methods will lead to further discovery of successful teaching strategies to keep pace with changes in the profession.

■ Examples of Innovation

Innovative teaching strategies can range from simple to complex. Innovations can be developed for an exercise within a course or for the method by which the entire course is taught. Teaching innovations can be developed for whole programs or even whole schools. They can be developed by one faculty member or by groups of faculty members. The prime objective is that the teaching strategies selected must address what needs to be learned in relation to the learning needs of students.

Think back to a favorite teacher or any strongly remembered event. Why does it stand out? What makes it unique among similar events? A major factor can be the realization that one object was completely different or out of its usually defined place, whereas the surrounding objects appeared normal. The teachers we remember often stood apart from our perception of others by only one or two details, but these details were out of the normal range. We remember the different much more than the normal, yet we can grasp only a small amount of the different and a large amount of the usual. The occasional nondigestible, completely different piece in the sea of the expected focuses our energies on analyzing not just the different piece, but also the other 99% rote material normally not given much attention and easily forgotten. Kirp, a professor of public policy, asked a former student, who had become a college professor, what she remembered about his teaching. He was astonished to hear that she remembered his baseball stories. She elaborated that the baseball anecdotes prodded her into thinking of him as more approachable and more human. Once she felt that way, she began to pay attention (Kirp, 1997).

Exhibit 3-1 provides an example of using something different in a lesson: an analogy of pain management to the sinking of the *Titanic*. The objective is to allow students to discover how what they know applies to other situations. Students will remember more if they can make the discovery.

Exhibit 3-1   Analogy: Pain Management and the Sinking of the *Titanic*

The aftermath of bone surgery, such as ankle fusion, is very painful for patients. To create a more dynamic understanding of a patient's experience with pain and the need for appropriate pain relief measures, an analogy was used to discuss the issues involved. The choice of the *Titanic* disaster as an analogy actually came from a patient's description of the pain he felt in the postoperative period and his feeling that the nursing staff needed to pay more attention to pain relief. He felt there were times when he was totally immersed with the pain, and relief could have been started sooner and put him on a more even keel.

The *Titanic* was constructed with six watertight compartments that were expected to withstand a breach and keep the ship afloat. The compartments had very high walls but, unfortunately, did not reach the ceilings. The design was appropriate for most possibilities, but not for the accident that actually happened. Students were told to think of the walls as the job of the pain medication and water as the pain. The wall of the pain medication isolates the water from the ship and the passengers' realization that they are surrounded by water. The pain is hidden. The danger lies in what happens if the water in the first compartment overflows its limit and then starts filling the second compartment. If up to three of these compartments fill with water (pain), it may not interfere with the ship's normal function; however, as the effect cascades into more of the compartments, the ship sinks by the bow until it's "all hands lost."

Patients initially don't understand that a sea of pain surrounds them. As the pain relief diminishes and they suddenly (perhaps by waking from sleep) find themselves immersed, a fear of this unexpected and uncomfortable situation is formed. This fear becomes a constant presence even after pain relief is restored, leading to anxiety and apprehension over the possibility of a repeat experience. In very painful procedures, this fear can result in clock watching over the medication schedule as well as a compulsion to do anything to stay ahead of the pain curve. Appropriate pain relief measures, timing of administration, and other nursing measures can be discussed, continuing use of the analogy (such as the use of lifeboats in the pain relief cycle). Students can also be taught to develop and share their own analogies to improve learning retention.

Art, literature, storytelling, humor, and technology-assisted learning can all be used in innovative ways. Whitman and Rose (2003) had students choose media to express their nursing philosophy. This technique required students to think differently about what they were doing and what they believed. One student used a guitar and song to express his philosophy of healing. Another painted a brain within a heart, which symbolized her need to incorporate compassion as well as intellect into patient care. A third wrote a poem to express her feelings and beliefs. This technique used sight, touch, and movement in addition to listening, which encouraged retention postclass for both the creator of the piece and the viewer.

■ Developing Innovative Strategies

Innovation can occur at all levels of an educational organization. Support for innovation in education may begin at the top of the organization or be developed and implemented at program or individual class levels. Success is enhanced when administrators and faculty members work side by side to plan strategically and implement changes to improve the educational milieu (Woods, 1998).

Innovation at the school level was demonstrated by a group of business school educators. These educators chose to focus more on entrepreneurship and to move away from the traditional management that prepared students to work in large organizations. This strategic innovation recognized the realities of the marketplace in a changing world. These schools set the pace for others to follow (They Create Winners, 1994). In working with social workers, Michael Chovanec (2008) recognized an educational need that wasn't being met. While group processes may be in the curriculum for social workers, they often need to work with involuntary groups, such as court-ordered programs in domestic abuse and chemical dependency. There is a very different process needed to work with people who do not want to be there but are forced to attend. Chovanec developed three innovative frameworks to teach social work students about this type of work. His article describes those frameworks as reactance theory for working with the reactions of those who do not want to be in the group, a stages of change model, and motivational interviewing, which encourages working with clients to improve their self-motivation. His model provides guidelines and exercises to model unpleasant experiences that students may be exposed to in their practice.

Nursing education has grown through innovation. Mildred Montag's introduction of the associate degree program in nursing, developed through research to meet an assessed need, changed the landscape of nursing education. The introduction of nurse practitioner programs also created a revolution in the profession. The physical therapy profession has endorsed the doctor of physical therapy (DPT) as the entry-level degree and strongly encouraged schools to provide transition programs for physical therapists currently in practice. The introduction of distance learning in all the health professions is the latest revolution and is growing rapidly, offering students different choices that are unfettered by the barrier of geography.

The Innovation Center for Medicare and Medicaid was established as a conse-quence of the passage of the Affordable Care Act (CMS Innovation Center, 2013). Trossman (2012) noted that nursing was long governed by rules, regulations, and rigid schedules, but times are changing, and 21 nurses were among the 73 healthcare professionals who were selected as innovation advisors in December 2011 through the CMS Innovation Center.

Successful innovation does not come easily and requires creativity, planning, and evaluation. **Exhibit 3-2** describes a process for educators to work through to develop innovative teaching strategies. Just as health professions call for patient assessments, the educational process calls for learning and program assessments. *Assessment* of a course requires a look at both strengths and problems. How can the strengths be

---

Exhibit 3-2 The Process of Innovation

Assessment
What is the content to be learned? What are the student learning needs? How are those needs being met? What is working and what is not?

Defining Options
How else can I look at this? Does the literature provide suggestions that would address the identified needs? Do students or other faculty members have sug-gestions that I could utilize?

Planning
1. Does this change require working with curriculum committees, collab-orating with other faculty members, or individual instructor planning? How should this change be approached?
2. Will there be a need to work with technical specialists in the use of computer technology? Do I need additional technological knowledge to carry out this change?
3. How can I best use change theory in this planning? Who are the stakeholders who need to be considered? How and where will I meet resistance? How will I develop support?
4. How will I plan to evaluate the effectiveness of this innovation?

Gaining Support for the Innovation
Which resources will be needed? How will they be acquired and funded? What is the level of administrative support required and available? Which strategies will I use to gain additional support if needed?

Preparing Students for the Innovation

Do I need written student instructions? If so, are they clear? Have I provided a mechanism for troubleshooting problems, and do students know how to address problems?

Preparing Faculty Members for the Innovation

If other faculty members are involved, do they need additional education? How will that be carried out? Is everyone in agreement as to how the strategy will be run? Is rehearsal time needed?

Implementing the Innovation

How much flexibility is available if the intervention is not going well? Will follow-up be needed?

Evaluating the Outcome

How will I measure the learning outcome? How have students reacted to the strategy, and can they provide input for change or improvement? If other faculty members are involved, can a consensus be reached about the direction for needed change and/or support for continuation?

enhanced? What needs to be changed? Educators must focus on what the expected learning outcome should be, with awareness of learning theory and student learning styles and needs. Specific content requirements change often in health care, as new techniques, technologies, and research bring new knowledge needs. With the overwhelming amount of information available in today's healthcare world, it will not be possible to include everything students need. They will need to have appropriate resources to supplement classroom or clinical learning. The instructor must decide what and how much content will be needed, a decision that is often difficult. While addressing the content to be learned, it is also important to consider student learning needs. An understanding of the diversity in learning needs provides a foundation for the development of effective strategies.

To ***define options,*** the literature should be searched for research, suggestions, or techniques that could address the identified needs. Asking students or other faculty members for suggestions can also be helpful. This is the place where creativity reigns. It is important to look at many different ways to address the learning objective before selecting one. Asking the question, "Is there another way to look at this?" can be fun and lead to additional options.

Once a strategy has been selected, ***planning*** is all important. Understanding who the stakeholders are and what their investment is in the status quo or in change can be helpful in planning strategies to bring them on board. Many stakeholders, including students, do not like change and will resist new approaches. Using change theory can assist in demonstrating need and provide information that can make resisters more amenable to change. Some strategies will require curricular change, which is a complicated process and one that needs to be started early to avoid implementation delays. It is important to take enough time to develop support for the strategy. If this is a simple change within a course, then the instructor will need the support of students to participate effectively and not sabotage the effort. In more complex strategies, it may be important to bring in other faculty members or administrators.

Some strategies will need help from technical specialists, who may be able to offer support and/or instruction for using the required equipment. Time must be allotted for adequate instruction to enable faculty members and students to reach a comfort level. Most importantly, the technical staff must be available to help solve problems, which are bound to occur. Planning strategies for troubleshooting and providing access for problem solving for both faculty members and students need to be thought out in advance of implementation.

Another phase of the planning process is planning for the evaluation of the strategy. This is the time to decide what needs to be evaluated and how it should be done. This phase can range from how the strategy will be used in student grading to evaluating learning outcomes for the class as a whole and needs to be developed to allow student and faculty input for future development. This can also be the time to develop an educational research project, if appropriate. Educational research and publication of results are needed and can assist all of us in understanding and applying an effective educational process.

Gaining support for the innovation is the next step. Some strategies require little or no resources to implement, whereas others require significant physical and/or financial resources. If resources are needed, then gaining support for acquisition of those resources is essential. Looking at alternative sources of funding is helpful. Grants can provide a good funding source but require time and effort to secure and may last for only a limited time. Administrative support may be required, but administrators may also be an excellent resource to tap to discuss potential funding or acquisition of physical resources. Once the project has been developed, it is important to validate the support of stakeholders.

Class preparation is a given in education. *Preparing students for the innovation* is an important step. Student instructions need to be clear and specific. This is the time for motivating students to want to try this process, and for gaining their support. Students need to know how to address problems, especially when technology is involved. There may be a learning curve required with some strategies. Students need to feel comfortable that they will not be punished for mistakes, but rather will benefit from those mistakes as part of the learning process. Evaluation methods or grading must be made clear.

Faculty members may also need preparation for the innovation. For some strategies, rehearsal time may be needed, or additional education may be required. Planning sufficient time for those activities will increase everyone's comfort level with the process. This is the time to be sure that everyone agrees about how the strategy will be run. Use of *perception, validation,* and *clarification* (the author likes to use the mnemonic *PVCs* when teaching students about this) can be valuable here. Health professionals are familiar with cardiac premature ventricular contractions as PVCs, but using this term in a different context can help students relate to the term and remember it better. Too often, people interpret statements differently. Checking that everyone has the same perceptions (validating) and clarifying differences can provide unity in approach to students and reduce problems of students playing one instructor against another. Saying, "Remember your PVCs," reminds us to think about this issue.

The best part of the process is ***implementing the innovation*** because it makes the innovation real for the innovator. It is hoped that things will go well, but flexibility may be required if problems arise. Sometimes, unintended consequences, such as surfacing of emotional issues, can occur. Instructors should be alert to the need for follow-up or referral if problems arise.

Evaluating the outcome is the final step in the process. Remember that learning can continue long after implementation of the strategy. It may be possible to measure short-term attainment of learning outcomes, but it may or may not be possible to explore long-term effects. For certain strategies that were developed to provide a foundation for other learning experiences, it may be possible to remeasure students at the end of their program. Students and faculty members should be able to provide input for future development and use of the strategy. A strong evaluation process provides an opportunity to participate in educational research. Even if a strategy is not suitable for research, it still may be appropriate for publication. Sharing teaching strategies presents the opportunity to improve the educational process. A catchword in health care today is *evidence-based practice*. We also need evidence-based practice in education.

■ Conclusion

Innovative teaching strategies must be based on both learning objectives and student learning needs. The wide diversity of student learning needs means that educators must recognize that, although most students will benefit from the new approaches, some will not. This perspective can be disappointing, but it is realistic, and educators must take pride in what they have accomplished. Problems that no one could foresee will occur despite adequate planning. These problems, although disturbing at the time, are often humorous memories later and can be addressed to improve future offerings. Developing effective teaching strategies is challenging and requires effort and persistence but can also be exceedingly rewarding and fun. Sharing those strategies with others will benefit students and faculty alike. We hope you will take advantage of the strategies presented in this book and go on to develop, implement, and share your own innovative strategies.

Interdisciplinary Case Study Analysis

An example of an innovative strategy at the school level was the introduction of interdisciplinary case studies to health professions students. Healthcare providers interact daily with members of other disciplines. The mission statement of the health professions school, with programs in nursing, physical therapy, and communications sciences disorders, included the following:

> While health professionals must be prepared to provide expert care within their respective disciplines, they contribute to evaluating and improving health care delivery by working in close cooperation with professionals from other disciplines. Students educated in an interdisciplinary setting, one that integrates academic and clinical pursuits, will be well-equipped to function as members of the health care team. The involvement of active practitioners from different fields in program planning, student supervision, and teaching supports such an integrated program. (MGH Institute of Health Professions, 2000, p. 13)

Faculty members and administrators felt the need to strengthen the manner in which that portion of the mission statement was being addressed. Although students were exposed to a few multidisciplinary courses such as research and ethics, there was overall agreement that they needed more useful exposure to other disciplines within a clinical context. An interdisciplinary faculty task force was developed to explore possibilities. The academic dean staffed the task force and provided administrative support. After much discussion, the task force settled on a series of four required interdisciplinary clinical seminars as the preferred method.

The mechanics of developing and implementing the program were daunting, but the group was committed to the project. They enlisted other members of their departments to develop four case studies—one for each seminar. The subject of the case study would require care from each of the three disciplines—nursing, physical therapy, and speech pathology. Thought was given to the need for students to be involved with different age groups and various clinical settings. Teams of faculty members with expertise in each area developed the following cases:

- *Seminar case 1*: Pediatric patient with cerebral palsy who is starting school.
- *Seminar case 2*: Elderly patient with cerebral vascular accident and dysphagia in an acute care setting.
- *Seminar case 3*: Middle-aged adult with HIV and family issues in the community (end stages of illness).
- *Seminar case 4*: Young teen with traumatic brain injury in a rehabilitation center.

The intensive involvement of many faculty members in the development of the cases had some very beneficial effects. Interdisciplinary cooperation was necessary as the cases were developed. Faculty members were able to learn from each other and appreciate the role of the other disciplines. The faculty members who developed the cases were invested in the project and were able to support and commend it to other faculty members and to students in their classes, which reduced some resistance.

Each program was responsible for determining which students would be required to attend the seminars. The nursing program selected students who were in the spring semester of the second year of an entry-level master's program and were enrolled in the Primary Care I course. Nursing students in this program held a baccalaureate in any field prior to entry into the program. They had completed the first year and second fall semester in the generalist level of the nursing program. They were in the process of taking the RN licensing exam during this semester (they all passed). They were then in advanced-level coursework that would lead to a master of science in nursing degree and eligibility to sit for certification as a nurse practitioner. Interdisciplinary seminar attendance was mandatory and counted as part of the clinical component in the Primary Care I course, so that students would not be required to add hours to the course. Compromise and negotiation were needed on the part of the course faculty to recognize and accept that the interdisciplinary seminar was a legitimate learning experience appropriate to the course.

Scheduling the seminars was a major problem. Coordinating three programs with students in different classes and in clinical sites was very difficult. The seminars were held in the late afternoon, and students in clinical placements were asked to leave their clinical site early enough to return to the school. There is no easy solution to this problem. Each student was sent a letter outlining the purpose of the seminars and given the dates and times. The letter explained that attendance was mandatory and that the seminar would count as class hours.

Approximately 60 students were expected to attend the seminars. Four faculty members from each department were recruited to facilitate each seminar. In smaller departments, this meant that department faculty members participated in more than one seminar. The case discussions were designed so that students had an opportunity to participate in multidisciplinary groups, meet with their own specialty, and meet as a total group. The sessions were planned to last 2 hours each.

The role of the faculty members was to facilitate but not to lead the discussion among students. Faculty members were available to correct wrong information, but the focus was to have students take responsibility for explaining their discipline's role in working with the patient. Faculty members were not expected to be experts in the area under discussion or to introduce new material. The faculty role was explained to the students at the beginning of the session.

Previously prepared case materials presented assessment tools used by each discipline and questions to be addressed. The goals of the seminar were presented and clarified to all of the students before breaking students into groups. Students presented their assessments and plans for working with the patients, defining priorities of care. Faculty facilitators encouraged participation by all. Each small group took notes to be presented to the entire group for general discussion.

Evaluations of the seminars from both faculty members and students were excellent. The time selected for the seminars was problematic for many participants and seemed to be the major concern of students. Some students had various excuses for not being able to attend. Snow forced the cancellation of one session. All students attended a minimum of one seminar, but most attended the sessions as scheduled. Students remarked that the discussions were excellent and that they had gained new knowledge from each

(continued)

other as the different disciplinary approaches were presented. Faculty members also benefited from the discussions, and interdepartmental communications were enhanced. Some faculty members were uncomfortable at first with the expectation of their role and were concerned that they did not know enough about specific cases; however, most soon realized that the objectives of the session were valid for the level of their expertise and the expectation of facilitation, not instruction. Overall, the project was deemed a strong success and was presented again, with minor changes.

The program has evolved, but the commitment to interdisciplinary education remains and has expanded. Students will have at least one interdisciplinary learning experience in each year. Each department is responsible for developing the experience for their students, and school-wide presentations will be carried out each semester.

REFERENCE

MGH Institute of Health Professions. (2000). Mission statement. *MGH Institute of Health Professions Self-Study, 13.*

REFERENCES

Chovanec, M. (2008). Innovations applied to the classroom for involuntary groups: Implications for social work education. *Journal of Teaching in Social Work, 28*(1/2), 209–225.

CMS Innovation Center. (2013). *About the CMS Innovation Center.* Retrieved from http://innovation. cms.gov/About/index.html

Kirp, D. L. (1997). Those who can't: 27 ways of looking at a classroom. *Change, 29*(3), 10–19.

Omachonu, V. K., & Einspruch, N. G. (2010). Innovation in healthcare delivery systems: A conceptual framework. *Innovation Journal, 15*(1), Article 2.

They create winners. (1994). *Success, 41*(7), 43–46.

Trossman, S. (2012, May/June). Nurses leading through innovation: Three nurses test strategies to improve care and reduce costs. *American Nurse,* pp. 1–7.

Whitman, B. L., & Rose, W. J. (2003). Using art to express a personal philosophy of nursing. *Nurse Educator, 28*(4), 166–169.

Woods, D. R. (1998). Getting support for your new approaches. *Journal of College Science Teaching, 27*(4), 285–286.

RECOMMENDED READING

Butell, S. S., O'Donovan, P., & Taylor. J. D. (2004). Educational innovations. Instilling the value of reading literature through student-led book discussion groups. *Journal of Nursing Education, 43*(1), 40–44. Abstract: With the desire to instill the value of lifelong reading, nursing faculty and a librarian developed a student-led book discussion group as an innovative teaching strategy for a senior seminar course. Inclusion of the librarian was unique and influenced the shape and rigor of the assignment. In this assignment, students chose one of the faculty-selected books, researched its author(s), read relevant professional book reviews, and developed questions for their peer discussion groups. Student and faculty responses were positive and clearly demonstrated the benefits of this assignment for students' personal development and professional growth.

Jesse, D. E., & Blue, C. (2004). Mary Breckinridge meets Healthy People 2010: A teaching strategy for visioning and building healthy communities. *Journal of Midwifery & Women's Health, 49*(2), 126–131.Abstract: In both midwifery and nursing education, it is essential to include innovative teaching strategies that address the health of communities. This article presents a creative learning activity for midwifery and/or nursing education that integrates Mary Breckinridge's historical example with today's national goals for building communities. The establishment of the Frontier Nursing Service in 1925 is an excellent example of the Mobilize, Assess, Plan, Implement, and Track (MAP-IT) framework for building health communities. Advanced practice nursing and midwifery students can use this historical template to implement their ideas for building healthy communities today.

Kirp, D. L. (1997). Those who can't: 27 ways of looking at a classroom. *Change, 29*(3), 10–19.

Nof, L., & Hill, C. (2005). On the cutting edge: A successful distance PhD degree program: A case study [Electronic version]. *Internet Journal of Allied Health Sciences and Practice, 3*(2). Retrieved from http://ijahsp.nova.edu/articles/vol3num2/nof.htm

Travis, L., & Brennan, P. F. (1998). Information science for the future: An innovative nursing informatics curriculum. *Journal of Nursing Education, 37*(4), 162–168.

Woods, D. R. 1998. Getting support for your new approaches. *Journal of College Science Teaching, 27*(4), 285–286.

CHAPTER 4

Finding Information: Teaching the Strategies for Searching

■ SHANTI FREUNDLICH ■

Educational approaches are constantly evolving and changing, as are student and educator expectations. The last decade has seen an elevation in our expectations regarding the availability and accessibility of information, as well as the sophistication of the search tools at our disposal. Students and faculty now not only expect all information to be available immediately online (Brantley & Pickard, 2010), but also tend to work from the starting assumption that their search skills are sophisticated enough to easily find all the information they're looking for, on any given subject (Dahlstrom, 2012). Finding relevant, high-quality information that can be the basis of evidence-based nursing practice is not as simple as the Google search that most students are comfortable using when they enter college or graduate school. Search skills can be learned, and this chapter will discuss strategies that will work regardless of search engine or interface design. These strategies are part of the mechanical skill set necessary for searching, as well as a larger critical thinking skill set concerning finding and evaluating the information that students will need throughout their nursing careers.

There is no one single correct search strategy, nor is there one single correct way to teach search strategies. Regardless of the teaching theory of preference for the professor or the learning style of the student, the keys for developing searching proficiency and confidence are repetition and a clear search topic. The more often students search for and find academically or clinically relevant information, the less intimidating the resources and strategies become. The teaching of search strategies and appropriate resources needs to be closely followed by opportunities for students to test them out via assignments that require finding information (Duke, 2011), and this type of assignment-based searching is a good way for students to become familiar with articulating topic concepts. As students become proficient in using search strategies and navigating the various resource interfaces, they can then focus their attention on critically evaluating the information they find. This chapter will discuss search strategies from two perspectives. First, it will discuss what librarians and other information professionals are doing to make information more easily discoverable; second, it will articulate strategies to make the search process more understandable, effective, and efficient. Being able to find, identify, and use high-quality information is an integral part of lifelong information literacy, and it speaks to the following teaching and learning core competencies:

- Nurse educators who incorporate teaching critical thinking about search strategies are working to meet the National League for Nursing Core Competencies of Nurse Educators (National League for Nursing, 2005): Facilitate Learning (Competency 1), Use Assessment and Evaluation Strategies (Competency 3), Function as a Change Agent and Leader (Compentency 5), and Function Within the Educational Environment (Competency 8).
- These skills also help students meet the Association of College & Research Libraries (ACRL) Information Literacy Competency Standards for Higher Education (2000)—specifically standards 1, 2, and 4: "The information literate student determines the nature and extent of the information needed (p. 8)," "accesses needed information effectively and efficiently" (p. 9), and "uses information effectively to accomplish a specific purpose" (p. 13).

▪ Current Issues in Searching

According to the 2011 Pew Internet Health Topics survey, 80% of Internet users, or 59% of U.S. adults, look online for health information (Fox, 2011, p. 5), and search engines have conditioned people, especially the younger generation to expect information to be easy to find (Purcell et al., 2012, p. 16). The 2012 Pew Internet survey titled "How Teens Do Research in the Digital World" found that teachers agreed that the amount of information available online can be discouraging or overwhelming to students (Purcell et al., 2012, p. 16). Even more importantly for healthcare professionals, there are the serious accuracy concerns for over half of all health information–related web resources (Chung, Oden, Joyner, Sims, & Moon, 2012). Unfortunately, while many students think that they have "Google-fu" (the ability to find anything with a Google search), the ERIAL Project and other research have shown that instead they have a rather "stunted understanding of how to finely tune a search in order to hone in on usable sources" (Kolowich, 2011, Exploding the "Myth of the Digital Native"). Students' mental models seem to primarily rely on typing whole questions into any and all search boxes, not inquiring how the results are generated or arranged, trusting the first few search results, and rarely scrolling past the first page (Duke, 2011; Pan, 2007). Students have limited experience utilizing advanced search features, and they sometimes compare academic databases to black holes. Thus, teaching search strategies must acknowledge students' existing models and processes, encourage them to embrace the search frustrations and failures that they regularly experience (Bain, 2012), explicate the personal benefit of altering their search strategies, and give them time to try out the new strategies on a topic of their choice.

■ The Information Landscape

The information landscape and the technology that shapes it continue to evolve rapidly; devices like smartphones that were uncommon 10 years ago are now central to web development and information access. Internet users have come to expect that all information will be immediately available at their fingertips; even the delay of making a photocopy or entering an additional password can be the difference between reading or skipping an article (Sathe, Grady, & Giuse, 2002). Researchers at every level admit that they would rather use a less relevant and less authoritative e-journal article than a more relevant and more authoritative print article (Sathe et al., 2002). In response, libraries and librarians are adapting rapidly and adopting new methods of access to, and the construction of, information.

Traditionally, libraries were gatekeepers to information, but in 2012, they were merely one gateway among many to information. Today's libraries use every tool at their disposal to connect students and faculty to the research they need, including interlibrary loans, patron-drive acquisitions methods, and e-resources. However, these gateways are limited by the licenses, contracts, and other costs associated with high-quality information. While the costs of serial subscriptions have been increasing exponentially for decades, they are now reaching a point where highly regarded research institutions, including Harvard University, are looking to alternative subscription models (Johnson, 2012). This sea change in the information landscape affects everyone doing research because the subscription difficulties that institutions face will affect which publications users can access, and therefore which search results they see; it may become not uncommon for faculty to be unable to access the published versions of their own research.

One of the reactions to the serials crisis (referring to the exponential price increase) has been the open access movement. This movement calls for publishing models of peer-reviewed research that distribute the costs and profits more evenly. As traditional publishing becomes increasingly unsustainable, the awareness of and interest in open access publishing is growing. It is on librarians' shoulders to increase awareness at their institutions about the costs of traditional publishing, the benefits of open access publishing, and ways that faculty, students, and researchers can shape the conversation and the information available for them to search.

As the number of resources available only through vendor-hosted platforms continues to increase, librarians are continuing to discuss whether simply being able to access this information is enough or if the ownership of information offers unique benefits to students and faculty. In the past, there was no gray area between access and ownership; a library purchased a physical book or subscribed to a print journal, and library patrons accessed (read) the information in it. But the advent of e-books, e-journals, and online point-of-care reference resources has blurred the line between access and ownership. Librarians and other information professionals are debating questions including:

> If a library is supporting an evidence-based nursing program, does it need to own the older, increasingly out-of-date physical texts, or is offering online access to current research and information sufficient?
>
> From a more long-term perspective, what happens if an increasingly larger number of libraries choose access over ownership? How does that affect libraries' negotiating position with publishers on licensing terms of agreement?

As the quantity of information available only through proprietary platforms increases, it becomes increasingly more challenging for end users to smoothly navigate all of the platforms. In addition to working to provide the highest number of high-quality resources as possible, libraries are working with vendors to improve the search experience and make it more straightforward. Discovery systems are an emerging technology on this front. These include proprietary platforms developed by database vendors like EBSCO and ProQuest that index all the resources that a library has access to or chooses to include, regardless of format or publisher, and allows patrons to search everything from a single search box. Discovery systems are still a fairly new technology with multiple kinks to work out, but they are being positioned as an answer to the intuitive search experience that users have come to expect and a means to connect little-known resources to the students and faculty who can most benefit from their use.

Libraries are working to increase faculty and student awareness of the factors that limit access, reach decisions on access versus ownership, and implement discovery systems. Meanwhile, faculty and students can empower themselves by becoming more effective and efficient searchers; technology may be constantly evolving, but a solid understanding of how to structure a search will lead to better search results regardless of the interface or indexed resources. An advantage of the myriad of vendor platforms is that their competition may push the development of friendly, faster, more responsive search functionality. As students tend to focus on only their own immediate information needs, it is important for teachers to be aware of the larger information landscape and understand the context in which their students are searching.

Librarians are also collaborating directly with faculty to develop more programmatic approaches to our teaching, so that it goes beyond the mechanics of getting the most out of an academic database and instead focuses on the critical thinking behind a search strategy and the evaluation criteria necessary to make informed choices, and it ties directly into the course curriculum. To do this, librarians must be up-to-date on the vocabulary and research concerns of the academic field and learning outcomes of the faculty member. Likewise, faculty must be up-to-date on the resources and services available and the limitations faced by their libraries.

■ Search Strategies

This section discusses methods to make searching more effective and efficient, especially where students face so much anxiety—finding research literature in academic databases. These strategies will also work in open search engines like Google, point-of-care reference sources like DynaMed, and general reference sources like Credo Reference.

A somewhat underappreciated but important part of the search process is translating a research topic into search terms. Without clear research concepts to start from, search strategies will never yield fully satisfactory results because there is no clear goal for the search. The search process combines articulating an initial topic, expressing it in search terms, picking where to search, and refining the results to only the relevant articles. Developing keyword search terms in many ways reverses the research question development process. That is, by necessity, a research question is narrow and highly focused, whereas the combination of search terms necessary to find relevant literature must start deliberately broad, encompassing alternate and related terms to describe the topic. Students tend to start their search with broad, long-form research topics of interest:

> "I'm interesting in comparing the Wong-Baker FACES Pain Rating Scale to nurses' judgment of pain in pediatric patients."
>
> "My topic is related to parent–nurse relationships and improved patient outcomes in the NICU."
>
> "What are the best practices around interdisciplinary nursing and medical education?"
>
> "We are hoping to improve communication between doctors and nurses in academic and clinical settings."
>
> "Our interest is to find out more about the attitudes of both healthcare providers and patients toward screening for domestic violence."

Once a students have an initial topic in mind, they can start translating it into keywords. Without instructions or an explanation of how databases use the search terms to produce search results, students will often try to type their whole question into a database's search box. When this fails to produce results, they become frustrated and revert to familiar Internet search engines. However, keywords can be explained simply and adopted quickly. Keywords express the concentrated essence of important concepts—the ideas that are core to the question. Any question complex enough to be a research question includes multiple concepts, and a good search strategy addresses all of them. Those different concepts are usually connected to each other using *AND*; expressed as keywords, the previous examples could look like this:

parent-nurse relationships AND patient outcomes
interdisciplinary nursing AND medical education AND communication AND clinical attitudes AND healthcare providers AND domestic violence

Most databases return articles that contain the literal search word or phrase typed, primarily in the title, author, abstract, or subject headings, although databases are becoming more flexible. Turning a question into keywords can be a challenge, but once students see the benefits to their search results, it can help them shift their mental models and adopt new habits (Bain, 2012).

Students are often reassured to hear that their search strategies are not being compared to a perfect search; the only ideal search is the one that returns the most relevant, accurate results. Search strategies and keywords are not precious; they are flexible tools to be changed or thrown away if the results aren't good enough. For the more anxious searchers, it may also be reassuring to hear that most databases and search engines will save their search histories, so previous keywords choices can be recovered. There is no correct number of keywords, and there is no perfect combination of keywords for each topic. That said, usually a range of two to four concepts with a keyword for each one will suffice for most searches, although there are exceptions, including for systematic reviews.

The advantage of expressing concepts as keywords is that students can express their ideas in their own words; there is no wrong keyword. However, this flexibility also means that there are an unlimited number of ways to describe a topic, and it can be challenging to align your keywords to the terms actually used in the literature. While a student might know exactly which concepts their keywords signify, it's quite possible that experts and researchers in the field might describe their work in different or more technical/medical terms. Adding alternate or additional keywords or using subject terms can help bridge this conceptual gap. Since a single concept can be described in many ways, adding alternate keywords expands the potential search results for a concept, so using the same example search topics as before, one might use the following criteria:

Parent-nurse OR family-centered OR parent-professional
Domestic violence OR intimate partner abuse OR spousal abuse

In our examples, the alternate keyword phrases describe the same core idea, so we're still searching for the same concept, only broader. Students sometimes assume that search boxes understand what they mean, rather than what they type. In reality, most research-focused resources still depend on literal words and phrases, so providing multiple terms for a core idea lets the database do more work for you. Brainstorming alternate terms to describe a concept indicates the ability to critically think about a problem from multiple angles, a core characteristic of the information-literate student (ACRL, 2000).

Teachers may recognize the connecting terms being discussed as Boolean operators, and they might realize that there is a third term: *NOT*. Similar to *AND* and *OR*, *NOT* defines the relationship between the concepts one is searching for in an electronic resource. However, *NOT* is an exclusionary term and removes concepts from the search, rather than broadening the concepts (OR) or narrowing the focus (AND). While it certainly can be a useful term, the author often hesitates to encourage students to build their initial search strategies based on *NOT*, because they tend to not know enough about their topic at the beginning to say with certainty that a given concept is definitely of not interest to them and is not crucial to the topic at hand. Assignment- and evidence-based projects will sometimes also ask for comparisons of topics, conditions, practices, and so forth, so to exclude a concept would remove relevant results. That said, as students become more experienced searchers, they can benefit greatly from excluding parts of the literature that they may have already explored, or those variations on a topic that are not part of their research question. An example of using *NOT* to exclude sections of the literature is a search for the latest research on cardiac risk factors; if a student is focusing on only nonsmoking patients, he could exclude research on the effects of smoking. This will be a more efficient search as it is getting the database to do more of the drudge work and gives the student more time to pick and choose from relevant research, rather than sorting through pages of article abstracts that he will not be able to use anyway.

Anyone who has tried to search for research literature in an academic database has experienced the frustration of a failed search and the moment of panic wondering if perhaps there just isn't any literature on the topic. Experienced faculty members know that a message of "no results found" is really just a message to try the search again, but students need to be prepared by their teachers for their search to fail. It is frustrating to labor through articulating a search strategy, only to be told there is no research matching the criteria. The truth is, there is almost always literature related to a research topic. The challenge, especially for students new to research, is to brainstorm additional search terms while still staying on topic; usually adding alternate terms gives a search enough flexibility to start returning results. For the students having difficulty reconceiving their topic in different terms, the subject heading and thesaurus functions built into most databases will give them hints and suggestions. However, for many initial student forays into the research literature, it is enough to simply broaden the keywords that represent the major concepts and remove keywords that represent minor concepts or demographic details. Suddenly seeing tens of thousands of results can reassure students that there are many potentially related articles, and the database has the tools to narrow down the list to the most relevant ones. The true challenge after a failed search is to figure out how to approach the same topic from a new direction but still maintain the same focus.

If approaching the topic with different keywords does not bring more relevant and satisfactory results, the issue may be where students are conducting their search. As we've established, students tend to expect that everything will be available from one search box. However, academic libraries still subscribe to a multitude of different databases because different content is available through each database. A student's search results can only be as relevant as the content he or she is searching; thus, while many students in health sciences field are content to return to Medline, PubMed, or CINAHL for search after search, they can truly broaden their searches by looking in a new place. Beyond the familiar resources, libraries will usually list and describe additional databases related to any given topic in research guides and on the library website.

As mentioned earlier, databases are built to assist with the mechanics of searching, and students are not required to think of every alternative term or search criteria on their own. In addition to the knowledge base students build through classroom and clinical learning, databases and other high-quality resources include tools to assist this process, including the thesaurus, or subject terms that students can use to find preferred and additional terms to use. Also, every search result article is a gold mine for additional keywords; titles and abstracts are full of clues as to how leading voices in a field are describing the current research. Those terms can be added to or even replace initial keywords, and altering search terms based on the language used by research in the field will help bring back more results that are current, relevant, and high quality. This stage of the process highlights that keywords are not precious, and as soon as a better or additional keyword is identified, it should immediately be incorporated into the search.

Mining article references is a long-standing method of enhancing a literature search and quickly gathering the significant, well-respected resources in a field. While in theory mining research article references is similar to following links in an online article, students new to the research process often need to be encouraged to see articles as dynamic tools that are more than just the sum of their research content. In addition to using an article's references, databases are starting to offer links to citing sources. That is, if an article was published in 2008, the citing sources are the articles published since then using the initial article as a reference. Mining these sources is a way for students to stay within their search topic but move forward into even more current research. This is a powerful search tool that can help students understand how past research informs future research, and how both of them inform practice.

Searching primarily with keywords is still a fairly recent development, and the subject heading searches previously depended upon are still the backbone of how articles, journals, and books are organized. This organization includes MeSH in Medline, CINAHL Headings in CINAHL, and the Library of Congress in most academic libraries. Simply put, subject headings are expertly applied tags that are pulled from a controlled list and are used to connect like research to like research. If you find yourself fascinated by the topic of subject headings and controlled vocabularies, then a career in cataloging, using metadata in connection to the semantic web, or information organization may be for you.

The advantages of a subject heading are that it is a term from a field of research (e.g., nursing, medicine) and that it has a consistent, specific meaning that has been applied by an expert. That is, every article with "Family Centered Care" as a subject heading is guaranteed to contain content on family-centered care, and a student can easily get to all the articles on family-centered care through that subject heading. Searching only via subject headings is possible and is often a useful exercise for graduate or PhD students who need to do an exhaustive literature search. Understanding the basics of subject headings can reassure students that they are not attempting to pull structure out of chaos, but that in fact databases are highly organized repositories designed to facilitate their search process. Understanding the underlying structure of information may help students shift their mental models about searching for and finding information to include keywords, subject headings, citation mining, and connecting terms (Boolean operators: *AND*, *OR*, and *NOT*).

■ Additional Search Strategies

Keywords are not limited to just topic concepts; they can also be used as a tool to roughly limit results to a specific type of literature. For example, adding *quantitative* can help limit the search results to only quantitative research. Similarly, adding *Cochrane* can be a quick way to limit to results indexed in the Cochrane Database of Systematic Reviews. That said, students are not solely dependent on the search box and keywords for narrowing down their results by relevancy. Instead, there are an almost overwhelming number of limiting tools built into databases to do the work of narrowing down the results for a student. There are limiters that can be used on any search for evidence-based literature, such as date range and peer reviewed; there are demographic options, such as age and gender; there are methodology-based limiters, including EBM review and randomized controlled trials; and there are a variety of others, including author or first author is a nurse, human subject only, inpatient, and language. None of these options is required for a search, but they will do some of the work of narrowing down the literature; they help the student researcher eliminate the information that is not relevant to the topic at hand and would have confused the issue rather than clarified it.

■ Conclusion

With everything else that faculty are being asked to integrate into their curricula and classrooms—meaningful assessment, active learning activities, social media, the latest technology, all on top of the increasing amount of actual content and up-to-the-minute research—it can sound like one additional element too many to ask faculty to teach search strategies as well. However, faculty can also choose to view search strategies as a skill set that empowers students to take responsibility for their own learning—both immediately in the classroom and in their long-term practice—and they can draw on their librarian colleagues for teaching support.

When students understand that research articles connect to practice guidelines and the everyday clinical choices they make, and when they are able to confidently search for the latest evidence, they will be empowered to take responsibility for their own learning. There is high-quality information available to support students through their learning process, but they need to develop confidence in their searching abilities, be willing to be flexible in their approach, and set high standards for the information they use. Teaching students to be empowered, confident searchers is the first step in training them to start thinking critically about the information they choose to use in their academic work, in their clinical practice, and throughout their everyday lives. The next step beyond finding information is confidently being able to evaluate it— weighing its strengths and weakness before consciously deciding how or if to use it as a foundation for evidence-based practice.

References

Association of College & Research Libraries (ACRL). (2000). Information literacy competency standards for higher education. Retrieved from http://www.acrl.org/ala/mgrps/divs/acrl/standards/standards.pdf

Bain, K. (2012, November). *What the best college teachers do—and how you can be among them.* Speech presented at the Colleges of the Fenway Teaching and Learning Collaborative Annual Fall Conference, Boston, MA.

Brantley, S., & Pickard, B. (2010). The ERIAL project at UIC: Understanding how students search for information. Retrieved from http://www.carli.illinois.edu/mem-serv/mem-train/100514pswg/Understanding_fromUIC.pdf

Chung, M., Oden, R. P., Joyner, B. L., Sims, A., & Moon, R. (2012). Safe infant sleep recommendations on the Internet: Let's Google it. *Journal of Pediatrics, 161*(6), 1080–1084.e1. doi: 10.1016/j.jpeds.2012.06.004

Core competencies of nurse educators with task statements. (2005). Retrieved from http://www.nln.org/profdev/pdf/corecompetencies.pdf

Dahlstrom, E. (2012, September). *ECAR study of undergraduate students and information technology, 2012* [research report]. Louisville, CO: EDUCAUSE Center for Applied Research. Retrieved from http://educause.edu/ecar

Duke, L. (2011). Search skills of the 21st century student. Retrieved from http://www.erialproject.org/wp-content/uploads/2011/04/ACRL-erial-results-presentation.pdf

Fox, S. (2011). Health topics. Pew Internet & American Life Project. Retrieved from http://www.pewinternet.org/Reports/2011/HealthTopics.aspx

Johnson, C. (2012, April 28). Harvard panel pushes benefit of free journals: Costly publications targeted. *Boston Globe.* Retrieved from http://www.bostonglobe.com/metro/2012/04/27/harvard-pushes-back-against-academic-publishers-pricing-encourages-open-access/9zKMiX3Qq0QJfuo2HI4pPL/story.html

Kolowich, S. (2011, August 22). What students don't know. *Inside Higher Ed.* Retrieved from http://www.insidehighered.com/news/2011/08/22/erial_study_of_student_research_habits_at_illinois_university_libraries_reveals_alarmingly_poor_information_literacy_and_skills

Pan, B., Hembrooke, H., Joachims, T., Lorigo, L., Gary, G., & Granka, L. (2007). In Google we trust: Users' decisions on rank, position, and relevance. *Journal of Computer-Mediated Communication, 12*(3), 801–823. doi: 10.1111/j.1083-6101.2007.00351.x

Purcell, K., Raine, L., Heaps, A., Buchanan, J., Friedrich, L., Jacklin, A., … Zickuhr, K. (2012). How teens do research in the digital world. Pew Internet & American Life Project. Retrieved from http://pewinternet.org/Reports/2012/Student-Research.aspx

Sathe, N. A., Grady, J. L., & Giuse, N. B. (2002). Print versus electronic journals: A preliminary investigation into the effect of journal format on research processes. *Journal of the Medical Library Association, 90*(2), 235.

RECOMMENDED READING

Blanchett, H., Powis, C., & Webb, J. (2012). *A guide to teaching information literacy: 101 practical tips*. London, UK: Facet Publishing.

Booth, C. (2011). *Reflective teaching, effective learning: Instructional literacy for library educators*. Chicago, IL: American Library Association.

Carpenter, J., Wetheridge, L., Tanner, S., & Smith, N. (2012). Researchers of tomorrow. Retrieved from http://www.jisc.ac.uk/publications/reports/2012/researchers-of-tomorrow

Gavin, C. (2008). *Teaching information literacy: A conceptual approach*. Lanham, MD: Scarecrow Press.

Gwyer, R., Stubbings, R., Walton, G., International Federation of Library Associations and Institutions, & International Federation of Library Associations and Institutions. (2012). *The road to information literacy: Librarians as facilitators of learning*. Berlin, Germany, & Boston, MA: De Gruyter Saur.

Kaplowitz, J. R. (2012). *Transforming information literacy instruction using learner-centered teaching*. New York, NY: Neal-Schuman Publishers.

Kvenild, C., & Calkins, K. (2011). *Embedded librarians: Moving beyond one-shot instruction*. Chicago, IL: Association of College and Research Libraries.

Palfrey, J., & Gasser, U. (2008). *Born digital: Understanding the first generation of digital natives*. New York, NY: Basic Books.

Walton, G., & Pope, A. (2011). *Information literacy: Infiltrating the agenda, challenging minds*. Oxford, UK: Chandos Publishing.

CHAPTER 5

Clinical Reasoning: Action-Focused Thinking

■ CHERYL A. TUCKER AND MARTHA J. BRADSHAW ■

Instructors in the health professions, who are also practitioners in their fields, are compelled to assist students in developing their clinical reasoning skills as beginners in the health professions and as novice thinkers. Sound reasoning is essential in preserving the standards of the profession and promoting quality patient outcomes. Health professions literature has long addressed this process as critical thinking. However, the critical thinking model is limited in that it does not move learners to the level of thinking about their thinking. Recent literature is addressing this awareness and the need to move to a deeper level of thinking. This process is *clinical reasoning*. Within the various health professions, many terms and models exist. With the call to interdisciplinary education and collaborative patient care, healthcare professionals need a shared model of clinical reasoning. This chapter provides an overview of what clinical reasoning is and why it should be taught in a purposeful way, and it presents a model that can be implemented across the healthcare disciplines.

■ Clinical Reasoning Framework

In 2003, the Institute of Medicine (IOM) published its report, *Health Professions Education: A Bridge to Quality,* which examined the need to transform health professions education. The IOM's vision for the education of health professionals is articulated in its core competencies, which assert, "All health professionals should be educated to deliver patient-centered care as members of an interdisciplinary team, emphasizing evidence-based practice, quality improvement approaches, and informatics" (IOM, 2003, p. 3). *The Future of Nursing: Leading Change, Advancing Health* (IOM, 2010) further addresses these core competencies and explores the necessity of transforming professional nursing education. The American Association of Colleges of Nurses (AACN) supports these core competencies as delineated in the *Essentials for Baccalaureate Education for Professional Nursing Practice,* which highlights such areas as "patient-centered care, interprofessional teams, evidence-based practice, quality improvement, patient safety, informatics, clinical reasoning/critical thinking, genetics and genomics, cultural sensitivity, professionalism, practice across the lifespan, and end-of-life care" (AACN, 2008, p. 35).

Various professional organizations use *critical thinking, clinical judgment,* and *clinical reasoning* interchangeably. A definition of clinical judgment is "an interpretation or conclusion about a patient's needs, concerns, or health problems, and/or the decision to take action (or not), use or modify standard approaches, or improvise new ones as deemed appropriate by the patient's response" (Tanner, 2006, p. 204). Clinical reasoning is the ability of the health professions student to use critical thinking skills in the practice environment. It should include the "context and concerns of the patient and family" (Benner, Sutphen, Leonard, & Day, 2010, p. 85). Clinical imagination and reflection are also part of clinical reasoning (Benner et al., 2010). The thought is that critical thinking is a snapshot in time while clinical reasoning can accommodate the changing nature in the clinical settings. Tanner (2006) acknowledges that problem solving, critical thinking, decision making, and clinical judgment are often used in the literature to mean the same thing.

In varying degrees, all students need guidance with transfer or application of knowledge to specific patient situations. This process, also called knowledge translation, is the means by which new knowledge is organized, given meaning or understood, and put in to action (Leahey & Svavarsdottir, 2009). As the teacher builds clinical reasoning abilities in the student, the individual student learns (or should learn) to recognize the meaning of knowledge (information) and then grasp how to use (apply) this knowledge. Transfer of knowledge is critical for success in the healthcare arena.

The IOM (2003) report, *Health Professions Education: A Bridge to Quality,* articulates the need for healthcare professionals to be amply prepared to address the healthcare needs of an ever-changing patient population. The IOM report calls for healthcare providers to collaborate on delivering individualized, yet comprehensive health care. This requires purposeful, thoughtful, analytical processing of information and deliberate communication of this process to other healthcare professionals. For this to happen, the educational process must be transformed into one that cultivates clinical reasoning.

What role does the health professions teacher play in the development of clinical reasoning in his or her students? Health professions teachers have been utilizing different tools in promoting clinical reasoning in their students. A few examples of various tools utilized in the thinking process include professional nursing's nursing process (assessment, nursing diagnosis, planning, implementation, and evaluation), medical education's SNAPPS (summarize, narrow, analyze, probe, plan, and select), and physical therapy's International Classification of Functioning, Disability and Health (ICF). These tools promote the student's thinking through various steps of the clinical reasoning process. When health professions students collaborate on patient care problems, the professionals must speak the same language as they develop their clinical reasoning skills. To develop those skills in an interdisciplinary manner, the students collectively should use a decision-making tree, based on the scientific method, as a clinical reasoning tool. Utilizing the clinical reasoning tool, students acknowledge the clinical problem and gather data; analyze the information, develop solutions or a plan, and make a decision; implement the decision(s); and evaluate the decision(s).

The scientific method of thinking, which uses problem definition, analysis, decision making, implementation, and evaluation, has long been used by healthcare providers. Every profession uses this method in some way but uses different nomenclature for the steps of the process. A proposed model for clinical reasoning (see **Table 5-1**) incorporates all of the analytical methods used by educators in the various health professions. The categories are similar in content, are sequential, and serve as a means for the novice to understand their thinking as they move through the process.

Health care continues to grow more complex and health professionals must be better prepared to utilize their clinical reasoning skills. Teaching clinical reasoning is difficult; it must be purposeful and can be both planned and spontaneous. The IOM report (2010, p. 544) states, "Faculty report spending most of their time supervising students in hands-on procedures, leaving little time focused on fostering the development of clinical reasoning skills" (McNelis & Ironside, 2009). It is essential that classroom and clinical experiences are interwoven with real-life clinical experiences. Health professions teachers assist the students as they make connections between gaining and applying knowledge, so that students stitch a strong tapestry of clinical reasoning skills for the diverse and complex healthcare environment (Benner et al., 2010).

■ Types of Learners

Teaching of clinical reasoning to the student will vary in style and depth depending upon the point at which the student is in the health professions program. Beginning students need a foundation based on the essential course work such as basic sciences, psychology, sociology, and the like. Furthermore, a fundamental condition for learning and practice in all health professions students is the ability to obtain and manipulate information from a variety of sources, organizing it in a meaningful way to bring about purposeful decision making. Students come to the learning environment with different learning styles and preferences. When faced with new knowledge, students gravitate to their dominant learning style and successfully assimilate new information when the teaching strategies utilized are in harmony with their preferred style. (Learning styles are discussed more thoroughly elsewhere in this text.)

Clinical practitioners also need the physical abilities to provide safe and competent care. To assist educators, the Americans with Disabilities Act (ADA) has defined

Table 5-1 A Clinical Reasoning Model for the Healthcare Professions

Healthcare Professions	Scientific Method[a]	Nursing[b]	Medicine[c]	Physical Therapy[d]
Clinical reasoning model	Scientific process	Nursing process	SNAPPS	The physical therapy clinical reasoning and reflection tool (PT-CRT)
Recognition				
Identify the clinical situation and collect relevant data	Define the problem; gather information (data)	Assessment (data collection): History taking, physical assessment, results of diagnostic tests	Summarize briefly the history and findings	Initial data gathering/ interview
Appraisal				
Analysis of findings and formulating conclusions	Analyze the information (data)	Nursing diagnosis: Consider assessment database and identify problems; choose nursing diagnosis	Narrow the differential to two or three relevant possibilities	Generation of initial hypothesis
Formulate Actions				
Develop interdisciplinary strategies to resolve clinical situation	Develop solutions; make a decision	Planning: Determine desired outcomes; choose interventions to achieve those outcomes	Analyze the differential by comparing and contrasting the possibilities Probe the preceptor by asking questions about uncertainties, difficulties, or alternative approaches	Examination/evaluation/ plan of care

Implement Actions				
Accomplish strategies using interdisciplinary collaboration	Implement the decision	*Implementation*: Carry out the interventions	Plan management for the patient's medical issues	Interventions
Clinical Judgment				
Evaluate decisions and outcomes and revise strategies as needed	Evaluate the decision	*Evaluation*: Assess the result of the interventions; determine if outcomes have been achieved; revise the plan if outcomes are not being met; terminate interventions no longer needed	Select a case-related issue for self-directed learning	Reexamination/outcomes

a. deWit, 2009, p. 50.
b. deWit, 2009, p. 50.
c. Wolpaw, Papp, & Bordaage, 2009.
d. Atkinson & Nixon-Cave, 2011.

core competencies, with the intent of clarifying minimal expectations for entry-level applicants (Americans with Disabilities Act, 1990). Each health profession then can develop specific criteria as appropriate for the benchmark of that profession. Examples of typical core competencies and the ways they are defined in nursing are displayed in **Table 5-2**.

Table 5-2   Example Core Performance Standards

Requirements	Standards	Examples
Critical thinking	Critical thinking ability for effective clinical reasoning and clinical judgment consistent with level of educational preparation	Identification of cause/effect relationships in clinical situations Use of the scientific method in the development of patient care plans Evaluation of the effectiveness of nursing interventions
Professional relationships	Interpersonal skills sufficient for professional interactions with a diverse population of individuals, families, and groups	Establishment of rapport with patients/clients and colleagues Capacity to engage in successful conflict resolution Peer accountability
Communication	Communication adeptness sufficient for verbal and written professional interactions	Explanation of treatment procedures, initiation of health teaching Documentation and interpretation of nursing actions and patient/client responses
Mobility	Physical abilities sufficient for movement from room to room and in small spaces	Movement about patient's room, work spaces, and treatment areas Administration of rescue procedures such as cardiopulmonary resuscitation
Motor skills	Gross and fine motor abilities sufficient for providing safe, effective nursing care	Calibration and use of equipment Therapeutic positioning of patients
Hearing	Auditory ability sufficient for monitoring and assessing health needs	Ability to hear monitoring device alarm and other emergency signals Ability to discern auscultatory sounds and cries for help
Visual ability	Visual ability sufficient for observation and assessment necessary in patient care	Ability to observe patient's condition and responses to treatments
Tactile sense	Tactile ability sufficient for physical assessment	Ability to palpate in physical examinations and various therapeutic interventions

Source: Retrieved from http://www.sreb.org/page/1390/the_americans_with_disabilities_act.html.

Prerequisite courses and core competencies assist beginning health professions students as they progress to clinical courses where their thinking about patient problems is transformed into clinical reasoning. There also are essential attributes of learners that will contribute to the development of clinical reasoning. These attributes are:

- *Motivation:* A willing learner who desires to become a health professional
- *Attention to details:* Recognize and use vital information to promote safe patient outcomes
- *Ability to formulate questions:* For the purposes of clarifying, acquiring, and processing information
- *Awareness of knowledge gaps:* Based upon known information, can identify what is not known and can identify resources for narrowing the knowledge gap
- *Awareness of own thinking:* Attention to own strategies for thinking through a problem and recognition of hindrances to effective problem solving
- *Ability to draw analogies:* Taking known information and applying it to new situations such as a challenging patient example

As learners gain more exposure in the clinical setting, they have more experiences and knowledge on which to draw on for their clinical reasoning. Individual students develop their own success strategies for developing clinical reasoning. Verbal learners, who process and absorb new knowledge through logic and sequence, are typical of left-brain thinkers. These left-brain thinkers will learn clinical reasoning best through a linear process as exemplified by nursing process care plans. Students who have a learning tendency toward right-brain thinking processes absorb information visually, holistically, and often intuitively. Right-brain thinkers prefer a more global approach such as the use of concept maps (Worden, Hinton, & Fischer, 2011).

■ Conditions for Learning

Effective Teaching for Clinical Reasoning

To cultivate clinical reasoning in the health professions student, the instructor should possess a comprehensive command of the subject and must facilitate thinking by the student rather than merely presenting information. Current practice knowledge is imperative and should include professional standards, guidelines, practice recommendations, and research evidence. The instructor's clinical practice background is beneficial in providing clinical scenarios that are realistic and promote retention of concepts that are useful in clinical practice. Furthermore, the instructor must possess the same attributes of the learner as listed in the previous section. Thus, the ideal teacher is one who can articulate and bring about clinical reasoning in his or her own self and in students.

A teaching style that incorporates Socratic questioning is ideal for developing clinical reasoning in the student. The questioning format stimulates clinical curiosity

("What would we expect in the patient when we see ____?"), and the process leads students to start thinking in the form of questions ("Why did this happen?"). The Socratic method also allows faculty and students to listen to each other's thinking processes and decision making (Rogge, 2001). When using Socratic questioning, the faculty member constructs questions purposefully to lead the student down a particular path of thinking. The process of moving through a scenario brings the student to outcomes the faculty wishes to reach. As the guide in this process, the faculty member redirects the student's thinking when needed, explores potential outcomes of the situation, challenges the student's clinical reasoning abilities by exploring options, and then discusses alternative actions. An example of this process is in **Figure 5-1**.

As can be seen in the example in Figure 5-1, the student's clinical reasoning is not enhanced when the faculty assumes control of the situation. Promoting clinical reasoning includes assessment, often through questioning, of the student's knowledge and potential knowledge gaps or misunderstandings. The instructor then can correct the student's thinking to bring about more accurate reasoning. Due to the nature of the clinical setting the instructor, at times, may need to be more directive in the approach with the student. In another illustration, in the teaching example at the end of this chapter, it would be easier for the faculty member to take action to correct the problem, but this does not promote the development of independent thinking and

---

On a routine clinical day, it was time for the student to give his patient an insulin injection. The student and the instructor met in the medication room to review pertinent information prior to preparing the injection. The student had all the correct information and began to prepare the insulin injection. During the process of drawing up the medication, the student drew up the wrong dose of insulin—50 units of insulin instead of 5 units. The instructor remained calm and thought about how to point out the medication error to the student in such a way that the student could learn from the experience, accept constructive criticism, and not lose self-confidence.

The instructor gave the student the opportunity to recheck each step in the process, in hopes that the student would identify the medication error. Unfortunately, the student did not realize he had prepared an incorrect dose. Using the Socratic method, the instructor began to ask the student questions concerning the medication in an effort to determine if a knowledge gap could be identified. If so, the instructor could provide additional direction and provide time for further review. Although the student knew the drug information, it became apparent that the student could not accurately read calibrations on a syringe. It was now time for the instructor to intervene. So the instructor asked the student to identify where on the syringe the 5-unit mark was for the correct dose. The student pointed to the 50-unit mark. The instructor directed the student to the correct calibration on the syringe. The student immediately realized his mistake and corrected the medication dosage. The instructor discussed with the student the potential outcome if he had administered the wrong dosage. Working through the steps of the clinical reasoning model, this situation became an opportunity for the student to explore the potential negative consequences to the patient. He then administered the insulin injection correctly.

As a follow-up, the instructor referred the student to the clinical skills lab for remediation.

■ **Figure 5-1** Case Example: Guiding a Student in Clinical Reasoning.

the student's clinical reasoning skills. Again, the role of faculty in developing clinical reasoning is to cultivate clinical reasoning in others.

Reflective practice serves as a basis for future action or as a guide in gaining understanding about an experience. Effective teachers can benefit from self-analysis through reflection prior to the teaching experience by asking such questions as "Where do I want them to demonstrate progress today?" "What are the clinical goals for the day?" "How can I promote clinical curiosity in my students?" "Is there anything about my teaching style that impedes the students?" Such self reflection by teachers will lead to beneficial effects in students, in the form of clinical reasoning.

Student Considerations That Promote Clinical Reasoning

An important condition that must be considered is that of student self-concept, which includes self-confidence. Learners who begin a program with limited self-concept or weak self-confidence lack the ability to trust their own judgment and feel good about their clinical decisions. Low self-confidence in a student will hinder initiating care or project to the patient and family a lack of competency. Thus the patient may have a lack of trust in the care provider, which jeopardizes the patient–care provider relationship. To guide the student in overcoming a lack of confidence, the instructor approaches the learning situation in progressive steps. A first step can be to identify a simplistic hurdle that can easily be overcome. An example is talking a student through improving a psychomotor skill such as sterile procedure. Oftentimes students need reassurance that they have the knowledge and skill to perform safely in the clinical environment. To assist the student in developing his confidence, the clinical instructor can talk through the steps with the student prior to entering the patient room. Also, the instructor can role play with the student the patient situation, anticipating questions the patient may have while care is being provided.

The goal of the educational program is to create a student who thinks like a health professional. In the skills practice lab, students prepare for clinical practicums, yet once in the patient care setting do not see themselves as the legitimate care providers. They do see themselves as students in an academic setting; therefore, the faculty member must elevate the student's concept of self as a health professional. Research by Etheridge (2007) addressed experiences students identified as beneficial in both their clinical nursing judgment and their role in making these judgments. Students stated that multiple clinical experiences helped them to increase self-confidence and learn responsibility for decisions and care outcomes. Also, students stated that having the opportunity to discuss clinical care experiences with their peers was helpful in validating decisions and gaining further insight. Active discussion assisted the students in learning to trust themselves and their thinking while developing collaborative care. Furthermore, students expressed personal growth through the support of the clinical instructor and through interactions with supportive professional staff. This evidence points to the value of the personal presence of the clinical teacher during student patient care experiences. The teaching example at the end of this chapter explains how the instructor guides the student through clinical reasoning to solve a clinical problem.

■ Potential Problems

For the student to develop clinical reasoning abilities, the student must be motivated to learn and apply information in the academic and clinical arenas. Preparation such as reading and completion of other assignments are fundamental for knowledge application and are essential in both the classroom and clinical settings. In fact, college students often do not read prior to class but wait to see what important content is covered in class, and then read that information (Starcher & Proffitt, 2011). However, the basis for clinical reasoning is core knowledge essential to the professional field. In the ideal learning environment, where Socratic questioning, active discussion, and case scenarios are used, it is assumed that at the time of class the student possesses preliminary information related to the topic of the day. Based on this assumption, learning outcomes are achieved and the student is equipped to use the information as a foundation for clinical decisions and actions. Without this fundamental information, the student will not be able to provide the appropriate level of care. Even though the faculty emphasizes the value of class preparation, the student may not appreciate this importance until after the first graded assignment. For those students who seek counseling after a failing grade, the instructor should explore time management and study strategies. If the student has been reading, the instructor can provide suggestions for more efficient reading. If the student has not been reading, the instructor can reiterate the benefit of reading and preparation.

In the clinical setting, the student who does not possess the fundamental information and skills will struggle with reasoned decisions necessary for safe and appropriate care. As can be seen in the example in Figure 5-1, the unprepared student would not be able to move through the thought processes to arrive at the correct conclusions. A student who is unable to process the information and display clinical reasoning has the potential to jeopardize patient care and his or her own success in the clinical course. As the student gains more knowledge and skill and increases in confidence, she or he should increase in independence. If this is not occurring, the student will not employ clinical reasoning and the instructor will need to have a conference with the student to determine the obstacle(s) and develop a remediation plan.

Many students are successful in the didactic portions of their academic programs but unable to demonstrate transfer of knowledge and concepts into the practice setting. Benner and colleagues (2010) indicate that this may be due to the type of teaching strategies employed. These strategies may be unidirectional, didactic, content-driven teacher-talk, with no opportunity for the students to manipulate and fully understand the information presented, much less apply it. Benner et al. further recommend that educators in health professions programs use strategies focused on the patient and care activities. Examples that can be found in this text include human patient simulation, case studies, and problem-based learning.

Educational programs must employ a continuous strategy that assesses a student's ability to transfer theoretical knowledge to the clinical practice. Part of this strategy should examine the learner's ability to overcome ethnocentrism and stereotypical thinking because these limit the learner's ability to be open to clinical reasoning that is unbiased and patient centered. In a similar fashion, some students enter their professional program with a work-related background that influences their thinking. A typical example is a student who has been a paramedic and enters medical school. This student likely has preconceived notions about his or her chosen field of study and his or her personal abilities related to the practice. Likely this is a misdirected self-concept in that the student sees himself or herself as competent and qualified to perform in the new clinical setting. The student may be competent in the previous field, yet not display clinical reasoning and skills appropriate in the new field. This can lead to overconfidence on the part of the student, which then leads to safety risks. It is the duty of the instructor to bring these erroneous notions to the student's attention and redirect his or her thinking.

■ Conclusion

Educators in the health professions are recognizing that successful patient outcomes call for more than critical thinking. Positive effects of patient care demand more than intellectual manipulation of content and critical analysis. The proficient healthcare provider fuses critical analysis with thoughtful, rational, and reflective deliberations. The healthcare professional faced with a clinical challenge must engage in clinical reasoning to process data from multiple sources, quickly synthesize the information to draw conclusions, and take action to bring about quality care. Teaching clinical reasoning calls for awareness of how students learn and think, and thus necessitates the use of a variety of teaching strategies. Effective teachers engage in self-reflection about their own teaching style, are willing to be flexible with students to accomplish learning on an individual basis, and are able to recognize and address barriers in the student that hinder clinical reasoning.

TEACHING EXAMPLE

It was the first day of clinical practice for first-semester nursing students. The students were prepared with care plans in nervous hands. A hundred thoughts raced through their heads. "Is my care plan good enough?" "Will my patient like me?" "I just have to get through this first day safely!" In preconference, the instructor discussed the student assignment for the day, which was to assist their patients with activities of daily living including bathing, toileting, and nutritional needs, as well as assessment of vital signs. As a part of the assignment, the instructor went with the students to each patient's room to validate the students' assessment of the vital signs.

(continued)

In one instance, as they entered the room, the instructor scanned the room and quickly noted two safety issues. First, the IV pump was blocking easy access to the bathroom for the patient. Second, the bedside table holding the patient's water, cell phone, and call light was across the room and out of the patient's grasp. Furthermore, the head of the hospital bed was pressed up against the wall, preventing easy access to the sphygmomanometer (blood pressure cuff) attached to the wall above the headboard.

The instructor knew she needed to guide the student in recognizing and correcting these safety issues. The first step was for the instructor to ask the student to take a mental snapshot of everything in the room; the instructor patiently waited while the student complied. Then the instructor asked, "What is wrong with this picture?" The student accurately identified the two safety issues and rectified them immediately. Then she proceeded with her assessment of the vital signs, which was her next priority. During this time, the instructor wondered how this particular student would reach the blood pressure cuff. It was challenging in this situation because this student had dwarfism and had abnormally short arms and legs for her age. The student successfully measured the patient's temperature, radial and apical pulse, and respirations. Then it was time to take the blood pressure. The student moved to reach the blood pressure cuff and was unable to reach the equipment. The student asked the instructor to please get the blood pressure cuff for her. The instructor paused and thought about a correct response. The instructor recognized the unique teachable moment of this opportunity and acknowledged that the greatest benefit would be for the student to use clinical reasoning to solve the problem rather than seek assistance. The instructor said to the student, "As you move through your nursing career, you will have many challenges. You will need to solve this problem on your own without my assistance." The student received this response positively and proceeded to discuss a solution with the instructor. The student's first action was to find a step stool. Using the stool, the student still could not reach over the patient to retrieve the cuff. She then reasoned that she needed to move the bed. After having done so, she realized she could reach the cuff without the step stool. She then proceeded with the rest of her assessments and completed her clinical assignment.

In this actual scenario, the student approached the problem using a reliable fall-back method (step stool) that did not solve the problem in this new setting. Therefore, the student *recognized* that she needed to approach a challenge with a new way of thinking, which is the first step in clinical reasoning.

This student had success in this and subsequent clinical courses and graduated from the program.

REFERENCES

American Association of Colleges of Nursing (AACN). (2008). *The essentials of baccalaureate education for professional nursing practice.* Washington, DC: AACN. Retrieved from http://www.aacn.nche.edu /education/pdf/BaccEssentials08.pdf

Americans with Disabilities Act. (1990). P.L. 101-336, *Federal Register, 42.* U.S.C. § 12101.

Atkinson, H. L., & Nixon-Cave, K. (2011). A tool for clinical reasoning and reflection using the International Classification of Functioning, Disability and Health (ICF) framework and patient management model. *Physical Therapy, 91,* 416–430.

Benner, P., Sutphen, M., Leonard, V., & Day, L. (2010). *Educating nurses: A call for radical transformation.* Stanford, CA: Carnegie Foundation for the Advancement of Teaching.

deWit, S. C. (2009). *Fundamental concepts and skills for nursing.* St. Louis, MO: W.B. Saunders.

Etheridge, S. (2007). Learning to think like a nurse: Stories from new nurse graduates. *Journal of Continuing Education in Nursing, 38*(1), 24-30.

Institute of Medicine. (2003). *Health professions education: A bridge to quality.* Washington, DC: National Academies Press.

Institute of Medicine. (2010). *The future of nursing: Leading change, advancing health.* Washington, DC: National Academies Press.

Leahey, M., & Svavarsdottir, E. K. (2009). Implementing family nursing: How do we translate knowledge into clinical practice? *Journal of Family Nursing, 15,* 445–560.

McNelis, A. M., & Ironside, P. M. (2009). National survey on clinical education in prelicensure nursing education programs. In N. Ard & T. M. Valiga (Eds.), *Clinical nursing education: Current reflections* (p.25). New York, NY: National League for Nursing.

Rogge, M. (2001). Transforming pathophysiology instruction through narrative pedagogy and Socratic questioning, *Nurse Educator, 26*(2), 66–69.

Starcher, K., & Proffitt, D. (2011). Encouraging students to read: What professors are (and aren't) doing about it. *Journal of Teaching and Learning in Higher Education, 23,* 396–407.

Tanner, C. A. (2006). Thinking like a nurse: A research-based model of clinical judgment in nursing. *Journal of Nursing Education, 45*(6), 204–211.

Wolpaw, T., Papp, K. K., & Bordaage, G. (2009). Using SNAPPS to facilitate the expression of clinical reasoning and uncertainties: A randomized comparison group trial. *Academic Medicine, 84,* 517–524.

Worden, J. M., Hinton, C., & Fischer, K. W. (2011). What does the brain have to do with learning? *Phi Delta Kappan, 92*(8), 8–13.

CHAPTER 6

The Teaching–Learning Experience from a Generational Perspective

■ LYN PESTA ■

"Each generation sees farther than the generation that preceded it because it stands on the shoulders of that generation. You're going to have opportunities beyond anything that we've ever known."

—*Ronald Reagan, 1981*

Much has been written in pedagogical and business literature about the learning differences among generations. Each generation is shaped in part by the cultural, technological, and political events that have transpired during the members' formative years. Therefore, each generation carries its own unique imprint from specific generational influences. Most of the college classrooms today are filled by generation X and Y (Xers and Yers) students, with the minority group being baby boomers. However, boomers have heavy influence on both of the younger generations as their parents and teachers.

Projection data for 2010–2020 from the U.S. Bureau of Labor Statistics (BLS) indicate that job growth is expected in all areas of healthcare occupations, and health care will generate more than 5.7 million new wage and salaried positions. There are currently 2,737,000 registered nurses in the United States. By 2020, the need is estimated to grow to 3,449,300 (BLS, 2012). Universities, colleges, and training centers that prepare people for health occupations may find several challenges in recruiting, admitting, and retaining a workforce prepared to meet the demand. Tension may arise between learners and educators of differing generations who may have conflicting expectations of each other.

■ Generational Perspectives of Faculty and Students

Several generations are bound together for the transference of essential knowledge, skills, and attitudes for the health professions. Faculty typically consist of three generations: the veterans/traditionalist/silent generation (veterans), who were born in the years between 1922 and 1945; the baby boom generation (boomers), who were born between 1946 and 1964; and generation X (Xers), who were born between 1965 and 1981. There is some overlap of years for each generation, depending on the source. Many healthcare programs, especially nursing, attract a wide group of students, including the traditional student who enters college after high school graduation, the slightly older student who has worked after high school or perhaps has a young family, and the seasoned individual who decides to pursue a career after raising a family or deciding to change professions. To help meet predicted needs for healthcare professions, recruitment efforts will remain focused on appealing to a younger demographic, fostering the idea throughout secondary educational settings that health care is an attractive career choice (Cohen et al., 2006). The majority of nursing students are either in generation Y, born between 1982 and 2001, or generation X. A minority of students today are boomers.

The Veterans

Cultural Setting

Most veterans experienced the effects of the Great Depression, where an estimated 25% to 30% of the U.S. population experienced unemployment or displacement. This ended when World War II broke out in 1941. Social programs such as Medicaid and Medicare were decades away. Credit cards had not arrived. Veterans are known for patriotism, loyalty, and duty. Many families were just beginning to afford a family car and the interstate highway system that linked remote areas of the nation had not been built. People listened to swing and the big band sounds of Tommy Dorsey and Glenn Miller on 78 rpm records. The whole family sat near the radio and listened to President Franklin Roosevelt's "fireside chats" or was spellbound by the *Shadow* series and other radio shows. Reel-to-reel tape recorders and televisions were new and extremely expensive. Any adult could correct a youngster and such behavior was not considered extraordinary by a parent. The virtues of frugality, thriftiness, and self-restraint were necessary for survival.

Rapid advances in health care came about during and after World War II. However, polio and tuberculosis killed or crippled thousands of people during this era. Many died from infection or sepsis from simple traumas. The widespread availability of penicillin during the 1940s reduced infection death rates (Smith & Bradshaw, 2008).

Despite the United States being the "melting pot" of the world, cultural diversity was not the norm or routine part of life for veterans, especially in smaller cities, towns, or isolated rural communities. Most Americans lived in homogenous neighborhoods that were segregated by cultural practice, religious belief, race, or ethnicity. Family farms were still a way of life and veterans were often isolated from outside influences. Life for the veterans was simpler, but they grew up in a formal and ordered society where manners and decorum were prized. They were taught not to question those in authority. Information from the outside world came from movie newsreels, *Life* magazine, newspapers, and postal delivery of handwritten letters. The digital age has made the world a smaller place, yet the veterans are not as accepting of cultural differences as are the younger generations.

Characteristics/Work Ethics/Learning Styles

Veterans are known to be disciplined, hardworking, patriotic, and loyal. Veterans are known to be team players. There is an almost universal belief within this generation in the motto, "All for one and one for all"—that is, the group good supersedes individual desires. Veterans believe that history has important lessons to be followed and used as bridges to the future. They have reached retirement age, but many work due to changes in retirement goals. Workplace stability and longevity in the work environment are prized by this cohort. Being raised in an environment that valued deference to established rules, veterans will usually follow the status quo. Veterans appreciate the wisdom of experienced leaders and elders, and they appreciate the mentor/mentee aspects in personal and professional relationships. Finally, veterans prefer a hierarchical structure in the workplace where lines of authority and responsibility are well defined. Veterans spent most of their lives without the convenience (or headaches) associated with personal computers, laptops, personal digital assistants (PDAs), instant messaging, e-mail, and Facebook. In fact, they often view technology suspiciously or as an intrusion. They put a higher value on face-to-face interaction, well-written notes, and telephone conversations.

The educational system in place during a veteran's upbringing placed a heavy emphasis on reading, writing, and arithmetic. Most learning acquisition occurred with an emphasis on process. Knowledge was obtained through sequential, step-by-step instruction and through memorization drills. Because of this, there may be a higher comfort level among veterans in using these strategies in teaching. There are few veteran faculty, but their influences persist in traditional healthcare curricula, policies, and teaching strategies.

The Baby Boomers

Cultural Setting

Boomers are generally classified as being born between the years of 1946 and 1964. During this time, the middle class was growing along with the economy.

Growth meant more resources to purchase goods. Automobiles, time-saving appliances, electronics, and store-bought clothing became the norm. The baby boomer generation learned that credit cards could provide more purchasing power and adopted a "buy now, pay later" mind-set with respect to homes, cars, and big-ticket items (Johnson & Romanello, 2005). Advances in medicine and health care meant that people lived longer. Health insurance was an anticipated benefit when one worked for a company or corporation.

Boomers were born prior to digital technology. Because veterans and boomers needed to learn these digital technologies, often as a result of employer mandates, they are sometimes called digital immigrants (Prensky, 2001). Boomers needed to adapt and catch up to the rapid changes brought about by the introduction of the public Internet in the early 1990s and the ubiquitous presence of personal computing, e-mail, distance learning, cellular telephones, and rapid information access through powerful search engines. Boomers learned that some of their previous prized skills of penmanship and spelling were antiquated. Predigital education placed an emphasis on punctuation, writing, spelling, drills, rules, and memorization. Learners were taught in a highly structured, teacher-centered educational system that called for obedience to the rules. Computers were behemoths and, because of their large size, needed entire rooms to house them. The average person could neither afford nor use a personal computer. Simple arithmetic could not be done on calculators. Manual typewriters created important documents. Correction fluid was considered a major time saver when correcting typed mistakes. Early television was not created as an educational tool but as entertainment that viewers watched on small, 9-inch screens in black and white with metal antennae. In the educational setting, challenging a teacher or parent was not usual or tolerated. Corporal punishment was not considered child abuse and was often used for a disobedient child.

Boomers used telephones to communicate when face-to-face encounters were not possible. Like learning a new language, they had to adjust to new technologies, such as e-mail and computer networks, as a necessity of work life and not a choice (Sherman, 2006). The boomers are not like the younger generations who are fascinated with new technology and often view these inventions as time savers and vital connections to significant others (Oblinger, 2003). For the boomer, Friday nights meant attending a chaperoned dance at school. London's Twiggy was the epitome of fashion. Boomers relied on eight-track tapes or AM/FM radios for music. Now digital MP3 players provide a wide variety of music in an instant to almost every Xer and Yer. Boomers were enthralled with a variety of musical styles, the most influential being rock. The energetic sounds from a multitude of rock and roll bands emerged. The Woodstock music festival was a celebration of youth and freedom but with a downside of a culture laced with the idealization of illicit drugs, anger sparked by the Vietnam War, and the promotion of casual sex.

Other events of the day also influenced the boomer generation. Following World War II, the tension between Russia and the United States escalated the threat of nuclear war. Other major events that shaped the attitudes of the boomers were the draft, the Vietnam War, the Kent State massacre, the civil rights movement, the assassination of Martin Luther King, Jr., the assassination of President John Kennedy, the feminist movement, and President Richard Nixon's Watergate scandal. Protests occurred in the street and on college campuses across the nation. Boomers are seen as idealists who want to right the wrongs of an unjust world (Gardner, Deloney, & Grando, 2007). The overall discontent of the era created an upheaval in the mores of society. Unlike their parents, many boomers came to mistrust authority figures and loudly questioned the wisdom of the institutions of organized religion, government, military, and marriage.

Characteristics/Work Ethics/Learning Styles

It is interesting that, as working adults, the boomers became known as the generation that put in long and hard hours—often at the expense of their families. Often referred to as the "me" generation, boomers sought individual accomplishment over the group good (Benedict, 2008). They often equate work with self-worth. In general, boomers crave positive acknowledgment for work performed and thrive on praise for their efforts. Boomers prefer a more casual style of dress than their predecessors and have an uneasy relationship with authority. The healthcare profession continues to have optimistic growth potential and many baby boomers dispossessed from another industry, job, or profession may find changing to health care both an attractive and challenging alternative. Boomers are known to be committed, lifelong learners and solve problems by action.

Generation X

Cultural Setting

There are differences among authors as to the exact years that define Xers. Some authors use the years between 1960 and 1977, while other ranges exist in the literature, such as 1965 to 1976 (Jones & Fox, 2009). The most agreed-upon years are in the range of 1965 to 1981. Regardless of the difference in defining age ranges, Xers comprise a much smaller group than the boomers who preceded them and the Yers who came after them. Culturally, this group was shaped by the important events of the time including *Roe v. Wade* (1973), which legalized abortion.

Xers were mostly raised by boomer parents. Demographic shifts meant many generation X children were not raised near extended family or even by both parents. Many children were raised by single parents or parents who both worked. Xers grew up with the experiment of the Children's Workshop Network, known as *Sesame Street*. Some of these children participated in after-school programs manned by unrelated adults. The term *latchkey kid* was coined for the Xer child who was left alone after school hours while a parent or both parents remained at work. Left home often without adult supervision, they entertained themselves with television shows, computer games, and videos.

Xer children were exposed to a higher level of violence in movies, music, and in video games. During this time, various musical styles emerged. Music Television (MTV) first aired in 1981. Musical influences such as grunge, heavy metal, and rap entered the mainstream American culture during the typical Xer's formative years. These musical styles and videos contained graphic violence and obscene material that needed close monitoring from busy parents. Xers grew up amidst both unprecedented economic prosperity and severe downturns in the economy. Middle-class children were exposed to more marketing commercialism for brand-name clothes, toiletries, and shoes than any other generation before them. Drugs such as ecstasy, heroin, and cocaine became prolific across the country. Major cities had increasing violence owing to gang warfare and violent initiation rites. Nationally, unwed teen pregnancy and divorce rates trended upward while marriage rates dropped (Boonstra, 2002; Stockmayer, 2004). The problems of acquired immune deficiency syndrome (AIDS) and homelessness were part of public discussions. Influential events included the Los Angeles riots of 1991, the *Challenger* space shuttle explosion, and the environmental disaster caused by the wreck of the *Exxon Valdez*. Overseas, the Tian'anmen Square protests of 1989, the unraveling of apartheid in South Africa, the Chernobyl nuclear accident, and the fall of communism helped shape this generation. Communication was instantaneous and brought to life in living color within moments after occurring. The Internet was introduced during this time. Xers became acclimated to learning on personal computers at school and during after-school hours.

Characteristics/Work Ethics/Learning Styles

There are many conflicting characteristics that are attributed to Xers. Generally they feel comfortable working alone and are considered independent. Due to their upbringing and isolation, it has been said that Xers have learned they can only rely on themselves. They readily identify friends as extended family. As a learning group, Xers receive instant gratification related to technological advances and from obtaining information at the click of a button. They tend to see themselves as consumers of education, and tend to mistrust authority figures, which could include faculty. Xers become bored in meetings where there is much discussion prior to making decisions (Sherman, 2006).

Leisure and time off to enjoy other interests are particularly critical to Xers. Unlike their parents who worked long hours, only to lose out on what their children consider to be the fun of living, Xers jealously guard their free time and view requests to work overtime as intrusions. Because of the higher value they place on personal time over the needs of their employers, they have been viewed as undependable. They highly value their individuality, but, as a group, widely adopted bizarre hair styles, tattoos, and body piercings as a sign of independence from the norm. This generation witnessed companies increasingly grow in international markets, thereby supplanting the local American worker for cheaper labor overseas. They realized that the years of loyalty their grandparents and parents gave in return for job security and a guaranteed pension no longer existed and, as a result, view government programs with skepticism and do not believe that social programs like Social Security will be available for them when they retire. Xers are described as cynical, ironic, clever, pragmatic, and resourceful (Johnson & Romanello, 2005). If there is a collective mantra that sums up the attitude of work versus leisure among Xers, it is "Work to live, not live to work."

Generation Y

Cultural Setting

Depending on the writer, there are many names and descriptions for generation Y. They are referred to as nexters, generation N, millennials, and digital natives. Collectively, Yers are usually placed as being born between 1981 and 2001. Despite variations in date, what is certain is that most Yers have never known a time before the age of digital technology. Culturally, Yers have been shaped by such events as the 1995 Oklahoma City bombing, the 1996 Summer Olympics bombing, the mass shootings at Columbine High School in 1999, and the terrorist attacks of September 11, 2001. The War on Terror, with efforts in Iraq and Afghanistan, continues to affect the paradigm of this generation. Generation Yers show a taste for diverse music by rap, alternative, and socially conscious groups such as Coldplay, Yellow Card, and Green Day. Music and videos from Yers' favorite groups can accessed digitally at an instant while the audience is simultaneously performing other tasks (Taylor & Keeter, 2010).

The U.S. birth rate continued to decline in this era. Most children born in this generation were planned and wanted. As a benefit of caring and involved parents, most millennials are secure and value family relationships. Parents who become too involved in every aspect of their child's life are known as helicopter parents because of their hovering tendencies—they are ready to swoop down to supply any need or rescue their progeny from any threat (Pricer, 2008).

Characteristics/Work Ethics/Learning Styles

Yers are thought to be more sociable than Xers. While veterans and boomers are referred to as digital immigrants because they were not exposed to the digital world until adulthood, Xers and Yers are comfortable with new technologies and are referred to as digital natives (Prensky, 2001). MP3 players, blogs, personal computers, Internet searches with Google or Yahoo, cell phones, instant messaging, text messaging, interactive gaming, video cameras, game technology such as Wii and PlayStation, wikis, Twitter, Flickr, YouTube, and Facebook/MySpace seem foreign to the digital immigrants. Digital natives, in contrast, were constantly exposed to the benefits of computer and digital technology and cannot remember a time before them. Many attributes have been assigned to Yers, including a high comfort level with computers and an insistence on being connected to family and friends technologically. There is no doubt that our world is becoming increasingly interconnected with wireless technology. Since Yers have never known a life without the presence of computers, cable, satellite radio, wireless connections, or cell phones, they are comfortable surfing the web, use digital music sources to download songs to MP3 players, and are usually experts in uploading or downloading videos through YouTube or other sources. Tweeting, texting, and using Facebook are activities that are as essential as breathing to the majority of the Yers.

Parents of Yers have been known to involve their children in a multitude of activities—sports, music, private tutoring, and group activities. Therefore, Yers often have multiple and diverse talents. Generation Yers generally are considered more optimistic than Xers. They have lived structured, scheduled lives and generally are much closer to their parents and feel more comfortable in a structured environment than their earlier X counterparts. They are known to be enthusiastic learners but want to know that "what they are learning is connected to the bigger picture" (Sontag, 2006). Most millennials were encouraged early in life to express and voice their opinions (Piper, 2012). They are known to be deeply committed to causes of justice, environmentalism, and volunteerism for the greater good. Of all the generations before them, they are the most ethnically and racially diverse generation and not only readily accept those who are different, but celebrate and prize diversity. They consider themselves to be global citizens (Johnson & Romanello, 2005).

The youngest generations have usually been exposed to a great deal of computer and digital technology in their formative years. Yers are comfortable in group settings yet feel isolated when unable to have instant access to friends through communication devices. They are more likely to treat technological innovations as integral to their lives, much like an appendage (Taylor & Keeter, 2010). It has been suggested that millennials may not have the verbal communication skills of their predecessors because they favor the use of digital communication media (Prensky, 2001).

There are similarities and differences among each of the generations. Although each generation is made up of individuals with unique characteristics, it is helpful to list some common characteristics that have been attributed to each generational cohort as outlined here. **Table 6-1** summarizes characteristics associated with each generation.

■ Generational Considerations for Educators

Changes in behavior, and thus learning, take place more readily when the student is fully engaged and can actively participate in the learning process. Faculty should plan teaching experiences carefully to achieve successful outcomes. With generational considerations in mind, an educator might ask the following questions:

Which factors influence each generation involved in educational settings? What are the typical characteristics for each generation?

How do my generational preferences and characteristics merge or differ from those of the newer generations?

What are the best teaching strategies to engage each generation of learners? How do generational differences affect communication?

Could generational differences simply be maturity issues? How does technology affect the new learner?

Who are digital natives and who are digital immigrants? Do digital natives think differently than other learners?

Which strategies can engage the new generation of learners?

Table 6-1 Generational Characteristics

Veterans, 1922–1945	*Boomers, 1946–1964*	*Xers, 1964–1981*	*Yers, 1982–2001*
Attributes/Characteristics/Interpersonal Relationships/Communication Style			
• Unselfish; group oriented; loyal; patriotic; will delay gratification; responsible; accepts line authority	• Self-seeking behaviors; "me" generation	• Confident; direct; assertive; fearless; adaptable; diverse; impatient; fun; informal; independent; pragmatic; outcome oriented	• Instant access to desires; technology integrated into life
• Prizes the group welfare over individual needs; honors tradition; formal and proper	• Inconsistent love–hate relationship with authority	• Challenges authority	• Assertive: ethnically diverse; optimistic; self-confident in most areas; embraces diversity; civic minded; consumer oriented; self-reliant; enthusiastic; easily bored; idealistic; patriotic; desires respect; optimistic; friendly; cooperative; open minded; talented; less mature; interested in others; collegial
• Prefers personal or written communication; not as comfortable with electronic style; prefers to communicate along established lines of authority	• Ambitious; challenges status quo; informal; casual; likes fewer rules; idealistic	• Body piercings and tattoos are popular forms of expression; pessimistic tendencies	• More respectful of rules and authority than Xers and boomers
	• Early wave accused of sacrificing family for work obligations	• Sees friends as extensions of family	• Closer to parents than predecessors
	• Prefers face-to-face communication; adapts to technology as a necessity	• Hesitant to commit to marriage and long-term relationships	• Enjoys face-to-face communication; craves social connections via technology
		• Prefers technology-driven over face-to-face communication	• Informal but schedule driven; being smart is cool; team players/collaborative

(Continued)

Table 6-1 (*Continued*)

Veterans, 1922–1945	*Boomers, 1946–1964*	*Xers, 1964–1981*	*Yers, 1982–2001*
Learning/Work Styles			
• Dependable; follows established rules; prefers hierarchy	• Prefers text over graphics; linear thinking; process oriented; step by step	• Education began in student-centered settings; processes quickly; multitasks; enjoys fast pace; focused; parallel/mosaic thinking; nonlinear thinking; concrete thinking	• Parallel/mosaic thinking; multitasks; expresses doubts about academic abilities; processes quickly; prefers graphics over text; likes to work in groups; curious; experiential; thrives on discovery; short attention spans; high incidences of ADD/ADHD diagnoses
• Educated in teacher-centered settings	• Likes contact with faculty		
• Values mentorship with established leader or experienced person	• Lifelong learning commitment; ties learning with life experiences; values rewards for work done; enjoys titles and accolades for achievements; willing to work long hours to get job done	• Prefers to work alone; needs safe environment to participate; experiential; embraces technology	• Enjoys interactive learning and games with immediate response; demands 24/7 access to learning/faculty; learns best by trial and error; prefers more structure than Xers
• Less likely to embrace newer technology than successors; more process oriented; seeks job security; very loyal to employer	• Seeks secure retirement; loyal to employer	• Little tolerance for extraneous information; dislikes assignments—does not view them as learning enhancements; discounts contact with faculty as important	• Likes creatively presented learning materials; enjoys entertainment aspect of learning; no tolerance for delays in class beginning and endings
	• Technology reluctant	• Desires work and school flexibility; seeks instant results for efforts; self-directed; entrepreneurial	• Has expressed concerns regarding academic abilities; enjoys mentoring relationships from experienced leaders; likes stories that are relevant to content; eager to learn new requirements for work/school
	• Does not enjoy games or being put on the spot	• Values free time over work hours; little loyalty to employer; wants success and ambition on his or her own terms; may overestimate contributions to an organization; wants rapid advancement without expending long work hours	• Prefers audio/visuals over reading; expresses higher reading comprehension than Xers

Educational Expectations of Teachers

Traditional teacher-centered learning has given way to a more student-centered approach (Brown, 2008). Within nursing programs, there are decades of separation from the authoritarian, quasimilitary chain-of-command programs that dominated the training for most of the veterans and boomers. The hospital-based apprenticeship model of nursing education has long since moved into colleges and universities, where students spend much of their time in the classroom but less time with actual patients providing care, yet nursing curricula haven't changed substantially (National League for Nursing [NLN], 2003). The challenges of a 21st-century acute care environment with shortened lengths of stays while maintaining a high degree of safe, ethical, skillful, and efficient care are emphasized. Increasingly, there are calls to reform nursing education into a model that espouses teaching in action (Benner, Sutphen, Leonard, & Day, 2010). A comprehensive study by the Institute of Medicine recommends that nursing curricula be reexamined, updated, and adaptive enough to change with the changing needs of society and technological advances (IOM, 2011).

A well-prepared professional must be educated and equipped to manage the complexities of the system or he or she will become overwhelmed by role performance demands. Faculty, armed with the knowledge and experience of the profession, challenge students through high ethical standards, self-discipline, professional development, and rigorous program curricula. Students who arrive late or do not attend class, communicate poorly, or appear to be inattentive in class are viewed circumspectly. Students who text message, shop online, do not keep appointments, talk in class, or use a disrespectful tone of voice are seen as uncivil by most boomer or veteran faculty. To maintain a positive rapport between faculty and students of different generations, the faculty member must clearly define behaviors that are acceptable in the classroom and clinical areas (Suplee, Lachman, Siebert, & Anselmi, 2008).

Educational Expectations of Students

Radical changes have occurred in primary, secondary, and postsecondary education among both parents and students in the past several decades. Advances in technology, the view that education is a commodity, developing maturity, tight schedules, previous life experiences, values, and cultural backgrounds have influenced learner attitudes. Education is no longer seen as a revered institution incapable of being criticized as much as it is a product—the result of a consumer-oriented culture. Whereas boomers appreciate a mentoring relationship with faculty, Xers believe they can teach themselves if given the right tools, while Yers view experienced faculty with admiration but not awe. Generation Y students, sheltered by doting parents, are said to be more grade conscious than their earlier counterparts. They are confident and not fearful of challenging faculty over a grade disagreement. They will quite readily voice dissent and demand their consumer rights. Younger students demand respect and to be listened to when their opinions are expressed. They prefer an egalitarian approach in the learning environment (Gardner et al., 2007). The newest generations want faculty who are not only experts in the field but have recent relevant clinical practice in the subjects that are taught (Oblinger, 2003). Students in today's environment want clear connections and rationales as to why subject matter is to be learned. This coincides with adult learning theory and is not a foreign concept to experienced educators. Students today like personal attention and immediate constructive criticism for their performance. Above all, students seek a connection with faculty (Gardner et al.2007). Younger generations seek 24/7 access to their instructors (American Association of State Colleges and Universities [AASCU], 2004). One study indicated that 64% of college students would be interested in communicating with faculty outside of the class schedule through postings created in blogs (Junco & Cole-Avent, 2008). Today, schools, colleges, and universities are striving to keep pace with these demands by putting the required technological infrastructures in place to support online access for students and faculty. Communication networks supported by colleges and universities enable communication methods to support the desire for increased learning activities or faculty support outside of the classroom.

Generation Yers anticipate support and nurturing from faculty (Gardner et al., 2007). Both the X and Y generations will adapt to a variety of teaching methods, with Xers being more comfortable with computer, online, and distance learning and self-paced modules. Experiential learning is preferred by both of these generations. Yers have a special penchant for hearing personal stories to illustrate points (e.g., analogies, humor, and wit) and seek an entertainment quality to teaching sessions. Despite their apparent addiction to new technologies, some studies indicate that nursing students actually prefer a well-designed and entertaining PowerPoint presentation with elements of multimedia embedded into the lecture material and a complete set of notes and slides over other methods (Paschal, 2003; Walker et al., 2007). Lecture and explanations are preferred for difficult content topics rather than group work. Undergraduate baccalaureate students younger than 25 years prefer to read about the subject first, followed by an expert's lecture, despite self-reports of reading comprehension difficulties (Walker et al., 2007). When attempting to learn a psychomotor skill, students in these cohorts favor demonstration over a lecture covering the material. Experiential learning fits easily within all three cognitive domains of nursing and is a valued methodology among all generations. Experiential learning is described as learning experiences (Kolb, 1984). Xers actually value doing over knowing, according to one author. Younger-generation learners have been reported to prefer to perform the skill first under the direction of the faculty and then independently, rather than hear a lecture on the material (Walker et al., 2007).

Barriers to the Teaching–Learning Experience

Education in a health professions program is challenging, especially for the incoming student. The sheer amount of reading and material can intimidate even the most scholarly student, yet it is clear that, to be successful in the program, one must be able to comprehend, analyze, and write well (Arhin & Cormier, 2007). The typical

Yers will have difficulty reading and studying for long periods of time (Gardner et al., 2007). Multitasking is second nature to the Yers, but sitting and reading for long periods of time is difficult. It is estimated that by the time students reach college, they will have spent 5,000 hours reading compared to 10,000 hours playing video games and 20,000 hours watching television (Prensky, 2001). There is no doubt that Yers have had more sensory input since childhood than earlier generations. Scientific evidence does support that environmental influences alter brain structures (Draganski et al., 2004; Sontag, 2009). It has also been suggested that the newer generations do learn differently from their predecessors because of the excessive amounts of visual stimulation they received throughout childhood.

Parallel/Mosaic Thinking Patterns

Mosaic thinking is a term coined by media theorist Marshall McLuhan (1978), who hypothesized that the electronic age sparked a revolutionary, or mosaic, way of processing information. Western civilization was formerly characterized by the dominance of reading and writing, which is now giving way to electronic media. Linear reasoning relies on a phonetic/alphabetical structure whose use is foundational to logical and sequential thought processes. Mosaic thinking is a consequence of visual symbols and images that are found in media today. According to McLuhan and others, this change in communication has radically altered the way information is processed and society functions. Similarly, parallel thinking is the ability to process information from a variety of sources simultaneously. These thinking/learning patterns have been ascribed especially to the newer generational cohorts who are comfortable in a fast-paced, technologically connected world.

Our newest cohorts connect with various digital technologies as they become available. Digital natives are said to gather information in parallel or a mosaic pattern. They process data quickly and have the ability to take in information simultaneously from various sources. Therefore, they do not always learn in a step-by-step sequential manner. Younger students have been exposed to endless hours of digitally enhanced games (Prensky, 2001). In gaming, trial-and-error methods meet with failure or reward. Quick motor reflexes for conquering spatial barriers and problem solving are rewarded and positively reinforced. A consequence of this is students' reduced tolerance for quiet reading, reflection, and listening. There is evidence that, because of changes in brain activity, technologically dependent students have a shorter attention span and poorer reading abilities than digital immigrants. As a result, boredom is not conducive to active learning.

Another downside to the reliance on instant feedback is the sometimes dubious accuracy of Internet sources. Easy distractibility due to the constant habit of multitasking is often observed in younger students. To engage today's learner, the experienced generations will need to understand their learners' preferred learning styles and adapt or enhance teaching strategies to help them connect with the material. The new generation prefers learning strategies that encourage exploration, discovery, and trial and error. Unfortunately, trial-and-error problem solving takes time and resources. It is not ideal in patient scenarios where the ultimate goal is to protect the patient's safety and comfort within limited time constraints.

Current nursing education may be outdated for digital natives as well as future generations of students. Curricula in health profession programs include a large demand for reading and sequencing. There is an emphasis on step-by-step processes to achieve learning outcomes. This method does not take into account new learners' propensity for a fast-paced, parallel, and mosaic thinking pattern. Online access, virtual reality, simulation, and computer games could solve these needs. Because of this, many nursing leaders question whether current nursing curricula are preparing a viable workforce. The American Association of College Nurses and the NLN have published position papers calling for major changes to incorporate the technology of this younger generation (NLN, 2008). More schools are going online to adjust to the ever-increasing demand from students for increasing class schedule flexibility. It is estimated that online and distance nursing programs will continue to rise and remain a viable option for many. Despite the plethora of options for students today, recent studies indicate boomers and Yers prefer face-to-face communication over distance learning–type arrangements.

Strategies for Teaching Among the Generations

To best serve our successors, it will be necessary for faculty to understand our personal biases, learning styles, and preferred methods of teaching (Pardue & Morgan, 2008). The methods used to teach students are going through a radical upheaval because of changes in societal expectations, technological advances, and increased access to information. Adult learning theory rests on the accepted principle that learners will retain and retrieve information when meaning is associated with it. Another important principle of adult learning theory is the idea that adults want to learn what is applicable to them at the moment (Knowles, 1973). Knowledge of the technological advances in a digital age and methods to employ them in the classroom, lab, or clinical site will become increasingly important over time. To say that it would be a necessity to engage the students would be an understatement. Foreknowledge of general attributes of the digitally engaged student is useful for nurse educators who have been a product of a different generation. For any generation, faculty creativity, an open and honest dialogue, and availability will help create a positive environment for students to thrive.

From a learning perspective, Xers jealously guard their time; they prefer the bullet point version of subjects. They want to know precisely what they need to know to pass to get good grades in the shortest way possible. They enjoy the presentation of specific information through e-mail, blogs, and instant messaging (Gibson, 2009). Xers have little tolerance for inefficiency and do not want their time wasted. They prefer brief learning episodes followed by group interaction and, because of their independence, will research information easily online (Gibson, 2009). They enjoy online courses because they provide more flexibility in scheduling. Xers are determined to complete tasks but see them only as a means to an end, not as learning for the sake of learning.

Yers learn best in an environment where there are multiple choices for obtaining the information, especially when the subject matter is difficult; choices include detailed notes, recordings of lectures, PowerPoint lectures, and videotapes of lectures that can be reviewed later. Yers enjoy the joy of discovery more than their older counterparts. They are known to enjoy hearing experiences from teachers whom they consider mentors. This trait may be especially heartening to the educator who has a rich history and experiences to share. Yers may need to be more directed by their educators than Xers (Gardner et al., 2007). Yers appreciate being asked for their opinions and relish opportunities to be part of a discussion. They are comfortable with technology and prefer peer collaboration, individual feedback, and interaction (Revell & McCurry, 2010). They demand respect from those who are in leadership roles. The Yer is more likely to be engaged when teaching strategies involve creative solutions (Gibson, 2009). The Yer prefers immediate feedback and instructors who are available beyond the classroom schedule.

The use of classroom clickers is a method to enhance classroom participation and may appeal to all generations within the classroom. They allow anonymous responses to classroom activities and provide immediate feedback to problems (Skiba & Barton, 2006). The risk for exposure is minimal and would appeal to a boomer student who chooses an incorrect response.

Technology and the role it plays in our lives will continue to expand, which may be sometimes intimidating and frustrating for the older generations but not so for the younger generations. In the workplace, the trend toward increasing reliance on electronic and digital equipment and electronic medical records underscores the fact that technology marches forward. It will be necessary to utilize the technology already in the workplace to prepare future health professionals. The Technology Informatics Guiding Education Reform (TIGER) initiative started in 2007 is a national plan to move nursing practice and education into the digital age. Members and experts from nursing education, informational technology, practice areas, and government agencies are collaborating to meet a 10-year strategic plan. The TIGER vision is twofold. First, it aims to "allow informatics tools, principles, theories and practices to be used by nurses to make healthcare safer, effective, efficient, patient-centered, timely and equitable" and, second, its goal is to "interweave enabling technologies transparently into nursing practice and education, making information technology the stethoscope for the 21st century" (TIGER, 2007, p. 6).

High-fidelity simulation (HFS) labs that use standardized patients and human-like computerized manikins to mimic real patient clinical situations are becoming more prevalent. This teaching methodology correlates with the preferences of the youngest generation to learn in an immersive and experiential approach that encourages important linkages between theory and practice. HFS fulfills the requirement to meet learning objectives, perform important skills, and develop clinical reasoning skills. Debriefing by faculty facilitators encourages students to analyze specific decisions and actions and reflect for future actions. Using a high-fidelity simulation lab requires dedication on the part of the program due to the added expense and time commitments (Garrett, MacPhee, & Jackson, 2010).

There are countless ways of involving and engaging students in experiential methods with or without technology enhancements. Virtual clinical experiences and lab practice are becoming more affordable, reliable, and evidence based. They may be essential educator extensions as the shortage of qualified educators in the health professions continues. They blend well with the traditional methods to assist the learner in gaining psychomotor skills. The power of multisensory experiences embedded in curricular teaching strategies cannot be overestimated because it increases the long-term memory retention and retrieval of the material for the learner. Increased networking with other faculty in distant universities through electronic mailing lists or blogs represent viable ways for faculty to network and increase their teaching method repertoires.

Computer-based video games have been part of entertainment and primary education for many years. Students are exposed to simulation experiences at increasingly younger ages. They become experts at manipulating objects in spatial environments repetitively throughout their childhoods. Applying trial-and-error methods in a safe environment allows the participant to practice necessary skills until perfection is achieved. Sources indicate that most younger students, especially digital natives, thrive on this type of learning. Older students may not embrace game playing as valuable, especially if they are not attuned to this particular modality. Fast-paced gaming may be threatening to an older student. There should be alternatives to this format if the class consists of multiple generations. Older students may need more time to practice or prefer a one-to-one, self-paced computer experience that focuses on decision making to enhance clinical reasoning skills. Simulation games have long been used for training purposes in aviation and the military. The learner plays out scenarios repetitively and receives immediate feedback for correct or incor-rect responses. Virtual reality games for the purpose of skill acquisition are in the beginning stages in nursing education (Kilmon, Brown, Ghosh, & Mikitiuk, 2010).

As the technology becomes more sophisticated and realistic, it is not hard to imagine the possibilities for all areas of the healthcare professions. Learning and creative expression can also be taken into the virtual world of Second Life (Junco & Cole-Avent, 2008; Linden Research, 2009). Second Life is a virtual reality world where players interact locally or across the world. With the combination of enhanced video games, role play, simulation, and case studies comes a potential new learning methodology using this system. The educational goals might be collaborative skill development, communication, reasoning abilities, and practicing complex psycho-motor skills. An exciting dimension to simulation learning has great potential in the healthcare professions. In 2005, Texas A&M University–Corpus Christi partnered with Breakaway Ltd., a gaming company, to launch a virtual reality simulation lab for training military and civilian emergency medical personnel in trauma care. This teaching modality immerses the learners in a high-fidelity, three-dimensional world that allows for multiple realistic patient scenarios to be played out in an emergency room setting. These experiential scenarios encourage critical thinking, psychomotor skill acquisition, and collaboration with other healthcare personnel—all in a low-risk, virtual environment (Breakaway, 2012). Educators should anticipate that virtual simulations will be more widely used as they become increasingly available and reliable (Schmidt & Stewart, 2009). It should be noted that students are more receptive when experiential learning takes place in a low-stress environment.

There are many teaching strategies that can be employed to engage the younger generations of learners. Narrative pedagogy is a way of interpreting information from different perspectives; using a deconstruction (analytical) approach may work in classes that welcome and encourage student participation, analysis, and dialogue (Diekelmann, 2001). Concept maps use parallel/mosaic thinking to promote clinical reasoning (Vacek, 2009). Reflection and critical thinking can be powerful and generationally relevant for promoting clinical thinking by experienced faculty. Students are guided in examining every angle through organized brainstorming techniques (Kenny, 2003). Another strategy that encourages clinical reasoning is engaging in Edward de Bono's six hat game (de Bono, 1999; Kenny, 2003). This encourages parallel thinking processes by looking at a problem from six different perspectives and discussing them.

Millennial students appear hardwired for action and engagement using web-based technology and resources. Educators identify lecture-based classes as transmitting low-level information that may actually reduce the ability to think critically. It is well known that learning is greater with an actively engaged learner than with a passive, bored one. In short, according to one expert in higher education, "class time is too valuable to spend time delivering content, which is, or can be, available elsewhere" (Taylor, 2010, p. 193).

■ Conclusion

Conflicts of younger generations with their elders have been documented for millennia. It may be debated whether the root causes of this conflict are student immaturity, undeveloped reasoning abilities, preferred learning styles, or alterations in brain structure.

Faculty reluctance to change or generational unawareness may also impact communication and learning. It will become increasingly requisite for healthcare curricula to change, modify, and adapt to strategies that coincide with technological advances and the societal expectations of the new generations. Whatever the causes, these changes must be reckoned with. The timeless determinant for true educational success will most likely remain the connections from teacher to learner and from learner to teacher that transcend generational differences.

REFERENCES

American Association of State Colleges and Universities (AASCU). (2004). *The key to competitiveness: Understanding the next generation learner—A guide for college and university leaders.* Washington, DC: Author.

Arhin, A. O., & Cormier, E. (2007). Using deconstruction to educate generation Y students. *Journal of Nursing Education, 46*(12), 562–567.

Benedict, S. I. (2008). How practitioners do and don't communicate: Part II. *Integrative Medicine, 7*(2), 54–59.

Benner, P., Sutphen, M., Leonard, V., & Day, L. (2010). *Educating nurses: A call for radical transformation.* San Franlsco, CA: Jossey-Bass.

Boonstra, H. (2002). Teen pregnancy: Trends and lessons learned. *Guttmacher Report on Public Policy, 5*(1). Retrieved from http://www.guttmacher.org/pubs/tgr/05/1/gr050107.html

Breakaway, Ltd. Retrieved from http://www.breakawaygames.com/serious-games/solutions/healthcare/pulse

Brown, S., Kirkpatrick, M., Mangum, D., & Avery, J. (2008). A review of narrative pedagogy strategies to transform traditional nursing education. *Journal of Nursing Education, 47*(6), 283–286. doi: http://dx.doi.org/10.3928/01484834-20080601-01

Bureau of Labor Statistics, U.S. Department of Labor. *Occupational outlook handbook, 2012–13 edition, registered nurses.* Retrieved from http://www.bls.gov/ooh/healthcare/registered-nurses.htm

Cohen, R., Burns, K., Frank-Stromborg, M., Flanagan, J., Askins, D., & Ehrlich-Jones, L. (2006). Educational innovation: The Kids into Health Careers (KIHC) initiative: Innovative approaches to help solve the nursing shortage. *Journal of Nursing Education, 45*(5), 186–189.

de Bono, E. (1999). *Six thinking hats.* Boston, MA: Back Bay Books.

Diekelmann, N. (2001). Narrative pedagogy: Heideggerian hermeneutical analyses of lived experiences of students, teachers, and clinicians. *Advances in Nursing Science, 23*(3), 53–71.

Draganski, B., Gaser, C., Busch, V., Schuierer, G., Bogdahn, U., & May, A. (2004). Neuroplasticity: Changes in grey matter induced by training. *Nature, 427*(6972), 311–312. doi: http://dx.doi.org/10.1038/427311a

Gardner, E. A., Deloney, L. A, & Grando, V.T. (2007). Nursing student descriptions that suggest changes for the classroom and reveal improvements needed in study skills and self-care. *Journal of Professional Nursing, 23*(2), 98–104. doi: http://dx.doi.org/10.1016/j.profnurs.2006.07.006

Garrett, B., MacPhee, M., & Jackson, C. (2010). High-fidelity patient simulation: Considerations for effective learning. *Nursing Education Perspectives, 31*(5), 309–313.

Gibson, S. E. (2009). Enhancing intergenerational communication in the classroom: Recommendations for successful teacher–student relationships. *Nursing Education Perspectives, 30*(1), 37–39.

Institute of Medicine (IOM). (2011). Committee on the Robert Wood Johnson Foundation initiative on the future of nursing. In *The future of nursing: Leading change, advancing health.* Washington, DC: National Academies Press. Retrieved from http://www.nap.edu/openbook.php?record_id=12956

Johnson, S. A., & Romanello, M. L. (2005). Generational diversity teaching and learning approaches. *Nurse Educator, 30*(5), 212–216. doi: http://dx.doi.org/10.1097/00006223-200509000-00009

Jones, S., & Fox, S. (2009, January). Generations online in 2009. Pew Internet and American Life Project. Retrieved from http://pewresearch.org/pubs/1093/generations-online

Junco, R., & Cole-Avent, G. A. (2008). An introduction to technologies commonly used by college students. *New Directions for Student Services, 124,* 3–17. doi: http://dx.doi.org/ 10.1002/ss.292

Kenny, L. J. (2003). Using Edward de Bono's six hats game to aid critical thinking and reflection in palliative care. *International Journal of Palliative Nursing, 9*(3), 105–112.

Kilmon, C., Brown, L., Ghosh, S., & Mikitiuk, A. (2010). Immersive virtual reality simulations in nursing education. *Nursing Education Perspectives, 31*(5), 314–317.

Knowles, M. S. (1973). *The adult learner: A neglected species.* Houston, TX: Gulf Publishing Company.

Kolb, D. (1984). *Experiential learning: Experience as the source of learning and development.* Englewood Cliffs, NJ: Prentice-Hall.

Linden Research, Inc. (2009). What is Second Life? Retrieved from http://secondlife.com/whatis/?lang=en-US

McLuhan, M. (1978). The brain and the media: The Western Hemisphere. *Journal of Communication, 28*(4), 54–60. doi: 10.1111/j.1460-2466.1978.tb01656.x

National League for Nursing (NLN). (2003). *Innovation in nursing education: A call to reform.* New York, NY: Author.

National League for Nursing (NLN). (2008). *Preparing the next generation of nurses to practice in a technology-rich environment: An informatics agenda.* New York, NY: Author.

Oblinger, D. (2003, July/August). Boomers gen-Xers millenials: Understanding the new students. *EDUCAUSE Review,* 37–47. Retrieved from http://net.educause.edu/ir/library/pdf/erm0342.pdf

Pardue, K. T., & Morgan, P. (2008). Millennials considered: A new generation, new approaches, and implications for nursing education. *Nursing Education Perspectives, 29*(2), 75–79.

Paschal, J. (2003). *Understanding generation Y: Expectations of nursing education* (Unpublished thesis UMI No. 1414800). Waco, TX: Baylor University.

Piper, L. E. (2012). Generation Y in healthcare: Leading millennial in an era of reform. *Frontiers of Health Services Management, 29*(1), 16–28.

Prensky, M. (2001, October). Digital natives, digital immigrants: Part II. Do they really think differently? *On the Horizon, 9*(5). Retrieved from www.marcprensky.com/writing/

Pricer, W. (2008). *Helicopter parents, millennial students an annotated bibliography* (pp. 93–108). Livonia, MI: Community College Enterprise. ERIC database (EJ837465). Retrieved from EBSCO.

Reagan, R. (1981, May 17). Address at commencement exercises at the University of Notre Dame. Retrieved from www.reagan.utexas.edu/archives/speeches/1981/517819.htm

Revell, S., & McCurry, M. (2010). Engaging millennial learners: Effectiveness of personal response system technology with nursing students in small and large classrooms. *Journal of Nursing Education. 49*(5), 272–275. doi: http://dx.doi.org/10.3928/01484834-20091217-07

Roe v. Wade (1973), 410 U.S. 113, 93 S. Ct. 705; 35 L. Ed. 2d 147.

Schmidt, B., & Stewart, S. (2009). Implementing the virtual reality learning environment Second Life. *Nurse Educator, 34*(4), 152–155. doi: http://dx.doi.org/10.1097/NNE.0b013e3181aabbe8

Sherman, R. (2006). Leading a multigenerational nursing workforce: Issues, challenges, and strategies. *Online Journal of Issues in Nursing, 11*(2), 1–13.

Skiba, D., & Barton, A. (2006). Adapting your teaching to accommodate the net generation of learners. *Online Journal of Issues in Nursing, 11*(2). Retrieved from CINAHL with full text database.

Smith, D., & Bradshaw, B. S. (2008). Reduced variation in death rates after introduction of antimicrobial agents. *Population Research and Policy Review, 27*(3), 343–351. doi: http://dx.doi.org/10.1007/s11113-007-9068-z

Sontag, M. (2009). A learning theory for 21st century students. *Journal of Online Education, 5*(4). Retrieved from http://www.eric.ed.gov/ERICWebPortal/detail?accno=EJ840530

Stockmayer, G. (2004, April). *Demographic rates and household change in the United States, 1900–2000.* Presentation at Population Association of America Annual Meeting, Boston, MA. Retrieved from http://www.demog.berkeley.edu/~gretchen/Stockmayer_Diss.pdf

Suplee, P., Lachman, V., Siebert, B., & Anselmi, K. (2008). Managing nursing student incivility in the classroom, clinical setting, and on-line. *Journal of Nursing Law, 12*(2), 68–77. doi: http://dx.doi.org/10.1891/1073-7472.12.2.68

Taylor, M. (2010). Teaching generation next: A pedagogy for today's learners. In *A collection of papers on self-study and institutional improvement* (Vol. 3, pp. 192–196). Chicago, IL: Higher Learning Commission. Retrieved from www.taylorprograms.com

Taylor, P., & Keeter, S. (Eds.). (2010, February). Millennials: Confident. Connected. Open to change. In *Millennials: A portrait of generation next.* Pew Research Foundation. Retrieved from www.pewresearch.org/millennials

Technology Informatics Guiding Education Reform (TIGER). (2007). Evidence and informatics transforming nursing: 3-year action steps toward a 10-year vision. Retrieved from http://www.thetigerinitiative.org/docs/TIGERCollaborativeExecSummary_20090405.pdf

Vacek, J. (2009). Using a conceptual approach with concept mapping to promote critical thinking. *Journal of Nursing Education, 48*(1), 45–48. doi: http://dx.doi.org/10.3928/01484834-20090101-11

Walker, J., Martin, T., Haynie, L., Norwood, A., White, J., & Grant, L. (2007). Preferences for teaching methods in a baccalaureate nursing program: How second-degree and traditional students differ. *Nursing Education Perspectives, 28*(5), 246–250.

CHAPTER 7

Esthetic Action: Creativity as a Collaborative Process

■ ELLEN LANDIS ■

Encouraging healthcare practitioners to share insights of sensory-emotional values, or esthetics, can contribute to more creative collaboration in the field. In the classroom or on location, the call to be creative often inspires feelings of excitement or something to be guarded against, as if a no-win outcome would inevitably occur. These responses make way for important conversations on personal, cultural, and institutional judgments based on deeply felt sentiments and corresponding actions. While research, theory, and protocol are of immense importance to practitioners, inevitably we are faced with the unexpected and a lack of apparent solutions. These junctures present the opportunity to develop new ideas, relationships, and practices.

Early in his career, the philosopher Gaston Bachelard (Thiboutot, Martinez, & Jager, 1999) adopted the prevalent attitude of the sciences at the onset of the 20th century: that creative imagination stood in the way of scientific objectivity. One needed to get beyond impulses to do scientific work. At that point, Bachelard thought imagination was important in intimate and informal settings but it was a hindrance in the workplace. He later replaced these essentialist views with the opinion that creative imagination joins together the opposites of self and other, mankind and nature, and what is and what is not. In doing so, he testified to the belief that creative imagination provides us with the capacity to unify our experience of living.

Approaches to collaborative creativity that help build reflexive practice and outcomes in health care can benefit the range of stakeholders. Why is it, then, that collaboration, and especially collaborative reflection, is considered a luxury by some and a burden by others? Generally speaking, we value the actions we perform over reflection on those actions. This focus on performance is linked to commerce and money making. *Time is money* and *time is not to be wasted* are familiar phrases encountered in the healthcare workplace. Look at all the time a mental health clinician works in isolation seeing clients and doing billing-related paperwork. Then, compare that with the time spent reflecting with colleagues on those actions. Some smart businesses build in time for group reflection. Google, for example, encourages people to spend time together in activities such as table tennis and pool during work as ways to support stress relief, relationship building, and, of course, creativity. This is based on an understanding that performance is enhanced in a collaborative–reflective work environment.

Findings from cognitive science demonstrate that emotional support is at the heart of educational processes. When people feel safe, listened to, and understood, their performance is enhanced. Professor Julia Byers, art therapist and family therapist at Lesley University, begins graduate school classes not with the expectations laid out in a syllabus, but rather with introductions, a process that bridges the gap between academic hierarchical knowing and cognitive/kinesthetic recognition and empathy. This immediately breaks down alienation among students who will be learning how to perform in the classroom and workplace together.

All too often, as new ideas emerge, they are credited to either a small number of people or an individual. Ideas have veins whose sources are vital, like fresh water springing up from the earth, whose underground sources may be hard to trace. For instance, everyone has had an experience of going unrecognized for a contribution that he or she made in resolving a difficult situation. We may also remember hiding our involvement in the development of an idea because of concerns about reverberations that may come with recognition.

People often seek health care when there is an acute situation—a crisis or emergency. Evidence-based, theory-driven, reflective practice can offer healthcare practitioners a work environment that brings the best out in people—either the patient or the professional. Collaborative creativity can bring forth unexpected resources from others. Despite our limited knowledge of what practitioners in health care will face in the coming years, we encourage students to explore the mystery of creativity as a collaborative process in school and at work.

■ Theoretical Rationale

The development of skills for creativity in the classroom includes personal agency, divergent thinking, and assessment of patterns. According to social philologist John Shotter (1993), to avoid becoming entrapped within the confines of narratives, metaphors, and theories about life, new practices for "multivoiced tradition(s) of argumentation" (Shotter, 1997, p. 10) must be invented. The extent to which someone is enmeshed in, or estranged from, a system can influence his or her ability to be effective in that system (Pearce & Cronen, 1980). Catherine Bateson (1994) believes that to emphasize a single activity, such as taking down an instructor's information, listening for diagnostic criteria from a client, or finding answers to specific questions, teaches us to devalue multisensory awareness. She emphasizes the learning potential of attending to relational as well as technical information. To this end, Barbara Vacarr (2001) approaches her role as an educator with a strategy that includes public expressions of vulnerability. By normalizing unexpected actions and self-revelations, she helps her students to become aware of transformational opportunities.

Any group in which the members listen to each other's perspectives on a given situation brings attention to variables that would otherwise be missed. Nursing educator Carol Picard believes that recognizing one's own patterns, making meaning of them, and considering their ramifications is especially important in turbulent times. Therefore, she invites healthcare professionals into partnerships with their patients.

Practitioners may find compassion to be a great asset to their work. They may also find a cost of caring (Figley, 2002), burnout (Maslach, 1982), compassion fatigue (Baranowsky, 2002; Joinson, 1992), or secondary traumatic stress (Stamm, 1999). These factors may include unwanted stressors, such as intrusive thoughts and nightmares about their patients, and distancing themselves from various sorts of intimacy. Maintaining high standards for client care while simultaneously attending to the costly impact of healthcare work on practitioners is a major concern for healthcare employers. Job-related stress and exhaustion are linked to extensive health challenges, including dysregulation of the hypothalamic-pituitary-adrenal axis and impaired immunity functions (Melamed, Shirom, Toker, Berliner, & Shapira, 2006; Toker, Shirom, Shapira, & Berliner, 2005). An evolving consensus suggests that rates of distress might be lowered by the use of collaborative–reflective practices (Landis, 2007b). Baldwin (2005) says:

> Collaborative creativity is one of the most powerful resources we have for transforming difficult situations into opportunities for growth. Yet, when we are overwhelmed by situations we feel we cannot resolve, we tend to lose this capacity, reacting, instead of responding reflectively, narrowing our range of behavior, often isolating ourselves from others. (p. 1)

Inherent to collaboration are clashing experiences with diversity, difference, and conflict. Circumstances that bring people to health practitioners can be thought of as social phenomena. Conditions arise in patterns of perception that demonstrate multiple social constructions, including economics, policy, tradition, law, environment, gender, ethnicity, race, religion, sexual orientation, and class. Anderson and Goolishian (1988, 1992) propose that practitioners facilitate problem-dissolving conversations rather than problem-solving ones. Instead of approaching clients with the aim of fitting them into preestablished hypotheses, they recommend that practitioners take a stance of not knowing.

Dance and health care have a shared history that offers an appealing example of this type of sensory-emotional healing. Pioneer dance therapist Marion Chace brought elements of her earlier dance career into working with psychiatric patients from the 1940s through the 1960s. She met with servicemen who had returned from war and were unable to speak, severely withdrawn individuals, and people who had schizophrenia. By observing their signature movements, she mirrored back to them in the gestures and emotions of their own expressions. These collaborative movement relationships Chace offered to her patients reflected her deep emotional acceptance and an ability to meet each person where he or she was and then move onward (Levy, 1988).

The invention of the reflecting team by Tom Andersen (1990) took the collaborative reflective process to a new level. Clients and practitioners would take turns listening to each other, highlight what was positive, and encourage each other. Katz and Shotter (1996) found that asking follow-up questions about arresting moments often suggests the social, as well as medical, explanations for which patients seek help. These practices are echoed in Hoffman's quote from Russian philologist Mikhail Bakhtin: "there is no knowledge of the subject but [the] dialogical" (2002, p. 161). Another proponent of this idea is the philosopher of reflectiveness, Donald Schon. Schon (1983) strongly states the case for becoming active learners through reflection-in-action. In order to engage in dialogue, we must be present with clients and use our senses to navigate the exchange. To all this, Hoffman writes, "it occurred to me that this communal perspective rests on a change in the definition of what needs to change . . . and since an environment is communally experienced, the antidote must be communal too" (2002, p. 271).

■ Sharevision: A Practical Example of Collaborative Creativity

The Sharevision approach is an example of creativity generated through collaborative reflection. It was developed by family therapy practitioners who were meeting families in their homes after the state had investigated charges of child neglect and abuse. This approach was facilitated by consultant Lynn Hoffman. Sharevision is currently being applied in graduate healthcare training and in healthcare facilities.

In 1987, Hoffman, a family therapist and social worker, brought her critique of the helping professions' flawed "power-over idea versus power-with" approach to working with teams of professionals and their clients. In meetings at the family services agency, People's Bridge Action in western Massachusetts, Hoffman was able to reduce ideological battles among staff by simply making time for each participant to speak and by honoring listening as much as speaking. Participants learned to value gestures and affect as much as words. The emphasis on hierarchy, reductionism, and convergent thinking was exchanged for personal experience, stories, and associative thinking. If the group was too large, participants were divided up into smaller groups. While there is a much larger conversation on the practice and theory of Sharevision (Baldwin, 1999, 2004a, 2004b, 2004c, 2006, 2008; Baldwin & Thompson, 1989; Fontes, 1995; Hoffman, 1993, 2002; Landis, 2004, 2005, 2006, 2007a, 2007b, 2008; Landis, Baldwin, & Thompson, 2004), a key premise is that, with more ideas on the table, better informed decisions would be made. It seems that the use of the model is linked to innovative programming, low staff turnover, and high morale.

■ Research on Collaborative Creativity

Research on Sharevision in hospitals and clinics was conducted with small groups of graduate interns and highly skilled clinicians who scored at extremely high risk for compassion fatigue on the Compassion Satisfaction/Fatigue Self Test for helpers and the Silencing Response Scale (Baranowsky, n.d.; Stamm, 1999). Sharevision research includes the integration of movement and arts activities based on their positive impact with people in resilience programs when trauma had been involved (Berrol, 2006; Fisher & Ogden, 2009; Kisiel et al., 2006; Milliken, 2004; Murrant, Rykov, Amonite, & Loynd, 2000; Newman & Holzman, 1999; Ray, 2006; Rothschild, 2006; Shapiro, Brown, & Biegel, 2007; Stokrocki, Andrews, & Saemundsdottir, 2004; Van dDer Kolk, 2006).

Part of the research on this collaborative-reflection approach includes an arts-integrated group social action project. Social action to interrupt the cycle of violence on behalf of oneself and others is effective in trauma recovery and building resilience (Freire, 1970; Golub, 2005; Harvey, 2007; Junge, Alvarez, Kellogg, & Volker, 1993; Kaplan, 2007; Powell & Marcow-Speiser, 2005; Schutzman & Cohen-Cruz, 1994). Choosing an arts-integrated group project stimulates sensory-emotional dialogue on values and aspirations, helping participants bridge their isolation to a community. This practice of Sharevision appears to correlate with a decrease in compassion fatigue, a decrease in silencing the responses of clients, and an increase in compassion satisfaction.

The Sharevision group project is called *Esthetic Action* (Landis, 2008). The term *esthetic action* emerged between Richard Baldwin, one of the originators of Sharevision, and the author of this chapter, the researcher, during a 2005 conversation about an early adaptation of Sharevision, which was focused on relieving compassion fatigue through arts and social action. Esthetic action is a process wherein the group examines existing patterns and builds ideas about new ones, then realizes these ideas through action in different contexts. Diverse communication media are used in this process to support nonlinear connections. The focus is to evolve a pattern that feels right or fits the group and the context. Once the esthetic action is accomplished, the group gathers and reflects on the results. In this way, an esthetic loop can be developed. These practices have roots in Gregory Bateson's ecological esthetics: "esthetics is this glimpse that makes us aware of the unity of things which is not consciousness" (Bateson & Bateson, 1987, p. 300).

■ Sharevision: Collaborative Reflection in the Classroom

In classroom adaptations of Sharevision, students have a chance to hear from each other about dilemmas they present in small groups. Sharevision can take place for 15–20 minutes during 2.5-hour classes. In large classes, students can miss opportunities to pose questions and hear from each other. Often, it is the more outspoken students who are the ones to regularly speak up. Sharing the time equitably provides each student with the opportunity to present her perspective. There is time for differing ideas and different ways of expressing oneself. Classroom practice in posing sensitive and concise questions and responses provides learning opportunities for developing listening and speaking skills that healthcare professionals need. When they are asked to identify their thoughts and feelings in front of a group, students also gain an awareness of the vulnerability patients have. The experience of receiving affirming responses from others in their small group can be crucial.

In smaller seminar classes, the teacher–student hierarchy is flattened in favor of timed periods of collaborative reflection. Students report that they:

- Like having a structure where everyone's issues can be addressed.
- Feel listened to.
- Feel safe enough to bring any questions and concerns about internship.
- Get lots of creative ideas from others on how to approach challenges during internship.
- Feel encouraged.

■ Creative Arts Learning and Collaboration in the Classroom: Practical Example

During a class on self-care for healthcare professionals, a collaborative, arts-integrated experience enriches the dialogue on the topic. Here is an example of a classroom activity that encourages collaboration. A class begins with a lecture on burnout prevention, addressing the risk and frequency of secondary trauma for professionals as well as thoughts and behaviors to watch out for in oneself and colleagues. An experience of self-care follows, addressing the elements of creating an environment that meets the needs of a multicultural workforce.

The class divides into small groups of four people. A box full of inexpensive supplies such as balloons, ribbon, colored markers, and paper and scissors is made available. The task is to create a safe place where students and professionals can decompress from the stress of their jobs. Their rich conversation about the range of possible priorities and ways to express their ideas using these simple supplies is limited by time. The goal is to create a performance piece that would include the development of this counterstress environment they have been asked to establish. Each group takes supplies, discusses the members' concerns, and comes up with a product that communicates their situation. This activity is followed by a group discussion. Themes that have emerged include bringing a spirit of fun to difficult work, feeling and emitting a sense of calm, being a good listener, offering new ideas to the discussion, and engaging conflict resolution skills.

TEACHING EXAMPLE

Developing Collaborative Creativity Skills

This activity by Ellen Landis was first used in a play therapy course for master's candidates in a variety of healthcare professions at Lesley University in Cambridge, Massachusetts. Most of these students had worked professionally in the healthcare field prior to returning to school or had experiences in the field through internships. The theme for the day was self-care for the professional. The class began with a lecture on burnout prevention and introduced the frequency and risk of secondary trauma for professionals as well as thoughts and behaviors to watch out for. An experience on self-care followed, addressing the sociocultural elements of creating an environment that meets the needs of a diverse workforce.

Landis brought out a box full of inexpensive supplies including balloons, ribbon, colored markers, paper, and scissors. The class divided into small groups of four people. They were all instructed to collaboratively create a safe place for them as students and professionals to decompress from the stress of their job. They needed to make decisions about their priorities and find a way to express their ideas using the simple supplies. They were asked to create a performance piece that could include the development of creating a safe place. Each group took supplies, discussed the members' concerns, and came up with a performance piece. The activity was followed up with a group discussion. Themes that emerged included bringing a spirit of fun to difficult work, bringing a sense of calm to the job, being a good listener, bringing ideas to the table, and bringing conflict resolution skills to the job.

Since people often seek health care when there is an acute situation, a crisis, or an emergency, students recognize the inherent stress related to their work. This trilogy of evidence-based, theory-driven, reflective practice brought students together in affirmation of their goal to be part of a work environment that brings out the best in people, whether that is the patient or the professional.

REFERENCES

Andersen, T. (1990). *The reflecting team: Dialogues and dialogues about the dialogues.* Kent, UK: Borgman Publishing, Ltd.

Anderson, H., & Goolishian, H. (1988). Human systems as linguistic systems. *Family Process, 27,* 371–393.

Anderson, H., & Goolishian, H. (1992). The client is the expert. In S. McNamee & K. Gergen (Eds.), *Therapy as social construction.* Newbury Park, CA: Sage Publications.

Baldwin, R. (1999). *Sharevision: A clinical group supervision model.* Amherst, MA: Sharevision, Inc.

Baldwin, R. (2004a). *Historical threads of Sharevision Inc.* Amherst, MA: Sharevision, Inc.

Baldwin, R. (2004b). *Reflective performance.* Amherst, MA: Sharevision, Inc.

Baldwin, R. (2004c). *Some ideas about the arts & clinical/educational practice.* Amherst, MA: Sharevision, Inc.

Baldwin, R. (2005). *Sharevision.* Hadley, MA: Sharevision.

Baldwin, R. (2006). *Sharevision: A story of its inception.* Hadley, MA: Sharevision.

Baldwin, R. (2008). *Sharevision: The process.* Hadley, MA: Sharevision.

Baldwin, R., & Thompson, L. (1989). *Sharevision: An alternative to supervision in clinical practice* (Unpublished paper). Hadley, MA: Sharevision Inc., Family Counseling Center & Consulting Group.

Baranowsky, A. (2002). In C. Figley (Ed.), *Treating compassion fatigue* (pp. 155–170). New York, NY: Brunner-Routledge.

Baranowsky, A. (n.d.). *Silencing response scale.* http://www.psychink.com/insite.htm

Bateson, M. C. (1994). *Peripheral visions: Learning along the way.* New York, NY: Harper Collins.

Bateson, G., & Bateson M. C. (1987). *Angels fear.* New York, NY: Dutton.

Berrol, C. (2006). Neuroscience meets dance movement therapy: Mirror neurons, the therapeutic process and empathy. *The Arts in Psychotherapy, 33*(4), 302 315.

Figley, C. (2002). *Treating compassion fatigue.* New York, NY: Brunner-Routledge.

Fisher, J., & Ogden, P. (2009). Sensorimotor psychotherapy. In C. Courtois & J. Ford (Eds.), *Treating complex traumatic stress disorders* (pp. 312–328). New York, NY: Guilford Press.

Fontes, L.A. (1995). Sharevision: Collaborative supervision and self-care strategies for working with trauma. *Family Journal, 3*, 249–254.

Freire, P. (1970). *Pedagogy of the oppressed.* New York, NY: Continuum.

Golub, D. (2005). Social action art therapy. *Art Therapy: Journal of the American Art Therapy Association, 22*(1), 17–23.

Harvey, M. (2007). Towards an ecological understanding of resilience in trauma survivors: Implications for theory research and practice. *Journal of Aggression, Maltreatment and Trauma, 14*(1).

Hoffman, L. (1993). *Exchanging voices: A collaborative approach to family therapy.* London, UK: Karnac Books.

Hoffman, L. (2002). *Family therapy: An intimate history.* New York, NY: W. W. Norton.

Joinson, C. (1992). Coping with compassion fatigue. *Nursing, 22*(4), 116, 118–119, 120.

Junge, M., Alvarez., J., Kellogg, A., & Volker, C. (1993). The art therapist as social activist: Reflections and vision. *Art Therapy: Journal of the American Art Therapy Association, 10*(3), 148–155.

Kaplan, F. (2007). *Art therapy and social action.* Philadelphia, PA: Jessica Kingsley.

Katz, A. M., & Shotter, J. (1996). Hearing the patient's "voice": Towards a social poetics in diagnostic interviews. *Social Science and Medicine, 43*, 919–931.

Kisiel, C., Blaustein, M., Spinazzola, J., Schmidt, C., Zucker, M., & Van der Kolk, B. (2006). Evaluation of a theater-based youth violence prevention program for elementary school children. *Journal of School Violence, 5*(2), 19–36.

Landis, E. (2004). *Sharevision: Looking through the lens of social construction theory.* Cambridge, MA: Lesley University Expressive Therapies Field Training Supervisors.

Landis, E. (2005). *Moving into family therapy: A collaborative approach.* Keene, NH: Annual New England Chapter of the American Dance Therapy Association.

Landis, E. (2006). *Building social action into group therapy with children.* Watertown, MA: Family Institute of Cambridge.

Landis, E. (2007a). *Concepts of wellness: Reflective performance builds resilience,* Northampton, MA: Northampton Veterans Affairs Medical Center.

Landis, E. (2007b). *Effects of a collaborative reflective model to ameliorate secondary trauma* (Unpublished paper). Cambridge, MA: Lesley University.

Landis, E. (2008). *A collaborative approach to eliminating secondary trauma: Pilot study findings.* Paper presented at the Lesley University Doctoral Student Conference, Cambridge, MA.

Landis, E., Baldwin, R., & Thompson, L. (2004). Expressive arts therapy: A voice from the USA. *Context.* London, UK: Invicta Press.

Levy, F. (1988). *Dance movement therapy. A healing art.* Reston, VA: American Alliance for Health, Physical Education, Recreation, and Dance.

Maslach, C. (1982). *Burnout the cost of caring.* New York, NY: Prentice-Hall.

Melamed, S., Shirom, A., Toker, S., Berliner, S., & Shapira, A. (2006). Burnout and risk of cardiovascular disease: Evidence, possible causal paths, and promising research directions. *Psychological Bulletin, 132*(3), 327–353.

Milliken, R. (2004). Dance movement therapy as a creative arts therapy approach in prison to the treatment of violence. *The Arts in Psychotherapy, 29*(4), 203–206.

Murrant, G., Rykov, M., Amonite, D., & Loynd, M. (2000). Creativity and self-care for caregivers. *Journal of Palliative Care, 16*(2), 44–49.

Newman, F., & Holzman, L. (1999). Beyond narrative to performed conversation ("In the beginning" comes much later). *Journal of Constructivist Psychology, 12,* 23–40.

Pearce, B., & Cronen, V. (1980). *Communication, action and meaning: The creation of social realities.* Westport, CT: Praeger.

Powell, M. C., & Marcow-Speiser, V. (2005). *The arts, education and social change: Little signs of hope.* New York, NY: Peter Lang.

Ray, S. (2006). Embodiment and embodied engagement: Central concerns for the nursing care of contemporary peacekeepers suffering from psychological trauma. *Perspectives in Psychiatric Care, 42*(2), 106–113.

Rothschild, B. (2006). *The psychophysiology of compassion fatigue and vicarious trauma: Help for the helper: Self-care strategies for managing burnout and stress.* New York, NY: W. W. Norton.

Schon, D. (1983). *The reflective practitioner: How professionals think in action.* London, UK: Temple Smith.

Schutzman, M., & Cohen-Cruz, J. (1994). *Playing boal.* New York, NY: Routledge.

Shapiro, S., Brown, K., & Biegel, G. (2007). Teaching self-care to caregivers: Effects of mindfulness-based stress reduction on the mental health of therapists in training. *Training and Education in Professional Psychology, 1*(2), 105–115.

Shotter, J. (1993). *Cultural politics of everyday life.* Buffalo, NY: University of Toronto Press.

Shotter, J. (1997). The social construction of our "inner lives." *Journal of Constructivist Psychology, 21*(1), 7–24.

Stamm, B. (1999). *Secondary traumatic stress: Self-care issues for clinicians, researchers, and educators* (2nd ed.). Baltimore, MD: Sidran Press.

Stokrocki, M., Andrews, S., & Saemundsdottir, S. (2004). The role of art for homeless women and survivors of domestic violence. *Visual Arts Research, 29,* 73–82.

Thiboutot, C., Martinez, A., & Jager, D. (1999). Gaston Bachelard and phenomenology: Outline of a theory of imagination. *Journal of Phenomenological Psychology, 30*(1), 1–17.

Toker, S., Shirom, A., Shapira, I., & Berliner, S. (2005). The association between burnout, depression, anxiety, and inflammation biomarkers: C-reactive protein and fibrinogen in men and women. *Journal of Occupational Health Psychology, 10*(4), 344–362.

Vacarr, B. (2001, Summer). Voices inside schools: Moving beyond polite correctness; Practicing mindfulness in the diverse classroom. *Harvard Educational Review, 71*(2), 285–296.

Van Der Kolk, B. (2006). Clinical implications of neuroscience research in PTSD. *Annals of the Academy of New York Sciences,* 1–17.

RECOMMENDED READING

Anderson, H., Gergen, K., McNamee, S., Cooperrider, D., Gergen, M., & Whitney, D. (2001). *The appreciative organization.* Chagrin Falls, OH: Taos Institute Publication.

Bradshaw, M. J., & Lowenstein A. J. (2007). *Innovative teaching strategies in nursing and related health professions* (4th ed.). Sudbury, MA: Jones and Bartlett.

Figley, C. (1997). *Burnout in families: The systemic costs of caring.* Boca Raton, FL: CRC Press.

Figley, C. (1995). *Compassion fatigue.* In B. H. Stamm (Ed.), *Secondary traumatic stress: Self-care issues for clinicians, researchers and educators* (pp. 3–28). Baltimore, MD: Sidran Press.

Figley, C. (1995). *Compassion fatigue: Coping with secondary traumatic stress disorder in those who treat the traumatized.* New York, NY: Brunner/Mazel.

Figley, C., & McCubbin, H. I. (1983). Looking to the future: Research, education, treatment, and policy. In C. R. Figley & H. I. McCubbin (Eds.), *Stress and the family, Volume I: Coping with catastrophe* (pp. 185–196). New York, NY: Brunner/Mazel.

Figley, C., & Stamm, B. H. (1996). Psychometric review of the Compassion Fatigue Self Test. In B. H. Stamm (Ed.), *Measurement of stress, trauma & adaptation.* Baltimore, MD: Sidran Press.

Gergerson, M. (2007). Creativity enhances practitioners' resiliency and effectiveness after a hometown disaster. *Professional Psychology: Research and Practice, 38*(6), 596–602.

Kakkad, D. (2005). A new ethical praxis: Psychologists' emerging responsibilities in issues of social justice. *Ethics & Behavior, 15*(4), 293–308.

Keeney, B. (1983). *Aesthetic of change.* New York, NY: Guilford Press.

Picard, C., & Jones, D. (2005). *Giving voice to what we know: Margaret Newman's theory of health as expanding consciousness in nursing practice, research, and education.* Sudbury: MA: Jones and Bartlett.

Stamm, B. H., & Figley, C. (1996). Compassion satisfaction and fatigue test. http://www.psychink.com/insite.htm

White, M. (2004). *Narrative practice and exotic lives: Resurrecting diversity in everyday life.* Adelaide, South Australia: Dulwich Centre Publications.

CHAPTER 8

Lighten up Your Classroom

■ MARIANA D'AMICO AND LYNN JAFFE ■

Humor is also a way of saying something serious.

—*T. S. Eliot*

He who laughs most, learns best.

—*John Cleese (Priest, 2007)*

Most educators take learning very seriously, especially those in health care. They overlook the fact that humor is a lifeline to sanity and reality. Humor is not a primary teaching strategy, and it is quite difficult to measure the educational effect of humor in isolation from other teaching methods. The judicious use of humor can influence the cognitive and behavioral aspects of learning by engaging at least six of Gardner's seven forms of intelligence (as identified previously in this text). Research on humor has been a multidisciplinary endeavor, including a focus on use in classrooms and health care (Adamle, Chiang-Hanisko, Ludwick, Zeller, & Brown, 2007; Chauvet & Hofmeyer, 2007; Garner, 2006; Wrench & McCroskey, 2001; Ziegler, 1998). Well-placed humor can make the classroom environment a safe, comfortable, and effective arena for cognitive and professional growth (Jutras, 2009; Mayo, 2010; Nesi, 2012; Purzychi, 2010). Educators have used humor to alleviate classroom stress and facilitate knowledge acquisition and application for decades. Humor contributes to a positive affect and, to that end, humor has been used as a teaching tool for generations. Effectively using humor in the classroom requires knowledge, art, and skill, all of which may be learned (Chiarello, 2010; Garner, 2005, 2006; Hellman, 2007; Zeigler, 1998). This chapter will highlight humor as an educator's tool and describe specific strategies for humor use in the classroom.

■ Definition and Purpose

Humor is a communication that induces amusement. Thus, it must be shared. It makes the learning environment a shared, pleasurable experience. In education, the most positive forms of humor are funny stories or comments, jokes, and professional humor. Sarcasm has been recorded as common in the classroom, but it tends to be a negative form of humor. Wit is the cognitive process that elicits humor. Mirth is the emotional reaction to humor, joy, and pleasure. Laughter or smiling is a physical expression of humor. With all these elements, the formal study of humor in the classroom has been a challenge. A decade ago, the literature on the use of humor in healthcare education was predominantly opinion pieces or reviews as opposed to actual evidence, although at least a dozen studies of humor were conducted in educational settings (Ziegler, 1998). Whether the evidence is as sound as it should be remains equivocal, but lately the majority of authors praise its contributions to the educational experience (Chauvet & Hofmeyer, 2007; Dormann & Biddle, 2006; Englert, 2010; Garner, 2005, 2006; Golchi & Jamali, 2011; Heitzmann, 2010; James, 2004; Makewa, Role, & Genga, 2011; Mayo, 2010; Nesi, 2012; Priest, 2007; Proctor, Maltby, & Linely, 2011; Southam & Schwartz, 2004; Symbaluk & Howell, 2010; Torok, McMorris, & Lin, 2004).

Humor has been studied and discussed from a variety of approaches—the physiologic, psychologic, emotional, and cognitive. Recent reviews have summarized these studies (Hart & Walton, 2010; Nesi, 2012; Purzychi, 2010; Southam & Schwartz, 2004; Torok et al., 2004) and confirmed that humor can promote health as well as learning through the physical benefits of reduced stress, increased productivity, and enhanced creativity. Humor has been deemed a primary vehicle for enhancing the learning environment through enlivening potentially dreary topics, keeping lectures engaging and enjoyable, and humanizing faculty in students' perceptions. The cultivation of the abilities to laugh at oneself and with others bridges many gaps between people and broadens the pathway from student to professional (Adamle et al., 2007; Chiarello, 2010; Field, 2009; Golchi & Jamali, 2011; Hart & Walton, 2010; James Andershed, Gustavsson, & Ternestedt, 2010; Lei, Cohen, & Russler, 2010; Makewa et al., 2011; Nesi, 2012; Priest, 2007; Procter et al., 2011).

The use of humor in the classroom can be productive, promoting comfortable, safe interactions between faculty and students. It has been shown to increase teacher credibility (Garner, 2006; Lei et al., 2010; Makewa et al., 2011; Symbaluk & Howell, 2010; Torok et al., 2004). The effective use of humor promotes creativity, learning, retention, and enculturation of professionals (Adamle et al., 2007; Chauvet & Hofmeyer, 2007; Chiarello, 2010; Dormann & Biddle, 2006; Flournoy, Turner, & Combs, 2001; Lei et al., 2010; Nesi, 2012; Purzychi, 2010; Southam & Schwartz, 2004). Counterproductive humor can cause fear and hostility, decrease self-esteem and motivation, and disrupt the community within classroom and work settings (Berk, 2009; Ciesielka, Conway, Penrose, & Risco, 2005; Laviosa, 2010; Shah & Inamullah, 2011).

Several studies (Chiarello, 2010; Golchi & Jamali, 2011; Makewa et al., 2011; Torok et al., 2004; White, 2001) compared perceptions regarding the use of humor between professors and students, whether students thought more favorably of professors who used humor, and which types of humor were preferred. Their findings had strong correlations with perceptions of the use of funny stories, funny comments, jokes, and professional humor. Students had mixed support for humor in testing. The use of sarcasm and derogatory humor was not supported. Shibles's (1989) analysis of humor declares that ridicule and sarcasm are used as a superiority differentiation or as a defense mechanism and therefore do not qualify as types of humor. Berk (2009) articulated the need to avoid derogatory and cynical humor in clinical teaching and the workplace by healthcare providers. He advocated the importance of maintaining professionalism, as these individuals are models for the next generation of providers. Educators need to be cognizant of this because such a misuse of humor will be counterproductive in the classroom and the clinic. Students often found positive humor facilitated attention, morale, and comprehension. Makewa and colleagues (2011) identified that affiliative humor and self-enhancing humor were most preferred by students. White's study identified agreement between professors and students regarding humor as a tool to relieve stress, create a healthy learning environment, gain attention, and motivate students. The item of greatest variation between faculty and student perceptions was the use of humor to handle unpleasant situations—students believed it could be used, but faculty did not. Laviosa (2010) and Nesi (2012) identified the importance of cultural awareness of humor and humor context when using humor in the classroom, especially with a culturally diverse student body.

■ Theoretical Foundations

Humor is a complex phenomenon with a long and rich history. While no one has been able to establish when the first joke actually occurred, we know the Greek theater used both comedy and drama to entertain and enlighten. Many authors, such as Dickens and Swift, used satire to comment on society. Theoretical foundations of humor are multiple (Shibles, 1989). They have been categorized by discipline (e.g., biological, cognitive, physiological, linguistic) and construct (e.g., incongruity, superiority, affiliative) (Ziegler, 1998). Boyd (2004) purports that humor and laughter relate to play theory and, therefore, create a sense of shared playfulness. He suggests that this sense of playfulness opens the participants to creative and critical thinking and action, while simultaneously alerting and disarming them in an environment of mutual trust and enjoyment. Effective use of humor may be a component of all learning theories. Humor and laughter contribute to all necessary principles of learning, which are enjoyment; creativity; interest; motivation; a relaxed, open, warm environment; a positive student–teacher relationship; and decreased tension and anxiety (Skinner, 2010). To be authentic is one of the most important qualities of an educator. Having a sense of humor is an aspect of authenticity (Hellman, 2007; Jackson, 2010; Lottes, 2008). Humor used constructively builds a positive self-image (Chauvet & Hofmeyer, 2007; Chiarello, 2010; Field, 2009; Garner, 2005, 2006; Golchi & Jamali, 2011; Hellman, 2007; Lei et al., 2010; Priest, 2007).

Cognitive and affective theories appear the most important for education, as they account for linguistic, intellectual, and emotional aspects of learning. Some humor theories state that laughter or amusement occurs as an intellectual reaction to something unexpected, illogical, or inappropriate in some way (Boyd, 2004; Mayo, 2010; Nesi, 2012; Purzychi, 2010 Shibles, 1989). Cognitive theory focuses on an understanding of language, knowledge, situation, and reasoning that addresses recognition of mistakes, incongruity, and wordplays. Research indicates that the recognition of incongruity begins in infancy (Boyd, 2004; Wild, Rodden, Grodd, & Ruch, 2003). Puns, irony, and satire require analysis and synthesis of words, knowledge, and context (Boyd, 2004; Wild et al., 2003). Without such understanding, students do not perceive the humor and may take affront or feel put down by the instructor. When students understand a concept well they can make jokes or funny remarks about it, indicating their synthesis of the material. Cognition is shaped by culture, and humor has been defined as culturally appropriate incongruity (Boyd, 2004; Chauvet & Hofmeyer, 2007; Purzychi, 2010; Wrench & McCroskey, 2001).

According to Bloom, affect is an important domain of learning. Those theorists who subscribe to affective theory stress emotional components of humor. However, it seems inadequate to treat affect as separate from cognition, because emotion is largely constituted by thought (Shibles, 1989). There has been extensive discussion regarding the emotional and physiologic benefits of releasing psychic energy through laughter. Because of this, humor is an invaluable contribution to the educational process. Its use creates an affirmation of shared understanding and experience (Boyd, 2004). Research supports its use to reduce anxiety and stress, build confidence, improve productivity, reduce boredom, heighten interest, and encourage divergent thinking and the creation of new ideas (Chauvet & Hofmeyer, 2007; Chiarello, 2010; Dormann & Biddle, 2006; Field, 2009; Golchi & Jamali, 2011; Makewa et al., 2011; Mayo, 2010; Nesi, 2012; Purzychi, 2010; Ziegler, 1998).

The affective component of humor engages the limbic system, thereby enhancing short- and long-term memory and increasing the willingness of the learner to apply knowledge and skills (Flournoy et al., 2001; Southam & Schwartz, 2004). Some believe the best time to deliver serious points to students when teaching is right after they laugh (Field, 2009; Hogue, 2010; Makewa et al., 2011). The expression of feelings, such as empathy and anger, can be more constructive when approached in a witty manner (James et al., 2010; Makewa et al., 2011; Nesi, 2012). Both sides of the brain are actively engaged during laughter and the perception of humor (Southam & Schwartz, 2004). The right side of the brain focuses on reading and interpreting the visual, nonverbal information of humor while the left side of the brain interprets the language nuances of humor. Novelty, imagination, and visualization help move information into long-term memory through the engagement of multiple brain cells firing simultaneously (Purzychi, 2010; Southam & Schwartz, 2004; Wild et al., 2003; Wrench & McCroskey, 2001). However, there is still much research to be done about the neuroscience related to humor and perceptions about what is humorous (Purzychi, 2010; Wild et al., 2003).

■ Types of Learners

Humor is a type of playfulness that spans multiple ages and venues. Developmentally and intellectually appropriate humor can be employed with all levels of learners. Classroom humor relevant to course content is more appreciated by the adult learner than is random humor. It also is necessary to be aware of students' cultural backgrounds because words and concepts may have different meanings and be misperceived, or worse, be taboo to discuss (Golchi & Jamali, 2011; Hogue, 2010; Jutras, 2009; Lei et al., 2010; Makewa et al., 2011; Mayo, 2010; Nesi, 2012).

Studies have provided mixed reviews about students' acceptance and appreciation of humor used by the teacher. Some studies have shown that gender impacts the acceptance and use of humor, as does the match between the educator's and students' sense of humor (Martin, Puhlik-Doris, Larsen, Gray, & Weir, 2003; Nesi, 2012). The associations found between intellectual ability and sense of humor suggest that educators need a firm check on the cognitive status of their students when employing wit, or they risk offending rather than amusing them (Boyd, 2004; LaFarge, 2004; Tallent, 2010; Wild et al., 2003). Gorham and Christophel (1990, as cited by Southam & Schwartz, 2004) found that learning outcomes of female students were not as influenced by teacher humor as were outcomes in male students, whose achievement was enhanced through the use of humor. Females, while not appreciably influenced by humor in that study, did prefer personal stories that illustrated pertinent points related to course content. Student reaction to humor has been differentially related to the gender of the educator as well, with female educators eliciting less overall appreciation of their efforts to be humorous (Golchi & Jamali, 2011; Nesi, 2012; White, 2001). Acceptance of humor in the classroom has been shown to be positively associated with a student's psychological health (Dziegielewski, Jacinto, Laudadio, & Legg-Rodriguez, 2003; Kuiper, Grimshaw, Leite, & Kirsh, 2004).

■ Conditions for Learning

Humor can be used judiciously throughout a class session or course and in all types of classroom situations, including lecture, lab, fieldwork, and various course assignments. Mood can enhance or inhibit the reception of humor (Heitzmann, 2010; Wild et al., 2003), making it imperative to read the class members accurately and create a positive and pleasant classroom experience. Positive and constructive humor can be used to put the learner and the teacher at ease with the subject matter (Garner 2005, 2006; Hellman, 2007; Lei et al., 2010; Makewa et al., 2011; Nesi, 2012; Purzychi, 2010). Humorous activities, or ice-breakers, that relate to the class session topic might begin a class. These activities can also be inserted at intervals to reaffirm the open, relaxed atmosphere that is most conducive to learning. Tension relievers before exams are usually helpful. As long as the humor remains embedded in the content, learners will internalize the new knowledge; otherwise, the flow of the lesson can be lost or misdirected (Weaver & Cotrell, 2001). Humor can be used to facilitate creativity and retention of material at any point in a lesson—from initial setup through final review (Chauvet & Hofmeyer, 2007; Garner, 2006; Hellman, 2007). Purzychi (2010) found using minimally counterintuitive ideas increased recall and retention of new concepts. These ideas challenge the students' current cognitive knowledge template about a topic by presenting an exaggerated or unexpected parallel idea related to topic content or knowledge application.

Relationship between class size and classroom size may impact the effective use of humor. Berk (2002, as cited by Torok et al., 2004) noted that laughter is likely to be greater in larger, more crowded classes than in smaller classes in larger rooms. Laughter, like yawning, is contagious, so once a large group gets going it may take time to bring them back to focus. Dziegielewski and colleagues (2003) encourage the group leader—the educator in this case—not to stop the laughter but to let it stop on its own accord. They perceive that this laughter helps reduce anger and tension and may build cohesion and well-being—both of which are essential to productivity and learning.

Humor is a part of communication and not dependent on the natural comedic ability of an instructor. It is an attitude and permission for enjoyment of the educational process (Adamle et al., 2007; Chauvet & Hofmeyer, 2007; Golchi & Jamali, 2011; Joyner & Young, 2006; Makewa et al., 2011; Nesi, 2012; Weaver & Cotrell, 2001). It can be spontaneous or planned. Weaver and Cotrell recommend inserting humorous breaks every 15 minutes. Golchi and Jamali (2011) recommend delivering the most important content or concept for learning just after a good laugh, when the mind is relaxed and opened to new learning. Essential to creating open communication and allowing humor within the classroom is the teacher's nonverbal communication and voice tone, as these can convey openness or constrict enjoyment of learning. If the humor style of the teacher and that of the class do not mesh, then the use of humor in the learning process will not be effective (Golchi & Jamali, 2011; Makewa et al., 2011; Nesi, 2012). It is important to understand your audience, which in this case is the class, and to know one's own sense of humor and be willing to experiment with others (Garner, 2006; Hellman 2007; Wild et al., 2003).

Humor is not necessarily universally appropriate. McMorris, Boothroyd, and Pietrangelo (1997) summarized studies that used humor in testing situations with mixed results. Positive results depended on the type of humor used. Some studies found humor to reduce tension, but others found it to be distracting in a testing situation. Humor with a strong linguistic base may also disadvantage international students (Lei et al., 2010; Nesi, 2012). Likewise, as mentioned previously, any use of sarcasm is seen as detrimental to learning (Berk, 2009; Garner, 2006; Hellman 2007; Nesi, 2012; Shah & Inamullah, 2011; Torok et al., 2004).

Humor can be very useful in the enculturation of novices into one's profession, especially when dealing with the elements of embarrassing intimacy and reality shocks that may occur in healthcare provision (Adamle et al., 2007; Chiarello, 2010; Hart & Walton, 2010; James et al., 2010; Southam & Schwartz, 2004). A healthy sense of humor is related to being able to laugh at oneself and one's life without degrading oneself. Those who enter the health professions must be able to cope with adversity and be able to help others cope as well (Adamle et al., 2007; Hart & Walton, 2010; James et al., 2010). The development of a healthy sense of humor, beginning in preservice classes and continuing through professional in-service educational programs, benefits everyone.

■ Resources

As with any teaching strategy, the effective use of humor needs to be learned and refined. Before using humor in teaching situations, educators may want to assess their own sense of humor using a humor profile such as the one developed by Richmond, Wrench, and Gorham (2001) (see **Appendix 8-1**). The score obtained on the humor profile reflects one's use of humor during communications. Completion of a humor profile is a preliminary step to learning one's current facility with humorous content.

Some ways to increase one's use of humor are exposing oneself to humorous experiences as found at comedy clubs; collecting humorous materials, such as comics, sitcoms, joke books; and even looking for the humor around oneself from everyday life. This may include viewing the world through exaggeration or broad, silly perspectives. Using exaggeration is a method to clarify concepts—the contrast assists understanding. Incongruity is another technique for promoting humor in the classroom, which Mayo's (2010) and Purzychi's (2010) studies found aided retention and recall of concepts and application. One such example is comparing a stripper and a corporate CEO regaining work skills (see the teaching example later in this chapter). Creating a top 10 list of teacher pet peeves or preferred learning behaviors can be a humorous way to share class performance expectations (Kher, Molstad, & Donahue, 1999). Using props in the classroom for role playing may also enhance the humor of a lesson (Joyner & Young, 2006; Polek, 2007; Priest, 2007). The cinema and YouTube are treasure troves of humorous situations waiting to be tapped by the healthcare professional looking for examples of exaggeration, incongruity, or basic fun (Polek, 2007).

Articles about infusing humor into online courses have suggested a number of techniques to promote a positive learning environment in the virtual classroom that mirror applications of humor in the regular classroom. Primary among these techniques is the use of humor to project an authentic representation of the educator. The humor used, by necessity, is primarily linguistic, although cartoons are readily available (James, 2004; Nesi, 2012). Being humorous online requires extensive commitment, time, and effort as it needs to be planned, personalized to the students, and monitored for receptivity (Boynton, as cited by James, 2004; Nesi, 2012). Listed here are a few choice resources for humor-related materials.

1. *Web resources (available as of publication; web addresses may change):*
   Humor Matters bibliography and resources: http://www.humormatters.com/bibindex.htm

Learning the art of using humor: http://www.humorproject.com/
2. *Sources for cartoon humor (some resources are paid services):*
Cartoons from the *New Yorker* magazine: http://www.cartoonbank.com
Single cartoons by Randy Glasbergen, often about business or family: http://www.glasbergen.com/
Variety of popular newspaper cartoon serials: http://www.gocomics.com/explore/comics
3. *Print resources:*
Print versions of cartoons (e.g., *Far Side, For Better or Worse, Calvin and Hobbes, Zits*), local newspapers, bookstores
Desk calendars such as *A Little Bit of Oy, The Far Side*, and *Peanuts*
Cathcart, T., & Klein, D. (2007). *Plato and a platypus walk into a bar: Understanding philosophy through jokes.* New York, NY: Penguin Group.
Tibballs, G. (2000). *The mammoth book of humor.* New York, NY: Carroll & Graf

Check the humor section of any bookstore.

■ Using the Method

The use of humor can be learned and there is a growing evidence base regarding its use in education, yet the use remains highly individualized. The Humor Project, developed in 1977, is one workshop venue for learning how to use humor effectively. Humor is often a skill picked up and used by healthcare professionals when assessing the health, recovery, and state of well-being of patients or residents in healthcare facilities (Hart & Walton, 2010; James et al., 2010; Proctor et al., 2011). Gender, culture, ethnicity, mood, and context impact the acceptance or rejection of this teaching strategy (Garner, 2005, 2006; Laviosa, 2010; Lei et al., 2010; Makewa et al., 2011; Nesi, 2012; Wild et al., 2003; Wimer & Beins, 2008; Ziegler, 1998). Nesi (2012) and Wanzer and Frymier (1999) found that witty, rather than funny, professors were considered interesting, entertaining, and motivating by adult learners. Robinson is often cited (Southam & Schwartz, 2004) as proposing the following four interrelated aspects to be considered in the area of education and humor: (1) enhancing the learning process itself through humor; (2) using humor to facilitate the process of socialization; (3) teaching the concept of humor as a communication and intervention tool; and (4) modeling the use of humor as a vehicle for facilitating the other three. Using humor in the classroom is not attempting to become a comedian. It is assuming an attitude of authenticity and comfort within the classroom (Garner, 2005, 2006; Golchi & Jamali, 2011; Hellman, 2007; Jackson, 2010; Lottes, 2008; Makewa et al., 2011; Nesi, 2012; Polek, 2007; Purzychi, 2010). Chiarello (2010) conducted a qualitative study of a clinical supervisor's deliberate use of humor for eight nursing students. Seven of the eight students were responsive to the humor and identified the use of humor as beneficial to their learning and growth.

The ability to learn to use humor has been questioned by a few authors (Wrench & McCroskey, 2001). These authors distinguish sense of humor, a culturally taught trait, from the act of being humorous, which may be a genetic trait. However, most authors promote the idea that the use of humor not only can be learned, but ought to be learned by educators to enhance the teaching–learning process (Adamle et al., 2007; Chauvet & Hofmeyer, 2007; Dormann & Biddle, 2006; Englert, 2010; Flowers, 2001; Garner, 2006; Mayo, 2010; Nesi, 2012; Priest, 2007; Skinner, 2010; Symbaluk & Howell, 2010; Trunfio, 2011). Employing humorous methods is within every educator's reach and will enhance the educational experience for students.

Using humor in the learning process can take several forms. It is easy for most faculty to use spontaneous storytelling by relating their own experiences to enhance the learning process. Other faculty may need to collect jokes, cartoons, movie excerpts, and humorous exercises to insert into their regular teaching activities to enhance the learners' receptivity to information and participation during content presentations. See **Figure 8-1** for some tips on using humor in the classroom.

Tamblyn (2003) highly recommends the frequent use of visuals such as cartoons, posters, and other images throughout an educational presentation to enhance the impact of the content. From a cognitive load perspective, the use of cartoons may enhance recall and retention due to the complementary effects of visual and verbal information processing, as long as the cartoon/text match is consistent with the course content and learning level of the student (Khalil, Paas, Johnson, & Payer, 2005; Makewa et al., 2011; Nesi, 2012). As has been mentioned, faculty must realize that what works for some people does not necessarily work for others (Boyd, 2004; Makewa et al., 2011; Mayo, 2010; Nesi, 2012; Tamblyn, 2003; Wild et al., 2003). Nesi (2012) found that some Asian cultures perceived humor used in the classroom as inappropriate.

---

1. Create a casual and safe atmosphere.
2. Smile; adopt a laugh-ready attitude.
3. Relax; use an open nonverbal posture; increase interpersonal contact through eye-to-eye and face-to-face contact.
4. Remove social inhibitions; establish a nonjudgmental forum for discussion.
5. Begin the class with a humorous example, cartoon, anecdote, or thought for the day.
6. Use personal stories, anecdotes, and current events related to class content.
7. Plan frequent breaks in content for application for humorous commercials or exaggerated examples; provide humorous materials.
8. Encourage give and take with students; laugh at yourself occasionally.

Sources: Adapted from Provine, 2000; Weaver & Cotrell, 2001.

■ Figure 8-1 Tips for using humor in the classroom.

Some specific techniques for including humor in a class situation include posting humorous situations on a bulletin board to teach interactive concepts (Flournoy et al., 2001). Using irony to contrast expected outcomes and actual occurrence enhances remembrance because of incongruity (Mayo, 2010; Nesi, 2012; Purzychi, 2010). Case studies with funny names related to topical content also enhance memory of the examples. (Example: Petunia Potter liked working in her garden. She needed some ergonomic changes to facilitate her participation in this avocation; how would you adapt this occupation for her?) Use of exaggerations and unusual professions increases awareness of people's needs in the healthcare arena. Personal stories about real-life experiences and challenges in one's role as a new professional or in unexpected circumstances (or embarrassing moments) can have teaching value. Sometimes when students are called on to do group presentations on a given topic, they will use humor (often in the form of mimicry or parody of the instructors) to engage their classmates and, possibly, to alleviate their own stress. Humor usage will be as variable as those using it (Chauvet & Homeyer, 2007; Garner, 2006; Hellman, 2007; Makewa et al., 2011; Nesi, 2012; Priest, 2007).

A picture's meaning can express ten thousand words
—Often misquoted Chinese proverb

■ Potential Problems

Not everyone gets a joke (Boyd, 2004; Wild et al., 2003). Some people are too serious. Some do not value humor in the educational process. Some find it too distracting to their learning. Using sarcasm, ridicule, and put-down humor can be counterproductive. Humor has the potential to be offensive, especially with ethnic, cultural, or gender issues. Incongruence between innate or cultural humor perceptions can be disruptive to the coordination of the learning environment. Besides potentially offending some members of a class, the use of deprecatory humor may affect students' perceptions of the faculty and undermine their effectiveness. Class clowns, who use humor for personal gain, also abuse the strategy and detract from the learning environment (Martin et al., 2003). It is essential for educators to remember that they are role models and exert power over students by their modeling (Berk, 2009; Shah & Inamullah, 2011); thus they should be cognizant of the type of humor used in their communications.

■ Conclusion

It has been said that Plato believed one could discover more about a person in an hour of play than in a year of conversation. The same could be said about the culture of a classroom, cohort, or department. Teaching–learning communities are built on engagement and communication amongst students and faculty. The development of respect and desire to learn can be facilitated with the thoughtful use of humor. See

Figure 8-2 for a humorous introduction to the concept of deductive clinical reasoning. All involved will find their creativity, enjoyment, and problem solving boosted by this cognitively stimulating and emotionally safe learning environment.

TEACHING EXAMPLES

At the beginning of a pediatrics class on toddler development, cartoons that related to the lecture topic were used as a starting point for discussion. The cartoons had been selected from the daily newspaper over a span of years, so there were many examples of toddler behaviors to choose from. Students who had their own children or younger siblings were able to immediately relate to the cartoon situations and discuss the behaviors depicted as well as other toddler behaviors and observations they had seen. Students without children and siblings participated in the discussion by asking questions of those with more experience. A lively discussion ensued. When presented with the accompanying reading material or tested on the material at a later date, students exhibited better retention and recall of the information and the discussion that occurred around the visual cue of the cartoon compared to nonhumorous content.

Another example of a humor-enhanced class discussion related to client-centered evaluation by using exaggerated comparison contrast of a stripper's and a CEO's daily activity routines, expectations, and needs. Students started discussing their perceived stereotypes of these exaggerated individuals and, as new elements of typical activities of daily living were suggested to the students to analyze for these individuals, another lively discussion occurred. When assessed for their understanding of activities of daily living evaluations, analyses, and syntheses for treatment plans, students exhibited a greater understanding of these processes related to individualized care with attention to details compared to standard examples typical everyday expectations.

Sherlock Holmes and Dr. Watson went camping. After a good meal and an excellent bottle of wine, they lay down and went to sleep. A couple of hours later, Holmes woke up and nudged his faithful friend.

"Watson, Watson," he said. "Look up at the sky and tell me what you see?"

"I see millions and millions of stars," replied Watson.

"And what does that tell you?" inquired the master detective.

Watson thought for a moment, "Well, Holmes, astronomically, it tells me that there are millions of galaxies and potentially billions of planets. Astrologically, I observe that Saturn is in Leo. Horologically, I deduce that the time is approximately 2:25. Theologically, I can see that god is all powerful and that we are small and insignificant. Meteorologically, I believe we will have a glorious day tomorrow. What does it tell you, Holmes?"

"Watson, you imbecile! Some thief has stolen our tent!"

Source: Tibballs, G. (2000). *The mammoth book of humor*. New York, NY: Carroll & Graf; joke 2470.

▪ **Figure 8-2** An example of a joke that may be appropriate for a class on clinical reasoning.

REFERENCES

Adamle, K., Chiang-Hanisko, L., Ludwick, R., Zeller, R., & Brown, R. (2007). Comparing teaching practices about humor among nursing faculty: An international collaborative study. *International Journal of Nursing Education, Scholarship, 4*(1), Article 2.

Berk, R. (2009). Derogatory and cynical humour in clinical teaching and the workplace: The need for professionalism. *Medical Education, 43*, 7–9. doi: 10.1111/j.1365-2923.2008.03239

Boyd, B. (2004). Laughter and literature: A play theory of humor. *Philosophy and Literature, 28*(1), 1–22.

Chauvet, S., & Hofmeyer, A. (2007). Humor as a facilitative style in problem-based learning environments for nursing students. *Nurse Education Today, 27*, 286–292.

Chiarello, M. (2010). Humor as a teaching tool: Use in psychiatric undergraduate nursing. *Journal of Psychosocial Nursing, 48*(8), 34–41.

Ciesielka, D., Conway, A., Penrose, J., & Risco, K. (2005). Maximizing resources: The S.H.A.R.E. model of collaboration. *Nursing Education Perspectives, 26*(4), 224–226.

Dormann, C., & Biddle, R. (2006). Humour in game-based learning. *Learning, Media and Technology, 31*(4), 411–424.

Dziegielewski, S. F., Jacinto, G. A., Laudadio, A., & Legg-Rodriguez, L. (2003). Humor: An essential communication tool in therapy. *International Journal of Mental Health, 32*(3), 74–90.

Englert, L. (2010). Learning with laughter: Using humor in the classroom. *Nursing Education Perspectives, 33*(1), 48–49.

Field, A. (2009). Can humour make students love statistics? *The Psychologist, 22*(3), 210–213.

Flournoy, E., Turner, G., & Combs, D. (2001). Critical care: Read the writing on the wall. *Nursing, 31*(3), 8–10.

Garner, R. (2005). Humor, analogy, and metaphor: H.A.M. it up in teaching. *Radical Pedagogy, 6*(2). Retrieved from http://radicalpedagogy.icaap.org/content/issue6_2/garner.html

Garner, R. (2006). Humor in pedagogy: How ha-ha can lead to aha! *College Teaching, 54*(1), 177–180.

Golchi, M., & Jamali, F. (2011). The effect of teacher's verbal humor on advanced EFL learners' classroom anxiety. *European Journal of Social Sciences, 26*(2), 185–192.

Hart, R., & Walton, M. (2010). Magic as a therapeutic intervention to promote coping in hospitalized pediatric patients. *Pediatric Nursing, 36*(1), 11–17.

Heitzmann, R. (2010, May). 10 suggestions for enhancing lecturing. *Education Digest*, 50–54. Retrieved from www.eddigest.com

Hellman, S. V. (2007). Humor in the classroom: Stu's seven simple steps to success. *College Teaching, 55*(1), 37–39.

Hogue, B. (2010). I'm not making this up: Taking humor seriously in the creative nonfiction classroom. *Pedagogy: Critical Approaches to Teaching Literature, Language, Composition and Culture, 11*(1), 199–205.

Jackson, J. (2010). On ethnic sincerity. *Current Anthropology, 51*(2), S279–S287. doi: 10.1086/653129

James, D. (2004). Commentary: A need for humor in online courses. *College Teaching, 52*(3), 93–94.

James, I., Andershed, B., Gustavsson, B., & Ternestedt, B. (2010). Knowledge constructions in nursing practice: Understanding and integrating different forms of knowledge. *Qualitative Health Research, 20*(11), 1500–1518. doi: 10.1177/1049732310376042

Joyner, B., & Young, L. (2006). Teaching medical students using role play: Twelve tips for successful role plays. *Medical Teacher, 28*(3), 225–229.

Jutras, P. (2009, November/December). Could we use a good laugh? *Clavier Companion*, 4–5.

Khalil, M. K., Paas, F., Johnson, T. E., & Payer, A. F. (2005). Interactive and dynamic visualizations in teaching and learning of anatomy: A cognitive load perspective. *Anatomical Record, 286B*, 8–14.

Kher, N., Molstad, S., & Donahue, R. (1999). Using humor in the college classroom to enhance teaching effectiveness in "dread courses." *College Student Journal, 33*, 400–404.

Kuiper, N.A., Grimshaw, M., Leite, C., & Kirsh, G. (2004). Humor is not always the best medicine: Specific components of sense of humor and psychological well-being. *Humor, 17*, 135–168.

LaFarge, B. (2004). Comedy's intention. *Philosophy and Literature, 28*(1), 118–136.

Laviosa, S. (2010). Deconstructing humour across languages and genres. *U.S.–China Foreign Language, 8*(7), 26–43.

Lei, S., Cohen, J., & Russler, K. (2010). Humor on learning in the college classroom: Evaluating benefits and drawbacks from instructors' perspectives. *Journal of Instructional Psychology, 37*(4), 326–331.

Lottes, N. (2008). FIRE UP: Tips for engaging student learning. *Journal of Nursing Education, 47*(7), 331–332.

Makewa, L., Role, E., & Genga, J. (2011). Teachers' use of humor in teaching and students' rating of their effectiveness. *International Journal of Education, 3*(2), 1–17.

Martin, R. A., Puhlik-Doris, P., Larsen, G., Gray, J., & Weir, K. (2003). Individual differences in uses of humor and their relation to psychological well-being: Development of the Humor Styles Questionnaire. *Journal of Research in Personality, 37,* 28–75.

Mayo, C. (2010). Incongruity and provisional safety: Thinking through humor. *Studies in Philosophy and Education, 29,* 509–521. doi: 10.1007/s11217-010-9195-6

McMorris, R. F., Boothroyd, R. A., & Pietrangelo, D. J. (1997). Humor in educational testing: A review and discussion. *Applied Measurement in Education, 10*(3), 269–297.

Nesi, H. (2012). Laughter in university lectures. *Journal of English for Academic Purposes, 11,* 79–89. doi: 10.1016/j.jeap.2011.12.003

Polek, C. (2007). The podium as a stage: A one woman act. *Nurse Educator, 32*(1), 8–10.

Priest, A. (2010). Learning through laughter. *Nursing BC, 39*(5), 8–11.

Proctor, C. Maltby, J., & Linley, P.A. (2011). Strengths use as a predictor of well being and health related quality of life. *Journal of Happiness Studies, 12,* 153–169. doi: 10.1007/s10902-009-9181-2

Provine, R. R. (2000). *Laughter: A scientific investigation.* New York, NY: Viking Penguin.

Purzychi, B. G. (2010). Cognitive architecture, humor and counterintuitiveness: Retention and recall of MCIs. *Journal of Cognition and Culture 10,* 189–204. doi: 10.1163/156853710X497239

Richmond, V. P., Wrench, J. S., & Gorham, J. (2001). *Communication, affect, and learning in the classroom.* Acton, MA: Tapestry Press.

Shah, J., & Inamullah, H. M. (2011). Social power of teacher. *European Journal of Social Sciences, 21*(4), 516–521.

Shibles, W. (1989). *Humor reference guide.* Retrieved from http://www.drbarbaramaier.at/shiblesw /humorbook/index.html

Skinner, M. E. (2010, October). All joking aside: Five reasons to use humor in the classroom. *Education Digest,* pp. 19–21.

Southam, M., & Schwartz, K. B. (2004). Laugh and learn: Humor as a teaching strategy in occupational therapy education. *Occupational Therapy in Health Care, 18,* 57–70.

Symbaluk, D., & Howell, A. (2010). Web-based student feedback: Comparing teaching-award and research-award recipients. *Assessment & Evaluation in Higher Education, 35*(1), 75–86.

Tallent, R. (2010, November/December). Education: What makes teaching worthwhile. *Quill,* 12.

Tamblyn, D. (2003). *Laugh and learn: 95 ways to use humor for more effective teaching and training.* New York, NY: American Management Association.

Torok, S. E., McMorris, R. F., & Lin, W-C. (2004). Is humor an appreciated teaching tool? Perceptions of professors' teaching styles and use of humor. *College Teaching, 52,* 14–20.

Trunfio, T. N. (2011). Navigate by the smiles [Letter to the editor]. *Journal of School Health, 81*(2), 53.

Wanzer, M. B., & Frymier, A. B. (1999). The relationship between student perceptions of instructor humor and students' reports of learning. *Communication Education, 48,* 48–62.

Weaver, R. L., & Cotrell, H. W. (2001). Ten specific techniques for developing humor in the classroom. *Education, 108*(2), 167–179.

White, G. W. (2001). Teachers' report of how they used humor with students perceived use of such humor. *Education, 122*(2), 337–347.

Wild, B., Rodden, F., Grodd, W., & Ruch, W. (2003). Neural correlates of laughter and humour. *Brain, 126,* 2121–2138.

Wimer, D., & Beins, B. (2008). Expectations and perceived humor. *Humor, 21*(3), 347–363.

Wrench, J., & McCroskey, J. (2001). A temperamental understanding of humor communication and exhilaratability. *Communication Quarterly, 49,* 142–159.

Ziegler, J. B. (1998). Use of humour in medical teaching. *Medical Teacher, 20*(4), 341–348.

Richmond Humor Assessment Instrument

The Richmond Humor Assessment Instrument (RHAI) was designed to be a self-report measure of an individual's use of humor in communication. Unlike some other similar measures, this instrument does not focus on a particular kind of humor (e.g., storytelling). Alpha reliability estimates for this measure have been near 0.90.

Directions

The following statements apply to how people communicate humor when relating to others. Indicate the degree to which each of these statements applies to you by filling in the number of your response in the blank before each item:

5 = Strongly agree; 4 = Agree; 3 = Undecided; 2 = Disagree; 1 = Strongly disagree

_____ 1. I regularly communicate with others by joking with them.

_____ 2. People usually laugh when I make a humorous remark.

_____ 3. I am not funny or humorous.

_____ 4. I can be amusing or humorous without having to tell a joke.

_____ 5. Being humorous is a natural communication orientation for me.

_____ 6. I cannot relate an amusing idea well.

_____ 7. My friends would say that I am a humorous or funny person.

_____ 8. People don't seem to pay close attention when I am being funny.

_____ 9. Even funny ideas and stories seem dull when I tell them.

_____10. I can easily relate funny or humorous ideas to the class.

_____11. I would say that I am not a humorous person.

_____12. I cannot be funny, even when asked to do so.

_____13. I relate amusing stories, jokes, and funny things very well to others.

_____14. Of all the people I know, I am one of the least amusing or funny persons.

_____15. I use humor to communicate in a variety of situations.

_____16. On a regular basis, I do not communicate with others by being humorous or entertaining.

Scoring

To compute your scores, add your scores for each item as indicated here. Recode items 3, 6, 8, 9, 11, 12, 14, and 16 with the following format:

1 = 5
2 = 4
3 = 3
4 = 2
5 = 1

After you have recoded the previous questions, add all of the numbers together to get your composite RHAI score.

Your score should be between 16 and 80. Scores of 60 and more indicate high degrees of humor usage; scores of 30 and less indicate low of humor usage; scores between 30 and 60 indicate moderate degrees of humor usage.

Sources

Richmond, V. P., Wrench, J. S., & Gorham, J. (2001). *Communication, affect, and learning in the classroom.* Acton, MA: Tapestry Press.

Wrench, J. S., & McCroskey, J. C. (2001). A temperamental understanding of humor communication and exhilaratability. *Communication Quarterly, 49,* 170–183.

SECTION II

Teaching in Structured Settings

This section focuses on teaching in structured (i.e., classroom) settings and calls for focused planning and preparation on the part of the teacher. Concept-based topics that are applicable in a variety of teaching situations, regardless of the level of the learner, the topic, or the class size, are presented. Themes evident in each chapter include flexibility on the part of the teacher, a specific manner in which information is conveyed, and the importance of active student involvement and responsibility for one's own learning.

The principles presented the previous section, Foundational Approaches to Teaching and Learning, are used in the traditional classroom environments addressed in these chapters. Application of teaching and learning theories and use of planned activities enhance critical thinking in the learner and lead to clinical reasoning in practice settings. Educators can use creative innovations with time-honored strategies, such as lecture, to bring a fresh approach to teaching.

CHAPTER 9

The Lecture: Long-lasting, Logical, and Legitimate

■ Barbara C. Woodring and Richard C. Woodring ■

■ Setting the Stage

Take a good look at your home entertainment center (e.g., voice-activated digital TV with 156 channels, DVD, CD, electronic game board) with its 120-inch, touch-activated, 12-window screen accompanied by surround sound. It is in front of such centers that most adults and children spend 6–8 hours per day. Huntley, an industrial chief learning officer, stated:

> Education is no longer enough. Learners expect to be engaged and entertained more than ever . . . [learners] are exposed to a variety of stimulating and on-demand media sources daily . . . learning modes need to be equally engaging. (Huntley, 2009, p. 32)

She identified a solution as *edutainment,* presenting knowledge in a way that engages and entertains.

Yet, with this concept of edutainment before us, we are reminded that the methodology that remains the backbone for transmission of knowledge in most educational settings is the lecture. How, then, can educators satisfy the need for interactive variety and edutainment, while implementing the most commonly utilized teaching method? The information in this chapter will assist in addressing this question.

The authors of other chapters in this text provide insight into creative and innovative teaching approaches that are currently used in higher education. The implementation and refinement of these strategies/methods during the last decade have often relegated lecture methodology to a lesser stature. Rather than revere what has previously been considered the educational gold standard, it became trendy to "lecture bash" (Woodring, 2006)—that is, to describe colleagues who used lecture techniques as old-fashioned and out of step with educational trends. Many educators add the term *lecture* to their list of unspeakable, four-letter words. A Carnegie Foundation publication suggested that for the sake of being PC (pedagogically correct), the honorable tradition of lecturing has been relegated to an "Index of Forbidden Pedagogies" (Burgan, 2006, p. 31). In reality, a lecture is only a means to an end. Intrinsically, it is neither good nor bad; its success depends on why and how it is delivered.

In practice, the lecture format is alive and well and remains one of the most frequently utilized teaching methods in the repertoire of postsecondary educators. When the objective is to communicate basic facts, introduce initial concepts, or convey passion about a topic, a well-prepared lecture is very useful (Cox & Rogers, 2005; Gleitman, 2006). In this chapter, readers will find a rationale for the long-term popularity of this teaching strategy and suggestions for becoming a better lecturer.

■ Definition and Purposes

The lecture is one method of presenting information to an audience. It should be a well-designed, instructor-led, interactive experience that engages students and supports diverse styles of learning. Acceptance of this description indicates how far the educational process has come. Prior to the invention of the printing press, when only scholars had access to handwritten information sources, the lecture was the primary means of transmitting knowledge. Learners would gather around the master-teacher and take notes related to what was said. The lecture remained the common mode of disseminating information until printed resources and technological advancements became available and affordable.

It would appear that when students were able to purchase their own textbooks, and then their own technology (e.g., PC, laptop, PDA, tablet), methods of presenting information would have changed. Interestingly, change has occurred slowly. Today, with e-books and technology galore, the lecture remains a commonly used technique. It is suggested that there are two major reasons for this longevity: (1) most current educators learned via the lecture format, and it is well known that individuals teach as they were taught unless they make a specific effort to alter their approaches; and (2) the lecture is the safest and easiest teaching method, allowing the teacher the most control within the classroom setting. Some of the common advantages and disadvantages of using the lecture method are listed in **Tables 9-1** and **9-2**. Whatever rationale is used, positive outcomes can be achieved when both the lecture and the lecturer are well prepared.

■ Theoretical Rationale

Few lecturers take time to contemplate the theoretical basis of their practice, but the lack of a theoretical or organizational framework may be one reason that learners perceive some lectures to be disorganized and/or difficult to follow.

Table 9-1   Advantages of Using Lectures as a Teaching Strategy

Advantages of a Lecture	*Secondary Gain in Use of Lecture*
Permits teacher maximum control of class.	Decreases teacher anxiety of entertaining unexpected questions (teacher sets the ground rules for when/if questions may be asked).
Creates minimal threats to students or teacher.	Lack of interaction or student participation may be desired and can be controlled by the teacher.
Clarifies and enlivens information that seems tedious in text.	Highlights enthusiasm/personality of teacher for topic.
Enables clarification of confusing/intricate points immediately.	May avoid frustration of time-delayed responses or clarification if teacher allows questions during the class time.
The teacher knows what has been presented.	Diminishes the "I never heard that before" comment by students.
Lecture material can become basis of publication.	Contributes to academic scholarship.
Students are provided with a common core of content.	May help students to prepare for testing.
Accommodates larger numbers of listeners at one setting.	High priority in weak economy and/or teacher shortage.
May be time saving.	Teacher can present key points in much less time than it takes to elicit the same points from text or an extensive list of references.
Provides a venue to become known as an expert in a specific topic.	Contribute to the scholarship of teaching.
Encourages and allows deductive reasoning.	Can support principles of critical analysis if desired.
Enthusiasm of teacher motivates students to participate and learn more.	Reinforces professional role modeling.
Allows addition of the newest information on a moment's notice.	Can support concept of evidence-based practice with just-in-time data.
Permits auditory learners to receive succinct information quickly.	Encourages higher-level learning, not rote memorization.
Enables integration of pro and con aspects of topic.	Encourages critical thinking and analysis.

Source: Adapted from Woodring, B., & Woodring, R. (2010). Lecture: Reclaiming a place in pedagogy. In M. Bradshaw & A. Lowenstein (Eds.), *Innovative teaching strategies in nursing and related health professions* (5th ed., pp. 113–115). Sudbury, MA: Jones and Bartlett.

Foundational principles for a lecture presentation may be derived from a variety of philosophical and theoretical processes. Three common approaches flow from theories related to communication, cognitive learning, and pedagogical/andragogical approaches to teaching and learning. The theories supporting effective communications should be common knowledge to all healthcare providers; therefore, they are

Table 9-2 Disadvantages of Using Lectures as a Teaching Strategy

Disadvantages of a Lecture	Suggested Remedy
Teacher may attempt to cover too much material in abbreviated time frame.	Elicit questions at the conclusion of segments of time or content (e.g., every 15 minutes).
Less effective when not accompanied by another teaching strategy.	Include at least one audio and/or visual aid or interactive activity per hour.
Eighty percent of lecture information is forgotten 1 day later, and 80% of the remainder fades in 1 month.	Provide visual reinforcement or active learning (gaming).
Presumes that all students are auditory learners and learn at the same rate.	Add at least one handout, visual, or activity to support various learning styles.
Alone, the lecture is not suited to higher levels of thinking.	Intersperse scenarios or activities requiring problem-solving principles.
Not conducive for personalized instruction.	Call several students by name during each class. Encourage use of scheduled office hours for personal clarification and reviews.
Encourages passive learners.	Use clickers/automated response systems to encourage engagement of all class participants.
Provides little feedback to learners.	Encourage online/threaded discussion boards; use automated response clickers to allow immediate feedback.
Student attention wavers in 30 minutes or less.	Alter voice tone, classroom environment, teaching method (even turning off/on PowerPoint slides); change direction of students' attention.
Not appropriate for children below fourth grade level.	Lectures for children must be brief an based on the child's cognitive abilities. This method is not recommended with children who have less than fourth-grade reading level and/or attention span; if utilized, lecture must be accompanied by other learning activities.
Consistent use inhibits development of inductive reasoning.	Be flexible; incorporate creative teaching strategies described in previous chapters.
Poorly delivered lecture acts as a disincentive for learning.	Practice before you present! Be a positive professional role model.
Viewed by students as a complete learning experience wherein the lecturer presents all they need to know.	Encourage outside research, reviews, and readings, and set aside 5 minutes during each class to discuss them.
Effective learning seldom occurs in a lecture-only format.	Integrate use of lecture recitation, expository lecture, and/or provocative lecture techniques (described in this chapter).

Source: Adapted from Woodring, B., & Woodring, R. (2006). Lecture is not a four-letter word. In M. Bradshaw & A. Lowenstein (Eds.), *Innovative teaching strategies in nursing and related health professions* (4th ed., p. 112). Sudbury, MA: Jones and Bartlett.

not discussed here. Healthcare educators should have an understanding of cognitive learning theory since it is the underpinning of developmental concepts found in most health-related courses. Pedagogical/andragogical approaches may not be as well understood and are addressed briefly.

Over the past few decades, graduate education for many health professionals has emphasized disciplinary skills. Nursing and physical therapy, for instance, have focused on advanced practice skills resulting in clinical nurse specialists (CNSs), nurse practitioners (NPs), and the professional doctorate degrees (DPTs/DNPs). This change has resulted in limited numbers of newer faculty members who are prepared in the areas of curricular design and learning theory. Pedagogy is a portion of learning theory that loosely refers to educating the chronologically or experientially immature. In a pedagogical approach, someone external to the learner decides who, what, when, where, and how information will be taught; the learner becomes a passive recipient of knowledge. Historically, professional health-related content and practice have been taught from a framework that has been based upon the medical model. Within the pedagogical context, the lecture strategy establishes the teacher as the one in command, the authority from whom answers come. This approach may provide a rationale for lecturing being viewed as traditional and out of step with innovation and creativity in the academy. Over the years, both the age and the experiential backgrounds of traditional college students have shifted, causing scholars to question the appropriateness of the previously used pedagogical methods. In response, educators such as Knowles (1970), Kidd (1973), and Cross (1986) introduced and refined the concept of andragogy. The principles previously utilized in teaching the young (pedagogy) were adapted and applied to mature learners (andragogy).

Those educators who ascribe to andragogical theory treat the learner as a mature individual who brings a variety of rich, valuable experiences to every learning situation. The who, what, when, and where of learning emanate from within the learner. Each model has value, and the needs of the learner should determine the singular or blended approach utilized. **Table 9-3** compares andragogy and pedagogy within the educational process.

■ Types of Learners

The information included in Table 9-3 emphasizes that the teacher must know as much as possible about both the learners and the topic before deciding on a specific theoretical approach/model and/or selecting the teaching strategy. The concept of "know thy student" has always been important; however, now it is not only important, it is critical. Classrooms are filled with students born after 1990 who have been raised in the wireless, techno age and who expect edutainment, while the faculty may be uncomfortable communicating electronically or using social media. To bridge this generational communication gap, the teacher must understand and acknowledge that many learners have a very short attention span, have an arsenal of electronic devices

Table 9-3 Comparison of Characteristics: Andragogy Versus Pedagogy

Characteristic	Pedagogy	Andragogy
Concept of learner	Dependent	Independent/autonomous
	Passive	Self-directed
	The learner needs someone outside self to make decisions about what, when, and how to learn.	The learner wants to participate in decisions related to his or her own learning.
		Students will increase effort if they are rewarded rather than punished.
Roles of learner's experiences	Narrow, focused interest	Wide range of experience, not just in nursing, that impacts life/learning
	Focuses on imitation	Focus on originality
	Past experiences are given little attention.	The learner has broad interests and likes to share previous experiences with others.
Readiness to learn	Determined by someone else (society, teachers)	Learners are usually in the educational process because they have chosen to be.
	Focus on what is needed to survive and achieve	The learner wants to assist in setting the learning agenda.
	The learner tends to respond impulsively.	The learner tends to respond rationally.
Orientation of teaching/learning	Needs clarity/specificity	Teachers are facilitators, providing resources and supports for self-directed learners.
	The learner looks to the teacher to identify what should be learned and to provide the information/process to learn.	The learner likes challenging, independent assignments that are reality based.
	The learner focuses on particulars concerned with the superficial aspects of learning (grades, due dates).	Evaluation is done jointly by the teacher, the learner, and/or peers.
	Evaluation of learning is done by the teacher or society (grades, certificates).	The learner tolerates ambiguity.

Source: Woodring, B., & Woodring, R. (2006). Lecture is not a four-letter word. In M. Bradshaw & A. Lowenstein (Eds.), *Innovative teaching strategies in nursing and related health professions* (4th ed., pp. 114–115). Sudbury, MA: Jones and Bartlett.

at their fingertips (including in the classroom), are used to multitasking (answering text messages and listening to e-tunes while reading about neuroanatomy), and are used to handling a rapid barrage of information. To address these different learning needs, the proficient teacher will accompany the lecture with adjuncts, such as electronic innovations like Second Life, video clips, electronic lecture retrieval (e.g., via MP3 players), lecture–discussion (addressed later in this chapter), realistic scenarios, questions/answers accompanied by automated audience response systems (the clicker) with real-time feedback (Caldwell, 2007), and other strategies presented in the chapters of this text.

A lecture can be used effectively with learners who represent a variety of developmental and cognitive levels. Adaptability is one of its most positive aspects. A teacher may, at a moment's notice, alter the teaching style, depth, sophistication, and level of the material being presented. These alterations can be made based on the needs, interests, and/or responses of the learners; new scientific revelations; or breaking news from the media. It is assumed that the lecturer has a sufficient command of the subject matter, as well as the presence of mind and the flexibility to alter the content and teaching plan; however, these assumptions may not be accurate with novice educators or when material is being presented for the first time.

Combining the lecture with pedagogical approaches can be especially useful in basic and beginning courses in a sequence, as well as in orientation to new clinical areas or agencies. Novice learners of any age tend to prefer the structure of pedagogy, rather than the more flexible andragogical approach; however, the more mature and secure teachers and learners become, the more they enjoy the flexibility and challenge of integrating andragogical concepts into the lecture format.

■ Types of Lectures

Lectures survive because, like most professional sports and the story line of *Gone with the Wind*, they continue to satisfy the need for dramatic spectacle and offer an arena in which psychological needs are met. A teacher may vary a lecture from a very formal presentation to a much more casual monologue. Although described more than a decade ago, Lowman's (1995) outline of three types of lectures is still accurate. He identified the formal, expository, and provocative formats as types most commonly used in higher education.

The *formal lecture* is sometimes referred to as an oral essay. In the formal setting, the lecturer delivers a well-organized, tightly constructed, highly polished presentation. The information provided primarily supports a specific point and usually is backed by theory and research. The presentation may be written and read to the audience, although recent data indicate that most learners do not like lecture materials to be read to them (Masie, 2006). Preparation of a formal lecture is time consuming; therefore, is not used for every class period during a school term. It may, however, be appropriate to tie things together either at the beginning and/or end of a course or to address a specified topical area. One of the major problems with a formal lecture is that it ignores the interactive dimension and sometimes fails to motivate learners.

A variation on the formal lecture is *lecture recitation*. This process may be integrated into the formal lecture. The lecturer stops and asks a student to respond to a particular point or idea by reading/presenting prepared materials. An example of this approach may be a formal lecture related to the pathophysiology of sickle cell anemia, followed by a student-presented case study about a patient experiencing that disorder.

The *expository lecture* is considered the most typical type of lecture. It is much less elaborate than the formal oral essay. Although the lecturer does most of the talking, questions from learners are entertained, or a critical thinking exercise may be introduced.

In the *provocative lecture*, the instructor still does most of the talking, but he or she provokes students' thoughts and challenges their knowledge and values with questions. This method is well suited for integration of video streaming or lecture capturing. Included in this category are lecture practice, lecture–discussion, punctuated lecture, and lecture–lab. *Lecture practice* utilizes props, illustrates the subject, and may include lectures with simulations, computer, or video integration. In *lecture–discussion*, the instructor speaks for 10–15 minutes and then stimulates student discussion around key points (the lecturer acts only as a facilitator to clarify and integrate student comments). In *punctuated lecture*, the presenter asks the students to write down their reflections on lecture points and submit them. In *lecture-lab*, the lecture is followed by students conducting experiments, interviews, observations, and other activities during the class period.

The introduction of automated audience response systems within the classroom has enhanced the interactivity, especially in large classes (Caldwell, 2007). Similar to a game show, each student has a synchronized response unit—a clicker—similar to a TV remote control. This allows the students to reply to the lecturer's questions and allows the presenter to immediately verify the connections and involvement of students (Harper, 2009; Mayer et al., 2009).

Keep in mind that a lecture, in and of itself, is neither a good nor a bad/inappropriate approach to teaching. It may be deemed the best method when dealing with certain groups; however, like any strategy, it is most effective when not used as the singular, exclusive technique. Eble (1982), in *The Craft of Teaching*, suggested that the lecture should be thought of as a discourse—a talk or conversation—not an authoritative speech. As a discourse, the lecture can be viewed as a planned portion of the art or craft of teaching. As such, lecturing becomes a learnable skill that improves with practice.

Since the utilization of the lecture as a best practice in teaching has been called into question, numerous research studies have been undertaken. Amare (2006) studied the experiences of students in PowerPoint-enhanced versus non–PowerPoint-enhanced lectures. She found that, for 84 engineering, humanities, and education majors in a technical writing course, the performance scores were higher in the non-PowerPoint section. However, the students preferred the addition of PowerPoint slides. PowerPoint presentations, podcasts, and other technological enhancements were found to support the lecture by (1) bridging direct and constructionist teaching methods (Clark, 2008; Read, 2005); (2) supporting class attendance (Hove & Cocoran, 2008); and (3) reinforcing difficult concepts (Guertin, Bodek, Zappe, & Kim, 2007; Young, 2008). However, when Costa, van Rensburg, and Rushton (2007) compared group discussion to the lecture presentation method, the majority of medical student participants found the interactive, group discussion style more popular, the retention of knowledge better, and the scores on written tests higher. Generally, educational research findings support the notion that the lecture is still a valid, appropriate teaching strategy that is most effective when accompanied by other thought-provoking interludes (Wiebel, 2010). In the "Sage on the Stage in the Digital Age," Chung (2005) presents a number of very salient points but concludes that both graduate and undergraduate online education would suffer if the lecture component were absent.

■ Preparing Oneself to Lecture

Do not underestimate the time needed for preparation regardless of how well versed you may be with the topic. When presenting an oral essay or formal lecture, preparation must begin well in advance of the presentation date. Planning, organization, and written preparation are essential and time consuming. Less formal forms of lecture may take less time, but their preparation should not be delayed by procrastination. If the lecture is one in a sequence (or within a course), the best time to add the finishing touches to the next lecture is at the completion of the preceding one. Significant ideas that need to be reemphasized are still fresh in the presenter's mind, as are the questions that were raised, or should have been raised, by the students. The lecturer can recall the presentation strategies that worked with a group of participants and those that did not. Changes that might have made the lecture more effective can be identified. Most lecturers, however, do not heed this advice, and lecture preparation is often relegated to a brief time immediately prior to the presentation.

To present an effective lecture, the speaker must invest in preparing for several crucial sections. Like the human body, a lecture is divided into specific parts, each with its own function. These parts include the first 5 minutes, the main portion or body of the lecture, and the last 5 minutes. In the following paragraphs, each part is reviewed briefly.

Lecture Introduction (First 5 Minutes)

During the first 5 minutes of the lecture, two significant things occur: (1) the speaker outlines the objectives, outcomes, and expectations held for the participants; and (2) the audience decides whether to trust the speaker to produce what has been promised (objectives/outcomes) and whether to invest energy in following the presentation.

> *"There is too much material to be covered within the time allocated, but I'll do the best I can."*

Once this statement has been made, the lecturer will have difficulty regaining the full attention of the listener. From a teacher's point of view, the statement is always true but it should *never* be said aloud to an audience. If a lecturer opens a session with such a statement, the listener is conditioned to expect less than a top-notch presentation. The participant internally asks, "Why should I bother to listen if I can't possibly learn what I need to know in this hour?" So, no matter how tempting it may be to use this statement, eliminate it from your repertoire. Instead, begin by identifying what the learner should gain from this lecture: *state the objectives* in clear, interesting, pragmatic, and achievable terms. Then, *make a solid connection* with the listeners by using an example of how the lecture material can be (or has been) used in practice or life in general. *Outline the key concepts* that will be addressed, and use your expertise and clinical experience to provide some background and rationale for this lecture. The key points should be limited in number. Research related to information retained following a lecture indicated that most students can absorb only three to four major points in a 50-minute lecture and four to five points in a 75-minute presentation (Lowman, 1995). Conclude the introduction by establishing an open atmosphere and *describing the rules of operation* (e.g., "feel free to ask questions at any time"; "I will be using the automated response system several times during class, so have it ready"; "there will be time at the end of the lecture for questions"). An open atmosphere can be established by posing a question, making a bold statement, using a controversial quote, using humor, or using a visual aid or cartoon. The better one knows the audience, the easier and more successful the introduction becomes.

Body of Lecture

The main portion, or body, of a lecture should begin with a definition of concepts or principles that are illustrated by pragmatic, personal/professional experiences. The speaker then conveys the critical information the learner needs to know. The body should be well organized, with smooth transitions between topics. The experienced presenter knows that a lecturer cannot carry the primary responsibility for conveying all information or imparting all skills. Readings or critical analysis assignments assist in accomplishing these goals, and students need to be apprised of this connection. The body of the lecture should contain (1) general themes that tie together related topics; (2) topics/concepts that are difficult for students to understand (e.g., fluid balance); (3) sufficient depth and complexity to retain the learners' interest; and (4) testimonies (e.g., quotes from cancer survivors), case-specific data (e.g., lab values from unusual patient diagnoses), and exhibits (e.g., charts/graphs of statistics) to support the outcome-related point being made.

The speaker's presentation style is most evident during the body of the lecture. Tips and suggestions contained in the Resources section later in the chapter will enhance your presentation style.

Lecturer Conclusion (Last 5 Minutes)

The lecture needs a definite stopping point. Closing a notebook, running out of time, or simply dismissing the class is not an acceptable conclusion. An effective communicator knows that any interaction deserves closure—a lecture is no exception to that rule. By focusing the learners' attention during the last 5 minutes of class, the lecturer is able to establish finality and make a link between what was taught and what the learner will be able to use in life, practice, and/or an upcoming test. A good conclusion ties the introduction and the body together in a manner similar to that of an abstract that precedes a well-written manuscript.

The objectives and outcomes statements that were used as a portion of the introduction should be reiterated, emphasizing those that have been accomplished and those that remain to be addressed. The conclusion should also contain a review of the key points or topics covered, and time should be included for elaboration, amplification, and/or clarification of issues presented. Offering suggestions related to the application and transfer of knowledge may be helpful to the participants, and the use of summative take-home points may provide additional reinforcement. Using this approach allows the learner to quickly rethink the content, stimulate continued interest, and consider further action. The participants will leave the lecture hall feeling a sense of accomplishment because they can summarize what has been learned. Since the introduction of podcasting, MP3 players, immediate lecture-capture techniques, and other technologies, a number of faculty have opted to discontinue technological transmission of the last 5 minutes' summarization at the end of the lecture. They reserve this summary and clarification for only those who attend class or are legitimately enrolled in distance transmission of the course (Young, 2008). That option, of course, is a faculty choice. Thus, each lecture should be carefully planned and presented with an introduction (first 5 minutes), a well-organized body, and a meaningful conclusion (last 5 minutes) (Woodring, 2010). An example of how this plan could be operationalized for a typical 50-minute lecture period follows (**Figure 9-1**).

■ Resources

The major resource needed to utilize the lecture techniques effectively is *you*, the well-prepared lecturer. Presenting an informative and interesting lecture is a craft and a learnable skill. Because the speaker is the key element for this strategy, some key points are identified in the following list to help polish your presentation skills with additional suggestions summarized in **Table 9-4**. Remember, participants want to believe that you are smart, interesting, and a good speaker (Germano, 2003)!

- *Conveying enthusiasm is the key element in presenting an effective lecture.* Enthusiasm is contagious and is demonstrated by facial expressions, excitement in the voice, gestures, and body language. A lack of enthusiasm on the part of the speaker is interpreted by the listener as a lack of self-confidence, lack of knowledge, a disinterest in the learner, and/or disinterest in the topic. If you do not have an effusive personality, practice adding a smile and small hand gestures to each lecture. Once these movements are comfortable, add other interactive methods.

Time Allowed	Teacher	Learner	Supports
Introduction			
5 minutes	–Personal introduction	Listen	*Visual No. 1:* Objectives
	–Today's objectives	Take notes	*Handout:* Skeletal outline for note taking
	–Overview of class process/handouts	Ask for clarification	
Body			
15 minutes	Lecture Part I	Look	Visuals No. 2, 3, 4
		Listen	
		Take notes	
5 minutes	Q & A	Q & A	
10 minutes	Ask two questions related to the topic	Divide into pairs, discuss then share responses with class	List common responses on board
10 minutes	Lecture Part II		Visuals No. 5, 6, 7
Conclusion			
5 minutes	—State objectives achieved in the class.		Have automated response system activated.
	—Ask three questions relate to topic presented that day.	Use clicker to respond	
	—Ask two questions related to evaluation of the lecture.	Use clicker to respond	

■ **Figure 9-1** Sample lecture plan.

- *Know the content.* Even a written, formal lecture will not hide the insecurity of being unprepared or underprepared. Be certain you clearly explain key points in a language understood by the audience; do not use jargon or attempt to impress with effusive speech.
- *Use notes.* The use of notes is generally the option of the speaker; however, to avoid the distress of losing your train of thought or incorrectly presenting complex information, the use of some type of handwritten or computer-based prompts is highly recommended. For ease of handling, record the notes on the computer or on pages/cards that are all the same size and sequentially numbered. If you are using PowerPoint slides to accompany the lecture, you may wish to operationalize the notation section and have your lecture notes or outline appear on the screen in front of you, with or without them being

visible to the participants. The depth and content of lecture notes should fit the lecturer's comfort level. Use of anything from a skeletal outline to a full manuscript is acceptable. Notes should be prepared by leaving white space that is easy for your eye to follow.

Major points should be highlighted so the eye can easily pick up a cue when scanning a page. Although the use of notes is perfectly acceptable, the verbatim reading of notes is *not* acceptable. Rehearse your presentation often enough to appear spontaneous and enthusiastic and to *complete it within the allotted time frame.*

■ *Speak to an audience of 200 as if it were a single student.* Speak clearly and loudly enough to be heard in the back of the room. The use of a microphone may be necessary if you are presenting in a large room or auditorium. Always use the microphone if there is any doubt that your voice will not be heard in the last row. It is sometimes helpful to have a friend sit in the back and signal if your voice is not being heard during the presentation. A small clip-on microphone is preferable to using a handheld or stationary microphone because it allows the speaker the flexibility to move away from the podium and frees the hands to handle notes and/or gesture. If a microphone is to be used, arrive in the assigned room early enough to try the equipment and to regulate microphone position and sound levels. If the lecture is being transmitted to multiple sites, as in distance/distributive education or videoconferencing settings, be certain to test the sound levels at all sites prior to beginning the lecture.

■ *Make eye contact.* Select a participant at each corner of the room with whom you plan to make eye contact. Slowly scan the audience until you have seen each of the designated participants. Smile at familiar faces. If needed, review information related to the process of group dynamics. If the lecture is being transmitted to multiple sites, be certain to make eye contact via the monitors with participants in the distant sites. You may wish to make a concerted effort to look into each monitor or screen as you visually scan the lecture hall, and address participants at each site.

■ *Use creative movement.* Movements of the speaker's head and hands in gesturing should appear natural, not forced. Be careful when standing behind a podium; do not grip the sides tightly with your hands or lock your (shaky?) knees. This action produces a circulatory response that could cause the speaker to faint. Occasionally step away from the podium and toward the listeners. This conveys an attitude of warmth and acceptance. Avoid distracting mannerisms such as pacing, wringing your hands, clearing your throat, or jamming your hands into pockets and jingling pocket change/keys.

■ *Avoid barriers.* The use of a stage or podium places an automatic barrier between the speaker and the listeners. This gulf needs to be bridged early and often during the lecture. Suggestions for bridging the gulf include the following:

1. Use note cards rather than a manuscript because they are more portable and allow freedom to move away from the podium.
2. Step out from behind the podium, especially if you are short in stature—the audience does not wish to see a talking head.
3. Walk toward the listeners, which is interpreted as a sign of warmth and reaching out to the audience.
4. Address the right half of the audience, the left half of the audience, and then the audience at each distant site (each monitor or screen), but do not turn your back to either side of the audience or to the transmitting cameras.
5. Call on at least one participant in the audience and at each distant site by name.
6. Use hand gestures to accentuate words, but be careful not to overdo this action (this is especially important if the lecture is being transmitted to multiple sites since large or exaggerated hand gestures are more distracting when seen on a monitor than when viewed live).
7. If given the opportunity to be seated on a stage/platform, be aware of the eye level of the audience, especially if you are wearing a skirt/dress.

■ *Create a change of pace.* An astute lecturer constantly assesses the audience and interprets participants' signals. Facial cues indicate agreement disagreement with what has been said and may express understanding/ misunderstanding of content. Another signal is given when listeners begin having side conversations or squirm in their seats. These signals call for intervention, response, or a change of pace by the speaker. The change of pace can be as simple as turning off the computer/projector, shifting to a new slide, adding sound or animation to your visual, or changing the lighting—any of these actions will cause the listener to refocus attention on the speaker or back to the visual. Shifting the focus from the speaker to a handout, using a humorous example, altering the tone or inflection of your voice, using automated interaction with feedback from participants, dividing into small groups for a brief discussion, or taking a "stand and stretch" break also can provide a needed change of pace. Keep this rule of thumb in mind: An individual's *optimal attention span is roughly 1 minute per year of age* up to the approximate age of 30 (e.g., a 5-year-old has a 5-minute attention span; a 25-year-old, 25 minutes) at which point it levels off. Therefore, plan a change of pace or break according to the average age of your audience. Bunce, Flens, and Neiles (2009) found that the attention of undergraduate chemistry students began to lapse within 30 seconds after the beginning of class but quickly returned, only to stray again within 9 minutes. These results cause one to question the necessity of more frequent breaks or change of pace within class sessions and more specific research into the topic. At any rate, the adage that "The mind can only absorb as much as the seat can endure" is a fairly valid and reasonable guideline. Know your audience.

■ *Distribute a skeletal outline to help the learners identify key points.* Emphasize principles and concepts. Do not copy charts, graphs, and materials that are found in the learners' texts. Handout information should supplement the lecture. The lecture should not be a rehash of basic information from the learners' textbook. If handouts are used, they should be clear and contain a limited amount of information so the learner is not overwhelmed. Handouts printed on colored paper stand out and are more likely to be read than those printed on white paper. The reproduction or web posting of the PowerPoint slides or lecture notes is a well-debated topic. Germano (2003) declares technology to be a tool, but notes that tools are not friends and are often rivals. Stewart (2006) suggests the distribution of full-text class notes or slides that contain a significant percentage of the lecture content truly discourages class attendance; however, students tend to request the maximum number of handouts related to the topic. The choice must be left to the individual lecturer.

Table 9-4 The Lecturer: Perceived Negative Factors and Suggestions for Improvement

Perceived Negative Factors	*Suggestions for Improvement*
Presentation disorganized or hard to follow	Spend time in practice and preparation.
Lack of outline or outline too detailed	Prepare and follow a brief outline for each lecture.
Presenter lacks professional appearance	Dress as a professional role model. If you are unsure what is acceptable for your role, consult a mentor or esteemed colleague.
Speaker lacks facial expression	Video one of your lectures; view the recording with a friend/colleague and establish goals for improvement.
Monotone voice or nervous/shaky voice	
Facial expression and/or voice lacks enthusiasm	
Reads lecture material; eyes do not meet those of listeners	Practice your lecture in front of a mirror until you know the main points by memory.
	Use only as many written notes as are absolutely essential; place cues in the margin for yourself. (Smile, walk, and relax!)
Remains behind podium to lecture (referred to as the talking head because that is all that students see)	Do not stand behind a podium unless you are 6 feet tall; request a shorter, lower lectern or table.
Uses no visual aids or visuals of poor quality	Avoid putting too much information in small print on slides and/or handouts.
	Ask a librarian, media center, or learning center personnel for assistance in preparing visuals.

(Continues)

Table 9-4 *(Continued)*

Perceived Negative Factors	*Suggestions for Improvement*
Too many PowerPoint slides	Use visuals to support, not replace content.
Does not acknowledge that adult learners like to participate	Review techniques for keeping adult learners engaged. See references by Cross (1986), Kidd (1973), and Knowles (1970).
Inconsiderate of learners' needs	Schedule breaks and/or implement change-of-pace activities every 30–45 minutes.
Distracting habits of presenter: Pacing, staring out windows, playing with objects (paper clips, rubber bands, change), using nonwords (*ah, um*) and repetitious phrases (*you know, like, well, uh*)	Use a video of your lecture to identify repetitive habits. Repositioning hands or holding notes may help the nervous hands problem. Make a list of alternate words that could be substituted for the frequently repeated pet phrases. Nonwords are a verbalization that allows your speech to catch up to what your brain is thinking; becoming aware of the use of nonwords may or may not be all you need to eliminate them. When they occur, stop, take a deep breath, and then go on.

Source: Adapted from Woodring, B., & Woodring, R. (2006). Lecture is not a four-letter word. In M. Bradshaw & A. Lowenstein (Eds.), *Innovative teaching strategies in nursing and related health professions* (4th ed., pp. 124–125). Sudbury, MA: Jones and Bartlett.

Several timely publications that may be of assistance in keeping the lecture process fresh are *The Teaching Professor, Change, Masie's Learning Trends, The National Teaching & Learning Forum,* and *Survival Skills for Scholars* series. In addition, websites maintained by most major universities offer guidance for teaching assistants and novice educators that are helpful.

■ Potential Issues

Factors That Contribute to a Successful Lecture

Nothing/no one is perfect. As with any method or technique, some problems exist when the lecture strategy is used. The key question to be answered is, "What makes lectures and lecturers successful or unsuccessful?" Over the past decade, Woodring has evaluated the response of nursing students to these questions, and each year responses have been consistent. The most frequently cited negative characteristics of lectures/lecturers focus on the person doing the presenting, *not* the method (Woodring & Woodring, 2006). In Tables 9-1 and 9-2, advantages and disadvantages of the lecture as a teaching method were outlined. Now we want to focus on the preparation and presentation of the faculty member as the implementer of the method. The teacher who consistently lectures without integrating other strategies into class time may be subjected to student-generated negative comments, such as "This class is so boring, all he does is lecture"; "It's awful, she reads to us right out of her book"; or "I can't learn to think critically if all she does is talk!" Based on comments such as these, lecturing is often identified as a poor teaching method, a last resort for instruction, when in fairness it is not the method (lecture) but the teacher who is generating the comments. Many lecturers, in fact, do not know how to impart information or stimulate interest effectively; consequently, their lectures are often poorly presented, badly organized, dull, and uninspiring (Gleitman, 2006) ... all of which lead to boredom among those expecting edutainment.

To present an effective lecture, one must prepare oneself, plan ahead, organize the content, and integrate at least one additional teaching method (e.g., discussion, video stream, audience response system, small-group interaction, role play, or demonstrative props/simulation) into each lecture session. This approach will increase self-assurance (O'Malley & Fleming, 2012) and student interaction and should increase both student and teacher satisfaction. Table 9-4 identifies attributes of lecturers that learners have perceived as negative and offers some suggestions for improvement.

Institutional Barriers That Lead to Negative Reactions to Lectures

There are certain physical, political, and situational barriers that exist within every institution—any or all of which may contribute to dissatisfaction with any instructional approach. The timing of a class offering is often a factor. Traditionally, teachers have disliked teaching, and students have disliked attending, classes offered at 7 AM or 9 PM. No one likes getting up that early or staying in class that late! Classes taught immediately after meal times are considered sleepers because blood leaves the brain and moves to the gastrointestinal tract, making everyone sluggish. Classes taught late in the afternoon or early evenings are difficult because the students and teachers are tired. Try as one may, short of one-on-one teaching or total reliance on online/asynchronous education, the perfect time to hold a class will never be found. Speakers must make their presentations stimulating and motivating at any time of the day! But changes of pace, interactivity, occasional webcasting, and other technologic media that engage students can help offset undesirable time placement of classes.

Another institutional barrier to be considered is the number of students relative to the size of the classroom and the number of students in proportion to the number of faculty (student:faculty ratio). Lecturers are often placed in small, crowded classrooms with large numbers of students or large, cavernous classrooms with small numbers of students. Often, geographical relocation of desks/tables could ease the space configuration and provide a more positive learning atmosphere. Should the lecturer have the option, it is most ideal to be able to clearly see and make eye contact with each participant. This may be accomplished by arranging seating in semicircles around the lectern or angling tables/seats. But if seating is fixed within the classroom, then it becomes the responsibility of the speaker to move away from the podium and make eye contact with as many learners as possible, as often as possible. Some of these logistical issues may be addressed as universities remodel or build new classroom facilities. The Masie Center's Classroom of the Future survey (Masie & Chen, 2011) found that despite the popularity of web-based and blended learning, classrooms are not going away. Eighty percent of the 654 respondents indicated plans for continued high usage of classrooms, plans for expanded classroom size, and plans for expanded classroom technologic capabilities (interactive whiteboards, video conferencing via webinar, audience response systems, cameras/ microphones, and flexible furniture).

The large student:faculty ratio within classes will probably not decrease in postsecondary education in the near future. Large classes, especially at the freshman and sophomore levels, are very cost-effective. The bottom line will continue to impose restrictions that are exacerbated by the increase in distance and multisite class sessions and faculty shortages in many health-related professions. The disproportionate student:faculty ratio will require lecturers to implement the tips listed in this chapter, as well as utilize technological support, teaching assistants for smaller group interactions, and other creative strategies to enhance student learning for material presented in large lecture sections. The results of a study of undergraduate students (Long & Coldren, 2006) reinforced the need for the lecturer to make personal connections with students in large classes. There was a positive correlation between the students' perception of interpersonal connection with the faculty and student success in the class.

Helping the Student to Remember Tomorrow?

The problem of retaining information gained from a lecture should be acknowledged and addressed. Although those educators who enjoy using the lecture method hate to admit it, research conducted in the 1990s found that 80% of information gained by lecture alone cannot be recalled by students 1 day later, and that 80% of the remainder fades in a month. Since minimal research has been done to alter that perception, one must still heed the results. Educational data indicate the more a learner's senses (taste, touch, smell, sight, and hearing) are involved in the learning activity, the longer the knowledge is retained. Therefore, if certain types of equipment are used to illustrate a point (touch, sight), a video clip is inserted into the midst of the lecture (sight, hearing), or any other active learning process (gaming, lab experiments, audience response activities) is introduced, the student's knowledge retention will increase.

In recent years, the use of *punctuated lectures* has also been viewed as a method to increase retention of information. The punctuated lecture requires students and teachers to go through five steps: (1) **listen** (to a portion of a lecture), (2) **stop**, (3) **reflect** (on what they were doing, thinking, and feeling during that portion of the lecture), (4) **write** (what they were doing, thinking, and feeling during that portion of the lecture), and (5) **give** (the written feedback to the lecturer) (Cross & Steadman, 1996). This approach provides the lecturer and the students with an opportunity to become engaged with the learning process, as well as to self-monitor their in-class behaviors. In addition, Brookfield (2006) suggests that students cannot read the lecturer's mind. Students cannot be expected to know what teachers expect, stand for, or wish them to value unless that information is explicitly and vigorously communicated to them. The reflective teacher, according to Brookfield, must continually work to build a case for learning, action, and practice rather than assume these values to be self-evident to the learner. Implementing these suggestions should enhance knowledge retention emanating from a lecture.

■ Evaluation

An evaluation of the lecture/lecturer must be completed in a timely manner. The most useful time to obtain this data is at the completion of an individual lecture. Obtaining this information need not be laborious. Ask the listeners to respond to a few specific questions and then allow them to provide additional comments or pose the questions and allow the automated clicker response before learners walk out the door. This type of feedback is especially helpful for the novice lecturer. The evaluation process should aim to provide constructive criticism and comments for improvement. One means of accomplishing this is to allow the students to make any comments they wish; however, a negative comment cannot be made without offering a suggestion for its resolution. When this evaluation technique is used routinely, the learners become accustomed to it. The process can be completed in 5 minutes or less, especially if automated response systems are used. Often, teachers are so interested in assessing whether the course objectives have been met that they forget to evaluate the means by which they were met. Lecturers will not improve without suggested change, and suggested change can best be obtained via the use of a planned evaluation tool/method that is completed by peers and/or class participants. The evaluation of a lecture or lecturer should not occur in isolation—it must be viewed as a portion of an overall evaluation and development plan—and should be conducted only when there are plans for growth, follow-up, and change. Rhem (2011) suggests that self-assessment and peer evaluation of even the most seasoned lecturer may result in improvement and professional reaffirmation. Be certain to provide feedback to your evaluators; let the class or colleagues know you have made a change in the way you are presenting some topic or how you have changed some assignment based on previous evaluative comments.

■ Conclusion

Presenting an effective lecture is more than a stand-and-deliver process. The lecturer must be knowledgeable, well spoken, organized, creative, and considerate of the learners' needs, abilities, learning styles, and cognitive/developmental level(s). The desired outcomes for the class and the individual objectives of the learners must be addressed. The lecture should be divided into the following three major segments: introduction (5 minutes), body, and conclusion (5 minutes). Each section should be planned and presented in an organized manner, never off the cuff. The prepared lecturer will be considerate, credible, and in control (not to be mistaken for rigid and controlling). Several factors enhance the presentation of a lecture, but none is more important than genuine enthusiasm. The lecture should not be considered a secondary teaching strategy. In many situations, it is the most appropriate methodology to be used. To elicit the best results, the lecture should be accompanied by at least one of the other effective strategies discussed in this text.

As we close this chapter on presenting a lecture, it is suggested that attention should be paid to the words of the wise elder: Select your words carefully, be sure your words are sweet, because you never know when you will be called upon them to eat! Happy lecturing.

References

Amare, N. (2006). To slideware or not to slideware: Students' experiences with PowerPoint vs. lecture. *Journal of Technical Writing and Communication, 36*(3), 297–308.

Brookfield, S. (2006). *The skillful teach* (pp. 100–101). San Francisco, CA: Jossey-Bass Publishers.

Bunce, D., Flens, E., & Neiles, K. (2009). Teaching is more than lecturing and learning is more than memorizing. *Journal of Chemical Education, 86*(6),674–680.

Burgan, M. (2006). In defense of lecturing. *Change: The Magazine of Higher Education, 38*(6), 30–34.

Caldwell, J. (2007). Clickers in the large classroom: Current research and best-practice tips. *CBE-Life Science Education, 6*(12), 9–20.

Chung, Q. B. (2005). Sage on stage in the digital age: The role of online lecture in distance learning. *Electronic Journal of e-Learning, 3*(1), 1–14.

Clark, J. (2008). PowerPoint and pedagogy maintaining student interest in university lectures. *College Teaching, 56*(1), 39–45.

Costa, M., van Rensburg, L., & Rushton, N. (2007). Does teaching style matter? A randomized trial of group discussion versus lectures in orthopaedic undergraduate teaching. *Medical Education, 41,* 214–217.

Cox, J., & Rogers, J. (2005). Enter: The (well-designed) lecture. *The Teaching Professor, 19*(5), 1–6.

Cross, K. P. (1986, September). A proposal to improve teaching. *AAHE Bulletin,* pp. 9–15.

Cross, K., & Steadman, M. (1996). *Classroom research: Implementing the scholarship of teaching.* San Francisco, CA: Jossey Bass Publishers.

Eble, K. (1982). *The craft of teaching.* San Francisco, CA: Jossey-Bass Publishers.

Germano, W. (2003). The scholarly lecture: How to stand and deliver. *Chronicle of Higher Education,* 50(14), 14b.

Gleitman, H. (2006). Lecturing: Using a much maligned method of teaching. In *Teaching at Chicago: A handbook.* Chicago, IL: University of Chicago Center for Teaching and Learning. Retrieved from http://teaching.uchicago.edu/?/ctl-archive/course-design-tutorials/in-the-classroom/gleitman.html

Guertin, L., Bodek, M., Zappe, S., & Kim, H. (2007). Questioning the student use of and desire for lecture podcasts. *Journal of Online Learning and Teaching.* Retrieved from http://jolt.merlot.org/vol3no2/guertin.htm

Harper, B. (2009). I've never seen or heard it this way! Increasing student engagement through the use of technology-enhanced feedback. *Teaching Educational Psychology, 3*(2).

Hove, M., & Corcoran, K. (2008). If you post it will they come? Lecture availability in introductory psychology. *Teaching Psychology, 35*(2), 91–95.

Huntley, J. (2009, June). Positioning the CLO. In B. Concevitch (Ed.), *The learning leaders fieldbook* (pp. 6–7). Saratoga Springs, NY: Masie Center. Retrieved from http://www.masie.com/fieldbook

Kidd, J. R. (1973). *How adults learn*. New York, NY: Association Press.

Knowles, M. (1970). *The modern practice of adult education: Andragogy versus pedagogy*. New York, NY: Association Press.

Long, E., & Coldren, J. (2006). Interpersonal influences in large lecture-based classes. *College Teaching, 54*(2), 237–243.

Lowman, J. (1995). *Mastering techniques of teaching* (2nd ed.). San Francisco, CA: Jossey-Bass Publishing.

Masie, E. (2006). *Learning Trends*. Saratoga, NY: Masie Center. Retrieved from http://trends.masie.com

Masie, E., & Chen, J. (2011). Classroom of the future & classroom of 2011 survey. Retrieved from http://masie.com/classroom2011

Mayer, R., Stull, A., DeLeeuw, K., Almeroth, K., Bimber, B., Chun, D., … Zhang, H. (2009). Clickers in college classrooms: Fostering learning with questioning methods in large lecture class. *Contemporary Educational Psychology, 34*(1), 51–57.

O'Malley, D., & Fleming, S. (2012). Developing skills for teaching: Reflections on the lecture as a learning tool for the novice midwife educator. *Nurse Education in Practice, 12*(2012), 253–257.

Read, B. (2005). Lectures on the go. *Chronicle of Higher Education, 52*(10), A39.

Rhem, J. (2011). Coaching and teaching. *National Teaching and Learning Forum, 21*(1), 8.

Stewart, E. (2006, February 6). Class-conscious: Teachers want tech to enhance—not replace—lectures. *Desert News (Utah)*. Retrieved from http://www.deseretnews.com/article/635181866/Class-conscious-Teachers-want-tech-to-enhance--not-replace--lectures.html

Wiebel, G. (2010). Interactive lectures I. *History Tech*. Retrieved from http://historytech.wordpress.com/?s=interactive+lectures+I

Woodring, B., & Woodring, R. (2006). Lecture is not a four-letter word. In M. Bradshaw & A. Lowenstein (Eds.), *Innovative teaching strategies in nursing and related health professions* (4th ed., pp. 109–130). Sudbury, MA: Jones and Bartlett.

Woodring, B., & Woodring, R. (2010). Lecture: Reclaiming its place in pedagogy. In M. Bradshaw & A. Lowenstein (Eds.), *Innovative teaching strategies in nursing and related health professions* (5th ed., pp. 109–130). Sudbury, MA: Jones and Bartlett.

Young, J. (2008). The lectures are recorded, so why go to class? *Chronicle of Higher Education, 54*(36), A1, A12.

CHAPTER 10

Problem-Based Learning

■ Patricia Solomon and Liliana Coman ■

Problem-based learning (PBL) is an educational process in which learning is centered on problems as opposed to discrete, subject-related courses. In small groups, students are presented with patient scenarios or problems, generate learning issues related to what they need to learn to understand the problem, engage in independent self-study, and return to their groups to apply their new knowledge to the patient problem. PBL is largely acknowledged as starting in the medical school at McMaster University in the mid-1960s in response to an educational environment that emphasized passive learning of large quantities of information that was quickly outdated and often appeared irrelevant. The emphasis in PBL is on learning all content in an integrative way through small-group, self-directed study of a problem with the assistance of a faculty instructor who is a facilitator of learning rather than an expert lecturer (Walton & Matthews, 1989). There is increasing support for the idea that PBL is effective because it encourages the activation of prior knowledge and provides the opportunity for elaborating on that knowledge in small-group settings (Hmelo-Silver, 2004; Schmidt, Rotgans, & Yew, 2011). While PBL is theoretically more effective in structuring knowledge, the most agreed-upon advantage is that it is more enjoyable than traditional learning methods.

■ Background and Definitions

Since being introduced, PBL has been adopted by many health professional programs worldwide (Neville, 2009). Schmidt, van der Molen, Te Winkel & Wijnen (2009) suggest that the literature includes at least three perspectives on PBL: PBL as a process of inquiry, as a learning-to-learn process, and as a constructivist approach to learning. Although many variants of PBL have been described, the following essential elements remain: (1) students are presented with a written problem or patient scenario in small groups; (2) there is a change in faculty role from imparter of information to facilitator of learning; (3) there is an emphasis on student responsibility and self-directed learning; and (4) a written problem is the stimulus for learning, with students engaging in a problem-solving process as they learn and discuss content related to the problem (Hmelo-Silver, 2004; Schmidt et al., 2011; Solomon,1994).

While PBL may be viewed as an educational methodology, it is most often associated with an overall curricular approach. PBL was originally viewed as an all-or-none phenomenon in which an educational program had to commit entirely to the curricular philosophy to attain the most benefits (Barrows & Tamblyn, 1980). Programs that had individual problem-based courses and more traditional courses running concurrently were thought to produce mixed messages in the student and devalue the problem-based components (Walton & Matthews, 1989). While there is still concern that isolated problem-based courses will not be successful (Albanese, 2000), there is greater acceptance of curricula that use mixed or partial PBL approaches. Fyrenius, Bergdahl, and Silén (2005) argue that lectures can be used as valuable tools for learning in a PBL curriculum.

There have been several attempts to define and classify PBL curricula. Barrows (1986) describes a taxonomy based largely on the problem design and role of the teacher. Charlin, Mann, and Hansen (1998) present an analytic framework to understand and compare PBL curricula that varies along 10 dimensions, such as the purpose of the problem and the nature of the task to be accomplished during study of the problem. Harden and Davis (1998) offer an 11-step continuum of PBL with theoretical learning and an emphasis on traditional lectures and textbooks at one end, and task-based learning (essentially learning in clinical practice settings with real patients) at the other. As one moves along the continuum, there is greater emphasis on the problem, activation of prior knowledge, contextual learning, and discovery learning. Solomon, Binkley, and Stratford (1996) provide a simple distinction between a problem-based curriculum, which they describe as "fully integrated" (with few or no subject-related courses), and a transitional PBL curriculum, which uses traditional curricular elements early in the curriculum and incorporates increasingly larger components of PBL as the students progress through their program.

■ Theoretical Foundations

Some of the original theoretical premises for PBL have not found strong support within the literature. Contextual learning, with roots in the constructivist learning theory, was an appealing rationale for the superiority of PBL. The rationale was that by learning all content (including basic, clinical, and social sciences) within the context of a problem, a learner would be able to recall information better when he or she encountered a similar patient within the clinical setting (Clifford & Wilson, 2000). But there is weak empirical support for this theory, and it is likely too simplistic to integrate the complexities associated with PBL (Colliver, 2000).

The information processing theory, proposed by Miller in 1956, incorporates aspects of contextual learning theory and provides more comprehensive theoretical support for PBL as it also considers activation of prior knowledge and elaboration of knowledge as core elements (Albanese, 2000; Schmidt et al., 2011). However, one theory may be insufficient support for PBL. Albanese (2000) outlines three others that are salient to PBL: cooperative learning theory, self-determination theory, and control theory.

Cooperative learning, based on Vygotsky's social development theory (McLeod, 2007), in which individuals are dependent on other group members to achieve their goals, is used extensively in small-group PBL. Learning occurs through mutual interaction and shared understanding (Dolmans, De Grave, Wolfhagen, & van der Vleuten, 2005). Additionally, accepting responsibility for learning as an individual and as a member of a group is thought to enhance intellectual development (Copp, 2002).

Self-determination theory identifies controlled, more maladaptive motivators of behavior and autonomous motivators that the learner finds more interesting and enjoyable (Williams, Saizow, & Ryan, 1999). Controlled motivators, which include external demands under which people act with a sense of pressure and anxiety, are more characteristic of traditional curricula. Autonomous motivators, which involve a sense of volition and choice, would be more characteristic of a PBL curriculum. Control theory states that all behavior is based on satisfying the five basic needs of freedom, power, love and belonging, fun, and survival and reproduction (Glaser, 1985). Instruction can fail if it does not meet these basic needs of the learner. PBL may be superior at meeting these needs. For example, fun, or enjoyment of learning, has been frequently associated with outcomes of PBL (Albanese & Mitchell, 1993).

Schmidt and colleagues (2011) summarized the evidence relevant to the mechanism by which PBL affects learning in terms of two hypotheses derived from cognitive psychology—the activation-elaboration hypothesis and the situational interest hypothesis. The authors concluded that elaboration in a small group (through self-explanation, discussion with peers, and practicing and responding to questions) facilitates the processing and adds to the long-term memorability of the knowledge gained. The situational interest hypothesis stems from the literature on psychology of curiosity and learning. The cognitively induced experience of knowledge deprivation (the gap between what one knows and what one wants to know) initiates information-seeking behavior intended to close the knowledge gap. As learning occurs, the situational interest decreases and knowledge equilibrium is achieved (Rotgans & Schmidt, 2011). It has been demonstrated that the presentation of the problem increased the level of situational interest significantly in the students in a PBL course, and this was maintained during the small-group discussion (Rotgans & Schmidt, 2011).

■ Types of Learners

PBL has been used extensively in many health professions programs. Health professions students at all levels can benefit from the use of PBL to simulate realistic clinical situations. It is important to note that students accustomed to more traditional ways of learning often experience stress and anxiety when adapting to this new student-centered style of learning (Solomon & Finch, 1998). Supports must be put in place to ease the students' transition to this type of learning.

■ Resources

PBL requires different resources to support its implementation. Unlike traditional programs in which one faculty member lectures to large numbers of students, learning occurs in small groups, necessitating additional faculty to support PBL. There also is a need for numerous small-group tutorial rooms and extensive library and other learning resources that enable self-directed learning. As elaborated upon next, there is an additional need for faculty who are well trained to assume the role of facilitators.

■ Role of Faculty

The instructor's role in PBL is different from that in a conventional class or tutorial setting. In PBL, the role of the instructor is to activate and facilitate learning in the group by encouraging participation of all members and to monitor the depth and breadth of knowledge and intervene when the desired quality of learning is not achieved (Barrows & Tambly, 1980; Maudsley, 1999). There has been significant debate in the PBL literature as to whether teachers with subject-matter expertise or teachers with good facilitation skills are preferable. Content experts are thought to be more likely to play a directive role in the learning process, speak more often, and supply more direct answers to students' questions, which may have a negative effect on the collaborative learning (Silver & Wilkerson, 1991). By contrast, Eagle, Harasym, and Mandin (1992) and Davis, Nairn, Paine, Anderson, and Oh (1992) suggest that instructors with content expertise are better at posing questions at critical moments, which positively influences students' learning. Although some debate remains (Kaufman & Holmes, 1998), it is generally recognized that a combination of content and process expertise is preferable.

Dolmans, Wolfhagen, Scherpbier, and Van Der Vleuten (2001) provide an excellent summary of issues related to instructor expertise. Not surprisingly, they conclude that faculty instructors initiate activities with which they are most familiar. Hence, content experts use their expertise to direct learner performance, and noncontent experts use their process facilitation skills to direct group dynamics. However, this relationship is not as simple as once believed. A teacher's performance is not likely to be stable and is influenced by contextual circumstances such as the quality of the written cases, the structure of the course, and students' prior knowledge. Thus, teacher expertise may compensate if the structure of the problem is low and/or the students have little prior knowledge of the case.

While the evidence suggests that there is not a simple distinction between expert and nonexpert teachers, the implications for faculty development are clear: faculty require training to assume more facilitative roles. Hitchcock and Mylona (2000) note that there has been little systematic study on effective ways to train faculty to assume PBL roles, although there have been many descriptions in the literature. They emphasize that while the most obvious training is in instructor facilitation skills, there are many other roles and skills that need to be developed. They quote Irby's sequence of steps of skill development: (1) challenging assumptions and developing understanding of PBL, (2) experiencing and valuing the tutorial process, (3) acquiring general teaching skills, (4) developing content-specific instructor knowledge and skills, (5) acquiring advanced knowledge and skills, (6) developing leadership and scholarship skills, and (7) creating organizational vitality.

It is clear that faculty members who possess a level of content expertise in the area under study are the preferred small-group facilitators. However, there is an equally important need for faculty who are well trained in PBL and the tutorial process. The skills needed to facilitate and evaluate the small-group process, to promote metacognitive skills such as self-monitoring of one's reasoning and decision-making skills, and to design curriculum and develop problems and other instructional materials to support self-directed learning are very different from the skills required in a traditional curriculum and require long-term faculty development initiatives.

■ Using Problem-Based Learning Methods

There appears to be no one best way to implement PBL. Although some maintain that fully integrated PBL is preferable, this curricular design may not be feasible for many institutions. Diversity in curricular design and approach is to be expected because different institutional structures and philosophies and faculty knowledge and skill development will influence the extent to which PBL can be incorporated into the curriculum.

Typically the process is as follows. Students are presented with a written problem as a stimulus for learning. Problems are carefully designed to facilitate discussion related to specific learning objectives. In groups of six to eight, students read the problem (either aloud or to themselves) and brainstorm about what they need to learn to better understand the problem or hypothesize potential causes of the problem. During this initial process, students generate learning issues or questions for self-study. Learning issues can range from factual knowledge (e.g., which nerves innervate the upper extremity?), to more complex physiological questions (e.g., what is the process of inflammation?), to questions that include broader psychosocial issues (e.g., how would I apply a model of ethical decision making to this patient?), or questions that require evaluation of the literature and integration of evidence-based practice (e.g., what is the effectiveness of ultrasound in the treatment of lateral epicondylitis?). The process of developing a high-quality learning issue that is researchable may be quite time consuming for the learner who is new to PBL. Generation of the final list of learning issues that will be researched and discussed at the next learning session constitutes the end of the first stage of the PBL process. Students can choose to independently research all learning issues that have been generated for that session or to divide up the learning issues among themselves for self-study. When students return for the next learning session, they discuss their findings and the implications for patient care. At the end of the session, students engage in a structured evaluation of the learning process and their performance. Each student provides a verbal self-evaluation of his or her performance that day, and both peers and faculty provide feedback.

During the learning session, the faculty instructor does not provide expert content information. Rather, his or her role is to establish the climate for learning, encourage problem solving, and promote debate and discussion within the group. The instructor also role models effective self-evaluation and provision of feedback. Barrows (1988) describes the faculty teaching role as going through the following three stages: (1) *modeling* of the thinking process for the students by questioning and challenging them; (2) *coaching* by the faculty when the students are off track or confused, which occurs as the group becomes more comfortable with the process; and (3) *fading* the role of the teacher, which occurs as students progress further and develop into a well-functioning and effective learning group, leaving the group to work more independently. Barrows suggests that groups should meet for at least 8 weeks to allow for progression of these three stages.

■ Potential Problems

The costs associated with the number of faculty required to deliver education in small groups is a key concern and potential barrier to implementation (Albanese & Mitchell, 1993). Other costs related to space requirements for small-group rooms and development of self-directed learning resources may also pose barriers (Solomon, 1994). Without institutional support for curricular change, many program leaders may find it difficult to engage successfully in curriculum reform.

An additional barrier to the implementation of innovative problem-based curricula relates to the lack of rigorous long-term data that demonstrate significant differences between traditional and PBL curricula. Consequently, debate about the effects of this method on learning when compared to traditional methods continues (Colliver & Markwell, 2007; Schmidt et al., 2011). The lack of evidence reinforces the concerns of critics who ask, "Why bother?" Some argue that PBL is worth implementing even if the only benefit of PBL is its more personal, humane, and enjoyable approach. Federman (1999) noted advantages of PBL that are not amenable to measurement and relate more to the personal and interpersonal aspects of practice. Even the most ardent of critics would agree that these benefits are desirable in health professional education. Some of these include: (1) the person-to-person contact inherent in a small-group learning process; (2) the positive regard that is fostered by the respect afforded to the beginning student; (3) the focus on patients that promotes relevancy of the curriculum from the early days; (4) increased opportunities to discuss moral and ethical issues and for the instructor to share his or her values; and (5) the positive effect on lectures because, with only a few lectures in the timetable, students are more committed to these lectures, which in turn has a stimulating effect on the faculty.

Recently, with the rise in popularity of online and web-based learning, there has been an interest in doing PBL online. Increased accessibility and opportunities for asynchronous learning are obvious advantages for distance and continuing education courses. In health professions educational programs, PBL online has inherent appeal as the number of facilitators required could be reduced, thus making it possible to implement in programs without sufficient resources to do face-to-face PBL. Although there have been a few descriptive articles (Bresnitz, 1996), few have examined the effectiveness of computer-based PBL. Some of the characteristics of PBL, such as using patient problems, sharing learning, promoting integration of knowledge, and self-directed learning, are relatively easy to transfer to online formats. Several authors (including Donelly, 2009, and Savin-Baden, 2007) consider PBL a pedagogical strategy that enables interaction, collaboration, discussion, and participation in the online environments. In an e-learning context, PBL requires specific tools enabling group synchronization, document management, discussion, and task assignment to engage students in the group learning process. However, the advantage of flexibility, related to the ability to access the course in an asynchronous manner, may not be realized in intensive, integrated professional curricula in which the students' timetables are more restricted. Face-to-face PBL allows for the development of communication and verbal skills related to the ability to clearly articulate and present information, provide feedback to others, and develop and evaluate group skills. In an online PBL experience, the communication skills that are central to professional practice would clearly not be developed in the same way as they would in a small-group, face-to-face PBL experience.

■ Conclusion

PBL is an increasingly popular teaching and learning strategy within the health professions. The clinical relevance, small-group interactions, and active learning provided make PBL an appealing curricular alternative. Faculty training and expertise are essential for successful outcomes.

REFERENCES

Albanese, M. (2000). Problem-based learning: Why curricula are likely to show little effect on knowledge and clinical skills. *Medical Education, 34,* 729–738.

Albanese, M. A., & Mitchell, S. (1993). Problem-based learning: A review of literature on its outcomes and implementation issues. *Academic Medicine, 68,* 52–81.

Barrows, H. S. (1986). A taxonomy of problem-based learning methods. *Medical Education, 20,* 481–486.

Barrows, H. S. (1988). *The tutorial process.* Springfield, IL: Southern Illinois University of Medicine.

Barrows, H. S., & Tamblyn, R. (1980). *Problem-based learning.* New York, NY: Springer.

Bresnitz, E. (1996). Computer-based learning in PBL. *Academic Medicine, 71*(5), 540.

Charlin, B., Mann, K., & Hansen, P. (1998). The many faces of problem-based learning: A framework for understanding and comparison. *Medical Teacher, 20,* 323–330.

Clifford, M., & Wilson, M. (2000). *Contextual teaching, professional learning, and student experiences: Lessons learned from implementation. Educational Brief, 2.* Madison, WI: Center on Education and Work, University of Wisconsin–Madison

Colliver, J. A. (2000). Effectiveness of problem-based learning: Research and theory. *Academic Medicine, 75,* 259–266.

Colliver, J. A., & Markwell, S. J. (2007). Research on problem-based learning: The need for critical analysis of methods and findings. *Medical Education, 41,* 533–535.

Copp, S. L. (2002). Using cooperative learning strategies to teach implications of the nurse practice act. *Nurse Educator, 27*(5), 236–241.

Davis, W. K., Nairn, R., Paine, M. E., Anderson, R. M., & Oh, M. S. (1992). Effects of expert and non-expert facilitators on the small-group process and on student performance. *Academic Medicine, 67*(7), 470–474.

Dolmans, D. H., De Grave, W., Wolfhagen, I. H., & van der Vleuten, C. P. (2005). Problem-based learning: Future challenges for educational practice and research. *Medical Education, 39*(7), 732–741.

Dolmans, D., Wolfhagen, I., Scherpbier, A., & Van Der Vleuten, C. (2001). Relationship of tutors' group-dynamics skills to their performance ratings in problem-based learning. *Academic Medicine, 76,* 473–476.

Donelly, R. (2009). Embedding interaction within a blend of learner centric pedagogy and technology. *World Journal on Educational Technology, 1,* 6–29.

Eagle, C. J., Harasym, P. H., & Mandin, H. (1992). Effects of tutors with case expertise on problem-based learning issues. *Academic Medicine, 67*(7), 465–469.

Federman, D. D. (1999). Little-heralded advantages of problem-based learning. *Academic Medicine, 74,* 93–94.

Fyrenius, A., Bergdahl, B., & Silén, C. (2005). Lectures in problem-based learning: Why, when and how? An example of interactive lecturing that simulates meaningful learning. *Medical Teacher, 27,* 61–65.

Glaser, R. (1985). *Control theory in the classroom.* New York, NY: Harper and Row.

Harden, R. M., & Davis, M. H. (1998). The continuum of problem-based learning. *Medical Teacher, 20,* 317–322.

Hitchcock, M. A., & Mylona, Z. (2000). Teaching faculty to conduct problem-based learning. *Teaching and Learning in Medicine, 12,* 52–57.

Hmelo-Silver, C.E. (2004). Problem-based learning: What and how do students learn? *Educational Psychology Review, 16*(3), 235–266.

Kaufman, D. M., & Holmes, D. B. (1998). The relationship of tutors' content expertise to interventions and perceptions in a PBL medical curriculum. *Medical Education, 32,* 255–261.

Maudsley, G. (1999). Roles and responsibilities of the problem-based tutor in the undergraduate medical curriculum. *BMJ, 318,* 657–661.

McLeod, S. A. (2007). Vygotsky: Social development theory. Retrieved from http://www.simplypsychology.org/vygotsky.html

Neville, A. J. (2009). Problem-based learning and medical education forty years on: A review of its effects on knowledge and clinical performance. *Medical Principles and Practice, 18,* 1–9.

Rotgans, J. I., & Schmidt, H. G. (2011). The role of teachers in facilitating situational interest in an active-learning classroom. *Teaching and Teacher Education, 27*(1), 37–42.

Savin-Baden, M. (2007). *A practical guide to problem-based learning online.* London, UK: Routledge.

Schmidt, H. G., Rotgans, J. I., & Yew, E. H. J. (2011). The process of problem-based learning: What works and why. *Medical Education, 45,* 792–806.

Schmidt, H. G., van der Molen, H. T., Te Winkel, W. W. R., & Wijnen, W. H. F. W. (2009). Constructivist, problem-based learning does work: A meta-analysis of curricular comparisons involving a single medical school. *Educational Psychologist, 44*(4), 227–249.

Silver, M., & Wilkerson, L. A. (1991). Effects of tutors with subject expertise on the problem-based tutorial process. *Academic Medicine, 66*(5), 298–300.

Solomon, P. (1994). Problem-based learning: A direction for physical therapy education? *Physiotherapy Theory and Practice, 10,* 45–52.

Solomon, P., Binkley, J., & Stratford, P. (1996). A descriptive study of learning processes and outcomes in two problem-based curriculum designs. *Journal of Physical Therapy Education, 10,* 72–76.

Solomon, P., & Finch, E. (1998). A qualitative study identifying stressors associated with adapting to problem-based learning. *Teaching and Learning in Medicine, 10,* 58–64.

Walton, H., & Matthews, M. (1989). Essentials of problem-based learning. *Journal of Medical Education, 23,* 542–558.

Williams, G., Saizow, R., & Ryan, R. (1999). The importance of self-determination theory for medical Education. *Academic Medicine, 74,* 992–999.

CHAPTER 11

Debate as a Teaching Strategy

■ Martha J. Bradshaw and Arlene J. Lowenstein ■

The debate is a strategy long recognized as a means by which to address a topic in which there may be more than one viewpoint. The value of a debate is not necessarily in the resolution of a topic or persuasive results, but rather the value as a teaching strategy lies more in the process and presentation of the viewpoints.

■ Definition and Purposes

A traditional view of debate may be that of argument for the purpose of persuading the audience toward a clearly identified position. To debate an issue is to consider or discuss it from opposing positions or arguments (Berube & DeVinne, 1982). Political debates are used as opportunities for candidates to make their perspectives known on key issues. This form of structured argument has long been used in philosophy, theology, law, and the sciences (Tumposky, 2004). Martin, Moran, and Harrison (2009) point out that debate is beneficial in cultivating critical thinking about salient issues in any discipline, including athletic education. Debate has been defined as "a systematic contest of speakers in which two points of view of a proposition are advanced with proof" (Barnhart, 1966, p. 311). Koklanaris, MacKenzie, Fino, Arslan, and Seubert (2008) noted that debate is useful to promote active learning because "debating inherently involves a variety of positive features: the impetus for intense preparation, active participation, and a forum ideally suited to controversial topics" (p. 235). Based on these definitions, debate becomes a useful teaching strategy.

Debate provides opportunities for students to analyze an issue or problem in depth and to reach an informed, unbiased conclusion or resolution. Debate encourages participants to identify quickly the essential nature of the issue as substantiated by evidence, to establish criteria for judging its successful resolution, and to weigh, compare, and contrast the merits of alternative strategies for resolution (Simonneaux, 2002). In addition, presentation of the debate allows students to practice oral communication skills, express professional opinions, and gain experience in speaking to groups and in working in groups when preparing the debates.

■ Theoretical Rationale

Two important components of the professional role are the analysis of significant issues and the ability to communicate in efficient and effective ways. Professional communication is seen in many forms; scholarly publication, oral presentations, and electronic networking are a few examples. Similar to other skills, the development of effective communication skills must be fostered by faculty. The ability to communicate one's thoughts clearly and concisely evolves from the formulation of a perspective on a topic, analysis of that perspective and other views, and development of sound conclusions. Debate enables students to participate actively in a meaningful communication exercise.

The college environment, especially in the health professions, is a time in which critical inquiry and analysis should be cultivated. The debate is particularly helpful in causing a student to examine the position juxtaposed to a personally held view. One of the purposes of debate is for the learner to go beyond merely identifying an issue. Learners must analyze the issue. What are its key elements? What historical precedents have contributed to the issue? Who are the key proponents and opponents of the issue? What is the future of the issue? Students can learn how personal values or emotions influence thinking and responses to issues. Students also can identify which factors influence their thinking, such as the views of news analysts, popular literature, or peers (Simonneaux, 2002). Analysis on this level leads to powerful learning, calling for the use of reasoning and other forms of higher-order thinking. The learner first becomes more aware of his or her own thinking, then broadens and purposefully adapts thinking (Tumposky, 2004).

In addition to exploring and analyzing a topic, debate is an excellent exercise in the power of live communication. Humans are highly affected by facial expressions, body language, and verbal inflections. Students can be taught to use these techniques to their advantage and how to analyze the techniques in others, apart from what is being said. Through this, students can learn that body language and related mannerisms can have a positive or negative effect upon the position the speaker represents (Karadag, Caliskan, & Yesil, 2008).

■ Conditions for Learning

Debate is most useful as part of a course or seminar in professional and academic settings. Because of the nature of this strategy, it should be employed in a course that centers upon issues or topics that raise debatable questions. Questions employed in a debate should be ones that can be addressed from more than one defensible perspective (Martin, Moran, & Harrison, 2009). Debate also is a means to validate and deepen content knowledge (Martens, 2007). This strategy can be used to facilitate students' ability to implement analytical skills, to systematically research and critique an issue, to arrive at salient points, and to demonstrate more professional development related to the group process (Candela, Michael, & Mitchell, 2003).

The learning goals for the debate strategy include improving oral communication and research-referencing skills, structuring and presenting an argument, and exercising analytical skills. The process for formulating and presenting the debate should facilitate these goals as much as possible; therefore, the faculty should provide a reasonable amount of freedom for the students to reach these learning goals independently. Students should be given enough structure or direction to help them plan and organize their work, but they also should understand the responsibility they must take for researching debate positions, scrutinizing key issues, and practicing speaking skills. In the debate strategy described by Lowenstein and Bradshaw (1989), students were encouraged to take the viewpoint opposite the one they (personally) held. This approach promoted an understanding of existing oppositional perspectives and enhanced the ability to respond to opposing views (Lowenstein & Bradshaw).

Preparation for the debate should begin early in the course to provide adequate opportunities for research of resources and exploration of issues. Faculty facilitation is an essential part of the learning process. Conditions central to use of debate as an effective strategy include that the students need:

- To be introduced to key issues in the course and to have been able to identify controversial points suitable for debate.
- To be familiar with one another in order to form working groups.
- Knowledge of existing resources to use in formulating debate. This includes increased familiarity with the faculty member(s) as a source of support and information.

■ Types of Learners

Debate can be used with all levels or types of learners, including undergraduate students, graduate students, and practitioners, because the learning goals of debate are suitable for all groups. Lowenstein and Bradshaw (1989) used debate with registered nurse students who were completing their BSN courses. Debate is a particularly successful strategy with this group because these students combine personal experience with actual patient or practice problems with the need to refine communication and analytical skills.

Swu-Jane and Crawford (2007) developed debate as a new component to an introductory core course for pharmacy students who were in their first professional year. Objectives were to facilitate the group process, improve critical thinking and communication skills, introduce controversial issues related to the U.S. healthcare system, enhance students' ability to analyze and evaluate evidence, help develop skills in formulating written arguments, and encourage tolerance of diverse points of view. Thus, debate provides a true opportunity for professional growth in this type of student. By immersing themselves in the topic, students have a better understanding of it than they would through other means of study.

By creating the need to objectively analyze an issue, debate is useful for a student who is strongly influenced by personal values or certain work experiences. An undergraduate who has not formed a worldview about sensitive ethical dilemmas, for example, can have the opportunity to examine the issues and how decisions are made. A practitioner who has been receiving negative influence in the work environment has the opportunity for objective analysis of the situation.

Debate is a strategy to be used when the instructor wishes to bring about active, rather than passive, learning, critical thinking, and creativity and wants to introduce the learners to the role of conflict in professional endeavors. Direct confrontation (i.e., face-to-face discussion) is particularly valuable in an educational environment in which students frequently converse in isolation through electronic means. Reliance upon technology hinders students from cultivating skills for professional, purposeful conversations. Furthermore, use of debate is an opportunity for a student to hone the ability to speak in front of a group, especially one that is not entirely supportive of the speaker's point of view.

■ Resources

Faculty members serve as an important resource by assuming the role of facilitator. Formal debate questions and positions can emerge from class discussion about important issues. Faculty members can assist students in formulating the debate question and can direct them to resources related to the issue. Clinical experiences and current issues in health care offer a wide range of debate topics. Faculty may wish to prepare the students early in the course by encouraging them to be alert to ethical dilemmas or patient care problems that are suitable for debate (Candela et al., 2003).

The electronic and traditional libraries offer many resources for debate preparation. By using the professional literature to support the debate position, students are introduced to a wide range of journals, books, and other printed material. Electronic information systems are extremely helpful to students as they identify debate issues and develop related positions. Database searches enable students to consider related topics and sources outside of their own professional field, which may generate additional support for a position. The electronic media access the most current information, which may be particularly helpful for students who have timely political topics. At the same time, faculty can guide students about the judicious use of electronic sites, many of which are sponsored by professional organizations, and some of which are suited for the lay reader. Electronic bulletin boards and other communication networks provide students with the opportunity to interact with individuals outside their own institution who are involved with the issue.

The debate can be presented in any planned classroom setting. The environment should be such that the debate teams can be seen and heard by the audience. The debate process can be used in online courses as well (Swu-Jane & Crawford, 2007). Through a process of informal forum, students use critical thinking skills to research and retrieve information, then compile it in a manner by which they can make informed decisions or develop opinions on the issue under discussion (Huang, 2007). Just like the traditional debate method, the informal forum is interactive between students, rather than being teacher directed. However, when conducted online, this approach does not provide the opportunity for face-to-face interaction and development of oral communication skills.

■ Using the Method

In the Lowenstein and Bradshaw method, faculty members define broad (topical) areas from the course outline and identify an advisor for each area. Students choose the general area in which they are interested and form groups of four or five members. At least one group is formed for each topical area to guarantee that course objectives or topics are addressed. Depending on student interest and enrollment, a second group may be formed in certain areas. For example, two groups may choose to address the area of professional roles and responsibilities. Specific debate questions are formulated by the group in keeping with the objectives or broad topics of the course and personal interests of group members. Many of the topics are those currently being debated by our colleagues in all areas of health care. Patient care delivery systems, healthcare reform, genetic screening, and euthanasia are a few examples.

Each group should meet with the faculty advisor as needed to organize the debate presentation, gain insight into the points being presented, and receive assistance with resources. The instructor may assist the groups by refining their reasoning approaches. Martens (2007) identifies several types of reasoning as part of the argument, as shown in the following list.

Reasoning by:

> Example
> Analogy
> Cause
> Cost benefit
> Evidence

Students are guided to consider the perspectives of all individuals or interest groups (Simonneaux, 2002). For each debate group, two students select the affirmative position, two select the negative, and the fifth serves as moderator. In groups of four, the faculty advisor serves as moderator. Each group develops a reading list of significant articles related to the issue under debate. The list is circulated to the entire class at least 1 week prior to the debate. Students not involved in the presentation are expected to be prepared to discuss the issues under consideration.

The debate consists of opening remarks by a moderator, two affirmative and two negative presentations, rebuttal, and summary. Following the presentation, the floor is opened to the class for discussion. Questions and comments based on the presentations and readings are generated by the class. The debate moderator facilitates discussion and provides a final summary of the issues and discussion. With some issues, it may be appropriate to develop a resolution plan upon conclusion of the formal debate. This plan can incorporate some ideas from both positions to encourage win-win negotiation. This process gives students experience in developing workable solutions to practice-related issues. Class members not participating in the debate are asked to evaluate each presenter based on a rating scale. Students evaluate the analysis of the issue, the evidence presented, supporting resources, organization of the presentation, the argument presented, interaction with the audience and opponents, and response to questions (**Figure 11-1**). An overall effectiveness score is given, and the evaluators indicate if their stand on the issue changed as a result of the debate. All faculty members participating in the seminar also evaluate the presenters. Debate grades are based on preparation, individual performance, and group efforts that were reflected in the effectiveness of the debate.

To reinforce the learning from the debate, students may be asked to write a formal paper on one of the professional issues discussed in the course. The paper can be evaluated on the presentation of the issue, arguments for both sides of the issue supported by literature, the student's position and rationale for selection of the position, application of ideas to practice, and use of references and format.

Validation of learning through debate has been assessed by use of a pre- and posttest quiz (Koklanaris et al., 2008). A group of students was given a quiz prior to

---

Date: _____ Subject/topic: _____

Evaluate each speaker using the following scale:

Superior = 5; Excellent = 4; Good = 3; Fair = 2; Below standard =1

Team A		**Team B**
1 2 3 4 5	Bibliography (4 max)	1 2 3 4 5
	Overview of problem (Debater 1 or 2)	
1 2 3 4 5	Representing side of debate (Debater 1 or 2)	1 2 3 4 5
	Opening remarks	
Debater		Debater
1 2 3 4 5		1 2 3 4 5
	Resolution plan	
Debater		Debater
1 2 3 4 5		1 2 3 4 5
	Response to opposing team	
Debater		Debater
1 2 3 4 5		1 2 3 4 5

▪ **Figure 11-1** Grading tool: Debate.

exposure to course content. Half of the students then received the content through a traditional lecture, and half of the students engaged in a debate over the same content. Student outcomes on the postquiz were statistically higher for the students who learned the content through debate. In addition to justifying debate as a learning strategy, the results of this study reflect that some students benefit from a different, more active form of learning. In the online format, Swu-Jane and Crawford (2007) developed a series of three debates over a 12-week term. Teams of 4 to 5 members were established and paired as pro (affirmative) or con (negative). Teams were encouraged to appoint a team leader to coordinate the work and communicate with an assigned teaching assistant. A forum was set up for discussion posts for the paired teams. Students were expected to post three arguments in an online forum that included two constructive arguments and one rebuttal and summary argument. Each group posted in 1-week intervals beginning with affirmative followed by negative; the second argument started with affirmative and was followed by negative; and the final argument started with negative first and then positive. A limit of 400–600 words excluding references was set to correspond to a speaker's time limit in an oral debate. Students were encouraged to read articles recommended by the instructors to provide an overview for both sides of the debate topic, and to search, use, and cite additional reference sources. An orientation to the debate process was provided with written materials to assist the students in understanding the expectations and flow. Three judges were appointed by the instructors to decide the winners of the debate.

■ Potential Problems

The debate strategy calls for significant student responsibility and preparation for both debaters and the audience. Debaters are required to thoroughly research the issue and the position taken for the argument. From this preparation, they formulate a succinct and effective presentation. Debaters are expected to practice speaking skills and to prepare supporting materials for the oral presentation. To promote class engagement, the debate group provides an appropriate reading list for the other class members. Those students take the responsibility to read about the issue prior to the presentation in order to understand the issue and participate effectively in discussion. Lack of preparation on the part of the team members leads to inadequate presentation of the issue and superficial discussion. On the other hand, students who are acquainted with the opposing team members might collaborate and develop a planned debate in order to maximize opportunity for a successful outcome. While this may be difficult to discover on the part of the instructor, it clearly is an example of academic dishonesty.

The debate causes students to clearly classify an issue as one that is right or wrong or answered "yes" or "no." Many topics have no conclusions or answers, and thus may impose a false dualism (Tumposky, 2004). Students may have to defend a position to which they are not clearly committed. Students with strong moral beliefs about an issue may have difficulty defending a specified position or accepting the views of others. Faculty may have difficulty presenting a neutral position when moderating the debate and guiding discussion (Simonneaux, 2002). At some point during the presentations, it must be made very clear that there is no right or singular answer to most issues.

Nervousness about speaking in public can be a major concern. Some students have had little or no public speaking experience, or they may have had negative experiences that generated anxiety. Students of certain cultural groups may have difficulty with open debate as a way to learn. Students need encouragement and need to view the debate as an opportunity to speak to an open, receptive group in order to gain experience. What some students look upon with apprehension often results in being uplifting and beneficial. For example, one student was timid about speaking in groups and was extremely nervous before and during her debate presentation. Her nervousness was manifested in physical symptoms, such as sweating, flushed face, tremulous voice, shaking hands, and rapid blinking. She received appropriate support from faculty and students, which encouraged her to work on this problem during the rest of her academic work. Three years later, she successfully defended her master's project in a dignified and professional manner. Her public speaking skills have now advanced to the point that she is able to address both groups and individuals effectively in her current employment as a clinical specialist.

The argumentative or confrontational nature of the debate may create anxiety. In addition, debate or public speaking may be a new strategy on which students are graded, thus heightening anxiety. Faculty and students must continually place emphasis on the debate as a learning experience. The excitement of defending a position, stressing key points, and deriving a workable solution should be presented as positive outcomes of the debate. Faculty members should stress that students will not be condemned or inappropriately criticized for taking unpopular viewpoints during the debate. Faculty members are prepared to handle strong emotional viewpoints and to help students understand that there is room for conflicting opinions in our society. In using debate as a teaching strategy, Candela and colleagues (2003) discovered that students liked the strategy and found it challenging but did not see how they would use the skill or strategy in their professional careers. It is possible that, as novices, students are not aware of potential situations in which there will be a need to defend a position regarding health care. Students also need to be encouraged to see the benefit of the opportunity to practice speaking skills, research skills, and group work.

■ Conclusion

Debate is a strategy that promotes student interaction and involvement in course topics. There are many advantages to using this strategy. Debate expands the student's perspective on a given issue, creates doubt about the existence of one clear answer, and requires much thought and further evidence before deriving a solution. Debate also increases awareness of opposing viewpoints. As an interactive strategy, debate develops techniques of persuasion, serves as a means by which students confront a controversial issue, and promotes collaborative efforts and negotiation skills among peers. This strategy promotes independence and participation in the decision-making process, as well as enhances writing and organizational skills. Debate allows for examination of broad issues that influence professional practice. Critical thinking is enhanced by the scrutiny of more than one position on the issue.

Selection of debate as a teaching strategy requires a strong commitment to preparation and guidance from faculty. Faculty members will have to deal with emotions that can be elicited by the arguments. Faculty members will need to provide support for students who take minority or unpopular positions and for those who have limited public speaking skills. Following the debate, those students whose ideas are not accepted by the majority should be encouraged to recognize those parts of their work that were of value, even if others disagreed with their position. Those students whose ideas reflected the majority view should also recognize that public consensus can change quickly, and, as more information becomes available, opinions may be swayed. Finally, faculty members can help students to recognize that the debate is just a start to exploration of professional issues. Students will need to be encouraged to incorporate their newly learned and practiced skills into their professional practice.

REFERENCES

Barnhart, C. L. (Ed.). (1966). *The American college dictionary*. New York, NY: Random House.

Berube, M. S., & DeVinne, P. B. (Eds.). (1982). *The American heritage dictionary*. Boston, MA: Houghton, Mifflin.

Candela, L., Michael, S. R., & Mitchell, S. (2003). Ethical debates: Enhancing critical thinking in nursing students. *Nurse Educator, 28*, 37–39.

Huang, G. H-C. (2007). Informal forum: Fostering active learning in a teacher preparation program. *Education, 127*(1), 31–38.

Karadag, E., Caliskan, N., Yesil, R. (2008). Developing the evaluation scale to determine the impact of body language in an argument: Reliability and validity analysis. *Journal of Instructional Psychology, 35*, 396–404.

Koklanaris, N., MacKenzie, A. P., Fino, M. E., Arslan, A. A., & Seubert, D. E. (2008). Debate preparation/participation: An active, effective learning tool. *Teaching and Learning in Medicine, 20*, 235–238.

Lowenstein, A. J., & Bradshaw, M. J. (1989). Seminar methods for RN to BSN students. *Nurse Educator, 14*(5), 27–31.

Martens, E. A. (2007). The instructional use of argument across the curriculum. *Middle School Journal, 38*(5), 4–13.

Martin, M., Moran, K. A., & Harrison, K. (2009). Utilizing debates in athletic training education. *Athletic Therapy Today, 14*, 31–34.

Simonneaux, L. (2002). Analysis of classroom debating strategies. *Journal of Biological Education, 37*, 9–12.

Swu-Jane, L., & Crawford, S. Y. (2007). An online debate series for first-year pharmacy students. *American Journal of Pharmaceutical Education, 71*(1), 1–8.

Tumposky, N. R. (2004). The debate debate. *Clearing House, 78*, 52–55.

SECTION III

Simulation and Imagination

The teaching–learning strategies in Section III are intended to encourage new ways of thinking, application of concepts, and use of imagination or visualization as applied in practice settings. By stretching their thinking, students realize that they can independently and successfully approach and solve problems. Games and communication exercises enable the students to visualize themselves in realistic settings and increase insight into individual responses to situations. Learning is most effective when students assume a participatory role, occasionally counter to roles held previously. The teacher assumes the part of a facilitator, encouraging interaction among students and holding an advisory, rather than leading, role.

Clinical experience has been the mainstay of a health professional's education. Students need foundational experiences specific to their practice roles, in some form of a skills lab, and then they need opportunities to combine or broaden use of both technical and communication skills. Chapters on simulation detail a prescribed amount of control of the learning environment, which is therefore safer than the clinical setting. Another advantage of a controlled setting is that it provides needed learning opportunities that are not always possible in practice settings. Simulation experiences bring together application of content, hands-on care, and professional, interdisciplinary communication, to represent the actual practice setting as closely as possible. Such learning opportunities strengthen students for future practice opportunities.

CHAPTER 12

Games Are Multidimensional in Educational Situations

■ LYNN JAFFE ■

> Games are central to human experience and an important way in which it is made meaningful.
>
> —*Dormann & Biddle* (2006)

In *Reality Is Broken*, Jane McGonigal expounds upon the failings of reality and how they might be repaired through games. It is not difficult to extend her arguments to education. Today's college students and adult learners are bored and underserved with lecture formats (Stanford University, n.d.) although they will cling to that format over having to teach themselves. Current technology has fostered reduced attention spans and reinforced students' reliance on instant gratification, immediate feedback, innovation, and novelty to sustain interest in learning situations (Greenfield, 2009; Oblinger, 2006a; Reiner & Siegel, 2008; Sauve, Renaud, Kaufman, & Marquis, 2007). Games can address these needs because they are experiential and can provide frequent feedback. Games used for educational purposes or serious games are a way to motivate, reinforce skills, and promote collaboration through their experiential format. There is extensive literature on games theory and gaming in multiple disciplines. This chapter is an introduction to the use of games as a teaching/learning tool within the classroom or clinical setting. It will also introduce the idea of "gamification" in education—the process of turning the entire learning experience into a multiplayer game (Sheldon, 2012). Definitions, evidence regarding practice, and the types of learning that will fit most easily within the various game structures will be described, as will the limitations of game use within the educational or clinical environment.

■ Definition and Purpose

A game is an activity often classified as fun, governed by precise rules that involve varying degrees of strategy or chance, and one or more players who cooperate or compete (with self, the game, one another, or a computer) through the use of knowledge or skill in an attempt to reach a specified goal (Beylefeld & Struwig, 2007; Sauve et al., 2007). In addition, and potentially the most salient feature of games, is that they have a fairly immediate feedback system (McGonigal, 2011). Educational or serious games are believed to provide learning benefits for all participants that last beyond the game itself, and evidence to that effect forms the basis of this chapter. Modern students expect and desire immediate feedback on the accuracy of the knowledge they are acquiring (Johnson & Romanello, 2005), and games may fulfill that desire. There are three major categories within the genre—games, simulations, and simulation games.

Game is a generic term that includes board, card, and skilled activities. Many simple educational games have popular formats, such as bingo, Jeopardy!, Trivial Pursuit, Monopoly, and Who Wants to Be a Millionaire?, that provide frameworks for inserting content and creating learning activities. These games typically involve a set of rules for player moves and termination criteria so that winners may be determined. The frameworks are easily adaptable to a wide variety of content and instructional objectives usually in the lower cognitive domain areas. These games have been described in the literature and examples are listed under *Recommended Reading*. Also see websites listed in the *Resources* section for templates of popular game shows for educational use.

Simulations, in this context, are role-playing games and are discussed in 13 other chapters. Simulation games are contrived reality-based conflicts that must be resolved within the constraints of the game rules and have been shown to enhance competency development among health professionals (Allery, 2004; Graham & Richardson, 2008; Sauve et al., 2007). They have the potential to attain new heights of efficacy in digital game formats where they can be used to enhance other aspects of the educational experience more than mere review of content. Within authentic contexts, students have the opportunity to get immersed in the game and call on past knowledge and experience to problem solve and make decisions (Oblinger, 2006b; Skiba, 2008).

Debriefing is an important aspect of the learning process that occurs after the game. It is a discussion focusing on the concepts, generalizations, and applications of the topics covered within the game (Gee, 2008; Graham & Richardson, 2008). This process assists learners in recognizing the learning that has occurred within the fun experience of the game and contributes to the learners' ability to use self-reflection, especially for the modern learner (Allery, 2004; Johnson & Romanello, 2005). Effective debriefing requires a good deal of skill and experience in the facilitator and should be allotted as much time as was spent actually playing the game (Blakely, Skirton, Cooper, Allum, & Nelmes, 2010).

▪ Theoretical Foundations

The use of games for educational purposes is a very old idea. The earliest recorded use was for war games 3,000 years ago in China, in the 18th century in Europe, and, within this century, by the U.S. military. Game use was brought to the business community by ex-officers to provide training in problem solving and decision making. It was considered a bridge between academic instruction and on-the-job training. In the 1950s and 1960s, as the theoretical focus of learning shifted from the instructor to the student, experience-based learning became prominent, and games were used to meet this goal. In health-related areas, psychologists and nurses made numerous contributions to the literature on game use in both academic and clinical education, although the research is still inconclusive when judging their effectiveness primarily due to small sample sizes, poor operational definitions, and other design flaws (Akl et al., 2010; Beylefeld & Struwig, 2007; Blakely, Skirton, Cooper, Allum, & Nelmes, 2009; Bochennek, Wittekindt, Zimmermann, & Klingebiel, 2007; Royse & Newton, 2007; Shiroma, Massa, & Alarcon, 2011).

Game use falls under the theoretical umbrellas of active learning strategies and cooperative learning described previously in this text and under the concept of flow coined by Csikszentnikhlyi, which refers to a psychological state achieved when learning and enjoyment coincide (Beylefeld & Struwig, 2007). The focus is on actual engagement with both the educational material and classmates, engendering positive attitudes that promote deep processing of the learning experience. It can be intense, absorbing, and motivating (Dormann & Biddle, 2006).

■ Types of Learners

Games are being used throughout the educational continuum, from preschool through graduate education. They can be used for students who like to compete or for those who prefer to cooperate. For learners with achievement needs, games motivate through competitiveness. Games may also be motivating for those with strong affiliation needs, such as millennial learners, because games can require team play and cooperation for completion. The element of luck within an educational game gives all students, not just the studious ones, a chance at winning and thereby keeps engagement higher. Educators must appreciate the different maturational stages students pass through. Adult learners have a particular need to engage meaningfully with content and apply it in a variety of methods, which can be accomplished through the interactive, immediate, and diverse format of gaming.

Games can be structured to require a degree of flexibility on the part of the student to adapt to changing circumstances, especially when addressing the development of interdisciplinary awareness, problem solving, cultural sensitivity, and empathy with clients (Graham & Richardson, 2008; Jarrell, Alpers, Brown, & Wotring, 2008). Finally, particularly with the use of digital simulation games, some degree of computer/technology comfort is required on the part of both the students and the faculty/trainer. Most millennial and postmillennial students arrive on campus equipped to use Web 2.0 technologies; some faculty need to increase their comfort level with this method.

■ Conditions for Learning

Games can be used to address all levels of cognitive objectives, from reinforcing the learning of basic facts, through developing application and analysis skills, and culminating in promoting synthesis and evaluation. They do this through the promotion of initiative, creative thought, and affective components within a safe forum for listening to others. Games are credited with supplementing rote memorization, providing useful organization of material, encouraging application of ideas, and providing comic relief from the otherwise anxiety-provoking task of preparing for exams.

Games are inherently student-centered and interactive, generating enthusiasm, excitement, and enjoyment. It has been found that students often prefer multiple methods, or styles, of learning (Lujan & DiCarlo, 2006; Wright, 2012). When new occupational therapy students are asked what their preferred learning style is, the predominant answer is usually hands on/experiential (M. D'Amico, September 12, 2012, personal communication). An experiential learning method, such as gaming, creates an environment that requires a participant to be involved in a personally meaningful activity using multiple styles of learning, such as visual, auditory, and kinesthetic styles. Fostering a match between teaching strategies and student needs is one of the key factors in effective education. In addition, learning has greater impact when it has an element of emotional arousal, takes place within a safe environment, and has a period of debriefing to provide a cognitive map for understanding the experience (Allery, 2004; Medina, 2008).

Board or card games tend to be most appropriate for skill-based knowledge and practice in the cognitive domain, such as memorizing or concept matching (Bochennek et al., 2007; Van Eck, 2006). Jeopardy! and Trivial Pursuit are quite popular in many disciplines for reviewing course information in such subjects as abnormal psychology and research methods because of the quick mobilization of facts or labels required. In health care, both would lend themselves to reviews in human development, clinical conditions, or other primary knowledge topics. These games are used to review facts, reinforce or test knowledge and understanding, and foster application (Patel, 2008). The games can be adapted in multiple ways—through the content and through the external attributes of the game itself, such as time limits and the degree of luck built into the format. Crossword puzzles, word searches, and bingo-style games have been used in nursing in-service training to review required materials as well as increase staff attendance and compliance. Games can also be created for the psychomotor domain; speed of manipulation, safety in transfers, and knowledge of intervention techniques could all be addressed through a game format that would reward an individual or a team.

Simulation games, referred to as adventure games when in digital format, are adapted to teaching problem solving, hypothesis testing, and the affective domain outcomes. Problem solving is best taught through practice and reflection. Within the format of the simulation game, especially in a computer or video game format, there is more opportunity for such repetition and practice than is available during limited classroom or clinical practice time (Reiner & Siegel, 2008). Video games also may offer consistent assessment of clinical reasoning skills in case study situations of home or clinic visits (Duque, Fung, Mallet, Posel, & Fleiszer, 2008). The potential is there for multiple users in these virtual environments, and professional exploration may be accomplished through digital simulation games. Serious game design works best when communication is built in through blogs, wikis, and other Web 2.0 technologies (Derryberry, 2007). The time/effort involved in creating such environments becomes more feasible when faculty are faced with overloaded clinical placements (Oblinger, 2006b; Skiba, 2008).

A recent academic development is to structure an entire class as a game, also referred to as gamification (Lee & Hammer, 2011; Sheldon, 2012). The concept employs elements of games, such as experience points for accomplishments as opposed to grades, levels that students rise through as they gain the experience points, and assignments that are structured as quests or challenges, to promote engagement in learning. One gamification approach is to have assignments that can be repeated until competence is achieved (challenges). These challenges are created for the student's current skill level and increase in difficulty as the student's skill level advances. Another approach is to have group-based activities (quests) that foster teamwork and critical thinking. The gamification approach sparks motivation and emotional engagement through the choices offered to students—choices to engage in select activities or not, and to plot one's own path through the course material (Lee & Hammer, 2011; Sheldon, 2012). The take-away message is to provide feedback often and keep the stakes low while initial learning is taking place, so that the repetition needed to actually master the material can be a positive emotional experience, rather than a punishment. It does not require a game format to accomplish this, but a game format can keep the focus on active, engaged learning that is within the learner's control rather than assignments being seen as an obstacle a professor is throwing in the path of perfect grades.

■ Resources

Creating games for the classroom usually takes time, imagination, and desire. The rewards can be great, although in this productivity-driven age, the tradeoffs must be considered. As has been described, the quickest resources are based on those games that are currently available in toy stores or on television. Using the frames of these games requires loading in course material, and then it is easy to introduce to the students because of their familiarity with the format.

As of the publication date of this text, the following websites offered templates for such games:

PowerPoint games at http://jc-schools.net/tutorials/PPT-games/
Game boards at http://jc-schools.net/tutorials/gameboard.htm

Crossword puzzles or word games at http://www.crossword-puzzles.co.uk/ or
Eclipse crosswords at http://www.eclipsecrossword.com/

WebQuest: http://www.webquest.org/index.php

A more challenging approach than using the aforementioned sites is developing
the entire game from one's own imagination, although if the educator engages small
groups from a class to create the game using some of the guiding principles in the
next section, this may become more feasible (Patel, 2008). Digital game developers
have been creating structures that may be available as frameworks for cognitive and
affective domain objectives. These frameworks range from addressing the lower/
moderate end of knowledge/awareness, as in a WebQuest search for specific information, through to the high-end evaluating/internalizing found in the Pod Game
(ZaidLearn), where one is making judgments and decisions under a time constraint.
The challenge for the educator is in finding and then using such formats because of
the technological knowledge required on top of the content application (Van Eck,
2006). Currently there are only a few such games that are directly applicable to
health care. It has been recommended that it is better to make teaching practices
gamelike than to try to develop whole games that may actually detract from the
educational intent because of the novelty or the development time involved (Begg,
2008). A key resource for gamification is a blog with many linked resources found at
http://gamingtheclassroom.wordpress.com/.

The *Recommended Reading* section at the end of this chapter has a variety of
articles and websites describing gaming used in classroom education and in-service
training. Some articles specifically target a greater use of technology, such as computer or web-based games. The references that describe active learning and cooperative learning are excellent background information for the new academician and are
available online.

■ Using the Method: Basic How-to

Many authors have described the methodology behind using games in the classroom,
and their advice is summarized in **Table 12-1**. To begin, games rarely succeed as
add-ons; they must be integrated into the overall educational strategy (Ridley, 2004).
A game pulled out of nowhere, just to be novel, will have no effect on outcome measures. In essence, when developing a game, the educator must determine the content
area, statement of the problem, and objectives of the game. After this, he or she must
determine the game format, number of players, time frame, and rules. If using a frame
game, the generic rules already exist and can be adapted for the topic within health
care. The next decisions regard roles players assume and scenarios in which play
occurs. These can be simple adaptations for frame games, or more complex if setting
up a game that is a simulation of a clinic. The scoring system and physical elements of
a frame game tend to remain consistent with the original game; for simulation games
they need to be created outright. The designer chooses the media used, whether they
are common materials or specially constructed components, based on available time

Table 12-1 Process for Game Development

Step	Element	Probes
1	Specific objectives for game.	Do they parallel and/or facilitate the course objectives?
2	Fit within the curriculum and the environment.	Are the concepts relevant? Is this for review or to move understanding forward? Is there adequate functional space for implementation? If digital, are there enough computers and technical support?
3	Employs conflict.	This could be a time limit, competition between teams, or competition with the manager, depending on the objectives. Does it provide a just-right challenge? Can the student alter the level of challenge?
4	Rules of play and criterion for closure are easily communicated.	Are all the rules known up front, or are they learned over time? If there are dead ends or eliminations, what happens next?
5	It is fun.	If not, stop and rework or discard.
6	Provides immediate feedback to the participants.	Do students know how they are doing at all times? Is uncertainty part of the game? Does the feedback assist the student in modifying beliefs or performance in order to improve?
7	Meets the needs of the students.	Does the game help organize the course material? Is it a reliable measure of students' comprehension, or will it mislead them? Does the game encourage the players to "laugh with" as opposed to "laugh at" one another? Is it inclusive in nature?
8	Field test to eliminate bugs.	Did it go as planned, or are there needed revisions?
9	Mechanism (such as pretesting and posttesting) that allows measurement of learning.	Other than student satisfaction, check to see if actual learning occurs.
10	Share it with colleagues.	Publish or post—there are many educational game websites.

and resources. The game needs to be tested on a small sample initially, critiqued, and possibly revised. Finally, it is beneficial to the community of healthcare educators if the game is then disseminated (Blakely et al., 2009).

Overarching elements that must be considered when using instructional games include the layout and amount of space in the classroom or availability of technology, to ensure equal opportunity to play. Time to be spent during the game with enough time for the debriefing must be planned. Also essential in planning are the method by which the students will become aware of the rules of the game and rewards for results, including whether the rewards are intrinsic or extrinsic. Remember that for best effect, the game must be integrated into the instructional strategy of the course and directly related to the subject. It must be challenging enough and not feel like work.

■ Potential Problems

Effective use of games in the classroom can be undermined in the ways most strategies fail—poor planning, lack of attention, and lack of follow-up. One example of inappropriate game use stemming from each of these obstacles was the use of a simulation game to evaluate treatment skills. There was a specific scoring sheet to test students on the use of a computer program for cognitive rehabilitation. The students were *therapists* with faculty *clients*. This experience was to provide feedback on the student's knowledge of the computer program, as well as provide valuable lessons on therapist–client interaction and use of the environment (e.g., paying attention to the physical environment even though they were intervening for a cognitive task). The main drawbacks to this experience were neglecting to emphasize the game nature of the simulation to reduce trepidation and having faculty be the clients, which increased anxiety. More planning would have improved the introduction of the activity. More faculty attention during the experience may have provided the impetus to revise the format so that there could have been *peer* clients. More knowledge about the use of educational games could have made this a more relaxed and appreciated learning experience.

Other potential pitfalls of game use require the instructor to be aware of:

- *Timing.* Monitor play, termination, and transition to the next learning activities. Fun activities can take on a life of their own. Simulations (especially) and games reduce control of the timing of the class period; the instructor must be comfortable with that reduced control or it will not work. While spontaneity and flexibility are admirable, there is also a need for planned sequences of activities and firm timekeeping.
- *Competition.* Motivation may be limited to those who win; losing may produce a failure experience that decreases self-esteem. Be conscious of all class members and monitor the degree of competition and cooperation required to achieve educational goals.
- *Initial high costs of developing and running a game.* It is quite time consuming to create or flesh out even a frame game. In some instances the task involves no more than developing more test questions/answers (as in Jeopardy! or Trivial Pursuit games), but that is often easier said than done. The outcome of a recent study found that educators did not have the time to develop appropriate games, and that class sizes made using games even more intimidating (Blakely et al., 2010). In the case of simulation games, a lot of thought is necessary to create an adequate situation and produce a complete cast of characters with goals and belief systems.
- *Unmet needs of participants.* Not all students' learning needs will be met within a simulation or game; therefore, instructors should not depend on these strategies as solo teaching approaches.
- *Closure.* Facilitate appropriate debriefing by allowing adequate time for this phase of the learning experience and being an active listener.

▪ Conclusion

Games are a suitable supplement for a variety of academic and clinical situations. They are a method of helping students recognize how much they know or how much they still need to study. Different types have been described, as has the appropriate usage within the wide variety of instructional objectives and content in healthcare curricula. The choice and time management required may seem daunting, but educators have found they enjoyed the respite from standard classroom practice while developing and implementing an educational game. It is well worth the effort.

TEACHING EXAMPLES:

Descriptions of Strategy in Use

The format of Jeopardy! lends itself for review of lots of material. One example involved preexam reviews in an undergraduate mental health class for occupational therapy students with categories covering such areas as theories, *Diagnostic and Statistical Manual of Mental Disorders,* fourth edition (DSM-IV), defense mechanisms, leadership techniques, and pharmaceuticals. The class was divided into three teams. The regular Jeopardy! and double jeopardy were employed, although final jeopardy was not. Each team had a person designated as the beeper, and the beepers could collaborate within the team to come up with the question that matched the answer on the overhead projector. Most of the class engaged in the spirit of the game. During the process there was time for discussion and clarification of the topic areas. There were errors made on the exam itself, despite the review, so the game did not lead to the degree of achievement expected. However, it was not formally evaluated or compared with other methods. The participation and apparent enjoyment of that review class were clear though.

An example of a simulation game used in a class on life span development employed the use of percentage dice rolls that each pair of students used to create families and newborns who would function throughout the semester to demonstrate typical human development from birth through adolescence. Each newborn had characteristics (e.g., motor skill, cognitive level, appearance, longevity, social environment, financial environment) that would be based on a limited number of dice rolls. The higher the dice roll, the better the performance or status of the attribute to which it was assigned. The students' first objective was to determine which combination of attributes would lead to the best life outcomes for their children. Was it more important to be very smart or to be very attractive? Could you be successful in life with poor motor skills? After these decisions, there were journaling assignments regarding the development of the children and lots of negotiation between the partners regarding a series of developmental issues, culminating in special dice rolls in adolescence that determined whether the adolescent engaged in smoking and/ or sexual activity, was involved in violence, and so on. Student feedback on this experiential assignment was mostly positive, although some did report that it was quite time consuming. The expected degree of learning regarding human development was demonstrated in the journals. However, the greater learning experience was attitudinal change based on the discussions between partners of differing backgrounds and how they managed to cope with some of the unexpected events of these simulated lives.

REFERENCES

Akl, E. A., Pretorius, R. W., Sackett, K., Erdley, W. S., Bhoopathi, P. S., Alfarah, Z., & Schunemann, H. J. (2010). The effect of educational games on medical students' learning outcomes: A systematic review. BEME Guide No. 14. *Medical Teacher, 32,* 16–27.

Allery, L. A. (2004). Educational games and structured experiences [Commentary]. *Medical Teacher, 26*(6), 504–505.

Begg, M. (2008). Leveraging game-informed healthcare education. *Medical Teacher, 30,* 155–158.

Beylefeld, A. A., & Struwig, M. C. (2007). A gaming approach to learning medical microbiology: Students' experiences of flow. *Medical Teacher, 29,* 933–940.

Blakely, G., Skirton, H., Cooper, S., Allum, P., & Nelmes, P. (2009). Educational gaming in the health sciences: Systematic review. *Journal of Advanced Nursing, 65*(2), 259–269.

Blakely, G., Skirton, H., Cooper, S., Allum, P., & Nelmes, P. (2010). Use of educational games in the health professions: A mixed-methods study of educators' perspectives in the UK. *Nursing and Health Sciences, 12,* 27–32.

Bochennek, K., Wittekindt, B., Zimmermann, S., & Klingebiel, T. (2007). More than mere games: A review of card and board games for medical education. *Medical Teacher, 29,* 941–948.

Derryberry, A. (2007). Serious games: online games for learning [White paper]. http://www.adobe.com /resources/elearning/pdfs/serious_games_wp.pdf

Dormann, C., & Biddle, R. (2006). Humour in game-based learning. *Learning, Media and Technology, 31*(4), 411–424.

Duque, G., Fung, S., Mallet, L., Posel, N., & Fleiszer, D. (2008). Learning while having fun: The use of video gaming to teach geriatric house calls to medical students. *Journal of the American Geriatric Society, 56,* 1328–1332.

Gee, J. P. (2008). Learning and games. In K. Salen (Ed.), *The ecology of games: Connecting youth, games, and learning* (pp. 21–40). Cambridge, MA: MIT Press.

Graham, I., & Richardson, E. (2008). Experiential gaming to facilitate cultural awareness: Its implication for developing emotional caring in nursing. *Learning in Health and Social Care, 7,* 37–45.

Greenfield, P. M. (2009). Technology and informal education: What is taught, what is learned. *Science, 323,* 69–71.

Jarrell, K., Alpers, R., Brown, G., & Wotring, R. (2008). Using BaFa' BaFa' in evaluating cultural competence of nursing students. *Teaching and Learning in Nursing, 3,* 141–142.

Johnson, S. A., & Romanello, M. L. (2005). Generational diversity: Teaching and learning approaches. *Nurse Educator, 30*(5), 212–216.

Lee, J. J., & Hammer, J. (2011). Gamification in education: What, how, why bother? *Academic Exchange Quarterly, 15*(2), 1–5.

Lujan, H. L., & DiCarlo, S. E. (2006). First-year medical students prefer multiple learning styles. *Advanced in Physiology Education, 30,* 13–16.

McGonigal, J. (2011). *Reality is broken: Why games make us better and how they can change the world.* New York, NY: Penguin Books.

Medina, J. (2008). *Brain rules.* Seattle, WA: Pear Press.

Oblinger, D. (2006a). Games and learning. *EDUCAUSE Quarterly, 29*(3), 5–7.

Oblinger, D. (2006b). Simulations, games, and learning. EDUCAUSE Learning Initiative. http://www .educause.edu/ELI/SimulationsGamesandLearning/156764

Patel, J. (2008). Using game format in small group classes for pharmacotherapeutics case studies. *American Journal of Pharmaceutical Education, 72*(1), 1–5.

Reiner, B., & Siegel, E. (2008). The potential for gaming techniques in radiology education and practice. *Journal of the American College of Radiology, 5,* 110–114.

Ridley, R. T. (2004). Classroom games are COOL: Collaborative opportunities of learning. *Nurse Educator, 29*(2), 47–48.

Royse, M. A., & Newton, S. E. (2007). How gaming is used as an innovative strategy for nursing education. *Nursing Education Perspectives, 28*(5), 263–267.

Sauve, L., Renaud, L., Kaufman, D., & Marquis, J. (2007). Distinguishing between games and simulations: A systematic review. *Educational Technology & Society, 10*(3), 247–256.

Sheldon, L. (2012). *The multiplayer classroom: Designing coursework as a game.* Boston, MA: Course Technology/Cengage Learning.

Shiroma, P. R., Massa, A. A., & Alarcon, R. D. (2011). Using game format to teach psychopharmacology to medical students. *Medical Teacher, 33,* 156–160.

Skiba, D. J. (2008). Nursing education 2.0: Games as pedagogical platforms. *Nursing Education Perspectives, 29*(3), 174–175.

Stanford University (n.d.). Center for Teaching and Learning: Lecturing. http://ctl.stanford.edu/handbook/lecturing.html

Van Eck, R. (2006). Digital game-based learning: It's not just the digital natives who are restless. *EDUCAUSE Review, 41*(2), 16–30.

Wright, K. (2012). Student nurses' perceptions of how they learn drug calculation skills. *Nurse Education Today, 32,* 721–726.

RECOMMENDED READING

Cowen, K. J., & Tesh, A. S. (2002). Effects of gaming on nursing students' knowledge of pediatric cardiovascular dysfunction. *Journal of Nursing Education, 41*(11), 507–509.

Dologite, K. A., Willner, K. C., Klepeiss, D. J., York, S. A., & Cericola, L. M. (2003). Sharpen customer service skills with PCRAFT Pursuit©. *Journal for Nurses in Staff Development, 19*(1), 47–51.

Dunn, J. (2012). The 100-second guide to gamification in education. http://edudemic.com/2012/09/the-100-second-guide-to-gamification-in-education/

Flanagan, N., & McCausland, L. (2007). Teaching around the cycle: Strategies for teaching theory to undergraduate nursing students. *Nursing Education Perspectives, 28,* 310–314.

Gifford, K. E. (2001). Using instructional games: A teaching strategy for increasing student participation and retention. *Occupational Therapy in Health Care, 15,* 13–21.

Jones, A. G., Jasperson, J., & Gusa, D. (2000). Cranial nerve wheel of competencies. *Journal of Continuing Education in Nursing, 31*(4), 152–154.

Masters, K. (2005). Development and use of an educator-developed community assessment board game. *Nurse Educator, 30*(5), 189–190.

Morton, P. G., & Tarvin, L. (2001). The pain game: Pain assessment, management, and related JCAHO standards. *Journal of Continuing Education in Nursing, 32*(5), 223–227.

Pearce-Smith, N. (2007). Teaching tip: Using the "Who Wants to Be a Millionaire?" game to teach searching skills. *Evidence Based Nursing, 10,* 72.

Persky, A. M., Stegall-Zanation, J., & Dupuis, R. E. (2007). Students' perceptions of the incorporation of games into classroom instruction for basic and clinical pharmacokinetics. *American Journal of Pharmaceutical Education, 71*(2), 1–9.

Smith-Stoner, M. (2005, September/October). Innovative use of the Internet and intranets to provide education by adding games. *CIN: Computers, Informatics, Nursing,* 237–241.

Stringer, E. C. (1997). Word games as a cost-effective and innovative inservice method. *Journal of Nursing Staff Development, 13*(3), 155–160.

Terenzi, C. (2000). The triage game. *Journal of Emergency Nursing, 26*(1), 66–69.

Ward, A. K., & O'Brien, H. L. (2005). A gaming adventure. *Journal for Nurses in Staff Development, 21*(1), 37–41.

CHAPTER 13

Role Play

■ Arlene J. Lowenstein and Micki Harris ■

■ Definition and Purposes

Role play is a dramatic technique that encourages participants to improvise behaviors that illustrate expected actions of persons involved in defined situations. A scenario is outlined, and character roles are assigned. The scenario can be scripted and rehearsed, but it is usually unscripted, relying on spontaneous interplay among characters to provide material about reactions and behaviors for students to analyze following the presentation. Those class members not assigned character roles participate as observers in the audience and provide feedback to contribute to the overall analysis. Role playing allows students to engage their imaginations to explore scenarios that target potential issues and stimulate team building. For the exercise to be productive, all the students must be committed to participating and feel comfortable and safe in the environment (Sasha, 2011). Role play exercises are an ideal way for the participants to practice skills and experience ethical or culturally sensitive situations. These learning experiences should be applicable to the actual context in which they will be used to be most effective in developing practical skills (Lane, Hood, & Rollnick, 2008).

Part of the category of simulation, role play allows participants to explore why people behave as they do. Participants can test communication skills, behaviors, and decisions in an environment that allows experimentation without risk. The scenario and behaviors of the actors are analyzed and discussed to provide opportunity to clarify feelings, increase observational skills, provide rationale for potential behaviors, improve communication skills, and anticipate reactions to decisions. New behaviors and communication techniques can be suggested and tried in response to the analysis.

Role play is used to enable students to practice interacting with others in certain roles and to afford them an opportunity to experience other people's reactions to actions they have taken. The scenario may be outlined to provide a background for the problem and the constraints that may apply. Defining the important characteristics of the major players establishes role expectations and provides a framework for behaviors and actions to be elicited.

The postplay discussion provides opportunity for analysis and new strategy formation. Repeating a role play after the debriefing session provides the students with the opportunity for a second chance or do over, thereby giving them confidence in handling tough situation(s) (Silberman, 2006). Although it is a dramatic technique, the focus is on the actions of the characters and not on acting ability. An actor plays to the audience; the role player plays to the characters in the scenario. The audience also has a role—that of observing the interplay among characters and analyzing the dynamics occurring. The instructor's role is that of facilitator rather than director. The impetus for the analysis and discussion belongs with the learners. The instructor's role is passive—clarifying and gently guiding.

The role play, regardless of its length, develops communicative competence. Throughout this creative process, the student group must work together to exchange information and polish the presentation as they both speak and listen. The peer feedback offered by the audience will be valuable in assessing how well the players adopted cultural roles and expressed opinions (Qing, 2011).

Clinical simulations often incorporate role play. Although the simulation computer and mannequin provide the physiological issues in the scenario, students or faculty members may play the human roles, such as the doctor or family members. The computer operator may also provide a voice for the patient, to which the healthcare provider needs to relate, and this technique allows for better assessment of a patient's response to issues such as anxiety or pain. The use of role play creates the opportunity to provide care to the simulated patient in a realistic environment and requires reactions to complexity in the situation. Smith-Stoner used high-fidelity simulation together with role play to provide a scenario where a student nurse, who was caring for a simulated patient who died during the scenario, needed to interact with the family member who was in the room. The exercise allowed the students in the class to explore their attitudes toward death and caring for dying patients (Smith-Stoner, 2009).

The use of the simulated patient has been effective to provide the practice and rehearsal necessary to increase competence in motivational interviewing, which is a method that works on influencing individuals to consider changing their behavior. Lane and colleagues found that experienced practitioners engaged in role play scenarios achieved the same level of competence in motivational interviewing whether they practiced with a peer or a simulated patient (Lane et al., 2008).

Role play can also be used in online courses. Although there may be no person-to-person drama, a scenario can be set up, parts assigned, and the conversation carried out via a chat room or discussion board. Riddle (2009) noted that online educational role plays engage students in the learning and can be an improvement over didactic teaching strategies alone. Online role play systems afford students the opportunity of acting and doing instead of only reading and listening.

Role play is a particularly effective means for developing decision-making and problem-solving skills (Hess & Giligannon, 1985). Imholz (2008) studied clinical research on psychodrama practice of role play, looking at the therapeutic activity that has both cognitive and emotional outcomes of the role play as change agent and also as a process that contributes to personal growth. Through role play, the learner can identify the systematic steps in the process of making judgments and decisions. The problem-solving process—identification of the problem, data collection, evaluation of possible outcomes, exploration of alternatives, and arrival at a decision to be implemented—can be analyzed in the context of the role play situation. The scenario can include reactions to the implementation of the decision as well as the evaluation and reformulation process (Alden, 1999; Domazzo & Hanson, 1997). Role play has also been used to increase student cultural awareness, aiding in the development of cultural competence in patient care (Shearer & Davidhizar, 2003).

Role play can be utilized to develop competence in overall communications as well as to increase students' intercultural awareness. Collaborative role plays, which are performed in groups, can be beneficial as the students create the entire story complete with the cast of characters and dialogue. This can be a long-term process where one or more cultural considerations are raised during each role play scenario and the interpersonal communication skills of the group develop. The group will rehearse the scenario and perform for the audience, followed by a peer feedback session (Qing, 2011).

Role play provides immediate feedback to learners regarding their success in using interpersonal skills as well as decision-making and problem-solving skills. At the same time, role play offers learners an opportunity to become actively involved in the learning experience in a nonthreatening environment. Role play is not limited to use in the classroom. Corless and colleagues (2004) successfully used role play as a student assignment that required the adoption of a persona of a person with HIV who was required to take a number of medications over a specific period of time. Students carried out the role play in their homes, taking placebos in place of medication over a specific time frame. Their experiences in following the HIV regimen were then discussed in class, leading to an awareness of the difficulties patients faced in following the regimen. Role play is also being used as a teaching strategy in online courses (Mar, Chabal, Anderson, & Vore, 2003).

Giving feedback to the role play performers, also called the debriefing, is a reflective process. Feedback is provided by peers, teacher, and a self-assessment. A feedback session is held at the conclusion of the role play exercise to engage all the students in reflective discussion. The teacher's observations and opinions are highly regarded, but the entire audience needs to provide productive comments. The class as a whole or small groups offer their reactions and feedback to the role play exercise. Prior to the feedback session, the teacher should instruct the students to offer positive and then constructive comments and to be specific. The teacher may assign specific students in the audience to attend to a player or group of players, a particular nuance (i.e., nonverbal behavior), and/or specific open-ended or closed-ended questions. The teacher seeks feedback from the players and the audience. What went well? What did not go well? What could be done to improve each player's performance? The teacher may offer observations or seek audience observations with a comparison to a benchmark/ideal script. Each role player is required to self-assess his or her performance and feelings about the experience (Silberman, 2006). Video-taping the role play exercise can be an effective debriefing technique if used to review specific points in the recording. The teacher should attempt to draw the problem solving and decision making from the students to facilitate long-term carryover and learning (Silberman, 2006).

Verbal and nonverbal communication must be considered. Students may experiment with various facial expressions; pace, volume, and tone of voice; body language and physical gestures; and use of humor or drama. Role play has the potential of creating an active atmosphere within the classroom that mobilizes the entire audience with enthusiasm (Qing, 2011).

▪ Theoretical Rationale

Role play developed in response to the need to effect attitudinal changes in psychotherapy and counseling (Shaffer & Galinsky, 1974). Psychodrama, a forerunner of role play, was developed by Moreno as a psychotherapy technique. Moreno brought psychodrama to the United States in 1925 and continued to develop it during the 1940s and 1950s (Moreno, 1946). In psychodrama, players may be required to recite specific lines or answer specific questions and may represent themselves, whereas in role play, players are encouraged to express their thoughts and feelings spontaneously, as if they were the persons whose roles they were playing (Sharon & Sharon, 1976).

Psychodrama provided a foundation for further development of role play as an educational technique. Corsini (1957) and other psychotherapists and group dynamicists began using role play to assist patients to clarify people's behavior toward each other. Further development led to the use of role play in sensitivity training, a technique that became popular in the 1970s. Human relations and sensitivity training events share a common educational strategy. The learners in the group are encouraged to become involved in examining their thought patterns, perceptions, feelings, and inadequacies. The training events are also designed to encourage each learner with the support of fellow learners to invent and experiment with different patterns of functioning (Gordon, 1970). Role play can be used to meet those educational objectives; it is often used in human relations and sensitivity training but has many other uses as well. DeNeve and Hepner (1997), in a study comparing role play to traditional lectures, found that students believed that the use of role play was stimulating and valuable in comparison to the traditional lecture method, their learning increased, and they remembered what they had learned.

In a study that looked at nursing students who role played with theater students and those who role played with other nursing students, Reams and Bashford (2011) noted that the students who played with the theater students gained confidence in their approach to patients and interdisciplinary colleagues by practicing repeatedly within a safe environment. However, when nursing students role played with a nursing student peer, they were inadvertently assisted by the peer. This assistance interfered with the nursing students' gaining confidence in their approach to patients, and it may be something for the instructor to watch out for.

■ Conditions

Role playing is a versatile technique that can be used in a wide variety of situations. One set of learning objectives might be role play dealing with the practice of skills and techniques, whereas another different group of objectives would use role play to deal with changes in understanding, feelings, and attitudes. Van Ments (1983) points out that role play is conducted differently for these two sets of learning objectives. The role play used for the practice of skills may be planned with the emphasis on outcome and overcoming problems. The second type of objective may be best met with an emphasis on the problems and relationships. This method explores why certain behaviors are exhibited and requires expertise from the instructor in dealing with emotions and human behavior. The teacher is responsible for helping the students to avoid the negative effects that could come from the exploration of their feelings and behaviors. In any scenario, there is potential for conflict. The students may struggle to control their feelings so as to clearly relay their message without emotion. To resolve disagreements, confusions, and obstacles, students will need to understand the motives behind their actions. The teacher helps the players stay focused on achieving the objectives (Sasha, 2011).

Role playing is a tool useful for developing communication skills. The role players assume personalities and act according to their understanding of their characters. The scenarios help prepare participants for future situations by allowing them to experience different perspectives. These lessons may be retained for long periods of time (Sasha, 2011).

Laughter can play a role in group communication and group dynamics even when the situation is not humorous. Laughter can be a tool, intentionally and strategically, to direct communication and affect group dynamics (Keyton & Beck, 2010). Keep in mind that a role play is an exercise, not a reality, so it should not be taken too seriously. Humor should be encouraged, as it can be effective in defusing tension or hostility provoked during the role play exercise, thus fostering positive attitudes (Bartle, 2007).

Role play exercises can be designed with more than one student playing a role to decrease the stress placed on an individual student. Two to four students can play one role, thereby allowing the shy students to feel more comfortable about actively participating in front of the audience. This technique also allows students to work as a team to create the dialogue, whether rehearsed or improvised. This collaboration is valuable training for what is required in practical healthcare situations where a team of doctors, nurses, therapists, nutritionists, and social workers provide patient care. Also, students in the audience have the opportunity to tap a role player on the shoulder and replace him or her as the character in the scenario so as to contribute something they feel is worthwhile. Likewise, a role player can tap an audience member on the shoulder and take that person's place as an audience member; thus all students are potential role players. This exercise may be set up in two rows facing each other, in a half circle, or in a full circle, which has been referred to as a fishbowl.

■ Planning and Modifying

Teachers who are new to the technique need to plan before class, but they should monitor the needs of the group as the experience progresses and be able to modify those plans if necessary. The situation developed should be familiar enough so that learners can understand the roles and their potential responses, but it should not have a direct relationship to students' own personal problems (McKeachie, 2002). It can also be effective to use two or more presentations of the same situation with different students in the roles if the objective is to point out different responses or solutions to a given problem. When that method is used, the instructor may choose to keep those students involved in the second presentation away from viewing the first presentation, to avoid biasing their reactions. The same role play scenario can be used throughout the semester to allow students to react to changing events within the same scenario (Rabinowitz, 1997).

Role play strategy qualifies as an adult-learning approach because it presents a real-life situation and tries to stimulate the involvement of the student. It has special value because it uses peer evaluation and involves active participation. However, it must be carefully guided to be sure participants have an understanding of the objectives and that feedback received from other players is congruent with outcomes that would exist in the real world (Mann & Corsun, 2002).

■ Types of Learners

Role play is appropriate for undergraduate and graduate students. It is especially effective in staff development programs because of its association with reality. It is used effectively to reach effective outcomes. Role play can be simple or complex, depending on the learning objectives. Regardless of the simplicity of the play itself, it is important to allow adequate time for planning, preparing the students for the experience, and postplay discussion and analysis. The actual role play may be as brief as 5 minutes, although 10–20 minutes is more common. Van Ments (1983) suggests that the technique be broken into the following three sections: briefing, running, and debriefing. Equal amounts of time may be spent in each session on simple objectives, or a ratio of 1:2:3, with most time spent on the debriefing or analysis for more complex learning objectives.

■ Resources

Role play can be used in most settings, although tiered lecture rooms may inhibit the ability of the players to relate to each other and to the observing students. In that setting, the theatricality of the technique is likely to be emphasized over the needed behavioral focus (Van Ments, 1983). Special equipment or props may be simple or not used at all, again depending on the objectives. An instructor may choose to use video or audio taping. This can be especially helpful to review portions of the action during the debriefing and analysis section. Reviewing tapes may also be helpful for participating students who, because of their roles, were not in the room to hear and see some of the interactions that occurred in other role plays. A checklist of specific observations may be helpful to the students when developing their debriefing skills, tone of voice, eye contact, response to constructive criticism, and other aspects of communication.

Outside resources are not usually needed for most role play situations, although additional instructors, trained observers, or specific experts may appropriately be used to meet certain objectives. The technique is best for small groups of students so that those not involved in the character parts can be actively involved in observing and discussing the action in the debriefing or analyzing portion. Van Ments (1983) found role play increasingly unsatisfactory as a technique in groups with more than 25 students, although there may be exceptions, depending on objectives and strategies for involving the audience. Creative role play methods to accommodate more than 25 students are discussed in the next section.

▪ Using the Method

When designing role playing exercises, start with the script, which consists of the roles to be played via improvisation, prescription, or rehearsal followed by the drama or situation. Improvisation, which promotes spontaneity, is often difficult and intimidating for some students. The teacher has the option of assigning the roles and instructing the students in how to behave. Although this approach is less intimidating to the students, it may be more challenging for the students to identify with their assigned characters. Some role plays involve a detailed description of the situation, but the students have the creative license regarding how to handle it. Student improvisations are risky, and the teacher's intended objectives may not be met (Silberman, 2006).

The situation may or may not be dramatic and may be a replay of a past situation or of a hypothetical event. Students may be most comfortable replaying a situation they have previously experienced. This can be performed informally as a conversation or with a rehearsed script. Realistic situations can provide valuable learning opportunities for all the students (Silberman, 2006).

Next consider the staging options, which include informal conversation between the teacher and a student that develops into a class discussion; formal setup with a pair or a trio in front of the group; simultaneous pairs acting out a scenario, which reduces anxiety as all the students are participating at the same time; rotational role play in front of the class, where the students tap in and out of the exercise; or one role played by three or four individuals simultaneously as a team (Silberman, 2006). These various models utilize more players, thereby accommodating groups of more than 25 students.

Planning is crucial to effective use of role play as a learning technique. It may be helpful to test the exercise before running it in the class situation to allow the instructor to anticipate potential problems and evaluate if the learning objectives can be met. Discussing critical elements of the role play with colleagues can be useful if full-scale testing is not feasible. A small amount of time going through the plans with someone else may prevent a critical element from going wrong and disrupting the exercise (Van Ments, 1983).

Selecting a scenario and deciding on character roles is an important part of planning. McKeachie (2002) cautions that situations involving morals or subjects of high emotional significance, such as sexual taboos, are apt to be traumatic to some students. He found that the most interesting situations, and those revealing the greatest differences in responses, are those involving some choice or conflict of motives. Student input into planning can also be effective.

To implement the role play, the scenario and characters need to be described briefly but with enough information to elicit responses that will meet the learning objectives. This planning is extremely important for obtaining good results. Spontaneity should be encouraged, so it is preferable to avoid a script, other than bare outlines of the action. Although spontaneity is valued in character dialogue, students need to have a clear understanding of their characters and their basic attitude and/or thought patterns. In some instances, spontaneity in the character description area could compromise the objectives and results, but if students understand the expected character, they can still be spontaneous within the character parameters. Allowing students in the character roles to have a few minutes to warm up and relate to the roles they will be playing is often helpful. Observing students absolutely must be briefed on their role. Enough time must be allotted for discussion and analysis of the action. The debriefing following the role play also allows for evaluation of the success in meeting the learning objectives.

In addition to the development of learning objectives and planning, the instructor is responsible for setting the stage for the role play, monitoring the action, and leading the analysis. Students need a clear understanding of the objectives, the scenario, the characters they are to play, the importance of the role of the observers, and the analysis as a vital part of the process. On occasion, the instructor may take a character role, but usually character roles are given to students.

When planning a role play session, the instructor needs to be concerned with the amount of time students may be excluded from the room while waiting for their turn to participate. This issue is especially important when two or more presentations of the same situation are to be used, or the role play has characters who should not be exposed to the dialogue that occurs before they appear in their roles.

In some instances, it may be appropriate to have students switch roles during the role play to provide them with an opportunity to see and feel different reactions to similar situations, thereby experiencing a new perspective. For example, to achieve the learning objective of how to conduct a group, students may benefit by playing a group member and then switching to the leader, or vice versa, during the exercise.

Students must practice their listening skills during role play exercises. Individuals must quiet their own thoughts when the characters are speaking. It is constructive for the students to prepare their thoughts before speaking, but listening is equally important. Players may jot down thoughts that pop into their minds on a notepad to ensure that they remain focused on other people's responses (Sasha, 2011).

The instructor needs to encourage students to respond to interactions in the role play in a spontaneous, natural manner, avoiding melodrama and inappropriate laughing or silliness. Effective use of role play focuses on student participation and interaction. The instructor, as facilitator, channels the discussion to meet the learning objectives but avoids monopolizing the play or discussion. The instructor must also be able to monitor and control the depth of emotional responses to the situation or interplay as needed, terminating the play when the objective has been met or the emotional climate calls for intervention.

Students need to understand the importance of playing the character roles in ways in which they believe those characters would act in a real-life situation (Mann & Cordun, 2002). Students in the observer role must be strongly encouraged to present their observations and contribute to the discussion and analysis. Students can also take part in the development of role play scenarios, identifying the learning objectives, issues, and problems they feel need to be explored, as well as scenarios that may provide that exploration.

Graduate schools are catering to the full-time worker market by offering online courses, provided either asynchronously without attendance on campus required or synchronously where there is a designated login time for class. Given that today's health care is team oriented and interdisciplinary with each member required to speak, whether it is to ask questions or defend his or her position in immediate time frames, the synchronous online course may be favored. Using real problem scenarios is an authentic learning approach that is effective in stimulating communication. Culley and Polyakova-Norwood (2012) had students work in teams to discuss and reflect upon their experiences and practice professional behaviors in a safe environment. Synchronous online role play was effective in fostering collaborative communication, which significantly improved their learning experience. Synchronous online role play requires coordination of all students' schedules and mastery of communication technology (i.e., Web cams and microphones to create a virtual meeting room) to be successful. Some students preferred to participate anonymously and thus were reluctant to engage in synchronous online role play (Culley & Polyakova-Norwood, 2012).

Role play in the online environment uses the same basic principles, but with some differences, since the characters will not be visible to each other or to the audience (Mar et al., 2003). A synchronous environment, where all parties are online at the same time, will allow for a written dialogue flow between parties, with more similarity to an actual conversation (Phillips, 2005). An asynchronous environment, where parties log on at different times, will take longer to carry out the scenario and may not have as much spontaneity, but can be as effective (Lebaron & Miller, 2005). As in all cases of role play, designing an online role play will depend on the learning objectives.

■ Potential Problems

Van Ments (1983) refers to the hidden agenda and warns that stereotyping may occur as roles are presented, often reflecting the expectations and values of the students or the teacher. This stereotyping may lead to unanticipated learning that can reinforce prejudices and preconceptions. Instructors need to be aware of this possibility and avoid writing in stereotypes. They should describe only functions, powers, and constraints of the role described. Roles should be rotated to avoid overidentification of one student with a specific role. In the debriefing session, the students are invited to question and challenge assumptions.

Students may not always make a distinction between an actor and a role. Criticism of the student playing the role must be avoided, while allowing for critique of the behavior of the role character. The instructor must be aware of the emotional tones involved in the role play and channel the emotions into activities that will lead to successful attainment of the learning objectives.

Planning and learning objectives should determine the course of the role play. Students may take the role play in an unexpected direction, possibly because they have a need to explore another issue or problem. If it is not appropriate to revise the learning objectives to accommodate student needs, then the play can be terminated. In that case, the postplay discussion can be used to assist students in recognizing why the technique was not effective. Students should advise how to improve the role play or develop a different teaching strategy. Repeating a scenario with the same or different characters can sometimes afford a more in-depth examination and add to the experience.

The instructor and students need to be aware that this is not a professional drama. Some students, because of stage fright, shyness, or other reasons, do not like participating (Middleton, 2005; Turner, 2005). Although at times it may be appropriate to change actors if the role play does not seem to be going well, it is important to not blame the students. In most cases, the teaching strategy needs changing, rather than the actors.

The environment must be arranged so all the role players can see and hear each other and the audience can see and hear all the players' verbal and nonverbal communication. Tone of voice and eye contact can affect how a verbal message is received. Some students multitask while participating in class. At times some students use social media site(s) while also attending to classroom presentations. Such incidents of divided attention displayed by the audience during a role play experience may be counterproductive to their ability to actively participate in the analysis portion of the exercise. Videotaping a role play exercise may be highly effective in providing a replay of specific sections of the exercise during the debriefing; however, the role player(s) may feel self-conscious being videotaped, thereby inhibiting their performance (Silberman, 2006). If these issues are understood and addressed, role play can be an effective and creative strategy to provide active student participation to meet specific learning objectives.

TEACHING EXAMPLES:

Group Dynamics—Conflict Resolution and Role Play Scenarios: Fishbowl

Micki Harris

These role play scenarios are a hands-on approach to engage the learners in the process of identifying a conflict early in its development, negotiating and implementing its resolution while using interpersonal skills to foster a positive working relationship and successful outcome. When conflict arises, work to be part of the solution, not part of the problem.

The fishbowl format enables multiple students to be actively involved in the role play activity while giving the players the comfort of playing the same role as several other classmates. The participants' comments build on each other while the audience observes and analyzes the role play as it evolves.

The content regarding identifying conflicts, strategies for negotiating, and reducing and resolving conflict(s) successfully utilizing an effective interpersonal approach will be presented after the role play is completed. The instructor may attempt to facilitate the objectives during the role play exercise.

Objectives

1. To use role playing to practice communication skills when in situations where conflict(s) arise so as to learn by doing.
2. To clearly identify a problem situation related to group dynamics.
3. To accurately state the problem identified in a nonemotional manner conducive to negotiation.
4. To establish a mechanism to clearly state a problem situation that has been identified.
5. To develop a process to deal with group situations involving a variety of personalities to foster relationship-building opportunities.
6. To effectively employ interpersonal skills when utilizing strategies for reducing conflict(s).
7. To efficiently implement steps to resolve problems to facilitate collaborative dynamics for students working in groups.
8. To establish boundaries for a group to work within to achieve an effective work product in a timely manner.

(continued)

ROLE PLAY FISHBOWL INSTRUCTIONS

The instructor divides the class into 4 groups with 10–12 students in each group as follows:

Group 1: Sally Slacker

Group 2: The four other students in Sally's group

Group 3: Carol Controller

Group 4: The four other students in Carol's group

Each group meets for 10 minutes to discuss its assigned role in the scenario. The students determine what the character they are assigned to play would say to explain or justify the character's behavior. Also, they must devise a plan of how to approach the situation in a manner to successfully resolve the conflict.

Each group chooses four students to enter the fishbowl.

SETTING: CLASSROOM

Setting up the Fishbowl

Two sets of four chairs are set up facing each other in the front of the classroom. (See **Figure 13-1** for classroom setup.)

■ **Figure 13-1** Classroom setup for Fishbowl

FISHBOWL RULES

The groups of students not sitting in the fishbowl act as the audience. Students can tap in and tap out of the fishbowl. Any audience member can tap in to verbalize something he or she feels needs to be said. When a student taps in, one of the students sitting in the fishbowl returns to the audience. Students in the fishbowl can tap out by picking a member of their group in the audience to take their place.

GROUP 1 AND GROUP 2 SCENARIO

Sally Slacker

You are working in a group of five on a project that is due at the end of a 12-week semester. Your group divides up the work evenly and sets deadlines for the work to be completed in increments. At each deadline, the group meets and reevaluates the progress of the project. Assignments are modified and the group produces the final project in phases. Sally does not complete her aspect of the assigned project on time and is not able to take on additional work during the group reevaluation sessions. During the final meeting, Sally reports she will complete her section and submit it to the group editor 24 hours before the final due date. When this 24-hour deadline arrives, there is silence from Sally. Twelve hours later Sally has still not responded to queries from the group editor. The group needs to decide how to approach Sally Slacker to obtain her section of the project so they can submit the project on time for the best possible grade. They schedule a meeting for 1 PM.

In the dialogue that follows, the characters are represented by letters and numbers as follows:

SS = Sally Slacker
SSG1 = Sally Slacker group member No. 1
SSG2 = Sally Slacker group member No. 2
SSG3 = Sally Slacker group member No. 3
SSG4 = Sally Slacker group member No. 4
SSG4R = Audience replacement for SSG4
SSG2R = Audience replacement for SSG2
A = Audience
I = Instructor

Role Play Dialogue

SSG1: Sally, we have called this meeting to discuss the section of the project you were assigned. I need to add your section into the document and submit the project by 5 PM today. Is your section ready to turn in?

SS: Well, there really isn't a problem; I am doing it and it will be finished by the time it is due.

SSG2: The project is due by 5 PM today!

SSG3: We all finished our sections 2 days ago!

SSG4: I finished my section last week. I need a good grade on this project and you are not taking this seriously!

(continued)

SS:	Well, I work better under pressure. I never finish a project a week early. I feel like you are all ganging up on me.
SSG4:	Maybe it is better if SSG1 speaks for the group so you won't feel like we are ganging up on you.
SSG1:	Sally, we respect that you work best under a deadline, but we are concerned that you have not turned in anything for the past 12 weeks and now the project is due in 4 hours and we still have nothing to add for your section. Are you okay?
SS:	You are all so organized and I know I haven't been able to keep up with the project. This has been a really tough semester for me. I couldn't afford my rent so I moved home, which is a 4-hour commute, round trip. I feel so disorganized. I never seem to have everything I need with me to work on my section.
SSG1:	I wish you had told us so we could have been supportive.
I:	As a group, how could you have handled this situation differently?
SSG4-2 (A taps in and replaces SSG4):	This meeting/conversation should have been initiated early in the semester during the group reevaluation sessions when it was clear that SS was not completing her aspect of the assigned project on time and was not able to take on additional work.
SSG2-2 (SSG2 taps out and is replaced with one of Group 2's audience members):	How do we, as a group, complete the project today? Do we discuss our problem with the course instructor? Do we request an extension?
I:	Let's open this discussion up to the audience.

Debriefing of Sally Slacker Role Play

Overall, good strategies for reducing conflict were employed, especially when SSG1 acted as the spokesman for the group. These strategies include the following:

Listen.

State the problem clearly.

Be respectful.

Consider other perspectives.

Be open to compromise.

When there was a problem, the group did not address it until hours before the project was due. When the group confronted SS, several members exhibited elevated emotions and anxiety level as they were concerned about completing the project on time to get a good grade.

Negotiation strategies were successfully employed by SSG1. These strategies include the following:

Call a meeting.

State the rationale for the meeting.

Give specific examples that illustrate the problem.

State why it is a problem.

Confirm the facts.

Listen to the other side.

This role play focused on the negotiation of the problem, whereas the active audience discussion focused on problem resolution, including the following:

Make suggestions for a solution.

Confirm feasibility of solution(s) and consider other solutions.

Achieve consensus regarding solution(s).

Offer help to make the changes.

Share responsibility for managing the outcome.

In discussing the interpersonal approach, it was noted that SSG1 effectively used *I/we* (versus *you*) when presenting the problem and focused on SS's behavior, not on her as a person.

GROUP 3 AND GROUP 4 SCENARIO

Carol Controller

You are working in a group of five, on a project that is due at the end of a 12-week semester. Your group divides up the work evenly and sets deadlines for the work to be completed in increments. At each deadline the group meets and reevaluates the progress of the project. Assignments are modified and the group produces the final project in phases.

Carol is the self-appointed leader of this group. Carol assigns each group member a section, and during the reevaluation meetings she determines the modifications needed. Carol Controller is out of control; she shoots down any ideas that the group members propose and is making all the decisions regarding the direction of the project. The group needs to approach Carol so that all ideas are heard and considered. In the dialogue that follows, the characters are represented by according to the following key:

CC = Carol Controller

CCG1 = Carol Controller group member No. 1

CCG2 = Carol Controller group member No. 2

CCG3 = Carol Controller group member No. 3

CCG4 = Carol Controller group member No. 4

CCG4R = Audience replacement for CCG4

CCG2R = Audience replacement for CCG2

A = Audience

I = Instructor

Role Play Dialogue

CCG1: Carol, we like the way you have organized the workload and moved the project along. However, we are feeling like our project is not a true reflection of our work. We would like to have a more democratic process for determining which aspects of the project make the final edit.

CC: I have always been a good leader. I am well organized and know what needs to be done to get assignments done on time.

(continued)

CCG2: We appreciate that you are organized and good at moving things along and getting things done. But, we would like to work together to fine-tune the final draft, choose the color schemes, and even choose the font that we feel make our project unique to our style as a group.

CC: We do work together. I always ask for input before I make changes.

CCG1: When I used a background color of green, you changed it to pink without even discussing it with me.

CC: I have taken courses with this teacher before, so I know what the teacher wants. I know pink is her favorite color, so we need to use pink.

CCG3: We have also taken courses with this teacher before, so we also know what she wants. There is more than one style and variety is not a bad thing. The goal is to produce a product that represents the whole group. We all need to participate.

CCG3: When we discuss the direction of the project, you don't seem to listen to us. No matter what we come up with, you shoot us down without even considering that our ideas were worth pursuing.

CCG3: And when you take my paper and change it so it is in your writing style, it makes me feel like you don't value my input and contribution. You should not change my words simply because you think your style is better.

CC: Why are you all being so sensitive? You should be happy that I am willing to carry this group.

CCG2: I see no point in putting hours into a product when Carol is going to edit all our work out and use only her ideas. Maybe we should be okay with Carol doing it all as long as we get a good grade.

SSG2R (A taps in and replaces SSG2): Let me just jump in here and say (to CC) that when you shoot down our ideas and edit out our words, it makes us feel like you do not value our contribution.

CCG4R (CCG4 taps out and is replaced with one of Group 4's audience members): Perhaps we should vote to pick someone else be the leader of the project and someone different to be the final editor.

CC: Well, I see no reason to change the way we are doing things, but if you don't care about getting a good grade, then I guess I don't have any say in this.

I: How can the group help CC reflect on the role of each group member so she can embrace the group's decision to restructure the way the project is being managed?

I: Let's open this discussion up to the audience.

Debriefing of Carol Controller Role Play

Overall, good strategies for reducing conflict were employed by the group. These strategies included the following:

Listen.

State the problem clearly.

Be respectful.

Consider other perspectives.

Be open to compromise.

CC, however, was resistant to seeing her role as a collaborative team player. CC's responses were indicative of poor self-awareness, which ultimately leaves the impression that her motivation to make changes is poor.

All the students want to get a good grade, and this group appreciates the importance making their project unique to their style as a group. CC is confident that she knows the teacher's preferences better than anyone else and even the color scheme is of utmost importance for her to dictate.

Negotiation strategies were successfully employed by most of the group members despite CC's inability to relinquish her control over any aspect of the project. The strategies included the following:

Call a meeting.
State the rationale for the meeting.
Give specific examples that illustrate the problem.
State why it is a problem.
Confirm the facts.
Listen to the other side.

This role play focused on the negotiation of the problem, followed by the discussion related to problem resolution, including:

Make suggestions for a solution.
Confirm feasibility of solution(s) and consider other solutions.
Achieve consensus regarding solution(s).
Offer help to make the changes.
Share responsibility for managing the outcome.

The group suggested changes in the management of the project and voted on the solution to employ. CC was not fully committed to changing the current structure of the project, so implementing the solutions chosen by the group may become an issue.

In regard to the interpersonal approach, it was noted that the group effectively used *I/we* (versus *you*) when presenting the problem and focused on CC's behavior, not on her as a person. However, CC appeared to take the message personally and denied all ownership of the conflict.

REFERENCES

Alden, D. (1999). Experience with scripted role play in environmental economics. *Journal of Economic Education, 20*(2), 127–132.

Bartle, P. (2007). Role playing and simulation games: A training technique. Retrieved from http://cec.vcn.bc.ca/cmp/modules/tm-rply.htm

Corless, I., Gallagher, D., Borans, R., Crary, E., Dolan, S. E., & Kressy, S. (2004). Understanding patient adherence. In A. J. Lowenstein & M. J. Bradshaw (Eds.), *Fuszard's innovative teaching strategies in nursing* (3rd ed., pp. 128–132). Sudbury, MA: Jones and Bartlett.

Corsini, R. J. (1957). *Methods of group psychotherapy.* New York, NY: McGraw-Hill.

Culley, J. M., & Polyakova-Norwood, V. (2012, January/February). Synchronous online role play for enhancing community, collaboration, and oral presentation proficiency. *Nursing Education Perspectives, 33*(1), 51–54.

DeNeve, K. M., & Hepner, M. J. (1997). Role play simulations: The assessment of an active learning technique and comparisons with traditional lectures. *Innovative Higher Education, 21,* 231–246.

Domazzo, R., & Hanson, P. (1997). Community health problems, apparent vs. hidden: A classroom exercise to demonstrate prioritization of community health problems for programs. *Journal of Health Education, 258,* 383–385.

Gordon, G. K. (1970). Human relations: Sensitivity training. In R. M. Smith, G. F. Aker, & J. R. Kidd (Eds.), *Handbook of adult education* (pp. 427–440). New York, NY: Macmillan.

Hess, C. M., & Gilgannon, N. (1985, April). *Gaming: A curriculum technique for elementary counselors.* Paper presented at the Annual Convention of the American Association for Counseling and Development, Los Angeles, CA (ERIC document no. 267327).

Imholz, S. (2008). The therapeutic stage encounters the virtual world. *Thinking Skills and Creativity, 3*(1), 47–52.

Keyton, J., & Beck, S. (2010). Examining laughter functionality in jury deliberations. *Small Group Research, 41*(4), 386–407.

Lane, C., Hood, K., & Rollnick, S. (2008). Teaching motivational interviewing: Using role play is as effective as using simulated patients. *Medical Education, 42,* 637–644.

Lebaron, J., & Miller, D. (2005). The potential of jigsaw role playing to promote the social construction of knowledge in an online graduate education course. *Teachers College Record, 107*(8), 1652–1674.

Mann, S., & Corsun, D. L. (2002). Charting the experiential territory: Clarifying definitions and uses of computer simulation, games and role play. *Journal of Management Development, 21*(9–10), 732–745.

Mar, C. M., Chabal, C., Anderson, R. A., & Vore, A. E. (2003). *Journal of Health Psychology, 8*(1), 161–173.

McKeachie, W. J. (2002). *McKeachie's teaching tips: Strategies, research, and theory for college and university teachers* (11th ed.). Boston, MA: Houghton Mifflin.

Middleton, J. (2005). Role play is not everyone's scene. *Nursing Standard, 19*(24), 31.

Moreno, J. L. (1946). *Psychodrama* (Vol. 1). Boston, MA: Beacon.

Phillips, J. M. (2005). Syllabus selections: Innovative learning activities. Chat role play as an online learning strategy. *Journal of Nursing Education, 44*(1), 43.

Qing, X. (2011). Role play: An effective approach to developing overall communicative competence. *Cross-Cultural Communication, 7*(4), 36–39.

Rabinowitz, F. E. (1997). Teaching counseling through a semester long role play. *Counselor Education and Supervision, 36,* 216–223.

Reams, S., & Bashford, C. (2011, Summer). Interdisciplinary role play: Nursing and theater students advance skills in communication. *Delta Kappa Gamma Bulletin, 77*(4), 42–48.

Riddle, M. D. (2009). The campaign: A case study in identity construction through performance authors. *Association for Learning Technology Journal, 17*(1), 63–72.

Sasha, I. (2011, May 3). Role play ideas for effective communication. Retrieved from http://www.livestrong .com/article/87296-role-play-ideas-effective-communication/

Shaffer, J. B. P., & Galinsky, M. D. (1974). *Models of group therapy and sensitivity training.* Englewood Cliffs, NJ: Prentice-Hall.

Sharon, S., & Sharon, Y. (1976). *Small group teaching.* Englewood Cliffs, NJ: Educational Technology Publications.

Shearer, R., & Davidhizar, R. (2003). Educational innovations: Using role play to develop cultural competence. *Journal of Nursing Education, 42*(6), 273–276.

Silberman, M. (2006). *Active training: A textbook of techniques, designs, case examples, and tips.* Malden, MA: John Wiley and Sons.

Smith-Stoner, M. (2009). Using high-fidelity simulation to educate nursing students about end-of-life care. *Nursing Education Perspectives, 30*(2), 115–120.

Turner, T. (2005). Stage fright. *Nursing Standard, 19*(22), 22–23.

Van Ments, M. (1983). *The effective use of role play: A handbook for teachers and trainers.* London, UK: Kogan Page.

RECOMMENDED READING

Alden, D. (1999). Experience with scripted role play in environmental economics. *Journal of Economic Education, 20*(2), 127–132.

Ashmore, R., & Banks, D. (2004). Student nurses' use of their interpersonal skills within clinical role plays. *Nurse Education Today, 24*(1), 20–29.

Chester, M., & Fox, R. (1996). *Role playing methods in the classroom.* Chicago, IL: Science Research Associates.

Goldenberg, D., Andrusyszyn, M., & Iwasiw, C. (2005). The effect of classroom simulation on nursing students' self-efficacy related to health teaching. *Journal of Nursing Education, 44*(7), 310–314.

Greenberg, E., & Miller, P. (1991). The player and professor: Theatrical techniques in teaching. *Journal of Management Education, 15*(4), 428–446.

Griggs, K. (2005). A role play for revising style and applying management theories. *Business Communication Quarterly, 68*(1), 60–65.

Kane, M. (2003). Teaching direct practice techniques for work with elders with Alzheimer's disease: A simulated group experience. *Educational Gerontology, 29*, 777–794.

Loprinzi, C. L., Johnson, M. E., & Steer, G. (2003). Doc, how much time do I have? *Journal of Clinical Oncology, 21*(9 suppl), 5S–7S.

Northcott, N. (2002). Role play: Proceed with caution! *Nursing Education in Practice, 2* (2), 87–91.

CHAPTER 14

Human Patient Simulation

■ CATHERINE BAILEY ■

Human patient simulations (HPSs), sometimes called high-fidelity patient simulations (HFPSs), have been used by health professional educators for more than 50 years (Rosen, 2008). In addition to HPSs, various other types of simulated experiences have supported the educational needs of healthcare professionals. Software-based simulations have been used to teach anatomy, physiology, pathophysiology, pharmacology, and clinical decision making. Task trainers or low-fidelity simulators, designed to represent specific anatomic areas of the body, have been useful for the acquisition and validation of complex psychomotor, assessment, and diagnostic skills (Decker, Sportsman, Puetz, & Billings, 2008). For example, task trainers have supported the development of technical skills associated with cardiopulmonary resuscitation, airway management, vascular catheter insertion, birthing, and various other invasive and noninvasive procedures. Virtual reality simulation (VRS) is a type of computer-assisted program that makes images appear real by projecting three-dimensional views and using stereo images to provide a sense of being in the environment (Jenson & Forsyth, 2012). VRS environments may be accessed on the World Wide Web and presented on an ordinary computer monitor or on multiple room-sized screens or through a head-mounted stereoscopic unit. VRS has been used to simulate real-life scenarios and provide nursing students with opportunities to practice nursing skills in an interactive environment. This technology has also been used for flight simulators and to support ship navigation through the oceans. For the sake of discussion, the focus of this chapter is on human patient simulations with the use of high-fidelity patient simulators.

■ Definition and Purposes

HFPSs are computerized, life-sized mannequins with complex, interrelated, multisystem physiologic and pharmacologic models that generate observable responses from the mannequin and allow students to interact with the simulator as they would with an actual patient in the clinical environment (Decker et al., 2008). The first human patient simulators were developed in the 1960s, and their use became widespread when anesthesia educators and researchers used simulators to improve education and study clinical performances (Gaba & DeAnda, 1988; Good & Gravenstein, 1989). By the late 1990s, the use of HFPSs evolved from the management of anesthesia to include other types of patient-related care within emergency medicine (Fritz, Gray, & Flanagan, 2008), Armed Forces medicine, pediatrics, surgery, trauma, cardiology, intensive care medicine, dentistry, and military medicine triage (Rosen, 2008). In 2005, computerized infant mannequins were introduced to assist with neonatal resuscitation. Applications of high-fidelity patient simulator use among healthcare providers have included procedure training, evaluation of individual responses to critical incidents, equipment evaluation, task analysis, and team training (Lupien, 2007; Merchant, 2012). Common educational applications of simulation have included theme-based workshops on ventilation, pharmacology, airway management, conscious sedation, disaster response, ongoing skills development, and the practice of clinical decision making.

The first nurse-specific uses of HFPSs were introduced to nurse anesthetists (Fletcher, 1995). After 2000, the use of HFPSs expanded to include the educational activities of prelicensure nursing students, licensed nurses returning to practice, and the validation of clinical judgment and competencies of nurses in the practice setting (Hoffman & Burns, 2011). Areas of focus have included the development of procedural skills, critical thinking, patient safety, the development of safer patient and nurse environments, competency testing of skills, and comprehensive models for the development of the graduate nurse from novice to expert and enhanced teamwork and crisis management skills of healthcare providers (Merchant, 2012; Nehring, 2010).

In the United States, HPSs are supported by the use of automated human patient simulators such as METIman, iStan, Human Patient Simulator (HPS), PediaSim, and BabySim from CAE Healthcare (CAE Healthcare, 2012); SimMan 3G, SimMom, SimBaby, and SimNewB from Laerdal (Laerdal, 2012); and various models of Hal (including preemie and newborn) and Noelle simulators from Gaumard Scientific (Gaumard, 2012). The simulators typically include the following four components: a lifelike mannequin, a freestanding enclosure that contains many of the simulator's components, a computer to integrate the function of the simulator components, and an interface that allows the user to control the simulation and modify physiologic parameters.

Depending on the sophistication of the specific high-fidelity patient simulator, features may include a functioning cardiovascular system with synchronized palpable pulses, heart sounds, measurable blood pressures (by palpation or auscultation), electrocardiographic waveforms, and invasive parameters such as arterial, central venous, and pulmonary artery pressures that may be displayed on a physiologic computer monitor (CAE Healthcare, 2012; Gaumard, 2012; Laerdal, 2012). Respiratory system components include self-regulating spontaneous ventilation, measurable exhaled respiratory gases, and breath sounds. Other simulator features include bowel sounds; speech; pharmacologic systems capable of responding to administered drugs; a urologic system; blinking and reactive pupils; tongue swelling; bronchial occlusion; jugular vein distention; and the ability to accept defibrillation, use of a transthoracic pacemaker, needle cricothyroidotomy, jet ventilation, needle thoracentesis, chest tube insertion, IV fluid administration, intraosseous infusion capability, and pericardiocentesis.

Examples of some modifiable physiologic parameters include changes in heart rates or sounds, respiratory rates or breath sounds, and the quality of bowel sounds. Most of the simulators have both a portable interface allowing instructors to control simulations from either the mannequin's bedside or a remote location where changes can be made without the students' knowledge. To initiate a simulation, the user selects a patient profile, such as a healthy adult male. If desired, a clinical scenario, such as a case that progresses to anaphylaxis, can be superimposed on the physiology of the healthy adult male profile. Once the scenario has been initiated, the instructor may allow the simulation to run as programmed or make on-the-fly modifications to individualize learning opportunities and emphasize specific teaching points.

A well-planned, simulated clinical experience allows the healthcare provider to practice nursing skills under realistic conditions in real time while using actual clinical supplies in a safe and controlled environment (Larew, Lessons, Spunt, Foster, & Covington, 2006). Observable practical advantages of simulation include the ability to replicate critical or common problems, to allow learner-driven management errors to develop, to provide multiple treatment options to be explored without injury or discomfort to a real patient, and to manipulate time as a factor in managing nursing care.

Educational advantages of simulation include opportunities for learners to improve skill performance and critical thinking, gain self-confidence, experience learner satisfaction (Jeffries, 2005; Monti, Wren, Haas, & Lupien, 1998), and gain feedback during debriefing or reflective sessions following the simulation (Fanning & Gaba, 2007). The simulated environment also has the potential of providing a cost-effective strategy to translate the real world of nursing into a standardized setting for testing critical thinking and decision making.

Disadvantages of simulation include the investment costs associated with the initial setup (including the purchase of the simulators and their associated support systems), maintenance of the simulation laboratory, and additional supporting lab personnel (Harlow & Sportsman, 2007; Parker & Myrick, 2008). Thus, the integration of patient simulations into a program's curriculum is resource intensive, as well as time intensive (Radhakrishnan, Roche, & Cunningham, 2007), because the process of preparing and facilitating a simulation is time consuming (Sittner, Schmaderer, Zimmerman, Hertzog, & George, 2009). Finally, the transfer of knowledge to actual clinical practice is not well documented as there remains a need to capture how a simulation experience influences a nurse's knowledge and clinical judgment on actual patient outcomes.

■ Theoretical Foundations

The landmark Flexner Report to the Carnegie Foundation in 1910 established the dominant paradigm for healthcare education in the 20th century (Beck, 2004).

Two key components of the model were to practice scientific medicine while the learner was also engaged in laboratory experimentation and hands-on care at the bedside. The scientific curriculum had historically featured lecture-based instruction during the first two years of training where students were passive recipients of factual scientific knowledge (Papa & Harasym, 1999). Information was imparted by domain experts according to a predetermined timetable. Although the lecture format assured that the important educational material had been disseminated, the learner was at risk of lacking the conceptual links that were necessary for retention of the information. By contrast, the clinical practicum involved students more effectively as active participants with a contextual experience for the facts that they had learned. (Clinical reasoning was discussed more thoroughly previously in this text.)

Achieving a successful balance between academic and clinical education has challenged educators who must prepare graduates for healthcare institutions with both broad-based knowledge and technologically current specialty clinical skills (Manuel & Sorenson, 1995). These expectations have in the past created a sense of placing classroom learning, viewed as the foundation of academic priorities, in competition with the need for clinical experiences, a workplace priority. From the perspective of situated cognition, both classroom and clinical experiences are equally necessary as knowledge is believed to be situated as a product of the activity, context, and culture in which it is used and not just something that happens inside of a person's head (Brown, Collins & Duguid, 1989). The principles of the situated cognitive framework include:

1. Thinking and learning as measures of knowledge make sense only within particular situations.
2. People act and construct meaning within communities of practice.
3. Knowledge depends on the use of a variety of artifacts and tools.
4. Situations make sense within a historical context (Paige & Daley, 2009, p. e99).

With the synthesis of the aforementioned situated cognition principles and the characteristic needs of nursing education, three interacting components may be used to support learners in their quest for knowledge (Paige & Daley, 2009). The interacting components of a situated cognitive framework may be viewed as people (including the community or more specifically patients, families, nurses, physicians, and ancillary personnel), ingredients or tools (including prior knowledge or concepts), and activity (including participation in real-life events). **Figure 14-1** shows a graphic representation of the situated cognition framework.

Learning that is structured within the situated cognition framework and the application of HPS offers nursing educators a strategy to bridge a student's advancement from theory-based knowledge to practice and social integration into professional nursing (Paige & Daley, 2009). For explanation purposes, Paige and Daley described a case of the care of a patient experiencing unstable angina. An HPS provided

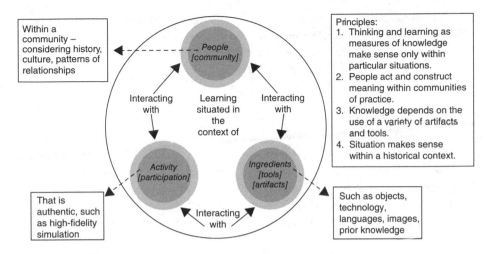

▪ Figure 14-1   Situated cognition framework.

Source: From Situation cognition: A learning framework to support and guide high-fidelity simulation, by J. B. Paige and B. J. Daley, 2009. *Clinical Simulation in Nursing,* 5 (p. e99). Copyright 2009 by Elsevier. Reprinted with permission.

students with opportunities to transfer knowledge that was enhanced by an environment, in which they needed to page the physician, provide a status report, take verbal orders, and prepare a drug for administration. The construction of meaning within the community of practice was exemplified by the necessity to meet the needs of the simulated patient, which included providing answers to the patient's questions about chest pain and interventions to reduce pain and anxiety. The ingredients or tools included the student's prior knowledge of the concept of pain that demanded an understanding of pain that was tailored to the unique needs of a patient with cardiac tissue ischemia. Finally, the principle of the historic context that encompassed cultural practices, values, and strategies of thinking and perceiving were viewed as inculturation into the healthcare environment with a review of the roles and responsibilities of professional nurses.

The simulated environment can promote the role of the teacher as an active participant and role model. Because clinical situations may be repeated as desired, the teacher can act initially as a role model by demonstrating a procedure or decision-making process and then allow the student to practice in an identical or similar situation. By contrast, in the actual clinical setting, the faculty member who actively models a procedure, such as insertion of an intravenous catheter, often provides the demonstration at the expense of the student, who may not be able to repeat the process with another patient. The timing of simulated experiences can be scheduled to reinforce recently introduced material from the classroom, with the level of difficulty adjusted to match the student's capabilities. The ability to create an active learning environment that has been customized for each student is a compelling argument for the addition of an HPS to the instructional armamentarium of nurse educators.

Simulation Framework for Nursing Education

Jeffries (2005, 2007) has developed a simulation framework for nursing education. The model provides guidance for the design and implementation of simulations as well as expected outcomes. Accordingly, variables of the model include the simulation design characteristics, teacher, student, educational practices, and outcomes, which include learning, skill performance, learner satisfaction, critical thinking, and self-confidence. **Figure 14-2** provides a graphic representation of the Nursing Education Simulation Framework.

A review of the literature indicates that the model has been recognized as a useful framework for the implementation of research designs in nursing education. Following a study that compared students who prepared for pediatric clinical experiences with simulation to those who did not, skill performance levels, such as therapeutic skills, documentation scores, and interpersonal communication, were significantly higher during the clinical rotation for those who prepared with simulation than for those students who did not (Meyer, Connors, Hou, & Gajewski, 2011).

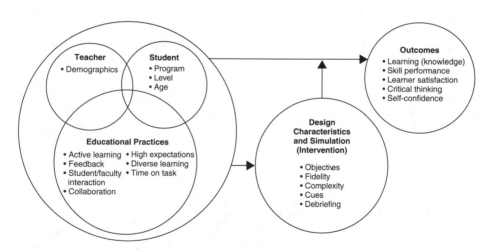

■ **Figure 14-2** The nursing simulation framework.

Source: From Simulation in nursing education: From conceptualization to evaluation (p. 23), by P. R. Jeffries, 2007, New York: National League of Nursing. Copyright 2009 by the National League of Nursing, New York, NY. Reprinted with permission.

Clinical Judgment Model

The Clinical Judgment Model (CJM) (Tanner, 2006) is an example of a conceptual framework that describes the variety of reasoning processes that nurses experience as they provide care in complex patient care situations (also discussed previously in this text). As clinical learning is one of the outcomes of clinical judgment, the model implies that nurses are continually learning as they develop their expertise through experiences and reflection. Components of the model include noticing, interpreting, responding, and reflecting. These components suggest that the nurse must be aware of the patient's needs, make sense of the situation, and respond with the best course of action, which will be submitted to reflection after outcomes are realized and evaluated. **Figure 14-3** displays the Clinical Judgment Model developed by Tanner (2006).

Lasater Clinical Judgment Rubric

Lasater (2007) developed the Lasater Clinical Judgment Rubric (LCJR) from the conceptual framework of the CJM (Tanner, 2006) in an attempt to provide a measure of clinical judgment skills. The four phases of the CJM—noticing, interpreting, responding, and reflecting—provided the basis for the rubric with 11 dimensions (Lasater, 2007). Effective noticing involves focused observations, recognizing deviations from expected patterns, and information seeking. Effective interpreting involves prioritizing data and making sense of data. Effective responding involves a calm,

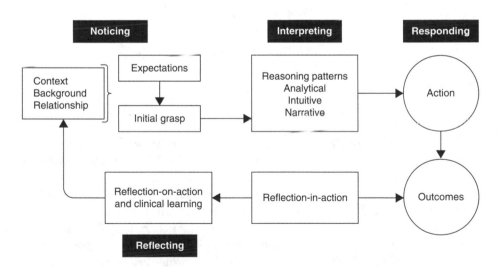

■ **Figure 14-3** Clinical judgment model.

Source: Reprinted with permission from Slack Incorporated, copyright 2009. From Thinking like a nurse: A research-based model of clinical judgement in nursing, 2006, *Journal of Nursing Education,* 45, p. 208.

confident manner, clear communication, well-planned intervention/flexibility, and being skillful. Effective reflecting involves evaluation/self-analysis and commitment to improvement. The rubric offers students an opportunity to reflect on their performance for each dimension and rate themselves as exemplary, accomplished, developing, or beginning following a simulation experience.

Through the efforts of three research teams, the LCJR has reportedly met the criteria for instrument validity and intrarater and interrater reliability during HPS (Adamson, Gubrud, Sideras, & Lasater, 2012). Adamson and Kardong-Edgren (2012) used a database of standardized, validated, video-archived simulations that depicted nursing students performing at three different scripted levels of proficiency, while nurse educator observers rated the student behaviors as below expectations, at level of expectations, and above expectations. Gubrud-Howe (2008) reported acceptable interrater reliability of observations with the LCJR during rater training and also following a pretest and posttest design when pairs of students working as registered nurses were observed during 50-minute-long simulations. Sideras (2007) demonstrated that four observers, who not informed of the educational levels of the nursing students, could apply the LCJR and accurately differentiate between the clinical judgment performance of graduating seniors and end-of-junior-year-level student abilities from three recorded simulation cases as a type of validity for known groups. Despite the reported achievement of instrument reliability, Adamson, Sideras, and Lasater (2012) suggested that researchers still need to (1) identify the locations of variability in reliability of the LCJR under different conditions of use, (2) identify the true ranges of students' clinical judgment abilities, (3) avoid cases of complex simulation scenarios where floor and ceiling effects influence rating responses, and (4) establish standards of rater training for the instrument.

■ Types of Learners

The Russian psychologist Vygotsky (1978) believed that learning was most effective when it occurred within the zone of proximal development, where the content of learning was just beyond the current knowledge level of the student. Thus, each simulation session can be adjusted to the optimal level of difficulty for a particular student or group, from beginner through expert and technical levels, by altering the delivery of care setting, patient history, clinical conditions, and patient sensitivity to therapeutic interventions. For example, beginning emergency and critical care students who are learning to recognize the signs of acute myocardial infarction may be asked to provide care for a patient with a robust cardiovascular system where signs of myocardial ischemia develop gradually without precipitating a cardiac arrest, whereas a more advanced student would be expected to recognize subtle physiologic clues quickly and initiate prompt, effective interventions. Nurse anesthetists, acute care nurse practitioners, respiratory therapists, or emergency care students who are learning basic principles of airway management can use the simulator as a task trainer to refine fundamental skills such as insertion of pharyngeal airways and bag-valve-mask ventilation in an apneic patient using oxygen saturation and respiratory gas measurements to guide ventilation. Alternatively, advanced students may be expected to perform sophisticated airway procedures to include tracheal intubation and needle cricothyroidotomy in simulated patients with an abnormal airway anatomy.

▪ Conditions for Learning

Because of the ability to create customized learning scenarios, HPSs can be used in a wide variety of situations for all types of students. Simulation may be useful to precede, complement, or replace actual clinical experiences. For example, prior to clinical experiences, simulation has been used to orient students to care on an unfamiliar unit. Meyer and colleagues (2011) prepared student nurses with a 6-hour curriculum over 4 days of caring for pediatric patients in an HPS setting prior to entering their clinical rotation. During the simulations, they practiced taking vital signs; administering medications; communicating with healthcare providers, the child, and the child's parents; and documentation. When compared to their peers who did not participate in these simulations, students who did participate demonstrated more significant and positive effects on therapeutic skills, scores in documentation, and interpersonal communication during their clinical rotations (Meyer et al., 2011).

Used concomitantly with clinical practice, simulation provides students and faculty with the opportunity to replicate real clinical experiences and then use the simulator for reflection to explore alternative strategies for managing the situation. Students also have the opportunity to create customized patients based on their knowledge of physiology and pathophysiology and then compare the responses of their simulated patients to patients observed in clinical practices (Register, Graham-Garcia, & Haas, 2003).

Although the fidelity of HPSs is not sufficiently developed to replace the practice of caring for human patients, simulation can be used to create learning opportunities that are not ordinarily available in most clinical environments. For example, students can practice high-risk technical procedures such as defibrillation, using actual equipment in real time, or provide patient care during cardiopulmonary resuscitation or anaphylactic reactions on the simulator.

Simulation has also been used to develop higher-order skills in ways that exactly parallel applications of simulation in commercial aviation. Aviation simulation has expanded beyond its use as a teaching/training tool for individual pilots to encompass team training through crew resource management (Helmreich & Foushee, 1993). Similarly, in the field of anesthesiology, programs such as Anesthesia Crisis Resource Management (ACRM) (Gaba, Howard, Fish, & Smith, 2001) and Team Oriented Medical Simulation focused on the actions of all members of a healthcare team with the goal of improving team performance (Baker, Gustafson, Beaubien, Salas, & Barach, 2005). Following an analysis of the documented effects of HPS in hospital-based education programs, Merchant (2012) concluded that simulation offered nurse educators enhanced learning opportunities with an ability to measure clinical performance during certain aspects of nursing care. Specifically, efforts that focused on teamwork-related competencies and crisis management demonstrated positive clinical outcomes that included error reduction, decreased mortality rates, cost reductions, and increased patient safety in high-risk circumstances.

In addition to its uses as an instructional tool, simulation has been recognized for its potential for formative and summative evaluation of student skills. Techniques for formative evaluation of student performances include using simulation as a mechanism for providing feedback on current skills and decision-making processes or to observe progression of a student's competencies. Instruments that are appropriate for formative evaluation offer insights into the pedagogy of simulation and measure students' self-perceptions about their learning and self-confidence, which can guide faculty decisions for future simulations (Cordi, Leighton, Ryan-Wenger, Doyle, & Ravert, 2012). The Simulation Effectiveness Tool (SET) is an example of a newly revised, 13-item, 3-point ordinal scale that has achieved an acceptable criterion (0.80) for reliability for its total simulation effectiveness score (Cordi et al., 2012).

Applications of simulation in summative evaluation are controversial because the relationship between the performance of the student in a simulated environment and the actual clinical setting has not been demonstrated, and descriptions of the psychometric properties to measure these relationships are limited. Adamson, Kardong-Edgren, and Willhaus (2012) have reported that the literature is full of low-level participant evaluations that address how learners reacted to a learning process. Adamson and colleagues stressed that there is a serious need to measure what really matters from a perspective of translational research and to identify how simulation affects not only learners and their behaviors, but also patient outcomes. These types of goals suggest that more researchers should focus on developing measurement instruments that are appropriate for the specific populations and activities that they are intended to measure in addition to having sufficient reliability and validity scores.

■ Resources

Although a design for best practices in simulation facilities has not been established, planners have been advised to focus on the intended function of the environment by integrating the concepts of clinical, educational, and theatrical environments (Seropian & Lavey, 2010). For example, types of rooms to consider would include an open learning area; a simulation theater; a control room; a room for debriefing, observations, or conferencing; a supply room; preparation areas; medication rooms; server rooms; rest rooms; offices; and reception areas. However, the most basic critical aspect of a successful simulation program is the designation of dedicated physical space for the simulator and its support equipment. To accommodate the simulator, instructor, and four to six students requires approximately 250 square feet of floor space. A sample floor plan for a simple simulation room is presented in **Figure 14-4**.

■ Figure 14-4 Sample floor plan for a simple simulation room.

Simulators require electricity and in the case of student anesthetists, gas sources, which could include oxygen, carbon dioxide, and nitrogen. Nitrous oxide is optional for simulation of general anesthesia. Electricity requirements include two to four outlets for the simulator plus additional sources of power for patient care equipment. Depending on the type of simulation selected, patient care equipment may include physiologic monitors, infusion pumps, ventilators, anesthesia machines, and a defibrillator. Support equipment includes airway devices, needles and syringes, dressings, chest tubes, intravenous and urinary catheters, scrub wear, gloves, surgical masks, caps, and gowns.

The efficacy of simulation can be enhanced through a video recording of sessions with subsequent debriefing. Recording systems range from a single video camera to complex recording systems that allow multiple camera views, superimposed physiologic waveforms, and audio recordings from participants and faculty. Dedicated simulation centers include a debriefing room where the videotapes can be reviewed. The debriefing room may also have the ability to receive live video and audio transmissions from the training room for the purpose of observation or simultaneous instruction of other students.

Simulation centers also include a control room adjacent to the training room. One-way glass windows between the rooms allow individuals in a control room to observe simulation sessions as the operator and faculty communicate via headsets with microphones. In this type of room arrangement, a technician or faculty member in the control room is responsible for monitoring the simulation, making adjustments to the scenario as necessary, and selecting video and audio sources for recording.

Because simulation is so resource intensive, adequate personnel support is essential. Depending on the type of simulators and the selected scenario, key faculty with moderate computer skills may be adequately prepared to support simulation activities on an as-needed basis, although many centers have found it beneficial to designate one faculty member or an associate to coordinate simulation activities and maintain the simulator.

■ Using the Method

The desire to promote the most appropriate and efficacious use of HPS associated with the education and evaluation of nurse-related health care has prompted a need to provide empirically supported guidance for these efforts. There are two major nursing resources that provide this type of support—the International Nursing Association for Clinical Simulation and Learning (INACSL) and the National League for Nursing (NLN).

The mission of the INACSL is to promote research and disseminate evidence-based practice standards for clinical simulation methodologies and learning environments (INACSL, n.d.). Its stated vision is to be nursing's portal to the world of clinical simulation pedagogy and learning environments. *Clinical Simulation in Nursing*, an international, peer-reviewed journal published online nine times annually, is the official journal for the INACSL. The INACSL has published standards of best practice for simulation that relate to the terminology used, professional integrity of participants, participant objectives, facilitation methods, the simulation facilitator, debriefing processes, and the evaluation of expected outcomes (INACSL Board of Directors, 2011). The website for the INACSL for informational purposes can be accessed at https://inacsl.org/.

The NLN promotes excellence in nursing education to build a strong and diverse nursing workforce to advance the nation's health (NLN, n.d.). The NLN has provided the Simulation Innovation Resource Center (SIRC), an online e-learning site where nursing faculty can learn how to develop and integrate simulation into their curriculum and engage in dialogue with experts and peers (NLN, n.d.). *Nursing Education Perspectives* is the research peer-reviewed bimonthly journal for the NLN. It provides an evidence base for best practices and a forum for the exchange of information regarding teaching and learning with simulation technology, among other issues important to nursing education. Online access to NLN-promoted courses and research for simulation strategies can be found at http://sirc.nln.org/.

Generally speaking, successful simulation sessions depend on carefully planned scenarios and clearly defined roles of the participants. The primary instructor is responsible for selecting the scenario, guiding students through the simulation, providing important information and clinical cues that are not immediately available from the simulator, providing transition cues to a simulator operator, modeling behaviors, monitoring student performance, and troubleshooting in the event of an unexpected simulator issue. In some situations, the faculty may be assisted by another faculty member or technician who may serve as the simulator operator. In this case, the operator's responsibilities would include activating the simulation system, starting the patient software, overlaying the clinical scenarios, monitoring the progress of a scenario, and adjusting the scenario as it was intended to be by the primary instructor. Depending on the expertise of the faculty, the complexity of the scenario, and the type of simulator, one individual may serve as both the faculty member and the operator. A complex scenario, however, may require not only an instructor and operator, but additional faculty, students, or assistants to role-play as members of the healthcare team and family.

Scenario Development

To develop and implement a new simulation scenario, the following seven-step process is recommended:

1. *Determine educational objectives or goals.* For example, the simulation may be intended to promote the advancement of technical, cognitive, or behavioral abilities or a combination of these competencies. The instructor should determine in advance whether the progression of the simulation will be constrained to unfold with a predetermined sequence or develop spontaneously.

2. *Construct a clinical scenario to facilitate attainment of educational objectives.* While the scenario should be clinically realistic, it should be customized to the student's level of expertise and designed to promote the student's successful progression toward a higher level of decision making and demonstration of competencies.

3. *Define underlying physiologic concepts to be manifested throughout the scenario as they relate to the patient's responses to various events as they occur.* The primary instructor determines which essential elements of the clinical scenario are to be represented in the simulation experience, which elements may be absent or overlooked, and which missing elements need to be integrated into the experience. For example, as a patient develops a progressive hypoxemia, tachypnea and decreasing hemoglobin saturation, as measured by pulse oximetry, are expected to occur. Although a real patient would also eventually become cyanotic, the instructor must decide whether the observation of skin color changes should be a necessary part of the educational objectives. When considering the accuracy of clinical situations, it is also essential to decide whether changes need to be technically accurate or sufficiently realistic and prominent to elicit the intended response from the learners.

4. *Modify programmed patients and scenarios, as necessary.* Program modification generally includes specifying the baseline physiology and clinical condition of the underlying patient, preparing the scenario to include optional modifiable states, and defining transitions between various patient states as the scenario evolves.

5. *Identify required equipment.* The instructor decides which devices will be displayed prominently or stored (as they might be in the clinical environment);

whether learners will have the opportunity to inspect, assemble, and test equipment prior to the experience; and if the student will have options among multiple devices for use in the simulation. The instructor also determines whether additional personnel will be required to implement the clinical scenario, the qualifications (both actual and the role played) of the additional participants, and how primary learners will be able to access/involve the supplemental personnel resources.

6. *Run program and collect feedback.* Prior to use with students, the scenario should be run to establish that the simulation scenario unfolds as designed, with the intended levels of instructor and faculty participation.

7. *Reiterate steps until satisfied.* The simulation scenario is continuously refined until it unfolds as intended, without unintentionally ambiguous details that distract from the attainment of the educational objectives, and the faculty is able to concentrate on observing and evaluating the student's performance while maintaining a positive effective learning environment.

Once the simulated scenario begins, the instructor may participate in a variety of ways. The instructor may function as a role model who demonstrates critical thinking, decision making, and therapeutic interventions; as a coach who is available to help students when necessary; or as a passive bystander observing the scenario with minimal involvement. Regardless of the level of participation during the simulation, one of the instructor's key responsibilities is to facilitate the debriefing session afterward to reinforce the objectives of the scenario and to ensure that the intended learning occurred. During an ideal debriefing session, through reflective thinking, the students should have opportunities to describe and interpret the scenario, clarify their thoughts and actions as they occurred during the simulation, critique their performance in a nonthreatening way, and generate alternative decisions and plans of actions that would improve future performances.

▪ Potential Problems

Perhaps the most significant potential problem with simulation is its dependency on faculty support and the time it takes to feel comfortable while using the technology for nursing teaching. Although issues revolving around the learning curve associated with faculty use of simulation have been recognized as barriers for its implementation, little has been reported in the literature. However, the concern for the estimated amount of time faculty members of undergraduate nursing programs perceived it would take them to plan, implement, and evaluate the use of SimMan to teach clinical skills was studied by Jones and Hegge (2008). The results indicated that a majority of faculty respondents estimated that they would need a 0.50 full-time equivalent release for one semester. Thus the researchers recommended a need for administrative support to identify funding mechanisms for faculty training and planning sessions.

A second limitation to HPS is its incomplete presentation of reality. Participants in a simulation are expected to suspend disbelief and respond to the patient according to what they observe. Although simulators provide lifelike representations of human beings, they are not capable of exhibiting a complete range of signs and behaviors. Thus, instructors need to be aware of the critical cues that are absent or that contradict the intended signs and provide missing cues that are necessary for the appropriate advancement of the scenario.

Another potential problem with simulation is controlling the overgeneralization of findings during HPS to the real world. At least two types of generalization errors can occur. The first type is generalizing an observed response in one situation to all patients. For example, whenever a baseline-healthy, 70-kg patient receives an intravenous bolus of 20 µg (microgram) epinephrine, the heart rate is raised approximately 20 beats per minute. Caution must be exerted to avoid the generalization that to increase any patient's heart rate by 20 beats, a dose of 20 µg epinephrine can be administered. To overcome this limitation, faculty can introduce the learners to a series of similar-appearing patients with slightly different physiologic parameters such as body weight, oxygen consumption, or baroreceptor responses. By using these similar patients interchangeably, students may see variations in drug responses.

The second error of generalization is an incorrect attribution of simulation responses. As an incomplete representation of a human patient, simulators do not represent a completely accurate or comprehensive clinical portrait. For example, the simulator patient, when breathing spontaneously, cannot create high negative pressures like a human is capable of generating. Therefore, using the simulator to practice measuring inspiratory effort would lead to inaccurate results. Faculty who understand how simulators function will quickly recognize which clinical findings are authentic and which are artifacts. Simulation sessions can then be designed to take advantage of areas where the simulator provides a reasonable portrayal of a real human and avoid involving students in activities that are different than would be expected under actual clinical conditions.

Finally, participants are sometimes hypervigilant during simulation sessions because they anticipate the onset of a clinical problem. This has been demonstrated by students during a scenario related to the care of a patient with anaphylaxis. Although hypervigilance cannot be avoided completely, its effect can be minimized by either mixing routine and critical event simulations or developing a series of potential events that evolve from a common scenario stem.

■ Conclusion

Simulation is an exciting application of advanced technology in healthcare education. Due to the ongoing refinements of simulators, enthusiasm for HPS has stimulated an interest in the development of new simulation applications in settings not possible 12 years ago. Lashley (2010) anticipates greater opportunities of HPS use as simulation centers become available to shared partnerships among the professions between educational groups and healthcare agencies. In addition to nursing education, the popular use of HPS has potential applications in the areas of nursing licensure, advanced practice nursing credentialing, orientation programs, and continuing education.

Before the previously mentioned anticipated uses of HPS become a reality, there is much work to be done. For example, Weaver (2011) reported a need for more study in areas of communication that address the feedback and support given to participants during and after simulation. In order to effectively bridge the gap between static classroom-based instruction and the dynamic, unpredictable clinical environment, there is a need to investigate the transfer of knowledge from the simulation environment to the clinical setting among students as well as newly graduated nurses. Although there is agreement associated with the importance of performance evaluations in nursing education, there is a need for researchers to develop specific measurement instruments that are useful for translating statistically valid HPS findings into the clinical setting (Adamson & Kardong-Edgren, 2012; Harder, 2010). Additionally, educational research methods must develop collaborative relationships between academia and the clinicians to provide data that support the validity and reliability of the many simulators available for clinical education and research (Schaefer et al., 2011).

With evidence that is supported by quality outcomes, Jeffries (2009) has suggested that simulation may eventually be used for the majority of the clinical time for nursing education to overcome the issues, such as "decreased numbers of clinical sites, patient safety issues, and the many rules and regulations required by clinical agencies' regulatory bodies and their effect on the amount and quality of education instructors can provide their students" (p. 71). The National League for Nursing has begun to lay the groundwork for use of a simulation-based assessment that may eventually establish a recommended simulation curriculum for nursing education (Holmboe, Rizzolo, Sachdeva, Rosenberg, & Ziv, 2011).

TEACHING EXAMPLE:

Using High-Fidelity Simulation in an Undergraduate Critical Care Nursing Course

This example[1] illustrates how simulation was used to reinforce concepts of respiratory assessment and nursing care as part of a critical care nursing elective for senior-level undergraduate nursing students. The course included 40 didactic hours and was designed to complement a 200-hour clinical practicum. The course focused on pulmonary, cardiovascular, and neurologic critical care; advanced hemodynamic monitoring; and critical care pharmacology. The respiratory care section of the course included lectures on respiratory gas exchange, advanced assessment techniques, arterial blood gas analysis, airway management, and ventilatory support. To complement the lectures, a seven-step process was used to develop a simulation session.

1. *Determine educational objective.* The simulation session was designed so that the student would be able to achieve the following objectives:
   - Complete and continuously revise the assessment of a patient who is acutely and dynamically ill.
   - Select appropriate oxygen therapy devices for a specified clinical situation.
   - Collect and prepare the appropriate equipment and medications for emergent tracheal intubation.
   - Administer appropriate medications to facilitate emergent tracheal intubation and assess the drug effects.
   - Perform airway management procedures, as indicated, to include bag-valve-mask ventilation, tracheal intubation, and insertion of an endotracheal tube.
   - Confirm appropriate placement of an endotracheal tube.
   - Prepare an unstable patient for transport from an inpatient unit to a critical care unit.
   - Initiate positive-pressure ventilatory support for an acutely ill patient and adjust ventilatory parameters (to include mode, FiO_2, tidal volume, respiratory rate, and positive-end expiratory pressure) as indicated by patient condition, arterial blood gases, capnography, and spirometry.

   Although the scenario involved only nursing students, it can be easily expanded to include respiratory and emergency care providers. The instructor was actively involved in the session as a coach who provided interactive feedback to students and helped them clarify clinical observations.

2. *Construct a clinical scenario.* Students were told that they were going to evaluate a patient with pneumonia hospitalized on an inpatient medical unit. A brief patient history was provided.

   Students were given the opportunity to assess the patient, including observation of respiratory effort, lung auscultation, estimation of arterial oxygenation by pulse oximetry, and measurement and analysis of arterial blood gases. At the time of initial contact, the patient demonstrated signs of moderate hypoxia to include rapid, shallow breathing, mild oxyhemoglobin desaturation, and rales on chest auscultation. Upon a signal from the instructor to the simulator operator, the patient experienced significant oxyhemoglobin desaturation.

   The scenario was designed so that the patient initially would require oxygen therapy and then required more aggressive treatment including tracheal intubation and positive-pressure ventilation using a bag-valve device with both face mask and tracheal tube. Once the patient was transferred to the critical care unit, ventilatory support using various modes such as assist control, intermittent mandatory ventilation, positive-end expiratory pressure, and pressure support ventilation could be explored.

(continued)

3. *Define underlying physiologic concepts to be manifested through the scenario—patient and events.* The physiologic concepts underlying pneumonia include decreased lung compliance and increased shunt. Manifestations of these alterations include an adaptive respiratory pattern with increased rate and smaller tidal volume, increased peak inspiratory pressure, hypoxemia, mild hypercarbia, rales, tachycardia, and cardiac dysrhythmias. Patient deterioration within the scenario resulted from progressive reductions in lung compliance and increases in shunt. For this exercise, it was determined that sufficient physiologic changes to induce learner critical thinking, decision making, and action were more important than technical accuracy.

4. *Modify programmed patient and scenarios, as necessary.* A geriatric model developed by faculty and master's-level nursing anesthesia students was used.[2] To exhibit signs of pneumonia, rales were introduced, lung compliance was decreased, shunt fraction was increased, and the CO_2 set point was increased slightly (to produce mild hypercarbia). Temperature was increased slightly to reflect an underlying infective process. As a result of these changes, tidal volume decreased automatically and respiratory rate increased to compensate for the reduced tidal volume. Physiologic alterations were also manifested automatically through changes in heart rate and arterial blood gases.

So that the patient would initially appear to be stable and then deteriorate upon the instructor's command, baseline and decompensation states were created. Although an automatic transition could have initiated the decompensation at a predetermined time, a manual transition was selected to assure that the destabilization occurred when intended by the instructor.

5. *Assemble required equipment.* Because the patient was not physically transported from the medical unit to the critical care unit, the simulation lab was originally configured with equipment available to acute care personnel. Items included a resuscitation cart with cardiac monitor and defibrillator, an oxygen source, oxygen therapy devices, various airway management devices such as a bag-value-mask device, pharyngeal airways, endotracheal tubes, laryngoscopes, and suction equipment. Once the scenario shifted to the critical care unit, a positive-pressure ventilator was also available for student use.

6. *Run program and collect feedback.* Prior to use with students, the scenario was run several times to observe the rate of change for physiologic variables and the effects of various therapeutic options.

7. *Reiterate steps 2–6 until satisfied.* Physiologic parameters were modified incrementally so that the patient would appear stable, but with sufficient respiratory compromise to entice the learner to initiate oxygen therapy. Once the deterioration sequence was initiated, the decompensation needed to be sufficient to warrant more aggressive therapy yet progress at a rate such that novice nurses with limited skills and therapeutic options could stabilize the patient.

To implement the simulation, the instructor selects the customized geriatric patient from the Patient Options menu of the user interface and respiratory exercise from the Scenario Options menu. The simulator immediately begins emulating the pneumonia patient in the stable baseline state. Progression to the decompensation state requires only one additional keystroke or mouse click.

Careful testing of the simulated patient and clinical scenario reduces the likelihood of unanticipated events during the educational session; however, the instructor should be prepared to help students with assembling and using unfamiliar equipment as well as performing advanced technical skills, such as effective bag-valve-mask ventilation and tracheal intubation. Careful coordination with the simulator operator will allow the patient to deteriorate at a rate appropriate for the experience of the learners with pauses in the deterioration, if desired, during specific teaching moments or as technical maneuvers are performed.

For this exercise, evaluation of the learner achievement was formative and informal. After the simulated patient's condition was stabilized, the faculty and students reflected on clinical signs observed and how the patient's condition, clinical setting, and events affected decision making and actions; medications, devices, and procedures used to stabilize the patient; and potential alternative solutions that would have led to more rapid or improved outcomes.

[1]Scenario developed by Beverly George-Gay, MSN, CCRN; assistant professor and coordinator of distance and continuing education: Department of Nurse Anesthesia, Virginia Commonwealth University, Richmond, VA.

[2]Development of the geriatric model was supported, in part, by a grant from the Division of Nursing, U.S. Department of Health and Human Services, Bureau of Health Professions.

REFERENCES

Adamson, K. A., Gubrud, P., Sideras, S., & Lasater, K. (2012). Assessing the reliability, validity, and use of the Lasater Clinical Judgment Rubric: Three approaches. *Journal of Nursing Education, 51*(2), 66–73. doi: 10.3928/01484834-20111130-03

Adamson, K. A., & Kardong-Edgren, S. (2012). A method and resources for assessing the reliability of simulation evaluation instruments. *Nursing Education Perspectives, 33*(5), 334–339. Retrieved from http://www.nln.org/nlnjournal/index.htm

Adamson, K. A., Kardong-Edgren, S., & Willhaus, J. (2012). An updated review of published simulation evaluation instruments. *Clinical Simulation in Nursing.* Advance online publication. Retrieved from http://dx.doi.org/10.1016/j.ecns.2012.09.004

Baker, D. P., Gustafson, S., Beaubien, J. M., Salas, E., & Barach, P. (2005). Medical team training programs in health care. In Agency for Healthcare Research and Quality, *Advances in patient safety: From research to implementation* (AHRQ publication No. 050021-4, pp. 253–267). Rockville, MD: Author. Retrieved from http://www.ahrq.gov/downloads/pub/advances/vol4/Baker.pdf

Beck, A. H. (2004). The Flexner Report and the standardization of American medical education. *Journal of American Medical Association, 291*(17), 2139–2140. Retrieved from http://jama.jamanetwork.com/journal.aspx

Brown, J. S., Collins, A., & Duguid, P. (1989). Situated cognition and the culture of learning. *Educational Researcher, 18*, 32–42. Retrieved from http://edr.sagepub.com/

CAE Healthcare. (2012). *METIman*. Retrieved from https://caehealthcare.com/0/eng/product_services /product_details/metiman#

Cordi, V. L., Leighton, K., Ryan-Wenger, N., Doyle, T., & Ravert, P. (2012). History and development of the Simulation Effectiveness Tool (SET). *Clinical Simulation in Nursing, 8*, e199–e210. doi: 10.1016 /jecns.2011.12.001

Decker, S., Sportsman, S., Puetz, L., & Billings, L. (2008). The evolution of simulation and its contribution to competency. *Journal of Continuing Education in Nursing, 39*(2), 74–80. Retrieved from http://www .slackinc.com/subscribe/jcen.asp

Fanning, R. M., & Gaba, D. M. (2007). The role of debriefing in simulation-based learning. *Society for Simulation in Healthcare, 2*(2), 115–125.

Fletcher, J. L. (1995). AANA journal course: Update for nurse anesthetists—Anesthesia simulation: A tool for learning and research. *Journal of the American Association of Nurse Anesthetists, 63*, 61–67. Retrieved from http://www.aana.com/newsandjournal/Pages/aanajournalonline.aspx

Fritz, P. Z., Gray, T., & Flanagan, B. (2008). Review of mannequin-based high fidelity simulation in emergency medicine. *Emergency Medicine Australasia, 20*, 1–9. Retrieved from http://onlinelibrary .wiley.com/journal/10.1111/(ISSN)1742-6723

Gaba, D., & DeAnda, A. (1988). A comprehensive anesthesia simulation environment: Recreating the operating room for research and training. *Anesthesiology, 69*, 387–394.

Gaba, D. M., Howard, S. K., Fish, K. J., & Smith, B. E. (2001). Simulation-based training in anesthesia crisis resource management (ACRM): A decade of experience. *Simulation & Gaming, 32*(2), 175–193. Retrieved from http://sag.sagepub.com/

Gaumard. (2012). *Simulators for health care education*. Retrieved from http://www.gaumard.com/

Good, M. I., & Gravenstein, J. S. (1989). Anaesthesia simulators and training devices. *International Anesthesiology Clinics, 27*, 161–166. Retrieved from http://journals.lww.com/anesthesiaclinics/pages /default.aspx

Gubrud-Howe, P. M. (2008). *Development of clinical judgment in nursing students: A learning framework to use in designing and implementing simulated learning experiences* (Unpublished dissertation). Portland State University, Portland, OR.

Harder, N. (2010). Use of simulation in teaching and learning in health sciences: A systematic review. *Journal of Nursing Education, 49*(1), 23–28. doi: 10.3928/014834-20090828-28

Harlow, K. C., & Sportsman, S. (2007). An economic analysis of patient simulators for clinical training in nursing education. *Nursing Economics, 25*(1), 24–29.

Helmreich, R. L., & Foushee, H. C. (1993). Why crew resource management? Empirical and theoretical basis of human factors training in aviation. In E. L. Weiner, B. G. Kanki, & R. L. Helmreich (Eds.), *Cockpit resource management* (pp. 3–46). London, UK: Academic Press.

Hoffman, R. L., & Burns, H. K. (2011). Using high-fidelity simulation as a teaching strategy with baby boomers returning to the RN workforce. *Journal of Nurses in Staff Development, 27*(6), 262–265. doi: 1097/NND.0b013e31823097e9

Holmboe, E., Rizzolo, M. A., Sachdeva, A. K., Rosenberg, M., & Ziv, A. (2011). Simulation-based assessment and the regulation of healthcare professionals. *Simulation in Healthcare, 6*, S58–S62. doi:10.1097/SIH.0b013e3182283bd7

INASCL. (n.d.). Mission and vision of INASCL. Retrieved from https://inacsl.org/about/mission

INACSL Board of Directors. (2011, August). Standards of best practice: Simulation. *Clinical Simulation in Nursing, 7* (4S), s3–s18. doi: 10.1016/j.ecns.2011.05.005

Jeffries, P. R. (2005). A framework for designing, implementing, and evaluating simulations used as teaching strategies in nursing. *Nursing Education Perspectives, 26*(2), 96–103.

Jeffries, P. R. (2007). *Simulation in nursing education: From conceptualization to evaluations*. New York, NY: National League for Nursing.

Jeffries, P. R. (2009). Editorial: Dreams for the future for clinical simulations. *Nursing Education Perspectives, 30*(2), 71.

Jenson, C. E., & Forsyth, D. M. (2012). Virtual reality simulation: Using three-dimensional technology to teach nursing students. *Computer, Informatics, Nursing, 30*(6), 312–318. doi:10.1097/NXN.0b013e31824af6ae

Jones, A. L., & Hegge, M. (2008). Simulation and faculty time investment. *Clinical Simulation in Nursing, 4*, e5–e9.

Laerdal. (2012). Patient simulators. Retrieved from http://www.laerdal.com/us/nav/207/Patient-Simulators

Larew, C., Lessons, S., Spunt, D., Foster, D., & Covington, B. (2006). Innovations in clinical simulation: Application of Benner's theory in an interactive patient care simulation. *Nursing Education Perspectives, 29*(1), 16–21.

Lasater, K. (2007). Clinical judgment development: Using simulation to create an assessment rubric. *Journal of Nursing Education, 46*(11), 496–503.

Lashley, F. R. (2010). Using high-fidelity patient simulation: What does the future hold? In W. M. Nehring & F. R. Lashley (Eds.), *High fidelity patient simulation in nursing education* (pp. 427–431). Sudbury, MA: Jones and Bartlett.

Lupien, A. (2007). High fidelity patient simulation. In M. J. Bradshaw & A. J. Lowenstein (Eds.), *Innovative teaching strategies in nursing and related health professions* (4th ed., pp. 197–214). Sudbury MA: Jones and Bartlett.

Manuel, P., & Sorenson, L. (1995). Changing trends in healthcare: Implications for baccalaureate education, practice, and employment. *Journal of Nursing Education, 34*(6), 248–253.

Merchant, D. C. (2012). Does high-fidelity simulation improve clinical outcomes? *Journal for Nurses in Staff Development, 28*(1), E1–E8. doi: 10.1097/NND.0b013e318240a728

Meyer, M. N., Connors, H., Hou, Q., & Gajewski, B. (2011). The effect of simulation on clinical performance: A junior nursing student clinical comparison study. *Simulation in Healthcare, 6*, 269–277. doi: 10.1097/SIH.0b013e318223a048

Monti, E. J., Wren, K., Haas, R., & Lupien, A. E. (1998). The use of an anesthesia simulator in graduate and undergraduate education. *CRNA: The Clinical Forum for Nurse Anesthetists, 9*(2), 59–66.

National League for Nursing (NLN). (n.d.). Mission/goals/core values. Retrieved from http://www.nln.org/aboutnln/ourmission.htm

Nehring, W. (2010). History of simulation in nursing. In W. M. Nehring & F. R. Lashley (Eds.), *High fidelity patient simulation in nursing education* (pp. 3–26). Sudbury, MA: Jones and Bartlett.

Paige, J. B., & Daley, B. J. (2009). Situation cognition: A learning framework to support and guide high-fidelity simulation. *Clinical Simulation in Nursing, 5*, e97–e103.

Papa, F. J., & Harasym, P. H. (1999). Medical curriculum reform in North America, 1765 to the present: A cognitive science perspective. *Academic Medicine, 74*(2), 154–164.

Parker, B. C., & Myrick, F. (2008). A critical examination of high-fidelity human patient simulation within the context of nursing pedagogy. *Nurse Education Today, 29*, 322–329.

Radhakrishnan, K., Roche, J. P., & Cunningham, H. (2007). Measuring clinical practice parameters with human patient simulators: A pilot study [electronic version]. *International Journal of Nursing Education Scholarship, 4*(1), Article 8.

Register, M., Graham-Garcia, J., & Haas, R. (2003). The use of simulation to demonstrate hemodynamic response to varying degrees of intrapulmonary shunt. *AANA Journal, 71*, 277–284.

Rosen, K. R. (2008). The history of medical simulation. *Journal of Critical Care, 23*, 157–166. doi: 10.1016/j.jrc.2007.1212.004

Schaefer, J. J., Venderbilt, A. A., Cason, C. L., Bauman, E. B., Glavin, R. J., Lee, F. W., & Navedo, D. D. (2011). Literature review: Instructional design and pedagogy science in healthcare simulation. *Simulation in Healthcare, 6*(7), S30–S41. doi: 10.1097/SIH.0b013e31822237b4

Seropian, M., & Lavey, R. (2010, December). Design considerations for healthcare simulation facilities. *Simulation in Healthcare, 5*, 338–345. doi: 10.1097/SIH.0b013e318ec8f60

Sideras, S. (2007). *An examination of the construct validity of a clinical judgment evaluation tool in the setting of high-fidelity simulation* (Unpublished dissertation). Oregon Health & Science University, Portland, OR.

Sittner, B. J., Schmaderer, M., Zimmerman, L., Hertzog, M., & George, B. (2009). Rapid response team simulated training for enhancing patient safety (STEPS). *Clinical Simulation in Nursing, 5*, e119–e127.

Tanner, C. A. (2006). Thinking like a nurse: A research-based model of clinical judgement in nursing. *Journal of Nursing Education, 45*(6), 204–211.

Vygotsky, L. S. (1978). *Mind in society: The development of higher psychological processes.* Cambridge, MA: Harvard University Press.

Weaver, A. (2011). High-fidelity patient simulation in nursing education: An integrative review. *Nursing Education Perspectives, 32*(1), 37–40. Retrieved from http://www.nln.org/nlnjournal/index.htm

CHAPTER 15

The Nursing Skills Laboratory: Application of Theory, Teaching, and Technology

■ DEBORAH TAPLER ■

Creating an effective skills laboratory can energize students and facilitate the transition from practice of required skills to delivery of direct care to clients. The skills laboratory, using multiple modes of teaching and learning, provides an atmosphere for students to acquire new skill knowledge and implement those new skills. With emerging restrictions on clinical placement of health-related students, the skills lab can be used as a learning environment without the presence of clients (Duffin, 2004). Nursing programs are debating proposals that would allow students to spend much more clinical time in practice labs instead of in actual hospital units. With unlimited hours of operation, the lab can provide needed opportunities to practice procedures, evaluate learning outcomes, and reinforce clinical reasoning objectives. As technology increases in complexity through the use of advanced human patient simulators, the skills laboratory can now provide almost true-to-life clinical situations.

■ Definitions and Purposes

Acquisition of new knowledge and skills is an important component of the educational curriculum for healthcare professionals. Nurses must be able to perform procedures such as wound care, intravenous therapy, and endotracheal suctioning. Through the use of a skills laboratory, these and other integral patient care skills are learned and practiced before implementation on patients. The instructor educating students about skills uses several sources for instruction.

The roles and responsibilities of the skills lab have changed with time and advances in learning technology. The skills lab takes on various labels based on its broad offering of services or purposes (Childs, 2002). Schools of nursing across the country suggest the following names: clinical skills laboratory, clinical resource center, learning resource center, clinical competencies learning laboratory, or, simply, nursing laboratory. Current laboratory facilities offer assessment labs, bed labs, static mannequins, simulation, training devices such as intravenous insertion simulators, video libraries, and computer services. Some universities support patient clinics associated with the skills lab for student experiences with actual patients. The skills lab offers a continuum of services depending on the school's interests, specific curriculum needs, and financial capability.

Theory-based practice guides the educator when preparing to teach new skills. Theory has a direct link to practice. Educational theories relate the instructor to students through the development of effective learning strategies appropriate for selected students. Theory also influences practice through theory-driven research that impacts patient care. For example, germ theory dictates the procedure of successful hand washing, which is a skill that every student must master to prevent infection. When learning in the skills lab, the student must progress beyond the how of a procedure to the more complex level of thinking to ask "why."

Evidence-based practice must also be used in the skills laboratory. Evidence-based practice is a systematic approach to problem solving that can be applied to patient care delivery as well as education (Pravikoff, Tanner, & Pierce, 2005). Teaching skills that are based on valid research provide students with state-of-the-art information for safe implementation of skills in actual clinical experiences. It is imperative to educate students about the process of accessing research evidence as part of a lifelong learning goal. Inviting students to participate in the evidence-based process is an important teaching opportunity to allow students to discover best practices regarding content reviewed in the skills lab. For example, students are assigned a particular topic, such as blood pressure monitoring or safe medication administration, to seek reputable best practice standards regarding the psychomotor skill. Elements of procedures and relevancy of skills change as knowledge and technology grow. The skills laboratory must reflect the most current information when educating nurses for the future.

The role of the skills lab is well suited for the development of clinical reasoning abilities in students representing all levels of the curriculum. From beginning students to students who are nearing graduation, specific planned activities in the skills lab can provide opportunities to learn, expand, and evaluate each student's ability to use clinical reasoning when delivering simulated patient care. Given a dynamic patient scenario in the lab, a faculty member may observe the student's ease of decision making and prioritization based on a set of simple to complex patient data. This type of evaluation, whether formative or summative in nature, is very effective when creating individualized goals to enhance student progress or success. In the lab, it is important that any teaching strategy be implemented with the purpose of promoting the progression of advancing levels of thinking (Billings & Halstead, 2011).

The purpose of this chapter is to explore the roles, diverse uses, and effectiveness of a skills laboratory. Based on current theory, valuable teaching modalities, and advanced technology, the skills laboratory can be an effective tool of education for a wide range of health-related disciplines.

■ Theoretical Rationale

Knowles's theory of adult learning has shaped the way that educators present information to adult learners (Knowles, 1989). Adults approach a learning situation differently than children. With life experiences to color the acquisition of new knowledge and skills, adults thrive in a learning environment that is open to creativity, values personal knowledge, and is relevant to immediate learning goals. Adult learners desire to make individual choices and decisions. Education in the skills laboratory is hands-on and relevant to direct patient care. Students are allowed and encouraged to self-evaluate their competence prior to clinical placement (Clarke, Davies, & McNee, 2002). They develop self-confidence as they learn psychomotor skills without fear of failure. After the students attend traditional learning presentations, such as lectures, the adult learners are motivated to learn those things in the skills lab that they know will be necessary to accomplish course objectives. Practice in the skills lab allows the students to cope effectively with future patient interactions. The skills lab can also provide academic assistance when a student has difficulty integrating knowledge regarding a psychomotor skill.

Benner's theory of skill acquisition plays an important part in the nursing education curriculum (Benner, 2001). Benner proposed a model for the nursing profession based on the Dreyfus model explaining that nurses function at various levels of skill from novice to expert. The novice level is characterized by a lack of experience of the situations in which the person is involved and is expected to perform. The beginning nursing student functions at the novice level. The nursing curriculum gives students entry to nursing situations and allows them to gain the experience through skills development. The skills lab acts as an instrument to transfer knowledge and skills to novice nursing students so that they may progress to increasingly more complex levels of understanding. The skills lab can be used to teach about situations in terms of "objective attributes" such as intake and output, blood pressure, and temperature (Benner, 2001, p. 20). These features of the task world of nursing have to be learned before the prospective nurse has actual situational experiences with patients. The behavior of the novice is rule governed and very limited and inflexible. Faculty members impart rules to guide performance before the information makes sense to students. Practice and rehearsal of new behaviors allow the students to gain confidence in their abilities despite little understanding of the contextual meanings of recently learned nursing concepts. Thus, the skills lab plays an important role in the learning process of new students who have no contextual cues. As the nursing student progresses through the nursing curriculum to graduation, the role of the skills lab can evolve and change to meet the expectations for learning dictated by the faculty and content objectives. According to Benner, students may progress from novice to advanced beginner, and then to the competent, proficient, and expert levels of nursing ability over the course of a career.

■ Conditions

The skills laboratory can be used effectively throughout the curriculum. According to Infante (1985), the purpose of a skills laboratory is to offer students the appearance of reality in an artificial environment where the setting is controlled and offers practical application. The students are encouraged to achieve a predefined level of skill competence (Clarke et al., 2002). As skills move from simple (such as bathing) to complex (such as suctioning), the skills lab can be a learning experience that provides for advancing levels of knowledge and abilities.

Faculty involved in undergraduate curricula should identify skills associated with each level of progression to ensure that all necessary content is reflected in the educational goals of the laboratory. In addition, identified skills should be appropriate to the skill level of the student. Typically, nursing education has utilized the skills lab to provide psychomotor skill acquisition at the beginning of the curriculum. However, with technologies used in the lab, such as computer-based interactive case studies and human patient simulators, new modalities have provided unlimited opportunities for knowledge as well as skill development. Clinical reasoning scenarios are appropriate and can be facilitated by skills lab experiences. Human patient simulation offered in the skills laboratory has positively impacted the level of clinical reasoning development in undergraduate students (Lapkin, Levett-Jones, Bellchambers, & Fernandez, 2010). The use of simulation appears to improve knowledge acquisition but may also enhance the decision-making process necessary to provide effective and competent patient care. With the high-stress, low-risk teaching situation of simulation, students have the opportunity to demonstrate clinical judgment abilities that are commensurate with the expected outcome of a course. Some professional disciplines, such as pharmacy, have reported the enhancement of clinical reasoning, problem-solving skills, and teamwork when implementing human patient simulation for students (Vyas, Ottis, & Caligiuri, 2011).

Faculty members using the skills lab should strive to teach a diversity of skills to students. Even though the skills lab typically provides an environment that lends itself to the training of psychomotor skills, other cognitive and affective domain skills can be developed by students. Students learn therapeutic communication and interpersonal skills through staged interactions with mannequins. Collaboration is instilled when students work in groups to deliver patient care through participation in simulation. Faculty-developed case studies used in the lab should be structured with a communication component to include telephoning the physician to clarify an order or suggesting strategies to interact with a distressed family member.

Learning situations can be enhanced by the contained setting of the skills laboratory. With close supervision and responsive interactions between students and faculty, the students learn in an environment of collaboration and inquiry. Questions about new procedures or concepts can be answered and discussed promptly without the constraints of a fast-paced patient care area. Faculty members act as facilitators and have opportunities to present information regarding advances in evidence-based practice. Students feel confident to try new skills in a low-risk situation without fear of harming patients. Mistakes are excellent sources of learning and do not have to result in penalizing consequences. However, if the skills laboratory is used for mastery performance evaluation of student abilities, the results can be recorded as a component of a course grade or used for remedial identification. Students who have weaknesses in psychomotor or clinical reasoning skills can use the environment of the skills laboratory for tutoring assistance from faculty. Through one-on-one interaction, the weak student can practice and receive immediate feedback from a qualified evaluator to gain knowledge and confidence.

■ Types of Learners

Undergraduate nursing students possess various learning styles. The skills laboratory can provide a rich learning experience for all types of learners. Whether the student learner is self-directed or takes a dependent approach, the faculty can individualize instruction based on each student's abilities and learning style. (Cognitive styles, learning styles, and learning preferences were discussed previously in this text.) Kolb's theory of experiential learning proposes cycles of learning along a continuum from concrete experience to abstract conceptualization of knowledge (Dobbin, 2001). Nursing students possess a concrete, active pattern learning style characterized by the need for dynamic involvement when learning new concepts and skills (Schroeder, 2004). According to Dobbin (2001), "learners also can have a preference for reflective observation (watching to learn) or active experimentation (learning by doing)" (p. 5). For example, tactile exploration by touching and manipulating syringes and needles is essential for the concrete learner. Lecturing has only limited ability to educate in regard to psychomotor skill acquisition. As the student learns new skills in the lab, questions arise and what-ifs are posed to enhance the learning experience. The use of return demonstration strengthens mastery and confidence.

Faculty must ensure that instruction in the skills laboratory is directed to students with a wide range of learning styles. Students may possess any one or a combination of the following learning styles: visual (spatial), aural (auditory-musical), verbal (linguistic), physical (kinesthetic), logical (mathematical), social (interpersonal), or solitary (intrapersonal) (Schroeder, 2004). Through the use of simulators, audio-visual software, graphs and diagrams, charts, pictures, demonstrations, practice, discussion, or even music, the skills laboratory can address the needs of all students when acquiring new nursing knowledge. The key to effective teaching in the lab is dependent on the faculty use of a varied and innovative approach to education.

Generational differences among students are addressed by the variety of teaching strategies that are offered by faculty in the skills lab. Whether a generation Xer, millennial, or baby boomer, each student approaches the learning environment with different characteristics and learning needs (Billings & Halstead, 2011). The skills lab offers an array of options to capture the attention of students in today's society. For example, the millennial student prefers to work with a team and be socially involved. According to Godson, Wilson, and Goodman (2007), third-year students working with first-year students in a nursing program proved very effective.

The third-year students were asked to teach a psychomotor skill related to patient care to the first-year students. The first-year students then practiced the skill that they had learned from their fellow nursing students. The mentors' support helped to comfort and ease the anxiety of learning a new skill experienced by the beginning nursing students. Each group described benefits of working together as a team. (Generational perspectives were discussed previously in this text.)

▪ Conditions for Learning and Resources

Opportunities for learning skills in the clinical environment continue to dwindle due to fewer clinical placements available in healthcare institutions. With often fierce competition among educational programs for optimal student assignments in hospital and community resources, the skills lab takes on an increased importance for all clinical courses in the curriculum. Skills, which were once discussed and practiced briefly in the lab and then performed on clients, may no longer be practiced in the clinical area due to patient availability, acuity level of patients in clinical agencies, and legal ramifications (McNett, 2012). Practice in the skills lab may be the only opportunity for learning many basic as well as complex skills needed after graduation. Therefore, skills taught in each course must be identified and additional time and supplies allotted for practice in the lab. Skills will not only be taught in isolation with low-fidelity simulators such as static mannequins, but can also become a part of scenarios with high-fidelity human patient simulators. These scenarios offer the students opportunities to interact with simulators with specific problems, and the skills learned are carried out as interventions become necessary, rather than in isolation. Thus, scenarios based on learning objectives for each course throughout the curriculum and embedded with increasingly complex skills become an important avenue for assisting the student in progressing from novice to higher levels of ability and clinical reasoning. As a student's professional knowledge increases in complexity with each course, clinical reasoning proficiency must also be increased through practice in the skills lab and refined through activities delivering direct patient care in the clinical area. Skills performed within scenarios also allow for the adult learner to apply knowledge and psychomotor ability to immediate learning goals.

Skills labs must take on a new look that mimics the hospital environment as simulators become patients and assist the student in the suspension of disbelief while practicing necessary skills. This environment includes not only sights, but also the sounds that are inherent in a busy clinical area. Labs must include the equipment, technology, and resources that are currently found in the clinical environment. The skills laboratory includes not only typical equipment, such as intravenous pumps, but also computers and laptops with evidenced-based resources that will be needed to assist students with problem solving and clinical reasoning as they work through scenarios. Informatics should be accessible as students must learn to work with databases and documentation software. Labs will need to be designed to provide rooms/bays that are essentially self-contained hospital units for scenarios to be carried out. Although the rooms may be used for a variety of scenarios, different rooms may need to be designed and equipped for areas such as obstetrics, emergency care, acute care, home care, pediatrics, and intensive care units in addition to ancillary units. As the hospital environment changes and innovations such as telenursing and eICUs become commonplace, skills labs will require design elements that provide multiple-screen workstations connected to multiple simulators.

■ Using the Method

Teaching within the new skills lab combines the best of the traditional methods of instruction with the new technological advances. Regardless of the complexity of the skill, acquisition begins with didactic instruction and practice in the lab on low-fidelity mannequins. Additionally, students may be provided with kits of equipment and supplies to continue practicing skills at home. These include such things as mock wounds for dressing changes and Styrofoam wig heads with tracheostomy tubes for practicing tracheostomy care. As mentioned previously, performance of skills at this time is rule governed and inflexible. These skills can then be embedded within a scenario accompanied by the complexity of care based on the course objectives. Three to five students can work through the scenario on a high-fidelity human patient simulator, identifying indicators for various skills, perhaps obtaining orders for the skill, collecting supplies needed, performing the skills, observing the effects, and documenting and reporting the procedure and effects. Although only one student actually performs any one skill, other students actively participate in the skill through discussion and support. The importance of the skill takes on a new meaning as it becomes a part of patient care for an illness and a patient with specific needs and responses. Communication and professionalism is fostered with other team members, such as healthcare providers, and among other members of the student's peer group. Debriefing following the completion of the scenario should be considered integral to the process. Discussions with the faculty as facilitators can assist the students in applying theory to practice, correcting mistakes, answering questions, identifying learning needs, and making connections to the real world.

The use of appropriate scenarios and all levels of human patient simulators and mannequins is invaluable for teaching skills in a safe environment where patient cooperation is not needed, where repetition is essential, and especially where skills could potentially cause harm to the patient. Clinical reasoning and problem solving, obtaining appropriate supplies, manipulating equipment, looking up resources, performing procedures accurately and safely, and communicating verbally and in writing are all activities that require considerable amounts of practice by the novice learner. In the fast-paced clinical environment, time is of the essence, and students are often expected to perform beyond the level of novice learner. Students can move beyond the novice level with the use of credible scenarios and simulated patients in the realistic, transferable environment of the skills lab.

Skills labs may include evaluation of specific skills as a part of outcome measurements at the end of the semester. Students are often evaluated while performing a specific skill or skills as the faculty observe and record their performance. Return demonstration to determine mastery of specified skills is an effective method to determine the safety of transition to patient care in the clinical setting. One type of summative evaluation is called objective structured clinical examination (OSCE) (McWilliam & Botwinski, 2010; Oranye, Ahmad, Ahmad, & Bakar, 2012). OSCE is a practical test that is used to determine proficiency of one or more skills. This strategy of evaluation has been used in the clinical field to evaluate undergraduate and graduate student competence in all areas of the health-related field. OSCE offers an effective teaching option for faculty to evaluate students at multiple stations using standardized patients. For example, a student may proceed through a series of skills stations to perform a particular skill, such as bandaging or interviewing, while being observed by a faculty member guided by a rubric of required actions to successfully complete the skill in a predetermined time frame. If students demonstrate a poor performance when evaluated, immediate remedial action can be taken to correct deficiencies before exposure to patients. Patient safety must be the overriding consideration when documenting student abilities. For example, if during a lab checkoff, a student draws up 10 mL of a medication instead of the required 3-mL dose, the faculty can reeducate the student immediately, validate that accurate knowledge is mastered, and avert a potential patient injury in subsequent clinical encounters.

Simulated patients also are used in effectively evaluating skills. The required skills are developed in a short scenario. Three to five students care for the patient using a mannequin and perform the skills as the intervention becomes necessary in the scenario. Students should be aware of the criteria and expected behaviors, having practiced all the skills to be evaluated previously. At the beginning of the scenario, students can draw from a hat for the skills they are to perform during the scenario. As the scenario progresses, students care for the patient together, except when a specific skill is needed. Peers then become observers as the student who was assigned a skill performs according to the criteria outlined and is evaluated by the instructor. Peer observers become active learners as they mentally rehearse and evaluate the skills as they are being performed. Once the skill has been completed, the scenario resumes until another skill is needed. The process is repeated throughout the scenario until all students have demonstrated their selected skills. Verbal and/or written feedback can be given to the students individually by the instructor following the scenario. Students may also give their peers feedback about their performance. This same strategy can be utilized for standardized or real human patients or actors as opposed to static mannequins. A standardized patient actor is paid by the institution to act like a patient with a specific disease state or case scenario as prescribed by the faculty.

According to McWilliam and Botwinski (2010, 2012), the use of faculty to play the role of standardized patients is not an effective model. Health professionals have a tendency to give clues and unintentionally assist the students who are being evaluated on a task. Lay persons are much more authentic in the role of a patient.

The skills lab is an essential environment to teach nursing skills. However, the space can also be used for teaching previously learned skills. After a long scholastic break, skills may be forgotten by students due to lack of practice (Roberts, Vignato, Moore, & Madden, 2009). Knowledge of psychomotor skills decreases after as little as 2 weeks and may need to be relearned after 2 months. Course faculty can schedule the lab space for skills reintroduction to the students. Having a daylong skills session before the semester commences is an effective strategy to refresh, practice, and critique skills in time for the beginning of actual patient care delivery. Skills must be sufficiently practiced to support retention of the skills and permit the student to gain the ability to transfer the skill knowledge to the clinical area competently (Oermann et al., 2011). These intensive skill sessions promote the performance of learned skills and also develop confidence in the nursing students.

Video recording may be used as an adjunct to learning or evaluation of skills. This method of assessment offers findings that are very objective when used for grading purposes. Students can learn by video recording and critiquing their own performance or viewing the video and discussing their performance with a faculty member. They can also video record and submit their video for evaluation and feedback by a faculty member. In a study by Brimble (2008), skills assessment using video analysis in a simulated environment was an effective evaluation tool. The nursing students completed a questionnaire before, during, and after videotaping a simulation in the skills lab. The most common positive theme that students expressed was the ability to learn from their mistakes by watching the reenactment of their performance on video. Subjects indicated that the visual feedback that they received from viewing their actual performance complemented the verbal critique offered by their faculty member. Negative themes included feelings of anxiety, being judged by others, and being embarrassed. However, Miller, Nichols, and Beeken (2000) found that students prefer faculty member presence during skill demonstrations and immediate feedback rather than video recording and delayed feedback.

■ Potential Problems

Major problems inherent in the development of the modern skills laboratory are the cost to provide the needed technology, supplies, and the physical space to house them. In order for students to practice with the equipment used in the profession, it must be purchased from medical vendors. Supplies are very expensive, especially when they are the most recent equipment used by the clinical agencies. Needles with integral safety devices are often more costly than traditional needle systems. Students must see and practice with the tools that they will use in their clinical experiences, which requires frequent equipment revision in the laboratory. As enrollment in schools of nursing increases due to shortage mandates, the skills lab provides space that is available from early morning to late in the evening for student use.

Skills labs have typically been large rooms with multiple beds and static mannequins. Large numbers of students often practice the same skill at the same time. Although this type of space and instruction present a good beginning, additional smaller simulation rooms are needed for the more costly high-fidelity human patient simulators with all of the equipment, technology, and added supplies needed for implementing simulations. In addition, some labs have a small control room with a one-way mirror attached to each simulation room.

Other problems include lack of faculty willingness to embrace new technology and other services offered by the skills lab. Implementation of high-fidelity simulation, evidence-based case scenarios, and the additional time it takes to have three to five students at a time complete the skills within the case scenarios requires dedicated faculty participation. Learning new simulation teaching strategies and management of the simulators requires additional faculty time and energy. Writing evidence-based scenarios that contain the necessary skills is another time-intensive faculty activity, unless these are purchased. According to Childs (2002), faculty and students must be interested and motivated to use the skills lab for the multiple teaching opportunities that are possible. Often, a core group of faculty members use the services of the skills lab on a routine basis, but all instructors should be informed about the applicability of skills lab services to augment the delivery of the curriculum content. In return, the skills lab must be responsive to the faculty and their needs to maximize the use of available technology.

Communication with faculty and students about the skills lab services is a critical element of an effectively functioning lab. This challenge is often addressed through the use of web-based software. Currently, most colleges and universities support a web-based framework such as Blackboard or WebCT. The skills lab should offer a website directed to students and faculty where policies and procedures, calendar events, and contact information for lab personnel are posted. A schedule of open lab times and remedial sessions should be easily accessible for students who need those services. Communication is an essential key to allow users to take full advantage of all the services offered by a well-equipped skills lab.

Every skills laboratory must be a safe environment for faculty, students, and staff. Skills labs are required to follow strict safety procedures to protect personnel and students in the lab from injury or spills. Needles, sutures, and performance of certain procedures pose daily threats. Adhering to federal and local government regulations may prove costly but is a necessary component of a safe and effective skills lab.

■ Conclusion

The skills laboratory provides an enriched teaching and learning atmosphere that encourages active and involved exploration and mastery of new knowledge and skills to develop competent graduate nurses. Theory is applied to practice and validated in the skills lab through teaching and technology. The faculty member can use unlimited strategies to educate students who have a spectrum of learning needs in order to foster clinical reasoning. In the protected environment of the skills lab, students learn, make mistakes, question conceptual ideas, practice psychomotor skills, and expand knowledge to a new level of understanding. Students learn by doing through experimentation that would be impossible and dangerous in direct patient care situations. Faculty members must engage in direct observation and supervision of all student activities, which is often difficult in a busy clinical agency. Transition to the role of graduate nurse is enhanced by effective and innovative use of the new skills laboratory.

TEACHING EXAMPLES:

Comprehensive Nursing Skills Experiences

In a fundamental skills course offered by various disciplines, skills are a primary focus requiring didactic instruction and demonstrations first given in lecture and then reinforced in the skills lab. Skills that are appropriate for beginning nursing students include the complex task of medication administration, which includes obtaining or understanding healthcare provider orders, learning the appropriate dosages and where to research information about the drug, calculating dosages from the correct amount of drug available, safely and competently handling the syringe during drawing up of medication, administration, disposal of the syringe, recognizing appropriate sites for administration (subcutaneous or intramuscular), performing the five rights prior to administration, and recording the medication in the permanent patient record. All these basic skills must be understood and practiced repeatedly by the student. To meet the wide range of learning styles, instruction should include verbal and written material as well as audiovisual demonstrations and one-on-one interactions and demonstrations with the students. Kinesthetic learning is provided by the use of different types of syringes, vials, and pills; and solitary practice is combined with discussion, reflective observation, and active experimentation.

Administering insulin and digoxin can be used as examples for student practice. Sliding-scale insulin orders could be written in a mock chart, and students could be given various blood glucose results so that different amounts of insulin would need to be drawn up. In the lab, students practice drawing up insulin, selecting an appropriate site, administering the medication on a mannequin, discarding the syringe, and documenting on the mock chart. They should also practice giving oral medications such as digoxin correctly, which would include auscultation of the apical pulse. Not only must they be able to perform the skill of giving the medication correctly, but they would also need to recognize that an apical pulse rate must be taken before administration, know under which circumstances the medication should be withheld based on current literature, and recognize when the healthcare provider must be notified for future actions.

Once the skills have been practiced, three or four students are introduced to the high-fidelity simulator. They are presented with the history and physical findings of a patient who

(continued)

is hospitalized with selected clinical problems. A mock chart is available with healthcare provider orders, which include treatment and medication orders. Medications are noted on the medication administration record, including insulin sliding scale, oral medication, and prn medication orders. The students are made aware of the time of day and results of lab studies such as blood glucose readings. Students at this point are assigned selected skills to perform, such as wound dressing change, urinary catheterization, administration of pain medication via the intramuscular route, application of bandages, or performance of a basic head-to-toe assessment. The skills are embedded in the scenario and must be performed according to patient need and healthcare provider orders. The students must prioritize their actions based on the dynamic events unfolding in the patient scenario. This complex situation cultivates clinical reasoning and problem solving to meet patient demands. The faculty member acts as facilitator to encourage competent participation by individual students and provides immediate feedback to correct problems in cognition and performance of skills. As the students progress in level of learning ability across the curriculum, the faculty member offers less prompting to increase the independence exhibited by the students. By applying adult learning principles, the students are allowed to demonstrate more creativity in a learning environment that supports personal knowledge and meets immediate learning goals.

Evaluation of required skills is an important function of the skills lab. The lab provides unlimited opportunities for faculty to observe and test acquisition of psychomotor skills as well as cognitive processing. For example, the evaluation process in the form of a formalized checkoff can be implemented at the end of a semester to determine mastery of required skills. Before the checkoff is completed, students receive detailed procedural (step-by-step) information or criteria regarding the skills that they must master. By knowing the exact expectation before the evaluation, the anxiety level experienced by the students is decreased, and the faculty member can more easily determine the skill level of an individual student unclouded by psychological barriers. Practice opportunities are provided to reinforce skills the week before checkoff. The lab is arranged to represent the hospital setting with a patient in bed, a medication room, and a supply area. The student receives an assigned skill, reviews the patient's mock chart, assembles the necessary equipment to perform the skill, and prepares the patient for the procedure. The interaction with the mannequin should appear as authentic as possible. This situation can be achieved by encouraging the student to communicate with the patient in a normal manner. The faculty member observes the performance of the skill based on the criteria previously provided to the student. A checkoff form is used to document and evaluate the student's actions in relation to the criteria. The faculty member does not interact with or prompt the student in any manner. If the student fails to follow the criteria, points are deducted, affecting the final score. The criteria contain selected critical behaviors that must be accomplished successfully to pass the evaluation. Examples of critical behaviors are contamination of a sterile field or recapping a used needle. If the student fails to acquire sufficient points or neglects to perform critical behaviors, the student fails the checkoff and is provided the opportunity for remediation and a repeated attempt. Failure of the course is possible if the student is unable to successfully master the performance of the skill. The skills lab is an excellent venue to assess competency and determine learning needs. By utilizing theory combined with innovative teaching approaches and technological advances in the skills laboratory, faculty members optimize learning opportunities.

REFERENCES

Benner, P. (2001). *From novice to expert: Excellence and power in clinical nursing practice.* Upper Saddle River, NJ: Prentice-Hall.

Billings, D. M., & Halstead, J. A. (2011). *Teaching in nursing: A guide for faculty.* St. Louis, MO: Elsevier Saunders.

Brimble, M. (2008). Skills assessment using video analysis in a simulated environment: An evaluation. *Pediatric Nursing, 20*(7), 26–31.

Childs, J. C. (2002). Clinical resource centers in nursing programs. *Nurse Educator, 27* (5), 232–235.

Clarke, D., Davies, J., & McNee, P. (2002). The case for a children's nursing skills laboratory. *Pediatric Nursing, 14*(7), 36–39.

Dobbin, K. R. (2001). Applying learning theories to develop teaching strategies for the critical care nurse: Don't limit yourself to the formal classroom lecture. *Critical Care Nursing Clinics of North America, 13*(1), 1–11.

Duffin, C. (2004). Simulated "skills labs" to ease pressure on training. *Nursing Standard, 18*(39), 7.

Godson, N. R., Wilson, A., & Goodman, M. (2007). Evaluating student nurse learning in the clinical skills laboratory. *British Journal of Nursing, 16*(15), 942–945.

Infante, M. S. (1985). *The clinical laboratory.* New York, NY: John Wiley.

Knowles, M. (1989). *The making of an adult education: An autobiographical journey.* San Francisco, CA: Jossey-Bass.

Lapkin, S., Levett-Jones, T., Bellchambers, H., & Fernandez, R. (2010). Effectiveness of patient simulation manikins in teaching clinical reasoning skills to undergraduate nursing students: A systematic review. *Clinical Simulation in Nursing, 6*(6), 207–222.

McNett, S. (2012). Teaching psychomotor skills in a fundamentals laboratory: A literature review. *Nursing Education Perspectives, 33*(5), 328–333.

McWilliam, P. L., & Botwinski, C.A. (2010). Developing a successful nursing objective structured clinical examination. *Journal of Nursing Education, 49*(1), 36–41.

McWilliam, P. L., & Botwinski, C. A. (2012). Identifying strengths and weaknesses in the utilization of objective structured clinical examination (OSCE) in a nursing program. *Nursing Education Perspectives, 33*(1), 35–39.

Miller, H., Nichols, E., & Beeken, J. (2000). Comparing video-taped and faculty-present return demonstrations of clinical skills. *Journal of Nursing Education, 39*, 237–239.

Oermann, M., et al. (2011). Deliberate practice of motor skills in nursing education: CPR as exemplar. *Nursing Education Perspectives, 32*(5), 311–315.

Oranye, N. O., Ahmad, C., Ahmad, N., & Bakar, R. A. (2012). Assessing nursing clinical skills competence through objective structured clinical examination (OSCE) for open distance learning students in Open University Malaysia. *Contemporary Nurse, 41*(2), 233–241.

Pravikoff, D. S., Tanner., A. B., & Pierce, S. T. (2005). Readiness for US nurses for evidence-based practice. *American Journal of Nursing, 105*(9), 40–52.

Roberts, S. T., Vignato, J. A., Moore, J. L., & Madden, C. A. (2009). Promoting skill building and confidence in freshman nursing students with a "skills-a-thon." *Journal of Nursing Education, 48*(8), 460–464.

Schroeder, C. C. (2004). New students–New learning styles. Retrieved from http://www.virtualschool.edu/mon/Academia/KierseyLearningStyles.html

Vyas, D., Ottis, E. J., & Caligiuri, F. J. (2011). Teaching clinical reasoning and problem-solving skills using human patient simulation. *American Journal of Pharmaceutical Education, 75*(9), 1–5.

CHAPTER 16

Innovations in Facilitating Learning Using Simulation

■ KIM LEIGHTON AND JUDY JOHNSON-RUSSELL ■

A decade has passed since faculty in the healthcare industry began facilitating learning with high-fidelity human patient simulation, a technique that continues to grow in sophistication. Educators are struggling with the realization that they are unable to prepare students adequately to assume the role of the healthcare provider. The vast amount of content, technical and interpersonal skills, and professional role expectations, coupled with the increased number of incoming students and decreased availability of clinical placements (Nehring, 2010), have created a frustrating and sometimes dangerous situation. Clinical sites, which once were the primary place of learning, now restrict student activities, leading to suboptimal experiences for content integration and mastery. Observational experiences and mentor-apprenticeship are not always beneficial as preceptors are frequently preoccupied with pressing patient problems and are not as invested in student learning. Using human patient simulation as a teaching strategy provides opportunities for educators to fill gaps in students' knowledge and experience that are a result of limitations posed by traditional clinical environments.

The use of high-fidelity simulators creates a learning environment that closely resembles the clinical setting and can present learners with almost any situation they might find in a patient care setting. Although the technology still intimidates many, the techniques of facilitating learning are at the essence of this pedagogy. For those who embrace this pedagogy, teaching with high-fidelity simulators using realistic scenarios is exciting and rewarding. This methodology provides an environment for educating students without risk to human life and helps learners transfer knowledge and skills into actual clinical practice (Morgan, Cleave-Hogg, Desousa, & Lam-McCulloch, 2006). This chapter is intended to present innovative ways of utilizing human patient simulation.

■ Definitions and Purposes

Simulation experiences and patient simulators are commonly referred to as low, medium, and high fidelity; however, there is no accepted classification that differentiates each from the other (Gaba, 2004). Fidelity of simulation follows a continuum beginning with low-fidelity simulation experiences, such as use of role-play, or may incorporate a static mannequin that does not respond to intervention. Medium-fidelity simulations build on the degree of realism presented and may involve task trainers or moderate-fidelity simulators that provide a degree of feedback to the participant. At the upper range of the continuum lie high-fidelity simulations that provide for more immersive simulated clinical experiences, using realistic and sophisticated computer technology to enhance the abilities of the patient simulator to provide feedback to learners (Decker, Sportsman, Puetz, & Billings, 2008; Hovancsek, 2007; Jeffries & Rogers, 2007b; Nehring, 2010). An overview on background and use of the high-fidelity patient simulator was presented previously in this text.

The purpose of integrating simulation into any curriculum is to provide students with beneficial learning experiences that will assist in meeting course and program objectives while promoting safe patient care. The focus of the simulated patient experience is on the needs of the learner, rather than being on the needs of the patient, as it must be in the hospital or other clinical environment. Carefully chosen simulated clinical experiences (SCEs) provide the opportunity for multiple objectives to be met by multiple learners at the same time.

Task trainers or low-fidelity trainers and mannequins provide for repeated skill practice, such as catheter insertion. The catheter is inserted and removed according to a defined order of skill demonstration. Higher-fidelity simulators challenge students to reach higher-level objectives by prioritizing care and promoting critical thinking and clinical judgment. Students must critically think about why the catheter is important to the patient's care, its correlation to the illness or disease process, and expected outcomes, as well as plan for additional care and safety needs of the patient as the scenario proceeds. The communication component is added as the patient simulator or the patient's family may question the student, asking for explanation of the procedure. Although the skill of catheterization is the same, it has not occurred in isolation, but in context as a part of the total care of the patient. As the simulation continues, students see the results of their interventions and the impact on the patient's condition (Leigh & Hurst, 2008).

An advantage to simulation is that an SCE can cover any desired time span to demonstrate the changes in the patient's condition. Students may take care of the patient upon admission to the emergency department and continue several hours later during admission to the patient care unit and as the patient's condition improves with intervention over time, and culminate with discharge planning and teaching. The time span of an SCE may cover anywhere from a few hours to days. Students experience the physiologic changes in the patient's condition over time, an advantage that is rarely available in the traditional clinical environment. Faculty control the progression of the SCE by changing from state to state as objectives are met or appropriate student behaviors are demonstrated. Each state represents a change in the patient's condition or situation. Students benefit from being able to experience and participate in the whole process of managing the patient's illness or condition.

When sufficient time is provided for simulation, students in nursing have the opportunity to work through the process of completing assessments, analyzing data, planning appropriate care, prioritizing care, providing interventions, and evaluating the responses to their interventions. Rarely is there time in clinical education experiences to proceed purposefully at this slower pace.

Another purpose of simulation is to enhance communication. Communication in the simulation laboratory can occur face to face, via the phone, or via written documentation in the electronic health record (EHR), which will be discussed in the *Charting* section of this chapter. Students can be provided opportunities to communicate face to face with the off-going nurse (role-played by faculty) during shift report, while being encouraged to ask questions or seek out additional patient information. Students communicate with each other as they determine priorities for care and problem-solve situations that arise.

Communication with the patient and any present family members provides for experiences that may not occur in the traditional clinical environment and can be tailored by faculty to present specific concepts that create a more holistic experience. For example, while receiving discharge instructions, the simulated patient may state that he does not have money to purchase his prescriptions. Perhaps as a simulated patient deteriorates, the student decides to call and notify the patient's family. It is at that point that the student learns that the phone has been disconnected because the bill has not been paid.

The simulation laboratory is also a safe place to practice communication with other healthcare providers, including physicians. Many, if not most, new nursing graduates have never been allowed to place a phone call to a healthcare provider while on the traditional clinical unit. Therefore, it is vital that an opportunity for communication with the healthcare provider be included in simulated experiences. This communication may occur face to face with a faculty person role-playing the provider or via phone. If the students place a call about early findings and the faculty wish to encourage further critical thinking, the caller can be told that the provider is not available because her cell phone is out of service range, she is busy in the operating room, or she is in a patient room at her office. Students should also practice communication with other healthcare providers by calling the laboratory, radiology, or other ancillary departments for test results.

It is important to make these exchanges as realistic as possible; however, it is equally important to not perpetuate stereotypes. For students who are novices at this type of communication, faculty should provide guidance and ask questions to promote critical thinking and organization. Using organizational tools such as SBAR (situation, background, assessment, recommendation) will help to arrange thoughts prior to initiating communication. As students progress through the program of study and become more proficient, the realism of the verbal exchange should increase accordingly.

Simulated clinical experiences provide numerous opportunities for faculty to observe intrapersonal, interpersonal, and communication among small groups of students, as well as with other professionals. It is often difficult to observe communication in the traditional clinical environment as clinical faculty attempt to meet the needs of all students. In the simulation laboratory, faculty can observe communication skills and provide immediate feedback (Pagano & Greiner, 2009).

There are many important skills that can be learned through interaction with other healthcare providers beyond communication. Interprofessional education has become a major focus of healthcare education, although it is challenging to achieve in single-purpose colleges. The Interprofessional Education Collaborative has developed core competencies for interprofessional collaborative practice to help guide educators in the development of interprofessional education, with the goal of strengthening teamwork and team-based care (Interprofessional Education Collaborative Expert Panel, 2011). More information on interprofessional education is presented later in this text.

The Institute of Medicine (IOM) identified five core competencies for integrating safety and quality into nursing education, all of which can be addressed in the simulation laboratory. The competencies are (1) provide patient-centered care, (2) work in interdisciplinary teams, (3) employ evidence-based practice, (4) apply quality improvement, and (5) utilize information (IOM, 2003). The goal is to decrease preventable patient deaths by improving education. Patient-centered care could include patient education and support interventions as patients learn to manage their health problems. Interdisciplinary teams can be formed with students working together to meet the scenario objectives. Nursing schools often collaborate with respiratory, pharmacy, social work, seminary, and medical students and together plan and carry out patient care. Evidence-based guidelines should be utilized to develop the SCE and to define interventions to be completed during the SCE. All SCEs can contain a safety issue so that students are able to identity hazards and take steps to prevent errors and accidents. Computers and personal digital assistants (PDAs) can be utilized in the simulation laboratory so that students experience working with computerized documentation systems and clinical decision support systems.

Policies and procedures from the traditional clinical environments should be available during the SCE, along with additional resources for students to reference prior to and during care provision. Students need to become expert seekers and processors of information in this ever-expanding healthcare environment. Having appropriate resources and references, as well as the time to utilize them, during the SCE will assist graduates to know where and how to find needed information.

A notable advantage to simulation is that it assists students in learning their role in emergency situations. When an emergency occurs in the hospital, generally students are not allowed to participate. However in the simulation laboratory, they can practice their role repeatedly without fear of harm to a patient. In addition, when incorrect decisions are made or the wrong interventions are completed in the simulation laboratory and the patient has a poor outcome, the opportunity exists to redo the SCE after debriefing occurs and correct patient management has been discussed. This allows the learner to see a better outcome and add experience.

Faculty often comment that participating with their clinical group of students in simulation activities provides them with knowledge of each student's strengths and limitations. This assists the faculty in individualizing clinical experiences and in providing focus for remediation and assignments. It is particularly helpful if an SCE is in the beginning weeks of the rotation. It is also possible to see growth and changes in behavior when an SCE is conducted some weeks later.

▪ Using the Method

Designing the Simulated Clinical Experience

Deciding on appropriate SCEs to include in any curriculum takes careful thought and planning. Above all, decisions should be made based on the objectives of the program, the course, and the particular class period that will use simulation. Major curricular threads should also be included when selecting SCEs to integrate. All clinical courses and some didactic classes, such as pathophysiology, pharmacology, and cultural issues, can incorporate simulation. A review of the program's specific strengths and limitations will assist in choosing SCEs that will best meet student needs. Concepts that seem hard for students to grasp or that are difficult to teach are excellent choices for SCEs. Test scores and item analysis, such as from the National Council Licensure Examination–Registered Nurse or Practical Nurse (NCLEX-RN; NCLEX-PN), Assessment Technologies Institute (ATI), Health Education Systems, Inc. (HESI), or faculty-developed tests for specific courses give indications of content and concepts students do not comprehend. SCEs that address these areas should be chosen to facilitate learning in weak areas.

When choosing SCEs, conditions or illnesses that are not readily available in the clinical agencies are beneficial, as all students then have the opportunity to care for that type of patient. SCEs that prepare students for specific clinical experiences, for high-risk situations, or for complex patients are also excellent choices. The timing of the simulation is another important consideration. Didactic material corresponding to the SCE should have been covered prior to the learning experience so that students have the necessary foundation upon which to base their decisions. Some schools incorporate simulation at the beginning of each course to assist with preparation for entering a new clinical rotation and again at the end of the rotation as a capstone experience. Test scores after simulation may reflect a deeper understanding of the content than before simulation. Each course within a program will have its own needs and objectives that can be addressed through carefully planned SCEs.

Scheduling Students in the Simulation Laboratory

Scheduling of simulated clinical experiences (SCE) is often a major hurdle for faculty to overcome. For most educational institutions, class scheduling is part of a complex process that includes many departments, faculty, resources, and buildings. Making one change can be very disruptive. Therefore, it is valuable to consider a variety of options when integrating simulation into the curriculum, beginning with a critical look at current teaching methods and clinical experiences.

Often health education programs have been challenged to increase enrollment but have limited clinical resources. As a result, clinical experiences that do not provide the best opportunity to meet learning objectives for the student may have been added to the curricula. The site's experiences may be too complex, or too easy, for a given level of learning. Available hours may not fit easily into the course schedule. Occasionally, professional behaviors at the clinical site do not mesh with those in the nursing program. Faculty are encouraged to critically review all clinical placement sites to determine if needs are being well met in those environments. If not, consideration should be made for moving the experience to the simulation lab.

A question is often raised about the number of hours that can be provided in the simulation lab. This is dependent upon the regulations of the program's licensing organization in each state and may be prescriptive as to the number of hours or percentage of hours. States vary widely on this issue; all allow simulation as a supplement to traditional clinical hours, while fewer allow for substitution of simulation for clinical experiences. In states where substitution is allowed, the percentages for nursing programs are as high as 30% (Utah). Other states leave discretion to the faculty as long as program outcomes continue to be met. A more difficult question is, "How many hours of simulation are needed to replace the same number of clinical hours?" This question is much more challenging to answer, and the answer needs to be supported by research. The National Council of State Boards of Nursing is currently supporting a multiyear, multisite study to determine the impact of simulation use and how outcomes vary when simulation replaces up to 50% of traditional clinical practice time.

Scheduling simulation throughout the curriculum is best achieved by using a variety of scheduling methods. This allows for increased simulation use with less disruption to the course schedule. Several methods can be utilized: stations in a lab, set blocks of time, post clinical conference, entire day, and class time. It is important to remember that the students will always take longer to make decisions and perform skills than faculty expect, as this is part of their learning process. To decrease frustration and catching up during the day, allow more time than thought necessary to schedule SCEs.

Stations

Using stations works well for integrating SCEs into assessment and fundamental skills courses. These courses are often designed so that students work in pairs and small groups to practice psychomotor skills, communication techniques, and critical thinking. Students often rotate through different learning activities during lab time. A short SCE that allows the students to apply what they have learned in the context of a patient situation can be added. Using this method may result in adding time to the existing lab, but more often, another learning station is deleted.

Blocks of Time

This method creates a set period of time for self-determined groups or faculty-assigned groups to participate in an SCE. All blocks of time might be together during a specific week of the course, or the blocks of time could be distributed throughout the semester until everyone has completed their time. Blocks of time must be long enough and filled with enough activity to make it worth the students' time to come to campus for the experience. For programs with set amounts of student contact hours, some faculty have decreased their clinical practice time by 10 minutes/week over a 15-week semester, resulting in the ability to reassign that time (150 minutes) to simulation.

Clinical Post Conference

A scheduling method involving a conference at the end of each clinical practice experience can be planned in advance or done impromptu based on activities of the clinical day. Typically, clinical post conferences last approximately one hour and occur at the end of the clinical day. They are designed to serve as a time to reflect on the day's activities, but they are often used for various other activities such as topical review of difficult theoretical concepts, as review prior to exams, or even as time to remain on the clinical unit to observe an unusual activity. This time frame is included in the schedule of the clinical day and some faculty facilitators have found that simulated clinical experiences, designed to include concepts unique to their clinical unit, are a valuable use of this time. For example, a postoperative unit may have several patients with chest tubes but not every student has the opportunity to care for those patients. Managing a chest tube patient in the simulation laboratory provides an opportunity for every student to care for that type of patient.

Entire Day

In this scheduling method, a clinical group participates in various simulated clinical experiences over an entire day. Rather than going to a hospital unit or clinical agency for a clinical experience, the students report to the simulation laboratory. The simulation laboratory is placed on the clinical schedule rotation instead of an agency site. A typical day's schedule should begin and end at the usual clinical times. Students can provide care for a variety of patient types, depending on the length of the scenario, or they can provide care to one patient over a simulated period of time, perhaps over days or even months. It is helpful to assign rotating roles to keep students engaged. Expectations for preparation, care, resource use, and documentation should be the same as on the clinical unit.

During Class

Simulators can be used during class time by either moving a portable simulator to the classroom or using video to transmit from the simulation laboratory to the classroom. Portable simulators are designed for ease of movement and can be placed in the front of the classroom to demonstrate various concepts. Students can be chosen to participate in caring for the simulated patient either randomly, based on skill level, or based on identified learning needs. Students remaining in the audience can participate in directing the care, prioritizing care, or observing for various aspects of care, such as communication techniques. Using video, especially two-way interactive video, provides the same in-class learning advantage without moving the simulator. Another learning opportunity is provided when both an adult and pediatric simulator are moved into the classroom, setting the stage for comparing and contrasting the care of an adult patient and pediatric patient with the same illness or disease process.

An additional in-class learning opportunity exists through use of the simulation software. The computer running the simulation software can be connected to the classroom LCD projector, allowing all students to see the patient parameters. After orienting students to the various parameters, the faculty member can demonstrate the hemodynamic changes that occur with hypervolemia, hypovolemia, pneumothorax, pericardial tamponade, different cardiac rhythms, and numerous medications. The simulator does not have to be connected to this computer in order to demonstrate these features. Further discussion of classroom use of simulation is provided in the *Implementing the Simulated Clinical Experience* section of this chapter.

Fidelity of the Simulated Clinical Experience

Realism of the simulated clinical experience is commonly referred to as fidelity. There is no consensus as to how much fidelity is necessary for learning to occur, but many believe that the closer to reality a scenario is, the more engaged students become and the more opportunities there are for learning to occur. Medley and Horne (2005) recommend that in a high-fidelity simulated clinical experience, the real-life situation be recreated in as realistic a manner as possible. Cantrell, Meakim, and Cash (2008) identified the theme, "the more real the simulation, the better the learning" (p. e1), when analyzing the qualitative portion of their study of student evaluations of a simulation experience. In a small pilot study, researchers found no statistically significant difference in pretest or posttest scores of a group learning with low-fidelity simulation and a group learning with high-fidelity simulation (Kardong-Edgren, Anderson, & Michaels, 2007). The literature is now replete with studies of fidelity levels within a variety of courses, with different levels of students, and its impact on characteristics such as anxiety and confidence. It is important to match the level of fidelity to the desired learning outcomes, as some simulated clinical experiences require higher levels of fidelity than others (Gaba, 2004).

The learning can be positive or negative, and while it is hoped that only positive learning is transferred to real patient care, the potential for negative transfer of learning also exists. Therefore, it is important that processes and procedures in the simulation laboratory mimic reality as closely as possible. The following four major areas of fidelity should be considered when creating the simulated clinical experience: the simulator, the physical patient, holistic aspects of the patient, and the environment. Simulator fidelity was addressed earlier in this chapter.

Physical Patient

Fidelity of the simulated patient's physical condition should impact as many of the student's senses as possible, including sight, smell, touch, and hearing. This involves significant creativity on the part of the faculty member but can often be accomplished at little cost. Creating this type of fidelity is often referred to as *moulage*. Examples of low-cost solutions to create physical conditions are provided in **Table 16-1**. Always test new moulage in an inconspicuous area if there is a risk for staining to occur.

Holistic Aspects of the Patient

Nursing care of the patient involves not only physical care, but developmental, cultural, psychosocial, and spiritual care as well. These important aspects are often left out of the simulated clinical experience. Undergraduate nursing students were asked their perceptions of how well their learning needs were met in the traditional clinical environment and in the simulated clinical environment (Leighton, 2007). Learning needs related to holistic patient care were better met in the traditional clinical environment ($p = 0.000$), revealing an area to be improved in the simulation lab.

Positively impacting these learning needs is easy to do in the simulation lab and costs little or no money to do so. In most cases, adding more information to the patient's story or health history can add this dimension. **Table 16-2** outlines several ways in which holistic patient care can be added to the simulated clinical experience.

Table 16-1   Physical Fidelity of the Simulated Patient

Sense	Physical Condition or Disease	Moulage
Sight	Vomit	Egg white whisked with fork; streak with yellow food coloring with toothpick tip
	Blood clots	Thick lumpy tapioca with red food coloring; partially gelled sugar-free red gelatin
Smell	Incontinence	Water with yellow food coloring and ammonia
	Vomit	Add grated parmesan cheese to vomit
Touch	Edema	Memory foam covered with ace wrap or antiembolism stockings
	Clammy skin	Spray with water bottle
Hearing	Hospital sounds	Loop MP3 recording and play back
	Hospital pages	Announce random overhead pages via microphone

Table 16-2 Holistic Care of the Simulated Patient

Aspect	Patient	Concern
Developmental	45-year-old male with heart attack	He and wife have five children, and he is unable to return to construction job.
	14-year-old with abdominal pain	Patient is sexually active and has contracted a sexually transmitted disease.
Cultural	26-year-old female speaks only Vietnamese	The only available person who knows Vietnamese is the hospital's maintenance man.
	88-year-old Native American patient who urgently needs medication	The patient prefers to wait for medicine elder.
Psychosocial	8-year-old boy requires appendectomy	Parents recently moved to the area and the family's health insurance has not yet taken effect.
	72-year old patient with COPD requiring several medications	The patient is unable to afford medications with current finances.
Spiritual	52-year-old female requires abdominal surgery	The patient refuses to remove jewelry with religious icons.
	66-year-old patient who was just diagnosed with cancer	The patient refuses treatment because he believes the illness is a result of past sins.

A variety of props can be added to the simulated patient's room to help prompt students to address holistic aspects of care. A picture frame with a family picture including several children might be placed at the bedside to see if students address the patient's role in the family. A Bible, Koran, or other religious book or icon can be placed at the bedside to shift the focus to spiritual aspects of care. It is helpful to have resources available to students to look up information about different cultural and religious beliefs while caring for the simulated patient.

Environment

Simulation centers or laboratories come in all shapes and sizes, from the corner of a skills lab to a large, free-standing space with individualized and very realistic-appearing patient rooms. No matter the space, it is important to make it appear as realistic as possible to the intended clinical environment. While this is typically a patient's hospital room, many simulated clinical experiences can occur in a patient's home, an outpatient setting, or in the recovery room. Having the equipment and props characteristic of the desired environment will help learners to be engaged and learn the use of appropriate equipment and supplies.

Obtaining supplies and equipment can be a costly endeavor. Consider discussing simulation needs with clinical nurse managers who may be able to divert opened sterile kits to the simulation laboratory if they cannot be used with human patients.

Many hospitals have warehouses where unused or overstocked equipment is stored. Simulation laboratories are often able to purchase at a discount or borrow equipment. Many pharmacies now return expired medications for account credit; however, simulation personnel may be able to obtain these medication vials or ampoules. Great care must be taken to dispose of real medications according to policy and to note that the fluid in the vials must not be used for real patients. Different regions of the country have differing rules and regulations as to disposal of expired items. Some simulation laboratories have reported obtaining syringes and expired intravenous fluids from veterinarians and from patients who no longer require home-care services. Be creative in seeking out solutions to supply and equipment needs.

Student Preparation/Professional Expectations

In the previously mentioned survey of undergraduate nursing students (Leighton, 2007), it was reported that students did not prepare to the same level for simulated experiences (0–1 hour) as they did for human patients (2–4 hours). Many reasons exist for this difference, such as the student may have already experienced caring for the type of simulated patient he or she expects in the simulation and therefore needs less preparation time, personal or social obligations limit preparation, or the student may perceive the simulated experience as less stressful and without consequence if performance is poor.

It is recommended that students prepare for simulated clinical experiences in the same manner and to the same degree as they do for traditional clinical experiences. Providing the students with focused preparation activities is also more efficient than the time spent seeking out information from the chart, the patient, the family, and other caregivers. Preparation activities contribute to learning and allow the simulation facilitator to answer questions, clarify misconceptions, enhance the knowledge base, and facilitate learning rather than teach. Time in the simulation lab is therefore likely to be focused and intense.

Professional behavior and dress are important to the learning experience in the simulation laboratory. In fact, observations have been made that students behave more professionally when in uniform than when in street clothes (Ravert, 2010). While learning to manage a variety of patient types and conditions, students are also learning professional behaviors and communication techniques. Providing an environment in which professional behaviors are modeled and practiced will likely enhance professionalism. At the same time, state boards of nursing are often being asked to consider human patient simulation as a replacement for traditional clinical experiences. If this is to occur, then efforts should be made to ensure that the experiences in the simulation laboratory are as realistic as possible.

Prebriefing

Many facilitators prefer to conduct a prebriefing to begin the SCE. During this time, assigned preparatory work may be reviewed and questions answered. Misconceptions are clarified, and facilitators determine whether students are prepared to provide care to the simulated patient. If not prepared, a student might be dismissed from the lab experience to return at another scheduled time when he or she has prepared better. After preparation is evaluated, the students will be given report on their patient, and they may be asked to determine which types of care are needed and how they will be prioritized. This ensures that students know where to begin upon entering the patient's room. Roles may be predetermined, and facilitators ensure that the students are oriented to the simulator and environment. As the students move from novice to advanced beginner, the facilitator may rely less on prebriefing to prepare the students.

■ Implementing the Simulated Clinical Experience

Faculty Roles

Faculty roles during simulation are primarily facilitative. Rather than being the sage on the stage, faculty become the guide on the side (Kardong-Edgren, Starkweather, & Ward, 2008). Although the role varies somewhat depending on the level of the students, the faculty may choose to provide the learners with prompts and cues. These are most often in the form of carefully crafted questions that stimulate critical thinking and problem solving and assist the students in taking necessary actions with appropriate interventions. As students progress through the program, fewer prompts and cues are required or are given. One way to manage cues is to stay in character and voice cues and questions via the patient's voice. For example, the simulated patients could ask, "Are there any side effects I should watch for?" when receiving a medication; or "I've heard I can get AIDS from a blood transfusion," requiring students to provide explanations. The facilitator can then evaluate the students' knowledge based on their responses.

In the absence of electronic health records (EHRs), critical thinking, problem solving, and planning care are aided in simulation when a large flip chart or white-board is utilized. One person is assigned to be the documenter/recorder for the simulation. Beginning with report, the documenter writes down pertinent information and continues to record as assessments, new data, and interventions occur. The information can then be easily viewed by all participants and is constantly referred to. This documentation can be utilized as the student calls the healthcare provider, as the faculty asks questions about the meaning of newly acquired lab data, or as students plan care based on new orders. If a flip chart is used, the paper can easily be removed and taken to debriefing for further evaluation and discussion of care. This method is also useful for concept mapping or nursing process development. The use of the EHR is further discussed later in the *Charting* section of this chapter.

The Dreyfus and Dreyfus model of skill acquisition (1980), adapted for use with nursing by Benner (1984), supports learning on a continuum beginning with novice and progressing through the advanced beginner, competent, proficient, and expert stages. This model has implications for faculty who facilitate sessions in the simulation laboratory. Learning the skill of facilitation is a new challenge for most faculty, and they begin at a novice level. It is important for faculty to recognize this and to not attempt a simulated clinical experience that is overly complex and detailed for their first efforts. They should begin with simple scenarios as they can often have as much impact as those that are complex. As the level of comfort with facilitation grows, so will creativity and willingness to attempt more complex scenarios. Trying to do too much at the beginning will only frustrate the facilitator and the students, making the next attempt at simulation more of a challenge.

The novice-to-expert approach has also been used to help determine the role of facilitators when interacting with students in the simulation laboratory. Novice students may experience increased stress or anxiety when placed in an unfamiliar environment and given new expectations to care for a simulated patient. They have little to no experience to draw from, and it may be of value for the faculty to be present at the bedside, assist in proper assessment techniques and respond to questions immediately.

As the students progress to advanced beginner, the facilitator can play the role of a family member. Continued presence in the room provides a level of comfort and reportedly decreases anxiety among students. The facilitator asks questions of students while in the family member role and is able to determine if students understand the care they are providing and can provide appropriate education and responses to the patient and family.

When learners reach the proficient stage, the facilitator becomes further removed, although depending on the laboratory setup, he or she might remain in the room with the students. However, at this point, the facilitator only observes unless it is essential to intervene and redirect the students. While some educators advocate for students to experience the results of their indecision or incorrect decisions, this must be weighed in light of whether the learning objectives will be met satisfactorily. At the expert stage, the facilitator is completely removed from the simulated patient room and observes through a one-way window or via technology such as Skype.

Student Roles

One of the biggest challenges facing faculty in the simulation laboratory is that of group size. Defining roles for each individual student brings focus to the experience and decreases confusion. A variety of roles can be utilized, depending on the simulated clinical experience. Roles can be assigned or chosen at random or purposefully assigned based on identified student weaknesses. Suggestions of roles and responsibilities utilized by many simulation laboratories are provided in **Table 16-3**.

Facilitators are encouraged to utilize roles that are nurse specific as outlined in Table 16-3. Assigning roles of other healthcare providers, such as laboratory technician, respiratory therapist, or physician, is often troublesome, as the students do not have the background to know the roles of those providers. It is also challenging to have students play the role of the family member, again because most lack that type of experience, but also because they have to perform in front of their peers.

Table 16-3 Roles for Students in the Simulation Laboratory

Role	Responsibilities
Primary nurse	• Assessment; final decision • Consider two primary nurses so one student is not responsible alone if a poor outcome is experienced
Secondary nurse	• Backs up primary nurse if two-primary-nurse system not used • Assists the primary nurse in assessment and decision making
Medication nurse	• Administers medications safely according to orders
Documentation nurse	• Documents on paper or electronically to maintain a patient record • Documents on flip chart or whiteboard to keep all informed of assessment findings and care provided
Healthcare communicator	• Provides information to healthcare provider in person or via phone calls; contacts ancillary departments for test results
Observer	• Provide focused role for the observer such as observing for communication between nurse and patient; identification of cultural care; patient education provided by nurse; recognition of psychosocial care; overall management of care

Those who are shy or introverted tend to struggle in these types of roles, while extroverts often go off script or break out in laughter at inappropriate times.

There often is concern expressed by facilitators that the students in the observation role will not learn as much as those actively caring for the simulated patient. In Phase III of the NLN/Laerdal project, *Designing and Implementing Models for the Innovative Use of Simulation to Teach Nursing Care of Ill Adults and Children: A National, Multi-Site, Multi-Method Study*, researchers reported that there were no significant differences in knowledge gain, satisfaction, or self-confidence based on the role of the student (Jeffries & Rizzolo, 2006).

Use of Resources in the Simulation Lab

Personal digital assistants (PDAs), phones with Internet service, and electronic tablets are being incorporated into simulation experiences. During the SCE, students can immediately access textbook information and can look up diseases, care plans, drug and laboratory guides, medical dictionaries, procedural guidelines, and literature databases. It is important in today's constantly changing healthcare environment that students learn where to access needed information rather than expecting to always rely on memory. Point-of-care access is vital so that nurses can rely on the latest evidence-based information to make decisions when needed. These electronic, Internet-based tools are invaluable as students move from performing skills to making decisions about care based on the latest knowledge available. Clinical calculators are also utilized in simulation laboratories to more safely determine drug dosing and intravenous drip rates, and for other physiological calculations.

The Joint Commission identified the leading root cause of sentinel events in the United States between 1995 and 2006 as a breakdown in handoff communication (World Health Organization & Joint Commission, 2007). These sentinel events resulted in unintended harm to patients and prompted the Joint Commission to recommend that hospitals standardize handoff communications. SBAR is being used by hospitals across the country to improve communication. During the SCE, students can have valuable practice in communication skills by giving handoff reports, by calling healthcare providers, and by interacting with the interdisciplinary team utilizing the SBAR format. Use of the format assists students in becoming more organized and confident in their thinking and reporting.

Charting

Types of documentation can range from paper charting, using blank forms obtained from a local facility or creating one's own, to electronic charting comparable to a full hospital-grade EHR. The level of complexity in the design of these documentation systems is up to the faculty. Some faculty create realistic systems using Microsoft Office products such as Word and Excel. There is no known research pointing to whether one method is better than another. The underlying principles and concepts of documentation are the important focus.

Charts and forms for all aspects of patient care should be constructed for each SCE. Additional forms that might be appropriate for the SCE, such as emergency department records, blood transfusion and blood bank forms, and incident reports, for example, should also be available. Documentation forms should be as similar as possible to those the students utilize in their clinical areas. Unfortunately, a large variety of documentation systems exist, and many students have to learn a different system at each clinical site.

Various methods are utilized in simulation laboratories to create documentation opportunities for students. While it is helpful to utilize a system as close to what students see on the traditional clinical unit as possible, many simulation laboratories do not have the resources to do this. There are several existing commercial products available, but many simulation facilitators create their own system.

Multidisciplinary/Interdisciplinary Team Simulations

As nursing faculty become more comfortable with simulation, they are beginning to incorporate SCEs that foster an interdisciplinary team approach with other healthcare students. The Institute of Medicine has said the "all health professionals should be educated to deliver patient-centered care as a member of an interdisciplinary team, emphasizing evidence-based practice, quality improvement approaches, and informatics" (IOM, 2003, p. 3). As the population ages and lives with multiple comorbidities and chronic health needs, the care for that population requires the collaboration of multiple healthcare professionals. Therefore, simulation provides the perfect opportunity for students to work together on complex patient care problems. Pharmacy, respiratory therapy, social work, seminary, and medical practitioners or students have all collaborated with nursing students during SCEs. Students learn the knowledge, roles, responsibilities, and frame of reference each brings to the patient situation. They learn to work together as a team, to share the information they have about the patient, and to communicate and resolve differences related to care.

Many hospitals and schools of nursing are utilizing the TeamSTEPPS program developed by the Department of Defense's Patient Safety Program in collaboration with the Agency for Healthcare Research and Quality (AHRQ). This program provides materials and a training curriculum for an evidence-based teamwork system to improve communication and teamwork skills. Information about this program can be obtained by going to http://teamstepps.ahrq.gov/. The goal of TeamSTEPPS and all intradisciplinary training is to assist in providing higher-quality, safer patient care through more effective communication among health professionals.

Classroom Use of Simulation

Most faculty think of a laboratory space when envisioning the use of human patient simulation in their courses; however, simulation can be added to the classroom experience as well. Three common methods of integrating simulation into classroom teaching follow.

Simulator in Classroom

Many patient simulators are portable and can be moved easily into a classroom. While this may seem overwhelming the first one or two times, it is not difficult to learn with repetition and can be accomplished in only a few minutes. Once the simulator is in the classroom, the instructor can place it at the front of the class and at the desired time, invite two or three students to care for the patient, who should be designed to facilitate learning of concepts currently being taught. Students often hesitate to volunteer for this role and may have to be assigned.

The simulated patient's condition or illness may be cared for to resolution during one time frame of the class, or the care can be divided into sections corresponding to the didactic material as it is presented. Another option is to simulate two different but similar conditions, such as heart failure and chronic obstructive pulmonary disease. Selected students care for each patient, and the subsequent patient management is subjected to contrast and comparison analysis.

Simulation via Two-Way Interactive Video

Some simulators and their environs are not designed for easy transport and cannot be removed from the laboratory. In such instances, simulation via two-way interactive video can be used. The simulated patient remains in the laboratory and the designated number of students leave the classroom to care for the patient there. This interaction is broadcast to the classroom using existing interactive video capabilities. Many schools do not have the resources for this type of equipment, but there are now many free or low-cost options, such as Skype, available via the Internet.

Simulation Software

The laptop that runs the simulation software can be connected to an overhead liquid crystal display (LCD) projector in the classroom in the same manner that a computer is connected to project PowerPoint presentations. Once the laptop is connected, the students are oriented to the instructor view and instructed on which visible parameters to monitor. Simple to complex material can be visually presented using the following examples:

- Administer the same medication and dose to a young, healthy simulated patient and to a simulated patient with cardiovascular disease. Observe changes in blood pressure and heart rate (novice students) or mean arterial pressure and central venous pressure (advanced students).
- Provoke a pneumothorax through the software and have learners monitor the respiratory rate and oxygen saturation levels for changes.
- Create a pericardial tamponade through the software and have learners monitor hemodynamic changes with various amounts of fluid.
- Remove 2–3 liters of blood through the software and have students monitor hemodynamic changes. Conversely, administer 2–3 liters of crystalloids and monitor the same hemodynamics.

■ After the Simulated Clinical Experience

Debriefing

Debriefing is essential to the simulation experience. It is during this time when students have the opportunity to reflect on the experience that much of the learning occurs. Faculty function as facilitators in the debriefing by stimulating students to consider what they were thinking during the simulation, how they were feeling, what they did, what occurred as a result, and how they can apply what they have learned to their care with real patients. It is important for students to be able to follow the fast-paced simulation with a quiet time away from the simulator where they can cognitively process and reflect on what occurred. Video clips may also aid in the understanding of what transpired (Fanning & Gaba, 2007).

Several different methods are popular with those facilitating simulation. Plus/delta places actions into a positive column and a column designated for actions or activities that could be done differently. Another method is advocacy/inquiry, which uses comments such as, "I saw you do _____ assessment and wondered what other assessments might provide more information," to provoke further discussion. One easy method of organization commonly used in nursing consists of the following four parts: the introduction, sharing of personal reactions, discussion of events, and the wrap-up (Johnson-Russell & Bailey, 2010). Although the first three are sometimes discussed simultaneously, all should be covered at some point in the debriefing.

The introduction sets the stage for the debriefing by letting students know that this is a safe place to discuss what went on during the scenario and that what they share about their feelings and behavior will not be discussed outside the room. Many faculty have students sign a confidentiality statement at this time. Another option is to treat confidentiality using the principles of the Health Insurance Portability and Accountability Act (HIPAA) that is in place at all clinical agencies and is designed to protect patient privacy. At this time, the faculty inform students about their expectations for the debriefing. All students are expected to contribute to the discussions by analyzing the simulation. Other expectations include making decisions, prioritizing, and capitalizing on opportunities for improvement, teamwork, and collaboration.

In the immediate postsimulation period, there is often excitement and/or anxiety from the tension built up during the simulation. Expressing these feelings or sharing of personal reactions is often necessary before students can cognitively process other aspects of the SCE. Assisting students to delve deeper into the events that led to these feelings may provide a new awareness of their functioning and thought processes. Generally, the focus of further discussion should build on the positive aspects of the experience and then move to challenges and areas for improvement. Students are often much harder on themselves and their performance than facilitators are. Focusing on the positive prior to the negative helps to keep the discussions in perspective.

The discussion of events focuses on the patient, the condition, the interventions, and the outcomes. The facilitator can segue into this part of the discussion using comments the students have previously made, or he or she can ask specific questions about the patient and his condition, anticipated outcomes, how the SCE unfolded, prioritization, and management of care. Review of the overall experience is also important. Use of resources, safety concerns, communication among team members, and accurate documentation should be reviewed. Questions about individual behaviors such as not listening to patient concerns or not wearing gloves when appropriate, difficulties in performing care, and how those concerns will be addressed should be asked.

Team functioning is important to discuss, especially in relation to communication with team members. Communication with family members and the patient may also need to be addressed. Debriefing is an excellent time to have students role-play and practice more effective communication. Students frequently have difficulty relating the events of the SCE to the real world since their experience is limited. It is valuable to spend time discussing how the SCE applies to the clinical setting and to patients they may encounter in the future.

Video clips may provide additional stimulation for discussions. They should be used as an adjunct in the debriefing to assist students in understanding those things that they might have missed or when there have been procedural problems, missed cues, or poor decision making. Viewing the videotape is an excellent way of helping learners understand the events that transpired in the SCE and their participation in them. Viewing segments where they performed well is also important in reinforcing appropriate behaviors and instilling confidence.

The summary or wrap-up can be accomplished using statements the students have verbalized about what they believed went well and what did not. Facilitators should remind students of areas they mentioned they need to improve upon. It is also valuable to have students identify which resources they will use to make those improvements. Some faculty prefer to have the students summarize the session by verbalizing what they learned from the SCE. Students appreciate hearing positive comments from the faculty about their performance or improvements that were observed. Additionally, some faculty post questions on their intranet, have the students reflect on the experience, and answer the questions within 24 hours of the SCE. Others ask students to journal their reflections.

Faculty may want to utilize the "Debriefing Assessment for Simulation in Healthcare (DASH)" from the Center for Medical Simulation to evaluate and develop their debriefing skills. Information about the rating forms can be found at the DASH website: http://www.harvardmedsim.org/debriefing-assesment-simulation-healthcare.php.

Students should complete evaluations of the entire simulated clinical experience at the end of the debriefing. These evaluations can provide valuable information about what was most helpful to the students and what might be changed to make the SCE an even better learning experience. Obtaining information about the design of the simulation, availability of resources, effectiveness of the facilitator, perception of learning outcomes, and suggestions for future simulated clinical experiences provides valuable insight to the facilitator (Horn & Carter, 2007). This information should be trended and adjustments to the scenario made as necessary. One frequently used tool is the Simulation Effectiveness Tool (SET), a 13-item evaluation tool with established reliability and validity (Elfrink Cordi, Leighton, Ryan-Wenger, Doyle, & Ravert, 2012).

After a Simulated Patient Death

Many simulation facilitators are fearful that simulated death experiences will cause the student to believe they killed the simulated patient or are responsible for its death, leading to feelings of guilt. There is also concern that buried feelings may rise to the surface, leading to psychological trauma. There is no literature to support these assumptions; however, the facilitator is charged with recognizing and managing psychological stress of participants (Leighton, 2009a).

The debriefing process is vital to managing this psychological stress as students are given the opportunity to talk about their feelings and explore the events that occurred during the simulated clinical experience in a safe, nonjudgmental environment. The facilitator may consider involving a chaplain or mental health practitioner in the scenario or during the debriefing. In some cases, the facilitator may need to refer the student for further psychological assistance (Leighton, 2009a). Anecdotally, many students have reported that experiencing death in the simulation lab helped them to better understand previous real-life experiences.

Evaluation/Testing/Assessment

Considerable discussion occurs at simulation conferences and informal meetings about evaluating students in the simulation laboratory. Several schools have developed rubrics to use for this process, while formal research protocols have created other methods to evaluate learning, critical thinking, or components of critical judgment (Lasater, 2007). Currently available tools have been outlined by Kardong-Edgren, Adamson, and Fitzgerald (2010), with an updated manuscript in press (2012). At this time, more nursing schools use simulation as a teaching strategy than do those who use simulation as an evaluation tool (Hovancsek, 2007).

A recent topic of focus is high-stakes testing and whether nursing education is ready for this. A roundtable discussion held at the 2009 International Nursing Association for Clinical Simulation and Learning (INACSL) conference was followed by an article created from the notes of that discussion. Generally, it was agreed that while it is a worthy goal, nursing education is not yet ready for high-stakes testing due to a variety of reasons, including the fact that all nursing programs are not teaching with simulation due to budgetary reasons. Another concern of significant proportions is the lack of consistent methods of facilitation and use of standardized scenarios (Kardong-Edgren, Hanberg, Keenan, Ackerman, & Chambers, 2011).

It is imperative that nursing programs identify their philosophy related to evaluation or assessment in the simulation laboratory. To begin, definitions must be determined. During meeting discussions, participants use a variety of different terminology to describe evaluation, assessment, and testing. It is clear that many of these conversations are attempting to compare apples to oranges.

Questions that should be considered during discussions about evaluation, testing, and assessment could include:

- "Is the simulation lab better suited for facilitating learning or for evaluating students? Is it possible to do both?
- Is it fair to test students if they have not had significant exposure to simulated clinical experiences?
- Are faculty all competent in their roles? How is this variable controlled for evaluation purposes?

- How do we account for the variety of student responses and interventions that are inherent in simulations?
- Are we sending mixed messages when we tell students that simulation is a safe environment to learn in and then use that same environment for evaluation?
- Do we test students in the traditional clinical environment? Is it then fair to test in the simulation lab?
- If the focus is on testing, will the experience become an experience about performing rather than about learning?
- What can you learn about your students in the simulation environment without formal evaluation or testing?
- If we say that most of the learning occurs in debriefing, can we fairly evaluate students before that debriefing occurs?" (Leighton, 2009b, p. e57).

If the decision is made to evaluate simulations, the faculty must determine the purpose of the evaluation, decide when to evaluate, create an evaluation plan, utilize instruments to collect the data, and interpret the data (Jeffries & Rogers, 2007a). Various instruments can be found in the education and simulation literature; however, the facilitator must consider the reliability and validity of the tool to be used.

Research and Advancement Opportunities

It should be clear to the reader of this chapter that a wide variety of research opportunities exist for the users of simulation. While simulation has been used in healthcare education for years, the use of high-fidelity human patient simulation is still in its infancy in nursing education. While it is often bemoaned that there is little research pointing to the efficacy of this teaching strategy, the research base has grown exponentially as facilitators have become more comfortable in their roles.

Conducting research in the simulation laboratory has several advantages over research in the traditional clinical environment—namely, there is no risk to patients. Facilitators are also able to control the scenario, patient responses, communication with healthcare providers, and equipment made available. However, those same faculty are also difficult to control as a variable. Faculty have different levels of education regarding the role of facilitator, respond in different ways to students' efforts to communicate, and often need to step outside of the planned script to respond to unpredictable student actions (Alinier, 2008).

There have been many obstacles to using research data to support increased use of human patient simulation or to justify the expense and time required to learn. A systematic research review, over a 34-year period ending in 2003, revealed wide variety in research design, methods of measuring outcomes, journal report structure, and use of small sample sizes (McGahie, Pugh, & Wayne, 2008).

It is a responsibility of each of us as simulation facilitators and proponents to help move the field forward through well-designed research studies and documentation of best practice and standards of excellence. It is no longer enough to document that students like simulation or that they prefer this method to another. The time has come to document that learning occurs and that it is equal to or better than the learning that occurs with our traditional teaching methods. As the competition for clinical sites continues to build, simulation will take a vital role in the future of nursing education.

Two international simulation organizations have taken the lead on furthering the competency of faculty and the overall management of simulation programs. The two organizations are the INACSL and the Society for Simulation in Healthcare (SSH). Both organizations include members of all types of healthcare educators, although the INACSL has a narrower focus to nursing in general. The two organizations affiliate with each other, and members can avail themselves to numerous benefits, including ongoing education, annual conferences, and academic journals.

The INACSL developed and published *Standards of Best Practice: Simulation* in the fall of 2011. There were seven standards developed, with plans for additional guidelines and biannual reviews. The first update and release of guidelines is complete and scheduled for publication in the fall of 2013. The seven standards include:

   I: Terminology
  II: Professional integrity of participant
 III: Participant objectives
 IV: Facilitation methods
  V: Simulation facilitator
 VI: The debriefing process
VII: Evaluation of expected outcomes (INACSL Board of Directors, 2011)

The Society for Simulation in Healthcare has created a certification program for simulation educators, that has completed the beta-testing phase and consists of a multiple-choice exam. In addition, SSH has developed an accreditation program for simulation centers and laboratories. Following a self-study and site visit, 22 centers have been accredited since the program's inception in 2010.

▪ Conclusion

This chapter has provided information intended to help those who take on the challenge of facilitating learning in the simulation laboratory. While many nursing programs have managed to obtain funding for simulation equipment, there has often been little forethought into how faculty will manage to learn this type of teaching strategy and where the time will come from for that purpose (Kardong-Edgren & Oermann, 2009). This chapter was intended to aid the process of faculty development by providing realistic ideas that can be easily implemented by facilitators of learning in simulation laboratories. The simulator and its features have little value if faculty do not know how to effectively teach with the technology.

TEACHING EXAMPLE

STRATEGY

The strategy involves the incorporation of fidelity, role of faculty, and holistic aspects of patient care for a beginning assessment course using a simulated clinical experience (SCE). Participants in the simulation laboratory include the course faculty member and up to eight students.

EXPECTATIONS

The students are expected to obtain subjective and objective assessment data and inform the healthcare provider of their findings. Prerequisite knowledge should include anatomy and physiology of the cardiovascular system and corresponding assessment techniques. The example involves a young, morbidly obese female patient whose symptoms are precipitated by a systolic heart murmur. Guidelines for the instructor follow.

SETTING

Place the simulator on a bed or stretcher and inform students the "patient" has not been seen by a healthcare provider. Place two individual breast models (often used to teach palpation for lumps) on the chest of the simulator. The patient's obesity can be simulated by placing a pillow over the abdomen and securing it with an elastic wrap or gauze roll. Put female clothes appropriate for the weather on the simulator (to make it easier to dress the simulator, cut the shirt up the back, leaving the collar intact; cut the pants along the back to the inseam) and add a woman's wig to the head. Makeup can be applied to the simulator after it is tested in a nonvisible place for staining. Personal effects such as a magazine, cell phone, and purse can be placed on the bedside table next to a bottle of sugary carbonated beverage.

SIMULATOR SETTINGS

Set systolic murmur (or other preferred abnormal heart sound). All other settings are normal.

FACULTY ROLE

If this is the first SCE for students, they are at a novice level and will need faculty assistance. It is preferable to orient students to the simulator and its features prior to starting the scenario. Only tell students what they need to know to care for this patient, as providing information on IV sites, defibrillation, or monitoring is above their knowledge level and will be extraneous information.

Begin outside of the simulator's room and brief students on the patient who has just arrived to the healthcare provider's office. Report is as follows:

"This is a 38-year-old female with complaints of fatigue, orthopnea, and palpitations. She is 5 feet, 2 inches tall and weighs 100 kilograms."

(continued)

Student Expectations

- Knock on the door and announce entry
- Introduce self and role to patient
- Wash hands
- Ask subjective questions to obtain more information from the patient, such as the following (with answers in parentheses):
  - How long ago did your symptoms start? (6 months ago; gradually worsening)
  - Any associated symptoms? (no shortness of breath or chest pain)
  - What makes the symptoms worse? (walking and exercise)
  - What makes the symptoms go away? (rest)
  - How many pillows do you use at night? (three)
  - Do you have any history of medical problems? (no)
  - Do you have any family history of medical problems? (no cardiac disease)
  - Do you smoke, drink alcohol, or use drugs not prescribed for you? (no)
  - How much do you exercise in a week? (none)
  - Has there been any change in your weight recently? (gained 40 pounds past 4 months)
  - What is your typical diet? (fast food, soda)
  - Do you take any medications? (ibuprofen as needed for back pain)
  - When was the last time you saw a healthcare provider?

Questioning may continue until the facilitator believes that enough data have been collected. The facilitator then prompts the beginning of the physical assessment.

Student Expectations

- Wash hands upon entering the room
- Explain what will be done to patient
- Conduct general survey
- Provide for privacy
- Head-to-toe physical assessment with emphasis on cardiovascular system
- Wash hands after assessment of the patient is complete
- Make sure personal items are in reach
- Ensure safe environment

During the physical assessment, the students will discover an abnormality in the heart sounds. Although it may be beyond their scope to recognize and define a heart murmur, they should be able to identify that an abnormality exists. All other findings, including vital signs, are normal.

Holistic Aspects (one or more may be included):

- *Psychosocial.* Patient does not have health insurance and voices concern about how to pay for office visit, follow-up tests, or prescriptions.
- *Spiritual.* Patient may be anxious and ask student to pray with her.
- *Cultural.* Patient may be from a culture other than that of most of the students.

- *Developmental.* Patient may blame weight gain on a recent life experience, such as a divorce.

ANTICIPATED AND UNANTICIPATED EVENTS AND CONSEQUENCES

NERVOUSNESS

As this is often the first SCE for the students, they are prone to nervousness and have trouble getting started. The facilitator may need to ask each student to pose a subjective question to the patient. The person responding as the patient should allow time for questions to be formulated, not rushing the students.

SCATTERED THOUGHT PROCESSES

Novice students tend to randomly ask subjective questions without organization. Following subjective questioning, the facilitator can help them to prioritize their completed assessment questions and findings.

INCORRECT ASSESSMENT TECHNIQUES

The facilitator is at the bedside with this novice group and can correct technique as problems occur. Unless the SCE is recorded, this level of learners may not recall what they did right or wrong by the time debriefing occurs.

FAILURE TO RECOGNIZE ABNORMALITY

This may occur in the novice student due to lack of experience to draw upon. If this is the case, the facilitator should point it out and have all students listen to the heart sounds. The respiratory rate may be lowered on the simulator and the heart sound volume increased to facilitate hearing of abnormal heart sounds.

EVALUATION OF LEARNER ATTAINMENT

The intent of this SCE is to provide an introductory-level experience for the student who has not yet interacted with a real patient and is just beginning to learn physical assessment techniques and concepts. The facilitator will often be surprised by the learner's inability to formulate subjective questions and conduct a basic physical assessment. Remembering that novice learners have no experiences to draw upon will keep expectations in perspective. Learners should be able to demonstrate physical assessment techniques learned in class; however, they often need help finessing their technique and need reassurance that they are doing the assessment correctly.

REFERENCES

Adamson, K. A., Kardong-Edgren, S., & Willhaus, J. (2012). An updated review of published simulation evaluation instruments. *Clinical Simulation in Nursing.* doi: 10.1016/j.ecns.2012.09.004

Alinier, G. (2008). Pitfalls to avoid in designing and executing research with clinical simulation. In R. R. Kyle, Jr., & W. B. Murray (Eds.), *Clinical simulation: Operations, engineering and management* (pp. 515–516). New York, NY: Elsevier.

Benner, P. (1984). *From novice to expert: Excellence and power in clinical nursing practice.* Menlo Park, CA: Addison-Wesley.

Cantrell, M. A., Meakim, C., & Cash, K. (2008). Development and evaluation of three pediatric-based clinical simulations. *Clinical Simulation in Nursing Education, 4*(1), e1.

Decker, S., Sportsman, S., Puetz, L., & Billings, L. (2008). The evolution of simulation and its contribution to competency. *Journal of Continuing Education in Nursing, 39*(2), 74–80.

Dreyfus, S. E., & Dreyfus, H. L. (1980). *A five-stage model of the mental activities involved in directed skill acquisition.* Washington, DC: Storming Media. Retrieved from http://www.dtic.mil/cgi-bin /GetTRDoc?AD=ADA084551&Location=U2&doc=GetTRDoc.pdf

Elfrink Cordi, V. L., Leighton, K., Ryan-Wenger, N., Doyle, T., & Ravert, P. (2012). History and development of the Simulation Effectiveness Tool (SET). *Clinical Simulation in Nursing, 8*(6), e199–e210.

Fanning, R. M., & Gaba, D. M. (2007). The role of debriefing in simulation-based learning. *Simulation in Healthcare 2,* 115–125.

Gaba, D. (2004). A brief history of mannequin-based simulation & application. In W. F. Dunn (Ed.), *Simulators in critical care education and beyond* (pp.7–14). Des Plaines, IL: Society of Critical Care Medicine.

Horn, M., & Carter, N. (2007). Practical suggestions for implementing simulations. In P. R. Jeffries (Ed.), *Simulation in nursing education* (pp. 59–72). New York, NY: National League for Nursing.

Hovancsek, M. T. (2007). Using simulations in nursing education. In P. R. Jeffries (Ed.), *Simulation in nursing education* (pp. 1–9). New York, NY: National League for Nursing.

Institute of Medicine (IOM). (2003). *Health professions education: A bridge to quality.* Washington, DC: National Academies Press.

International Nursing Association for Clinical Simulation and Learning (INASCL) Board of Directors. (2011). Standards of best practice: Simulation. *Clinical Simulation in Nursing, 7*(4 suppl), S1–S20.

Interprofessional Education Collaborative Expert Panel. (2011). *Core competencies for interprofessional collaborative practice: Report of an expert panel.* Washington, DC: Interprofessional Education Collaborative.

Jeffries, P. R., & Rizzolo, M. A. (2006). Final report of the NLN/Laerdal simulation study. In P. R. Jeffries (Ed.), *Simulation in nursing education* (pp.145–158). New York, NY: National League for Nursing.

Jeffries, P. R., & Rogers, K. J. (2007a). Evaluating simulations. In P. R. Jeffries (Ed.), *Simulation in nursing education* (pp. 87–103). New York, NY: National League for Nursing.

Jeffries, P. R., & Rogers, K. J. (2007b). Theoretical framework for simulation design. In P. R. Jeffries (Ed.), *Simulation in nursing education* (pp. 21–33). New York, NY: National League for Nursing.

Johnson-Russell, J., & Bailey, C. (2010). Facilitated debriefing. In W. M. Nehring & F. R. Lashley (Eds.), *High-fidelity patient simulation in nursing education* (pp. 369–385). Sudbury, MA: Jones and Bartlett.

Kardong-Edgren, S., Adamson, K. A., & Fitzgerald, C. (2010). A review of currently published evaluation instruments for human patient simulation. *Clinical Simulation in Nursing, 6*(1), e25–e35.

Kardong-Edgren, S., Anderson, M., & Michaels, J. (2007). Does simulation fidelity improve student test scores? *Clinical Simulation in Nursing Education, 3*(1), feature 4.

Kardong-Edgren, S., Hanberg, A. D., Keenan, C., Ackerman, A., & Chambers, K. C. (2011, January). A discussion of high-stakes testing: An extension of a 2009 INACSL conference roundtable. *Clinical Simulation in Nursing, 7*(1), e19–e24. doi: 10.1016/j.ecns.2010.02.002

Kardong-Edgren, S., & Oermann, M. H. (2009). A letter to nursing program administrators. *Clinical Simulation in Nursing, 5*(5), e161–e162.

Kardong-Edgren, S., Starkweather, A., & Ward, L. (2008). The integration of simulation into a clinical foundations of nursing course: Student and faculty perspectives. *International Journal of Nursing Education Scholarship, 5*(1), Article 26. Retrieved from http://www.bepress.com/ijnes/vol5/iss1/art26

Lasater, K. (2007). Clinical judgment development using simulation to create an assessment rubric. *Journal of Nursing Education, 46*(11), 496–503.

Leigh, G., & Hurst, H. (2008). We have a high-fidelity simulator, now what? Making the most of simulators. *International Journal of Nursing Education Scholarship, 5*(1), Article 33.

Leighton, K. (2007). Learning needs in the simulated clinical environment and the traditional clinical environment: A survey of undergraduate nursing students. *ETD Collection for University of Nebraska–Lincoln.* Paper AAI3271929. Retrieved from http://digitalcommons.unl.edu/dissertations/AAI3271929

Leighton, K. (2009a). Death of a simulator. *Clinical Simulation in Nursing, 5*(2), e59–e62.

Leighton, K. (2009b). What can we learn from a LISTSERV? *Clinical Simulation in Nursing, 5*(2), e57–e58.

McGahie, W. C., Pugh, C. M., & Wayne, D. B. (2008). Fundamentals of educational research using clinical simulation. In R. R. Kyle, Jr., & W. B. Murray (Eds.), *Clinical simulation: Operations, engineering and management* (pp. 517–528). New York, NY: Elsevier, Inc.

Medley, C. F., & Horne, C. (2005). Using simulation technology for undergraduate nursing education. *Journal of Nursing Education, 44*(1), 31–34.

Morgan, P. J., Cleave-Hogg, D., Desousa, S., & Lam- McCulloch, J. (2006). Applying theory to practice in undergraduate education using high fidelity simulation. *Medical Teacher, 28*(1), e10–e14.

Nehring, W. M. (2010). History of simulation in nursing. In W. M. Nehring & F. R. Lashley (Eds.), *High-fidelity patient simulation in nursing education* (pp. 3–26). Sudbury, MA: Jones and Bartlett.

Pagano, M. P., & Greiner, P. A. (2009). Enhancing communication skills through simulations. In S. H. Campbell & K. M. Daley (Eds.), *Simulation scenarios for nurse educators: Making it real* (pp. 43–51). New York, NY: Springer.

Ravert, P. (2010). Developing and implementing a simulation program: Baccalaureate nursing education. In W. M. Nehring & F. R. Lashley (Eds.), *High-fidelity patient simulation in nursing education* (pp. 59–74). Sudbury, MA: Jones and Bartlett.

World Health Organization & Joint Commission. (2007). Communication during patient hand-overs. *Patient Safety Solutions, 1*(3), Solution 3. Retrieved from http://www.who.int/patientsafety/solutions/patientsafety/PS-Solution3.pdf

CHAPTER 17

Interprofessional Communication Skills Lab

■ Jeanine Salfi and Patricia Solomon ■

As the delivery of health care becomes more complex and challenging, it is essential that all healthcare professionals communicate and collaborate effectively as a team. The ability to communicate in a respectful manner facilitates connectedness among members of a team, as it allows for an awareness of equal power and fosters shared decision making, responsibility, and authority (Sele, Salamon, Boarman, & Sauer, 2008). Interprofessional education is a critical step in preparing a collaborative, practice-ready workforce that is better prepared to respond to the challenges and complexities of the current health care system (World Health Organization, 2010).

■ Interprofessional Education

Interprofessional education (IPE) occurs when students of two or more professions learn with, from, and about one another to improve collaboration and the quality of care (Centre for the Advancement of Interprofessional Education [CAIPE], 1997). CAIPE (2008) uses the term *interprofessional education* to include learning in both academic and clinical settings, before and after qualification, certification, or licensure. Some of the benefits of exposing prelicensure students to IPE are that it helps to cultivate mutual trust and respect, confronts misconceptions and stereotypes, and dispels prejudice and rivalry between professional groups (CAIPE, 2010).

Effective Interprofessional Education

A few key points should be upheld when designing and implementing activities and opportunities for IPE. Effective IPE (1) reinforces and provides the opportunity for students to develop and refine essential team-based skills; (2) provides students with the opportunity to learn about their own scope of practice, while learning the skills, languages, and perspectives of others' professional roles; and (3) is grounded in mutual respect, honoring the distinctive experiences and expertise that all participants bring to the healthcare team from their respective backgrounds (CAIPE, 2010). Embedded within these principles of effective IPE are several competencies (knowledge, skills, and behaviors) that are required for interprofessional collaborative practice. The number and specificity of interprofessional competencies may vary across academic institutions, but overall they can be summarized into four core areas:

1. Knowledge of and the ability to clearly articulate one's professional role and responsibilities.
2. Knowledge of the roles and responsibilities of other health professionals, and knowing when to refer and/or collaborate with others, in order to provide optimal person-centered care.
3. Possession of the skills required for collaboration, and the ability to collaborate with others to establish common goals (i.e., demonstrates effective communication, shared decision making, collaborative leadership, problem solving, and conflict resolution).
4. Contribution to team functioning by consistently exhibiting the following behaviors: sharing information, listening attentively, respecting others' opinions, demonstrating flexibility and the ability to trust others, using a common language, and providing and responding to feedback from others, among others.

These four competencies are embedded in three levels of IPE: exposure level, immersion level, and mastery level (Charles, Bainbridge, & Gilbert, 2008).

Exposure Activities

Exposure activities are primarily knowledge based, relating to the first two competencies, and focus on describing roles and responsibilities and demonstrating awareness of the scope of practice of other health professions. These activities are generally of short-term duration, and examples include interviewing and shadowing experiences and observing multidisciplinary panel discussions.

Immersion Activities

Immersion activities are typically of longer duration than exposure activities and require higher levels of interaction between the health professional students. All four competencies may be addressed through these activities. Students will be required to collaborate with other health professional students, make decisions, and solve problems together. Some examples of immersion activities include interactive e-based learning modules and the communication skills labs (which will be described in greater detail later in this chapter).

Mastery Activities

The mastery activities group is the most complex and integrative group of activities. Students will integrate their interprofessional knowledge and skills in a team environment. Typically, this will be of longer duration, and students will build relationships in a team environment and be actively engaged in team decision making around client care. Although mastery activities are primarily clinical practice experiences, some extended courses or student projects may also be considered mastery-level activities.

■ Theoretical Foundation

IPE introduces a pedagogy with its own classification that aims to recontextualize traditional and distinct bodies of professional knowledge into the knowledge of collaborative practice. Most prelicensure education is uniprofessional, in which students learn together as a single group and do not learn with or alongside other professional groups. IPE attempts to sensitize students to the roles of other healthcare professionals and teach the delivery of interprofessional care (Schmitt, 1994).

Social psychology theories such as contact theory (Carpenter & Hewstone, 1996) have been used in the interprofessional literature. Originally developed by Allport (1954), contact theory proposes that the most effective way to reduce tension between groups is to bring them together. Allport (1954) believed that simply placing people together was not enough to effect positive change, so he proposed the following three conditions: (1) equality of status between groups; (2) groups that work on common goals; and (3) cooperation of the groups during their contact.

This form of teaching can overcome the traditional ways of knowing about how to be a professional practitioner, and it has the potential to result in more effective relations within the healthcare team. The most predominant philosophical argument for IPE is that when IPE is offered at the prelicensure level, improvements will be made in interprofessional communication and collaboration in practice and, ultimately, will result in improved delivery of care and health outcomes for patients (Salvatori & Solomon, 2005).

■ Types of Learners

Some prelicensure programs are at the undergraduate level (e.g., nursing). The introduction of IPE at the undergraduate level remains controversial. One of the arguments against the introduction of IPE at the undergraduate level is that most students at this level have not acquired a sense of their own professional characteristics or sufficient practical experience to be able to experience the full benefits of IPE (Fraser, Symonds, Cullen, & Symonds, 2000). Some believe that premature introduction of IPE could have negative repercussions on undergraduate students because it might interfere with the establishment of a distinct professional identity (Miller, Ross, & Freeman, 1999). Conversely, students at the postgraduate level are able to take full advantage of the learning opportunities available through IPE because they possess background professional knowledge and practical experience on which to base their insight and discussions (Barr, Freeth, Hammick, Koppel, & Reeves, 2000).

Currently, there are no studies demonstrating that early exposure to IPE hinders the ability to acquire or develop one's professional identity. Some advantages associated with integrating IPE within undergraduate curricula include the opportunity to overturn negative stereotypes at an early stage in an individual's professional social-ization (Barr et al., 2000), and to improve the student's confidence and ability to communicate with other members of the healthcare team. It also introduces the concept of teamwork in the healthcare setting and the importance of collaboration among a variety of professionals to enhance patient care.

▪ Interprofessional Communication Skills Lab

One example of IPE at the immersion level is the communication skills lab, which was originally developed in 2004, and designed to address core IPE competencies (Salvatori, Mahoney, & Delottinville, 2006). Each lab session is 3 hours in dura-tion, beginning with an introduction/orientation to the session, followed by a team meeting in which the students review a patient scenario and an interview with a standardized patient (an actor/actress who has been specially trained to portray the patient in the scenario). It has been suggested that students need to be challenged with complex, realistic, healthcare problems using cooperative learning as part of the learning process, such as using a paper-based healthcare scenario or, better yet, a simulated patient (D'Eon, 2004).

Developing the Scenario

The scenario provides the starting point for learning in a communication skills lab. Well-constructed scenarios provide a focus for learning, stimulate interest in the content, and provide a meaningful context within which prior learning is activated and new knowledge is gained (Drummond-Young & Mohide, 2001). The design and development of a patient scenario are composed of several steps. Using a design sim-ilar to that of Drummond-Young and Mohide (2001), the following framework was constructed to illustrate the steps of development used to create a scenario for an interprofessional communication skills lab.

Figure 17-1 shows the cyclical nature of developing a scenario. There are multiple steps involved in creating a scenario for an interprofessional communication skills lab.

1. *Identify the who, what, why, and how of the scenario.*
    a. *Who will be the audience experiencing the scenario? Make sure the scenario has something to offer each profession.* In creating the scenario referred to in this chapter, the author had to first identify who the audience was going to be, so that the scenario could be designed to offer each student (profession) opportunities for learning in terms of knowledge, skills, and dispositions (Drummond-Young & Mohide, 2001). A scenario involving an older adult in the community setting was chosen for its complexity, and for the number of health and social care professionals who could potentially be involved in the delivery of care.
    b. *Why is this scenario being developed? What is the purpose?* The scenario was being developed for an interprofessional communication skills lab. The main

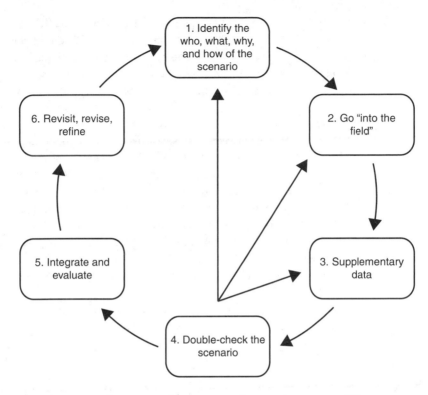

■ **Figure 17-1** Development of an interprofessional scenario. There are multiple steps involved in creating a scenario for an interprofessional communication skills lab.

purpose of this scenario was to provide an opportunity for communication and collaboration with other students (from other professions). Effective communication skills (sharing information, listening attentively, respecting others' opinions, demonstrating flexibility, using a common language, providing feedback to others, and responding to feedback from others) are critical in a healthcare team and are the main focus of these interprofessional labs.

c. *What are the main concepts/issues of the scenario?* A scenario about an older adult in a community setting could present several issues for exploration, but being cognizant of the target audience and the purpose of the communication skills lab, the author chose to focus the scenario on these two main issues: caregiver burden and long-term care placement. Effective communication and efficient collaboration within a team of healthcare professionals is critical in order to deliver a holistic plan of care that is person centered.

d. *How will it play out? What is your vision for execution?* The author wanted to develop a scenario that would mimic a common situation in the community setting—caregiver burden and long-term care placement. The vision for the scenario involved a recently widowed woman and a very tired and worried daughter, whose relationship had become very tense since the daughter suggested assessment for long-term care placement. To play out the scenario, there would be two standardized patients—a mother and daughter dyad—so that the students could gain practice assessing and communicating with both individuals, as well as observe the dynamics of the relationship and communication patterns between an older adult and her daughter.

2. *Go into the field.* If possible, go into the field and retrieve/develop a scenario based on a real clinical case(s). To further enhance the authenticity of the scenario, have a professional who has had experience with a similar case provide detail and feedback. Authenticity and customization of an interprofessional event so that it reflects relevant healthcare delivery and settings are important for a positive experience for the participants (Hammick, Freeth, Koppel, Reeves, & Barr, 2007).

3. *Provide supplementary data.* The scenario itself should be brief, with enough detail to offer some focus for discussion, but open enough to stimulate critical thinking and encourage hypothesis generation. Previous research dictates that students prefer and appreciate a complex scenario (Salvatori et al., 2006). Create supplementary resource material—for example, lab results or chart data—to offer additional details of the scenario.

EXAMPLE OF A SCENARIO:

The Case Manager's Home Visit

Mrs. Cooke is a 74-year-old woman who lives with her small dog in a one-bedroom apartment.

Recently widowed, her community case manager came to reassess her ability to function on her own. Prior to this visit, Mrs. Cooke was receiving one hour of personal care per week to assist with her bath. Upon the case manager's arrival, the door to the apartment was wide open, Mrs. Cooke was wandering around without stockings, and her blouse was half-open. Bruises were visible on her legs.

Her wallet sat open on the kitchen table, next to an empty medication dosette.

A community case manager was selected as the lead professional in this case, as case managers are the individuals who primarily assess and coordinate home care services, and potentially initiate the process for long-term care assessment. They also tend to be one of a variety of healthcare professionals (i.e., nurse, physical therapist, occupational therapist, social worker, dietician, or speech-language pathologist).

The previous scenario was created with enough information to steer the interprofessional group of students toward the author's intended focus for the scenario: an older woman with a decreased ability to function safely at home—and

possibly a potential candidate for long-term care placement. However, the scenario also included a few added details to augment discussion. For example, the following topics could be explored from this scenario:
- What is the cause of her current state?
  - Polypharmacy?
  - Disease?
  - Other sources of confusion: Diabetes? Urinary tract infection?
- What else could be going on?
  - Depression? Grief and bereavement?
  - Was there an intruder?
  - Falls? Other safety concerns?
  - Is she able to stay in own home with increased home care service?

4. *Double-check the scenario.* After the scenario has been created, seek evaluative feedback, preferably from other healthcare professionals with similar experiences. Once feedback has been received and adjustments made as necessary, recruit and train standardized patients for the scenario. Standardized patients are individuals who "are specially trained, by a specific yet not complex method similar to 'method acting' to simulate an actual patient in every detail" (Barrows & Tamblyn, 1980, p. 63). In the example provided previously, there were two standardized patients trained—an older woman as the mother and another woman as the daughter. In training this dyad, the author simply narrated her vision of the scenario, describing in detail the personalities of each individual, the relationship between the mother and daughter, and the communication (verbal and nonverbal) techniques to be acted out by each individual. Another detail that was included in the author's vision for the scenario was the appearance of the standardized patient; in this case, the elderly woman was to appear a bit disheveled, indicating probable difficulty in completing activities of self-care.

   Once details and plausibility of the scenario have been checked out and the standardized patients have been trained, test the scenario to observe how it unfolds. Does it unfold as you had envisioned it? Does it meet the objectives of the skills lab and have something to offer each discipline in the group? Does the scenario promote communication, teamwork, and collaboration? Make adjustments and add information to the scenario as necessary.

5. *Integrate and evaluate.* Integrate the scenario into the program, and continue to evaluate the content and process of the scenario. Gather feedback on a regular basis from multiple sources, including faculty, students, and standardized patients. Students, faculty, and standardized patients all bring a unique perspective to the scenario, which can elicit valuable comments and suggestions for change.

6. *Revisit, revise, and refine on a regular basis.* Scenarios grow old and outdated, so to remain current in the field of health care and to continue to offer exciting new challenges for the students, scenarios must be revisited on a regular basis. Review the scenario and determine whether it needs to be refined, revised, or re-created.

Small-Group, Problem-Based Learning Approach

The communication skills lab unfolds similar to a small-group, problem-based learning class. Small-group learning allows students to develop a sense of responsibility for their learning progress. Small-group learning in an interprofessional environment further enhances learning as students develop a sense of responsibility for accurately representing the knowledge and skills base of their profession. Furthermore, students in a group environment learn about human interaction, develop interpersonal skills, and may become more aware of their own emotional reactions and moral standing. Learning how to listen and provide and receive evaluative feedback, which are all essential in a healthcare environment, are also skills that small-group learning helps to cultivate (Neufeld & Barrows, 1974).

The composition of a small group in a communication skills lab may vary from week to week (depending on the availability of students), but generally consists of five to eight students, with representation from at least three professional groups (Salvatori et al., 2006). A week prior to class, students are asked to complete some key readings to provide some context for the IPE event. They are also asked to review their scope of professional practice, because this is information that they will be required to share during the lab.

The initial interview with a standardized patient is 20–30 minutes in duration. When the interview is over, the patient leaves the room, and the student team meets to discuss its findings and treatment and/or discharge plan. Once this task has been completed, the patient returns to the room, and a follow-up meeting is conducted to discuss the interprofessional plan of care. The entire session typically runs for approximately 3 hours in length, with a 15- to 20-minute break midway.

The interprofessional nature of the group provides an opportunity to learn about each other's roles and skills set, and the students learn to respect the distinctive experiences and expertise that each participant brings from his or her individual professional fields (CAIPE, 2008). Mutual respect is fundamental in collaborative work and may also promote the level of confidence in working with other healthcare professionals. Finally, the experiential learning associated with the communication skills labs reinforces the importance of communication and teamwork in providing quality care in the healthcare setting (Barnsteiner, Disch, Hall, Mayer, & Moore, 2007).

Role of Faculty

The main roles of faculty are to observe the interprofessional group of students from behind a one-way mirror, intervene (if necessary), and provide feedback using a standard observational guide (Salvatori et al., 2006). At the completion of the interaction with the patient, there is a 60-minute debriefing and feedback session where the faculty facilitator provides individual and team feedback to the student group. Ideally, the faculty will be familiar with the small-group, problem-based approach to learning so that they can quickly distinguish the group's dynamics and identify individual roles within the group. The faculty should also be efficient in providing evaluative comments, specifically constructive feedback, so that the students can grow from the experience.

Role of Students

The role of the students is very similar to that of students in a small-group, problem-based learning class. Students need to demonstrate behaviors in critical inquiry, effective team functioning, and professional conduct. They need to be well aware of their role and scope of practice because they will need to represent their profession in this multidisciplinary environment.

Students also may assume one of two functional roles as described by Sampson and Marthas (1990)—task roles and maintenance roles. Task roles are actions such as initiating, clarifying, informing, sharing information, and evaluating whether or not group goals are being achieved. Setting up an agenda at the beginning of a group session is a common example of a task role (Uys & Gwele, 1999). Maintenance roles are behaviors that act to strengthen the group and maintain harmony—for example, offering encouragement and support, open and effective communication strategies, and compromising (Sampson & Marthas, 1990).

The role of the student in a communication skills lab is comparable to that of a member of an interprofessional team. Working in student teams establishes mutual respect and enhances collaboration, and the relatively equal status of students contributes to a sense of safety, allowing them to take risks that they normally would not be ready to take in clinical practice (O'Neill & Wyness, 2004).

Evaluation of Interprofessional Communication Skills Labs

Interprofessional activities are generally well received by participants, especially when the context for learning reflects the students' current or future practice (Hammick et al., 2007). One study revealed that students enjoyed their experience in the communication skills lab—in particular, interacting with students from the other health science programs. Students reported an increased awareness of other professional roles and agreed that the feedback provided on their individual communication skills and overall group performance was informative (Salvatori et al., 2006). In a recent mixed-method study, students from a variety of health professional programs ($n = 96$) rated their satisfaction with the communication skills labs as high. Students enjoyed the opportunity to interact with colleagues from other professions in an intensive, yet realistic educational event. It was revealed that the students learned about each other's scopes of practice and became more confident in their communication skills. The skills of the facilitator and preparation for the experience were perceived to promote the success (Solomon & Salfi, 2011).

■ Potential Problems

There are many barriers to interprofessional activities, despite the many benefits associated with this style of learning. IPE is "complex and time consuming to arrange and sustain" (Kilminster et al., 2004, p. 719). It can be very challenging to identify available time for IPE initiatives within preregistration professional courses (Hammick et al., 2007). Incompatible clinical shifts and timetables as well as rigid curriculum were identified as the most significant barriers in establishing IPE (Morison, Boohan, Jenkins, & Moutray, 2003).

Another barrier to the delivery of IPE in health science programs includes faculty interest and expertise in IPE. As identified by Hammick and colleagues (2007), a key mechanism for effective IPE involves faculty development. Faculty need to be knowledgeable, competent, and confident if they are to be effective in implementing interprofessional core competencies into the health sciences curricula. Faculty also need to be proficient in applying principles of adult learning, as this has also been cited as essential for well-received IPE (Hammick et al., 2007).

Student numbers can also affect the ability to deliver effective IPE. Care is often taken to balance groups with representation from at least three professional groups, to avoid experiences that are dominated by any one profession. Some health science faculties have only a few professions to choose from, affecting the ability to create balanced groups of at least three different professions.

Even though skills and content may be similar across professional programs in health sciences, there is generally minimal interaction between the students in each professional program and few opportunities for faculty development in the area of IPE. This lack of attention to IPE could lead to undervaluing or misinterpreting each profession's contributions, with the potential of impairing communication, collaboration, and teamwork in the clinical environment after graduation. Thus, in order to address the calling for enhanced communication and collaboration among healthcare professionals, IPE can be used as a mechanism to enhance professional practice and improve the delivery of healthcare services (Hammick et al., 2007).

■ Conclusion

Students in health professional programs do not acquire interprofessional competencies from sitting side-by-side in lecture halls, and they do not develop skills in communication and collaboration by simply observing or shadowing a different health professional. A learning experience that involves authentic scenarios, standardized patients, an opportunity to work with students from other professional programs, and peer and faculty feedback enhances the interprofessional learning experience, which can develop students' competence and confidence in team environments. The communication skills lab provides the opportunity to communicate and collaborate with students from a variety of health professions, which has been shown to promote role understanding and the importance of working together as a team, which is a critical step in preparing a collaborative, practice-ready workforce.

REFERENCES

Allport, G. (1954). *The nature of prejudice*. Reading, MA: Addison-Wesley.

Barnsteiner, J., Disch, J., Hall, L., Mayer, D., & Moore, S. (2007). Promoting interprofessional education. *Nursing Outlook, 55*(3), 144–150.

Barr, H., Freeth, D., Hammick, M., Koppel, I., & Reeves, S. (2000). Evaluations of interprofessional education: A United Kingdom review for health and social care. Retrieved from http://www.caipe.org.uk/publications.html

Barrows, H., & Tamblyn, R. (1980). *Problem-based learning*. New York, NY: Springer.

Carpenter, J., & Hewstone, M. (1996). Shared learning for doctors and social workers: Evaluation of a programme. *British Journal of Social Work, 26,* 239–257.

Centre for the Advancement of Interprofessional Education (CAIPE). (1997). *Interprofessional education: A definition*. London, UK: CAIPE.

Centre for the Advancement of Interprofessional Education (CAIPE). (2008). *Interprofessional education: A definition*. London, UK: CAIPE.

Centre for the Advancement of Interprofessional Education (CAIPE). (2010). Defining IPE. Retrieved from http://www.caipe.org.uk/about-us/defining-ipe/

Charles, G., Bainbridge, L., & Gilbert, J. (2008). *The college of health disciples and the UBC model of interprofessional education*. Vancouver, BC: UBC.

D'Eon, M. (2004). A blueprint for interprofessional learning. *Journal of Interprofessional Care, 19,* 49–59.

Drummond-Young, M., & Mohide, E. A. (2001). Developing problems for use in problem-based learning. In E. Rideout (Ed.), *Transforming nursing education through problem-based learning* (pp.165–193). Sudbury, MA: Jones and Bartlett.

Fraser, D., Symonds, M., Cullen, L., & Symonds, I. (2000). A university department merger of midwifery and obstetrics: A step on the journey to enhancing interprofessional learning. *Medical Teacher, 22*(2), 179–183.

Hammick, M., Freeth, D., Koppel, I., Reeves, S., & Barr, H. (2007). A best evidence systematic review of interprofessional education: BEME Guide No. 9. *Medical Teacher, 29*(8), 735–751.

Kilminster, S., Hale, C., Lascelles, M., Morris, P., Roberts, T., Stark, P., . . . Thistlethwaite J. (2004). Learning for real life: Patient-focused interprofessional workshops offer added value. *Medical Education, 38,* 717–726.

Miller, C., Ross, N., & Freeman, M. (1999). *Shared learning and clinical teamwork: New direction in education for multiprofessional practice*. London, UK: English National Board of Nursing Midwifery and Health Visiting.

Morison, S., Boohan, M., Jenkins, J., & Moutray, M. (2003). Facilitating undergraduate interprofessional learning in healthcare: Comparing classroom and clinical learning for nursing and medical students. *Learning in Health and Social Care, 2*(2), 92–104.

Neufeld, V., & Barrows, H. (1974). The "McMaster philosophy": An approach to medical education. *Journal of Medical Education, 49*(11), 1040–1051.

O'Neill, B., & Wyness, M. (2004). Learning about interprofessional education: Student voices. *Journal of Interprofessional Care, 18*(2), 198–200.

Salvatori, P., Mahoney, P., & Delottinville, C. (2006). An interprofessional communication skills lab: A pilot project. *Education for Health, 19*(3), 380–384.

Salvatori, P., & Solomon, P. (2005). Interprofessional education. In P. Solomon & S. Baptiste (Eds.), *Innovations in rehabilitation sciences education* (pp. 95–111). Berlin, Germany: Springer.

Sampson, E., & Marthas, M. (1990). *Group process for the health professions*. Albany, NY: Delmar.

Schmitt, M. (1994). USA: Focus on interprofessional practice, education, and research. *Journal of Interprofessional Care, 8,* 9–18.

Sele, K., Salamon, K., Boarman, R., & Sauer, J. (2008). Providing interprofessional learning through interdisciplinary collaboration: The role of modelling. *Journal of Interprofessional Care, 22*(1), 85–92.

Solomon, P., & Salfi, J. (2011). Evaluation of an interprofessional education communication skills initiative. *Education for Health, 11,* 616. Retrieved from http://www.educationforhealth.net

Uys, L., & Gwele, N. (1999). A descriptive analysis of the process of problem-based teaching/learning. In J. Conway & A. Williams (Eds.), *Themes and variations in PBL* (pp. 169–179). Callaghan, Australia: PROBLARC.

World Health Organization (WHO). (2010). *Framework for action on IPE & collaborative practice*. Geneva, Switzerland: Author.

SECTION IV

Educational Use of Technology

Educational technology continues to grow by leaps and bounds and has changed the complexion of the world of education. The technology can be as simple as communicating by e-mail, or as complex as presenting full degree-granting programs by distance learning. Classroom teaching is utilizing more and more technology, from PowerPoint presentations and student- and faculty-made videos to blended learning, a combination of in-class and asynchronous discussions. Online courses are now using learning management systems (LMS) that allow both synchronous and asynchronous technologies. Social media include blogs, wikis, Twitter, and YouTube. Libraries have become accessible to distance learners by use of technology, and full-text articles are now available online. The Internet has opened a new and extensive world of information that was not previously available, and both faculty and students need to learn not only how to take advantage of what is out there, but also how to use it with caution. Students are increasingly involved in social technology, where they communicate with wide audiences. Teaching in a technological world requires faculty collaboration with academic information technology specialists, a specialty field in itself, to learn how to use the ever-changing systems, as well as to keep abreast of new resources as they become available and provide technological support for students.

The discussion in these chapters provides a look at different ways of utilizing available technologies and discusses strengths of the systems and problems that may occur. As technology has grown in the past few years, the technology discussion in this edition has increased as well. Social media are included in teaching strategies as discussed in the chapter "Social Media as a Context for Connected Learning." Distance learning techniques have moved into the classroom in blended or hybrid classes, and faculty need to learn to incorporate these strategies as a way to better achieve their learning objectives. Distance learning can be asynchronous, meaning students can access the material and discussions at any time, or synchronous, meaning students are online together regardless of where they are. A chapter about synchronous learning is included to discuss the various ways this can be carried out.

Technology may be used to assist learning, but it does not replace the instructor. Teaching methods require adaptation to be effective in this new environment and should be evaluated for that effectiveness. The amount of Internet information may be overwhelming, and it is critical that faculty and students begin to cull the material to a reasonable amount, and validate its accuracy. The use of educational technologies may require extra time and effort from faculty, but can be very effective in enhancing learning and can be rewarding for students and faculty alike.

CHAPTER 18

Multimedia in the Classroom: Creating Learning Experiences with Technology

■ KAREN H. TEELEY ■

Health professions educators have new roles to fill in an era of increasing technology. Multimedia has grown from simple A-V (audio-visual) to a never-ending, ever-growing list of technological opportunities. The challenge for the instructor is not just to master new, complicated technology, but also to find more meaningful ways to engage the students. Expectations are higher with each succeeding generation as students are exposed to technology at earlier ages. Today's students have grown up with technology; they have been raised on the Internet, they use Google or other search engines for information, they have thrived in online communities, and they are connected 24/7. John Sener addresses the "cyberization" of education as now being mainstream and unlikely to change (Sener, 2012). Students expect educators to be adept with the current technology and its applications (Prensky, 2001).

With increasing student enrollments in the health professions, the additional challenge is to be able to reach more students, with more content, yet maintain that all-important student–teacher relationship so vital in educating health professionals. Aside from technological sophistication, today's students are skilled in the art of multitasking or parallel processing (Prensky 2001) and lose interest quickly if the learning environment is not dynamic or interesting or both.

How can instructors use technology to reach and engage students and create opportunities for students to apply what they learn? This chapter will look at multimedia and multidelivery formats including web-based course tools, the Internet, and other learning activities designed to create meaningful learning experiences.

■ Definition and Purpose

There are numerous definitions of *multimedia*, but for the purposes of this chapter, multimedia simply means using more than one type of media and integrating the use of multiple technologies for teaching and learning.

Barr and Tagg (1995) describe paradigm shifts taking place in higher education from teacher-centered to learner-centered education. Weimer (2013) notes that while learner-centered education has become more popular, it has distinct characteristics that are more than active learning and student engagement, and is still in the process of developing.

Educators are no longer the experts; teachers have become "persons with expertise." Since students have access to volumes of information via the Internet, the instructor can no longer possibly keep ahead of the abundance of information, but instead must guide the student into making the information meaningful. Students struggle with prioritizing information and organizing it in meaningful ways. The instructor's role changes from the traditional "sage on the stage" to the role of the "guide on the side" (Collison, Elbaum, Haavind & Tinker, 2000).

Educators must be knowledgeable in new and emerging multimedia technology to be able to reach and engage students in ways the students are willing to learn. With increased competition for students, institutions must reach more students more effectively. Multimedia technology and a variety of delivery methods provide the flexibility for faculty and institutions to engage students both in the classroom and online.

■ Theoretical Foundations

Creating learning environments through multimedia technology has roots in our knowledge of adult learning. Components of adult learning are described by Malcolm Knowles (1990), who emphasizes that adults are self-directed, are interested in topics that are relevant to their lives, like to be actively involved in the learning process, and have control over where and how they learn so they can learn at their own pace. Knowles's theory of andragogy makes the following assumptions about the design of learning: (1) Adults need to know why they need to learn something; (2) adults need to learn experientially; (3) adults approach learning as problem solving; and (4) adults learn best when the topic is of immediate value (Knowles, 1990).

It is important that the instructor know the learner's needs and design learning activities that are relevant to those needs. The student should be actively involved in learning, with the instructor acting as a facilitator or guide. The instructor who recognizes that adults have different learning needs can tailor his or her instruction design to the characteristic ways adults prefer to learn.

Adult learning theory is important in multimedia instructional design for several reasons. First, it is important to tailor the content specifically to the learner's level or it will not be effective (Lee & Owens, 2000). Second, learner goals and objectives must utilize a variety of learning activities if adults are to be engaged in the learning (Fink, 2003). Last, by engaging in meaningful activity, students feel like they are making significant, sustainable contributions (Teeley, Lowe, Beal, & Knapp, 2006).

Educators are familiar with Benjamin Bloom's taxonomy of educational objectives, as they have been a standard framework since the 1950s (Bloom, 1956). Educators generally refer to the cognitive domain most frequently. These educational objectives include, from the lowest to the highest:

- Knowledge
- Comprehension
- Application
- Analysis
- Synthesis
- Evaluation

L. Dee Fink (2003) responded to the changing needs of students and educators by introducing a new taxonomy, called a *taxonomy of significant learning,* in his 2003 publication, *Creating Significant Learning Experiences* (**Figure 18-1**). He addressed needs that are not easily met by Bloom's taxonomy, such as learning how

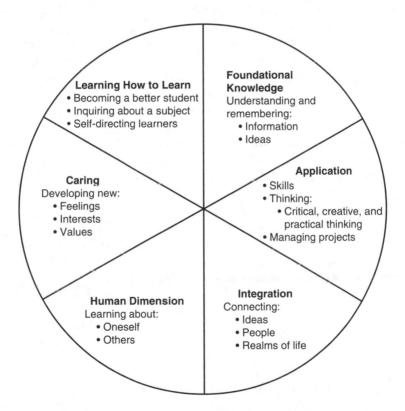

▪ **Figure 18-1** The taxonomy of significant learning

Source: Fink, L. D. (Ed.). (2003). *Creating significant learning experiences.* San Francisco, CA: Jossey-Bass, p. 31. Used with permission.

to learn, leadership and interpersonal skills, ethics, communication skills, character, tolerance, and the ability to adapt to change (Fink, 2003). Fink defined learning in terms of change, stating that, "For learning to occur, there has to be some kind of change in the learner. No change, no learning. And significant learning requires that there be some kind of lasting change in the learner" (Fink 2003) (**Table 18-1**).

■ Types of Learners

Students enter the health professions in different stages in their lives. While some are traditional college students, most students have very busy lives with jobs and children and other additional family obligations. With the added expense of college tuition, it is a rare student who does not have to work in addition to attending school and fulfilling clinical placements. This changing profile of the learner suggests that most students fulfill the pedagogical requirements of the adult learner (Jairath & Stair, 2004). The more flexible and self-paced the course delivery is, the more likely the students will be able to fit it into their schedule and be successful.

Web-based courses using a learning management system such as Blackboard or Moodle require a comprehensive orientation to the format. Students must quickly become proficient in navigating the tools and knowing how to troubleshoot common problems such as disabling pop-up blockers and mastery of e-mail and attachment functions. Most importantly, students need to know how to access help.

Students in higher education in the first decade of the 21st century fall into the generation called millennials (Howe & Strauss, 2000). Millennials were born between the years of 1982 and 2002. They are global, connected, and interactive. Although they grew up in a media age, they will undoubtedly have varying levels of proficiency that will require access to support functions.

Marc Prensky (2001) differentiates *digital natives* from *digital immigrants*. He describes digital natives as the students today who are *native speakers* to the digital language of computers, video games, and the Internet; those who are not native to the digital language (most instructors) are said to be *immigrants*. Immigrants have to learn a new language and adapt to a new environment. "Digital natives are used to receiving information really fast, they like to parallel process and multi-task and they function best when networked" (Prensky 2001, p.1). He suggests that it is unlikely that digital natives are going to learn the immigrants' language, so in order to reach these students, immigrant instructors must learn to communicate in the language style of the students.

Conditions for Learning: Blended Learning

A web-based or blended design course requires that the students are self-directed and are accustomed to working independently. A blended design is a combination of on-site and distance learning. It is separate from web-based learning and may also be called hybrid learning. Although beginning college students may do well with the

Table 18-1   Fink's Major Categories in the Taxonomy of Significant Learning

Foundational Knowledge

At the base of most other kinds of learning is the need for students to know something. Knowing, as used here, refers to students' ability to understand and remember specific information and ideas. It is important for people today to have some valid basic knowledge, for example, about science, history, literature, and geography. They also need to understand major ideas or perspectives—for example, what evolution is (and what it is not), what capitalism is (and is not), and so forth. **Special Value:** Foundational knowledge provides the basic understanding that is necessary for other kinds of learning.

Application

This familiar kind of learning occurs when students learn how to engage in some new kind of action, which may be intellectual, physical, social, or some other type. Learning how to engage in various kinds of thinking (critical, creative, practical) is an important form of application learning. But this category of significant learning also includes developing certain skills (e.g., communication, playing the piano) or learning how to manage complex projects. **Special Value:** Application learning allows other kinds of learning to become useful.

Integration

When students are able to see and understand the connections between different things, an important kind of learning has occurred. Sometimes they make connections between specific ideas, between whole realms of ideas, between people, and/or between different realms of life (e.g., between school and work or between school and leisure life). **Special Value:** The act of making new connections gives learners a new form of power, especially intellectual power.

Human Dimension

When students learn something important about themselves and/or about others, it enables them to interact more effectively with themselves or with others. They discover the personal and/or social implications of what they have learned. What they learn or the way in which they learn sometimes gives students a new understanding of themselves (self-image) or a new vision of what they want to become (self-ideal). At other times, they acquire a better understanding of others—how and why others act the way they do, or how the learner can interact more effectively with others. **Special Value:** This kind of learning informs students about the human significance of what they are learning.

Caring

Sometimes a learning experience changes the degree to which students care about something. This may be reflected in the form of new feelings, interests, and/or values. Any of these changes means students now care about something to a greater degree or in a different way than they did before. **Special Value:** When students care about something, they then have the energy they need for learning more about it and making it a part of their lives. Without the energy for learning, nothing significant happens.

Learning How to Learn

This occurs when students learn something about the process of learning itself. They may be learning how to be a better student, how to engage in a particular kind of inquiry (e.g., the scientific method), or how to become self-directing learners. All of these constitute important forms of learning how to learn. **Special Value:** This kind of learning enables students to continue learning and to do so with greater effectiveness.

Source: Fink, L. D. (Ed.). (2003). *Creating significant learning experiences.* San Francisco, CA: Jossey-Bass. Used with permission.

technology, the discipline and organization required means that the more mature student will be better prepared and ultimately more successful.

The course must be well planned out in advance since the students will have access to the entire course once they are registered and enrolled. Clear instructions and troubleshooting guides should be readily available and included in a course orientation or overview.

Blended design is the best of both worlds; it allows for the development of independent study style and self-discovery in the online portion, yet the classroom component provides the intimacy found in the face-to-face classroom environments. The design promotes community building both online and in the classroom. Multimedia delivery formats have the potential to better engage the students by creating self-directed, lifelong learners.

Goals for multimedia/multidelivery format:

- Create a positive learning environment
- Provide for greater interactivity and increased engagement in the course
- Address different learning styles
- Retain information after the course
- Develop an ability to transfer knowledge
- Make information meaningful
- Develop self-directed learners
- Develop a love of knowledge and lifelong learners
- Create collaborative learners
- Promote community building

■ Resources

Personnel

The most essential resource for a blended or web-based design is the availability of experienced faculty facilitators to manage the smaller discussion groups of 6–12 students. A group that is too small does not have the diversity of input and opinions to make it interesting, but a group that is too large becomes unwieldy for both the students and the facilitator, especially if there are multiple postings and responses are required within a short time frame.

Technology

Students and faculty need access to Internet-enabled devices. Classrooms must also have computers and Internet access plus projection equipment for CDs and DVDs. Faculty must be proficient in the use of the classroom technology. If the educational setting offers training for faculty, it is advised that they take advantage of not only emerging technologies, but also learning the basics of the classroom podium. Nothing seems to diminish the important role of the faculty more quickly than stumbling through the technological setup in front of a class.

Faculty Development

Faculty development for online course development is essential in addition to ongoing design support and technology support.

■ Using the Method

There are numerous *how to* texts available for Web design courses, and many of these are listed in the *Recommended Reading* section at the end of this chapter. This section will look specifically at developing a blended course and incorporating within the course design multiple media types aimed at engaging the student in the learning experience.

The key to successful implementation of a blended course is allowing sufficient time for planning the course itself as well as allowing time to train faculty facilitators. See **Table 18-2**.

Planning

Taking an existing course and adapting it for use online requires *reconceptualizing* the learning material (O'Neil, Fisher, & Newbold, 2004). Each module or learning section needs to be reassessed in light of new available options. How are the module's objectives best met given the skill level of the faculty and the available technology? Can the content be packaged and available online for viewing at the student's own pace? Does the content lend itself to small-group discussions that can be facilitated on a discussion board? If the students read or view material online in preparation for the next face-to-face class, then can class time be better spent in classroom activities and discussions instead of simply imparting content? Does the use of technology allow for "flipping" the classroom (Bergman & Sams, 2012). Flipping the classroom is a method that provides online material for students that includes the class content that would have been given in lecture. Students are expected to view and read this material online and complete any exercises that go along with the content. Classroom time is then used for activities and discussions around the content that students bring to the discussions. Which activities, case studies, and discussions are better suited for an online discussion or a face-to-face class? For integrated planning, use a course design worksheet based on goals and learning objectives; see Table 18-2.

Feedback and Assessment

How will the students receive feedback? And how will they be assessed and graded? Discussion questions need to be carefully constructed to elicit thoughtfully researched responses. Clearly defined rubrics are helpful for the students as well as the faculty facilitators to assure uniform grading criteria.

Table 18-2 Taxonomy Design Worksheet

Goals	Fink's Taxonomy	Learning Activities: In Class	Learning Activities: Outside Class	Types of Media/Delivery	Feedback and Assessment
1. Describe basic elements of the financing of health-care delivery including Medicaid, Medicare, and managed care options	Foundational knowledge	Lecture Textbook CD interactive game	Online vignettes Self-paced PowerPoint Clinical setting	Instructor-led lecture CD interactive game PowerPoint Web-CT	Preclass online quiz Midterm or final exam 1-minute papers
2. Evaluate opportunities for disparities in present-day system	Application Integration Caring Human dimension	Discussion Debate Case studies	Clinical setting Online discussion question Online reflection Literature/stories	Web-CT Text-based case studies Discussion board Internet audio Internet video	Discussion grade Weekly reflection Project presentations
3. Investigate resources for eliminating disparities	Integration Caring Learning how to learn	Discussion Debate	Clinical setting Links to websites	Self-directed Internet exploration	Project presentations

Expectations

In addition to the traditional course content with objectives and outcomes, the online and blended faculty need to clearly set the tone and the expectations. The students will most likely have access to the online component of the course before they meet face-to-face (which is optional). What the students see on their first visit will most likely determine their first impressions of the class. Will it be visually appealing and friendly, or chaotic and hard to navigate? A friendly welcome from the professor with the blended course expectations clearly explained will ally fears and set the tone for a positive learning experience.

Dispel the myth that less class time means less work. Clearly define the students' expectations for workload plus the expectations of the new role for the faculty facilitators. When can the students expect responses from the faculty and how will their grades be communicated? Develop a list of course frequently asked questions and add to it as the course evolves.

Training and Orientation

New roles and expectations for faculty facilitators must be clearly defined, as this is most likely a brand-new role. Time involved should not be underestimated and should be agreed upon at the start of the course to prevent any unwelcome surprises. Rubrics for grading as well as timelines and sample responses to the student's discussion postings are helpful for new faculty. How-to resources for moderating online discussions will help support the faculty as they grow in this new role.

Group faculty training with hands-on Internet and Web course access is ideal for introducing the faculty facilitators to the course design and to hear concerns and questions before the class begins. Practice discussion questions help the faculty work together to anticipate student issues. Once the training period is over, it is helpful to establish a private discussion area on the course's website just for faculty to communicate with each other; they will undoubtedly have common questions from students and it will be helpful to have a *community* as a resource.

Student orientation to the blended design needs to be just as thorough as the faculty orientation, especially if this is a new way of learning. In addition to online resources, the first face-to-face class should be spent going over required technology skills, course layout and navigation tips, expectations for timely assignment submissions, organization tips, appropriate communication strategies (netiquette) and, most importantly, how much time will be expected to complete the assignments (see **Table 18-3**).

Potential Problems

For Students

The most challenging problem is for the students to embrace a new way of learning. Although the students may be accustomed to the technological features, this blended course requires a lot of independence and self-direction, and the student who is not

Table 18-3 Course Development Workflow Checklist

1. Outline the course into teaching modules.
2. Identify online and face-to-face segments.
3. Define learning objectives for each module.
4. Outline module content.
5. Define feedback and assessment strategies.
6. Identify integration link each week between online and classroom.
7. Identify resources for content support.
   a. Websites, books, articles
8. Determine teaching/learning activities to address course content and objectives.
9. Determine assessment tasks.
   a. Quizzes/tests
      i. Develop test questions based on objectives.
      ii. Provide rationale for answers.
   b. Discussion board questions/case studies
      i. Develop questions based on module objectives.
      ii. Clearly define instructions for posting and responding including length and deadlines (visual chart).
      iii. Provide rubric for correct answers.
      iv. Communicate rubric to other course faculty.
      v. Design method for weekly faculty communication with course coordinator.
   c. Other written assignments
10. Develop grade plan based on assessment tasks.
11. Communicate all of the above in the course syllabus.
    a. Include time management expectations for students (3 hours prep per hour class)
    b. Include help desk resources and academic technology support
12. Communicate all of the above to clinical faculty in a faculty orientation/training session.
    a. Develop clinical faculty training materials.

ready for this different way of learning can feel lost and resentful. Poor organizational skills and impaired time management can also derail a student if he or she gets behind. Students who are not Web savvy need to get up to speed quickly. Varying computer skills and access to the Internet can also be problematic in this course style. Online quizzes are a particular challenge for varying Internet speeds, and students can experience a high degree of frustration on top of the quiz anxiety when the Internet is inaccessible or slow.

For Faculty

Course development takes a considerable time commitment just in the planning stages. Once the course is implemented, the first few iterations need continued tweaking and modifying to work out unforeseen bugs. Because of the nature of technology, plus the addition of new areas of content, the course will never be finished, but will always be evolving.

▪ Conclusion

Students entering the health professions in the 21st century are different learners than their instructors were. Internet access to new information and the convergence of technology is a way of life and must be an integral part of the classroom if the goal is to be meaningful engagement and lifelong learning. Instructors need to learn to reach students in ways that will cause students to use the material and foster a love of learning. A successful student is one who knows that learning will not end with graduation but will graduate with the necessary tools and skills to make lifelong contributions to the profession.

TEACHING EXAMPLE:

Community Health Nursing—A Blended Course

The decision to use a blended model emerged from growing class sizes and increased need to deliver more content in less time. A creative way was needed to better engage the students in learning and increase the connectivity between the students and the faculty in light of the larger class sizes.

The course coordinator/designer met with instructional designers and Web course experts from the college's academic technology department. Goals and timelines were established with an 8-month planning time frame. In addition, the first blended model was scheduled to run as a pilot project with only three modules online. Once some of the bugs were worked out of the pilot, the full blended course had five modules online with seven face-to-face classes.

The community health nursing class content was already organized in modules and posted online in a Web-enhanced format; most of the documents, such as the syllabus, handouts, and forms were already online, as was the test question database. This reduced some of the redesign time.

The course modules were reevaluated, taking into consideration the best way to engage the students with the material. Online and web-based activities were selected with multiple learning styles in mind. The class was scheduled to meet every other week online, alternating with face-to-face classes.

One of the major hurdles in online course management is the increased faculty time required for the reading and responding to multiple discussion posts. With a class size of 70-plus students and 2–3 posts per week, it quickly becomes unmanageable to respond to more than 200 posts each week.

Since the course already employed clinical faculty for a student/faculty ratio of six to seven students per faculty member, it seemed logical to include the clinical faculty in the course

(continued)

design as *faculty facilitators*. As the students were assigned to their clinical groups, the same groups were used in the classroom, and the clinical faculty/facilitator was responsible for managing the discussion posts for his or her groups. This worked out especially well by engaging the clinical faculty in the classroom portion and provided much-needed continuity for the students, connecting the classroom and the clinical settings. For the online component, the students had assigned readings and activities followed by two-part discussion questions and responses due on specific dates. The responses were important as they were designed to engage the students in an online community and promote a back-and-forth discussion as opposed to just posts. Faculty facilitators were guided in their role as *facilitators* and were encouraged to not jump into the discussion but rather let the discussion flow among the students. The facilitators graded the students' posts individually but responded to the groups' postings as a whole once all the posts were complete. Once the faculty facilitators posted their response to the student group, they were encouraged to share their response with other faculty members on a private (faculty only) faculty forum discussion board. The faculty forum was also available to faculty to share ideas and concerns throughout the class.

In order to keep the classroom times interesting by leaving time for activities and discussions, the students were required to read the assignments *before* class and complete an online quiz based on the material. Because this was structured as a learning experience rather than a test, the students could take the quizzes multiple times. This worked well because the students came to class with questions and were already engaged in the material. The students also liked this because they received immediate feedback from the online quizzes.

Academic misconduct was minimized as much as possible by stating up front that the quizzes and tests were *open book*. The questions were designed to be higher level—that is, *application* and *integration* rather than simply *knowledge based* (Fink, 2003)—and required fuller comprehension of the material. Midterms and final exams, while also online, were built on Learning Management Systems' (LMS) feature of a computerized random selection of questions so that no two tests were alike. Misconduct is always a concern with online tests, but by enabling the students to take the quizzes more than once and enabling the random selection feature for the tests, the opportunities were minimized.

One of the most successful features of the course was the students' presentation project based on reading current literature about a selected vulnerable population group (Leffers & Martin, 2004). The learning goal was to evoke a caring response by immersing the reader into the personal struggles of the population. This goal is consistent with Fink's *taxonomies of significant learning* (Fink, 2003) for both the caring and human dimension taxonomies.

The students presented their project as a group to the class utilizing creative Multimedia methodologies. Their presentations included formats such as video production, VoiceThread conversations, a Jeopardy! game, and others that engaged the rest of the class and communicated the message of heartfelt vulnerability.

The best way to keep up with new and meaningful delivery methods is to take notes from the students; they will let instructors know how they like to learn. Feedback for the blended delivery method was elicited from both students and the clinical faculty facilitators. The responses were organized into the following four themes: time management, participation, learning opportunities, and technology. The results were favorable for the blended style in general, as most students like the flexibility and opportunities to participate. Some students still would prefer to sit in class and be passive learners, but for the most part the students enjoyed the learning experience and students and faculty alike benefited from the increased engagement in the discussions. See the survey results in **Table 18-4**.

Table 18-4 Feedback for Blended Learning

	Student: Advantages of Hybrid Model	Student: Disadvantages of Hybrid Model	Faculty Facilitator: Advantages of Hybrid Model	Faculty Facilitator: Disadvantages of Hybrid Model
Time/ Schedule	"Fits schedule better" "More flexible—less stressful" "Quizzes can be taken in a relaxed environment" "More time for readings" "Less commuting time" "Lets me organize my time better"	"Writing out the discussions is time consuming" "Seems to be more work involved, too much time researching answers to discussions" "Hard to keep organized, the time management is difficult" "Very time consuming, makes you prefer classroom lectures"	"The students seem to manage their time better"	
Participation	"More engaged with material" "Really enjoy learning others' opinions" "More communication with classmates" "Students who don't speak easily in class, speak up online" "More time for a better prepared response" "More feedback from peers" "Smaller groups, more attention" "Good for someone like myself who does not speak up in class yet has a lot to say"	"Don't like sharing with other students" "Feel disconnected from the classroom professor" "Miss the classroom interaction with other students" "Online discussions feel like busy work" "Online doesn't feel 'real'; hard to take it seriously" "I would rather sit in class for 2 hours and listen to the professor than to read on my own and share my thoughts on the Internet" "Too much computer screen time, would rather more face-to-face time" "Others' discussions are too long to read"	"Very interesting discussions, I love reading them!" "Allows the students to clearly express their thoughts" "I learn a lot about the students from their postings; I would never get that otherwise" "Would love to see more of the course online!"	"The students don't like reading all the discussions and responses" "I worry that the students view the online sessions as an 'off' week"

(continues)

Table 18-4 (continued)

	Student: Advantages of Hybrid Model	Student: Disadvantages of Hybrid Model	Faculty Facilitator: Advantages of Hybrid Model	Faculty Facilitator: Disadvantages of Hybrid Model
Learning Opportunities	"Forces you to look things up and learn more" "Like the independent learning—I learn more on my own" "Enables students to learn in different ways" "Need to really read to participate in class" "I am learning more through the discussions and quizzes than I am in the classroom" "The discussions allow us to think about what we read" "The Internet connectivity leads us to different websites with a lot of new information" "The discussions make you really think about the readings instead of just memorizing" "Ties in the clinical practice with class" "The discussions revealed whole new areas of interest for me"	"Feel different instructors grade discussions differently; it's not fair" "Find the different assignments confusing" "We have to learn quite a bit on our own"	"The students did great research in preparation of the discussion questions" "The discussion questions seem to cover a great deal of material" "The students seem to learn more from the assignments" "The students seem to be able to organize their thoughts better by putting them in writing" "The students seem better at tying together the classroom and the clinical"	"Hard to give feedback—at this level students still need feedback on basic grammar and APA format; I find it hard to use this format to make comments"
Technology	"Improves my technology skills by forcing me to use the WebCT features"	"If the Internet is down, participation is difficult" "The technology is confusing" "Frustrating to work on an old PC" "Culture shock compared to other nursing classes"		"I don't like correcting online; I would rather have a Word document I can print out and make comments on"

REFERENCES

Barr, R. B., & Tagg, J. (1995). From teaching to learning:A new paradigm for undergraduate education. *Change, 27*(6), 12.

Bergman, J., & Sams, A. (2012). *Flip your classroom: Reach every student in every class every day.* Alexandria, VA: International Society for Technology in Education.

Bloom, B. S. (Ed.). (1956). *Taxonomy of educational objectives: The classification of educational goals handbook I: Cognitive domain.* New York, NY: McKay.

Collison, G., Elbaum, B., Haavind, S., & Tinker, R. (2000). *Facilitating online learning: Effective strategies for moderators.* Madison, WI: Atwood Publishing.

Fink, L. D. (Ed.). (2003). *Creating significant learning experiences.* San Francisco, CA: Jossey-Bass.

Howe, N., & Strauss, W. (2000). *Millennials rising: The next greatest generation.* New York, NY: Vintage Press.

Jairath, N., & Stair, N. (2004). A development and implementation framework for web-based nursing courses. *Nursing Education Perspectives, 25*(2), 67.

Knowles, M. (1990). *The adult learner: A neglected species* (4th ed.). Houston, TX: Gulf.

Lee, W. W., & Owens, D. L. (2000). *Multimedia-based instructional design.* San Francisco, CA: Jossey-Bass.

Leffers, J., & Martin, D. C. (2004). Journey to compassion: Meeting vulnerable populations in community health nursing through literature. *International Journal of Human Caring, 8*(1), 20.

O'Neil, C. A., Fisher, C. A., & Newbold, S. K. (Eds.). (2004). *Developing an online course: Best practices for nurse educators.* New York, NY: Springer.

Palloff, R. M., & Pratt, K. (2001). *Lessons from the cyberspace classroom.* San Francisco, CA: Jossey-Bass.

Palloff, R. M., & Pratt, K. (2003). *The virtual student.* San Francisco, CA: Jossey-Bass.

Prensky, M. (2001, October). Digital natives, digital immigrants. *On the Horizon, 9*(5).

Sener, J. (2012). *The seven futures of American education: Improving learning and teaching in a screen captured world.* CreateSpace Independent Publishing Platform.

Teeley, K., Lowe, J., Beal, J., & Knapp, M. (2006). Incorporating quality improvement concepts and practice into a community health nursing course. *Journal of Nursing Education, 45*(2), 65–71.

Weimer, M. (2013). *Learner centered teaching: Five key changes to practice* (2nd ed.). San Francisco: Jossey-Bass.

RECOMMENDED READING

Bonk, C. J., & Zhang, K. (2008). *Empowering on-line learners.* San Francisco, CA: Jossey-Bass.

Bozarth, J. (2008). *From analysis to evaluation.* San Francisco, CA: Pfeiffer.

Brookfield, S. (1986). *Understanding and facilitating adult learning.* San Francisco, CA: Jossey-Bass.

Clark, R. C. (2008). *Building expertise* (3rd ed.). San Francisco, CA: Pfeiffer.

Clark, R. C., & Mayer, R. E. (2003). *E-learning and the science of instruction.* San Francisco, CA: Pfeiffer.

Collison, G., Elbaum, B., Haavind, S., & Tinker, R. (2000). *Facilitating online learning: Effective strategies for moderators.* Madison, WI: Atwood Publishing.

Conrad, R., & Donaldson, J. (2004). *Engaging the online learner.* San Francisco, CA: Jossey-Bass.

Fink, L. D. (Ed.). (2003). *Creating significant learning experiences.* San Francisco, CA: Jossey-Bass.

Fink, L. D. (2013). A self directed guide to designing courses for significant learning. http://www.deefinkandassociates.com/resources.html http://www.docsearch.in/view/d3d3LmR lZWZpbmthbmRhc3NvY2lhdGVzLmNvbS9HdWlkZXRvQ291cnNlRGVzaWduQXVnMDUuc GRm/a-self-directed-guide-to-designing-courses-for-significant-learning.html

Garrison, D. R., & Vaughn N. D., (2008). *Blended learning in higher education.* San Francisco, CA: Jossey-Bass.

Horton, W. (2006). *E-learning by design.* San Francisco, CA: Pfeiffer.

Howe, N., & Strauss, W. (2000). *Millennials rising: The next greatest generation.* New York, NY: Vintage Press.

Krug, S. (2006). *Don't make me think: A common sense approach to Web usability* (2nd ed.). Berkeley, CA: New Riders.

Matthews-Denatale, G., & Cotler, D. (2005). Faculty as authors of online courses: Support and mentoring. Retrieved from http://www.academiccommons.org/commons/essay/matthews-denatale-and-cotler

Novotny, J. M., & Davis, R. (Eds.). (2006). *Distance education in nursing.* New York, NY: Springer.

O'Neil, C. A., Fisher, C. A., & Newbold, S. K. (Eds.). (2004). *Developing an online course: Best practices for nurse educators.* New York, NY: Springer.

Pacansky-Brock, M. (2013). *Best practices for teaching with emerging technology.* New York, NY: Routledge.

Palloff, R. M., & Pratt, K. (2001). *Lessons from the cyberspace classroom.* San Francisco, CA: Jossey-Bass.

Palloff, R. M., & Pratt, K. (2003). *The virtual student.* San Francisco, CA: Jossey-Bass.

Palloff, R. M., & Pratt, K. (2005). *Collaborating online: Learning together in community.* San Francisco, CA: Jossey-Bass.

Pink, D. H. (2006). *A whole new mind.* New York, NY: Riverhead Books.

Prensky, M. (2001, October). Digital natives, digital immigrants. *On the Horizon, 9*(5).

Wiske, M. S. (2005). *Teaching for understanding with technology.* San Francisco, CA: Jossey-Bass.

Web Resources

Blended Learning at Simmons College. http://at.simmons.edu/blendedlearning/

Faculty Resources. http://www4.uwm.edu/ltc/hybrid/faculty_resources/index.cfm

Illinois Online Network. http://www.ion.uillinois.edu/resources/tutorials/id/index.asp

University of Calgary: Teaching and Learning Centre Resource Library. http://tlc.ucalgary.ca/resources/library/

University of Michigan: Center for Research on Learning and Teaching. http://www.crlt.umich.edu/tstrategies/tsot.php

University of Minnesota Center for Teaching and Learning. http://www1.umn.edu/ohr/teachlearn/

CHAPTER 19

E-Communication That Fosters Connections Between People and Ideas

■ GAIL MATTHEWS-DeNATALE AND ARLENE J. LOWENSTEIN ■

This chapter provides a pedagogical analysis of options for electronic communication (e-communication), along with a recommended process for selecting the e-communication strategy that best suits a given situation or learning scenario. With the advent of personal computers and the Internet, technology has become integral to all aspects of academic life and work (Green, Brown, & Robinson, 2008; Mitra & Steffensmeier, 2000). E-communication has brought about dramatic changes in the interactions between students, faculty, and staff, because many, if not most, of our interactions now take place in digital format. E-communication takes many forms. In addition to well-established technologies such as e-mail, we now have the following:

- *Learning management systems (e.g., Blackboard, Pearson eLearning, Moodle).* These provide educators with a bundled set of tools for communication, including instant messaging, threaded discussions, chat rooms, and "live classroom" webinars.
- *Personal response systems.* These allow students to respond to a poll or survey question in the classroom with a clicker and then see the results displayed on a projection screen. This provides the professor with real-time information about the strengths and gaps in student understanding. This information is arguably more reliable than a verbal poll, because the anonymity of clickers creates a sense of safety in admitting confusion or misunderstanding (Weerts, Miller & Altice, 2009).
- *Texts and tweets.* These brief communications provide quick rounds of near-real-time interaction. This format is useful in getting a message out quickly—for example, about a course location or time change—or connecting with a colleague at a conference. Another benefit is that texting is the preferred format for communication among most youth,

The authors wish to thank Doug DeNatale for his review and contributions to this piece.

many of whom believe that "email is for old people" (Carnevale, 2006, p.1). Texting can be both a blessing and a bane because it sets up expectations for immediate response and some students have difficulty knowing when it is appropriate to use text shortcuts (for example, *r* instead of *are*).

■ *Lecture capture and screencasts (e.g., Camtasia, Jing, iTunes podcast).* These systems record audio and the computer screen so that students can listen to or view lectures at a time and place of their convenience or see a video demonstration of the steps required to perform a computer-based task.

■ *A host of free, easy-to-use social media apps and tools.* These apps include blogs, wikis, YouTube, VoiceThread, Google Apps, LinkedIn, and Facebook.

With all of these options readily at hand, some educators understandably feel overwhelmed by the myriad possibilities. As educators in the age of the Internet, we are challenged to explore the possibilities associated with new technology and to reinvent ourselves as teachers. Research conducted at Memorial University in Newfoundland concludes, "the [online] medium itself changed the dynamics of class interactions, not only those between students and professor, but also the interaction between students themselves" (Reid, 2009, p. 1).

Effective use of this technology depends on a clear understanding of the type of communication that will best further goals for learning in a given situation. For example, student blogs, including comment tool feedback from faculty, may be most appropriate for individualized and reflective learning, while threaded discussions or wikis may be more appropriate for learning that improves collaboration and group analysis. This forces us to reexamine our fundamental assumptions and sometimes our misconceptions about communication in general.

Communication is not just a back-and-forth between one student and the instructor. Communication can take place between the instructor and groups of students, or between group members, with the instructor acting as a guide on the side, rather than as the sage on the stage (Collision, Elbaum, Haavind, & Tinker, 2000). According to Reid (2009), "Online courses are a disruptive technology in the sense that it requires different pedagogical methods which may not yet be fully understood. In many ways it is a break with the past and requires professors to rethink their teaching practices" (p. 1). Successful integration of e-communication into the course plan requires a thoughtful process of learning design that sets the stage and provides appropriate resources for learning. The teacher is able to transition into a facilitative role because the plan for learning is well conceived, clearly articulated, engaging, resource rich, and so generative that students are equipped to take responsibility for their own learning. Sarah Haavind describes this as "front loading" learning (2008, p. 1). If the learning design has fostered a culture of respect and engagement, students can also be charged with researching, developing, and facilitating their own discussions. Student-led discussions increase engagement and also provide a window into student thinking that is less visible during teacher-led discussions.

People who are unfamiliar with this constructivist approach to teaching some-times wrongly assume that it is completely spontaneous and unplanned. On the contrary, educators need to think very carefully about the goals for learning and desired interactions as they design assignments that involve collaborative meaning making. Discussion does not automatically add up—it needs to be focused and facilitated through the use of guiding questions. Discussion also serves a purpose that can vary according to the phase of learning. For example, the *Talk Science* dis-cussion facilitation materials developed for the NSF-funded Inquiry Project outline these four distinct purposes for scientific discussion or academically productive talk: eliciting ideas, discussing data, consolidating learning, and explaining why (TERC, 2011). In addition to this typology, *Talk Science* offers a compendium of talk moves, verbal strategies for expanding and deepening discussion (Michaels & O'Connor, 2011). These materials can be valuable in crafting questions for discussion and providing guidance in posing follow-up responses that engage all learners in deep learning, even though the *Talk Science* framework is intended for face-to-face discus-sions among younger learners.

Not all communication takes place within groups. Sometimes communication is an intimate affair that involves internal dialogue, peer-to-peer feedback, or dialogic meaning making between the student and teacher. E-portfolios provide students with a personalized Web space in which they can store and reflect on their work, with commenting tools that allow feedback from faculty and peers. Because this space exists independent of a course, the e-portfolio helps students make intellectual connections between life and learning throughout their program of study, and many e-portfolio systems allow students continued access beyond graduation. Reflecting on e portfolios as a tool for enhanced meta-cognition, Trent Batson has observed, "If we in higher education wish to learn the most and leverage the most during this knowledge revolution, we have to recognize the active agent in the revolution. The active agent is humanity" (2008, p. 2).

Not all communication takes place in written form. Recent research indicates that learning can be enhanced through the juxtaposition of words, sounds, and images. E-portfolios support this process of multimodal meaning making. However, the use of multimedia needs to be carefully guided. Media need to be relevant, substantive, and thoughtfully constructed so that the mix of text and other media enhances instead of distracts from understanding (Clark & Mahyer, 2003).

Even though the portfolio process can be a powerful strategy for integrative learning, students do not automatically achieve this goal. Honest reflection is dif-ficult, and the process needs scaffolding. Students need to be mentored through teacher–student conversations about their e-portfolios. Rubrics and exemplars can provide guidance, and peer feedback is also helpful for increasing student engage-ment with their e-portfolios. E-portfolios are different from journals in which stu-dents record generalized thoughts about their learning, because the e-portfolio is evidence driven and grounded in the examination of work samples (also known as learning artifacts). This process is sometimes described as "collect, select, reflect, and connect." Students *collect* many samples of their work, *select* the ones that they deem most representative of their development, *reflect* on their strengths and areas for growth (in writing), and *connect* course-based learning with the learning that has taken place during other courses and life experiences. Because this process often spans the program, it is useful to provide students with online resources to guide their e-portfolio work (Matthews-DeNatale, 2013).

Communication is not inevitable; it takes practice. In the same way that faculty should read and understand a book before assigning it to their students, instructors should also spend time using technology in their own lives as learners to "discover in themselves what talents and abilities come forward" (Batson, 2008, p 2.). Ruth Reynard extols the virtues of "getting your hands dirty" (p. 1), testing ideas to solicit student input, and making sure that the technical implementation strategy is explicitly aligned with learning goals (Reynard, 2008).

The teacher is also responsible for introducing students to the resources available, providing guidelines for their use, and troubleshooting with the student when technical problems occur or referring the student to appropriate technology support. The teacher should experiment in advance with the electronic tools and strategies under consideration to develop personal mastery and ensure that they function as anticipated. The course design process may begin months or even semesters before the course is launched, and it may involve collaboration with one or more instructional designers or instructional technologists.

▪ Theoretical Foundations

In the face-to-face classroom setting, decisions about verbal communication are relatively straightforward, and there is also a commonly held understanding among students and faculty about the forms and conventions of communication. For example, issues that are of general importance are raised during class, whereas communication with individuals takes place during office hours, before class, or after class. Seasoned educators develop an intuitive sense for appropriate formats: when to lecture, convene small-group discussions among students, or host a question-and-answer session.

The advent of e-communication greatly increases options for dialogue, offering the opportunity for enhanced interaction between teachers and learners through text, images, audio, and video. With this opportunity comes a new set of responsibilities to:

- Reflect on the goal and desired effect of each act of communication.
- Understand the range of options available, as well as the advantages and constraints of each tool.
- Select a communicative strategy and tool that is appropriate to the goal.
- Consider issues of access, including the needs of students with disabilities.

To make pedagogically sound decisions about communication with students, it is helpful to first take a step back and consider how communication happens among people. Although communication is fundamental to everyday life, communications experts will tell you that it is deceptively complex. From Aristotle's time to the present day, academics have grappled with the challenge of developing a theoretical model for communication that captures the nuances of the process. Early models described a linear process that involved the transmission of information from a sender (e.g., speaker, writer) to a receiver (e.g., listener, reader) (Shannon & Weaver, 1949).

But communication, particularly e-communication, is anything but linear. Contemporary theorists describe communication as a multidimensional process that can take place over extended periods of time, for distinct purposes (e.g., persuasion, inquiry), and within complex systems in which the specific context can dramatically alter perceived meaning (Littlejohn, 2002).

For example, a single instructor (sender) can record a presentation for download by hundreds or even thousands of people, yet each person (receiver) will probably listen to the recording in a different context (e.g., in the car, at the gym, while cooking supper), stopping and starting to complete the process of listening in different increments of time. At first glance, this might appear to be problematic, but listener control over time, place, and pacing is central to the dramatic rise in podcast popularity (Read, 2005). Anxieties that podcasting might contribute to increased absenteeism have proved to be irrelevant. In a recent study conducted by the University of Washington, 84% of student respondents in UW's podcasting pilot initiative reported the same or increased levels of attendance, and faculty reported that even if attendance did decline, in podcast-enhanced courses, "those who were there were truly present" (Lane, 2006, p. 8). This is yet another example of the ways in which e-communication challenges educators to rethink assumptions about teaching.

▪ Conditions

If possible, gather information about the conditions under which students will access the course. For example, if many of students will be accessing the course through a slow connection, bandwidth-intensive strategies such as video are not advisable. Likewise, some institutions set limits on storage and file upload. Sometimes the limits for teachers differ from those for students, so do not assume that your students will have the same privileges that you enjoy. Research institutional policies beforehand to ensure that your strategy is viable and that course materials are within file size limits.

Wherever possible, build technology orientation into the learning experience well in advance of the time that it will be needed. For example, in the first week of class, require that students complete an online scavenger hunt that uses key technologies. In addition to the scavenger hunt, provide self-based tutorials, quick-start guides, and practice areas so that students can experiment, troubleshoot, problem solve, and self-teach. Include information about where to go for technical support in the syllabus and in the support materials. These resources will help students resolve technical glitches before they have a chance to compromise the learning, and you are less likely to be inundated with technical questions.

Internet users are increasingly concerned about the loss of privacy that can result from uninformed interaction online. Parents often wonder about the safety of their underage children, and adolescents learn too late that youthful indiscretions have considerable staying power online. As an instructor, it is your responsibility to keep students apprised of privacy laws and to take steps to provide a safe learning environment whose privacy is appropriate to the learning scenario. Whenever possible, provide explicit instruction to the students on how to set permission privileges in the online tools that they use for your course. Instructors also are responsible for ensuring that course materials and assignments do not result in copyright infringement.

Some projects may be appropriate for public consumption (e.g., a vetted online poster presentation that presents original student research), but the vast majority of coursework should be password protected. If a password-protected learning management system is used, many privacy concerns become moot. However, security measures in cutting-edge, free technologies will vary, and the stability of these platforms should be carefully considered as well. Should a company go out of business midcourse and shut down its servers, student work may be at risk if there is no offline copy of the files. Familiarize yourself with FERPA and TEACH Act regulations so that you can be mindful about how privacy laws relate to electronic communication in the classroom. For more information, see the privacy and copyright links listed in the *Resources* section of this chapter.

■ Types of Learners

When thoughtfully designed and judiciously implemented, e-communication improves a teacher's ability to meet the needs of heterogeneous learners as follows:

- Personal response system clickers engage people who prefer kinesic learning.
- Lecture capture recordings are helpful for students who prefer to listen, and English-as-a-second-language learners often appreciate the opportunity to review a presentation several times.
- Threaded discussions are a boon to introverts who need time to reflect before contributing to a discussion.

However, a strategy that opens doors for one type of learner may also be a strategy that presents a barrier to entry for another. For example, lecture capture recordings may not be accessible for students who are hearing impaired. Ideally, coursework is offered in a range of formats using a variety of strategies, embodying the principles of differentiated learning and universal design (Burgstahler & Cory, 2008).

According to the Americans with Disabilities Act (ADA), all communication that takes place via image, video, or audio must also be made accessible, upon request, to students with learning disabilities. Do not wait until a sight- or hearing-impaired student requests formal accommodations. Develop the habit of providing alternative means of access, such as closed-captioning or video/image-thick description.

New media tools such as YouTube can create captions on the fly, and most online word processors provide the option of including alternate text (an image or video description) when embedding media in a webpage. The Center for Applied Special Technology (CAST) also provides a host of resources and information about accessibility and universal design on its website. If you need assistance in converting course content into an accessible format, contact your institution's academic support center or office of instructional/academic technology to request help. Explain that you want your course materials to be brought into Section 508 ADA compliance.

■ Resources

Although most faculty members and students use computers and mobile devices, many are uncomfortable with unfamiliar programs, and few are expert users. Training and technical support follow-up must be made available (Bates & Poole, 2003). E-communication can be extremely frustrating and stressful for novices unless an adequate system of support and encouragement is in place. Coordination with the center for learning, academic technology, or information technology department will help you arrange for adequate support and avoid the frustration of underestimating the need for assistance. In addition to resources on your campus, you may want to consult the following:

- The New Media Consortium Horizon Project (http://www.nmc.org/horizon)
- The Educause Learning Initiative (http://www.educause.edu/eli)
- *Innovate*, an online journal dedicated to the creative use of technology in education (http://innovateonline.info)
- Resources on privacy and copyright law
  - FERPA (http://nces.ed.gov/forum/ferpa_links.asp)
  - The TEACH Act (http://www.nea.org/home/35377.htm)
  - The TEACH toolkit (http://www.educause.edu/library/resources/teach-toolkit-online-resource-understanding-copyright-and-distance-education-0)
  - *Campus Guide to Copyright Compliance* (http://www.copyright.com/Services/copyrightoncampus) http://www.copyright.com/Services/copyrightoncampus/intro/
- Universal design
  - CAST (Center for Applied Special Technology) (http://www.cast.org/publications/UDLguidelines/version1.html)

■ Using the Method

The choice of which technology is to be used depends on the learning objectives, the need for synchronous or asynchronous processes, and the resources available.

The following questions are designed to guide readers through a pedagogically grounded process for integrating electronic communication into teaching and learning.

1. What are the overarching goals for student learning? Consider goals for the course as a whole, because that helps inform the suite of tools to be used during the entire semester. Unless your course has technology as its focus (e.g., an informatics course), it is advisable to be judicious in your selection of technology. It is better to use a few tools extremely well than to overwhelm students with different technologies each session. If your learning management system allows you to hide tools that are not in use, doing so will make your course easier to navigate and less overwhelming.

2. What are the session- or unit-specific goals for student learning? Some tools lend themselves particularly well to specific tasks. For example, clickers are particularly good for polling large classes to get a snapshot of student learning in the aggregate (persistent misconceptions, concepts that have been mastered), and then to involve students in personalized discussions with neighbors or with the group as a whole.

3. Which evidence (artifacts of student work) will be needed so that the instructor and the students can assess and improve progress toward learning goals? Polls provide evidence of aggregate learning, and discussion posts provide evidence of individual learning (also known as learning artifacts). This evidence is easier to assess if it is viewed in relationship to a rubric, and students can also use rubrics in conjunction with artifacts to self-assess and improve the quality of their work.

4. To what extent should a given act of communication be public (e.g., discussion and debate) or private (e.g., reflection and self-assessment)?

5. What is the desired level of interactivity (give-and-take) associated with the act of communication? Is it a one-way broadcast (content delivery) or is it an open-ended question that is best understood by hearing from a range of perspectives?

6. How complex is the act of communication? Text messages and chat rooms are great for simple questions (e.g., "Did you mean for us to read Chapters 3 *and* 4?"), but they are inadequate for following a nuanced thread of extended discussion among multiple participants.

7. How collaborative is the assignment? Do you want students to work as a team to produce a product, report, or analysis? If so, then choose a tool that can provide each group with its own work space (e.g., wikis, live classroom breakout rooms).

8. What are the learners' time constraints? If class members live in different time zones, it could be disastrous if students are required to log in at a given time for synchronous interaction.

After you have considered these questions, use **Table 19-1** to identify the e-communication strategies best suited to your needs and pedagogical purposes.

Table 19-1 E-Communication Strategies

Use	Texting and Twitter	Chat	E-Mail	Online Journal (Private)	E-Portfolio	Blog (Public)	Wiki	Threaded Discussion	Lecture Capture and Screen cast	PRS Clickers	Live Classroom Webinar
One to self				x	x						
One to one	x	x	x		x						
One to many	x	x	x (list, cc)		x	x		x	x		x
Many to one							x			x	
Many to many	x (list)						x	x		x	x
Presentation and content delivery					x	x	x		x		x
Can embed or attach media (visual/auditory)	x		x	x	x	x	x	x	x	x	x
Short questions and clarification	x		x					x		x	x
Reflection and individualized interaction			x	x	x						
Collaboration and group work						x	x	x			x
Synchronous		x								x	x
Asynchronous	x		x	x	x	x	x	x	x		

PRS = Personal Response System.

■ Potential Problems

Technology changes and evolves rapidly. Cell phones quickly gave way to smart mobile devices that can take pictures and videos, gather data, provide access to text messages, and interface directly with social media. Many of the major learning management systems also provide apps that allow users to log in directly from a tablet computer, smartphone, or other mobile device. It is important for faculty to be aware of new apps and devices, but there should be a clear rationale for using them if they entail expense on the part of students.

Instructions for use must be clear, particularly the expectations for standards of communication. For example, students might believe that e-mail messages and discussion posts can be more informal than student papers. Some educators believe that typos, spelling, and grammar do not need to be corrected in e-mail messages, as long as students understand that good grammar, spelling, and proofreading are required for paper assignments, while others believe that all communication should be thoughtfully composed, grammatical, and error free. It is important to make your expectations for communication clear, because your students may have been operating under a different understanding in another class. Many schools have ethical policies for computer usage and e-mail. Course syllabi should inform students of those policies and lay out clear expectations for adherence.

Although younger students have grown up with computer technology, graduate-level academic programs may attract older students who have not had that advantage. Conversely, a tech-savvy student whose smartphone is always at hand may have no idea how to use technology for academic learning. Students' computer literacy should not be taken for granted. It is helpful to assess student experience and comfort level with technology before introducing an assignment that hinges on e-communication. The results will help you to spot people requiring extra help, to pair more experienced users with novices for the purpose of peer mentoring, and to direct struggling students to institutional resources for more support.

As noted previously, privacy is an important concern. E-mail messages are not private and can be retrieved even after they have been deleted. Both students and faculty need to be aware of this and consider e-mail to be a durable form of communication. Likewise, seemingly evanescent communications like chat and text messages can be saved, or the sender and receiver can take a screenshot of the interaction.

Reading e-mail and discussion board messages can be a time-consuming task for both students and teachers, especially if the task involves one-on-one student/ instructor dialogue. Strategies for meeting this challenge include collecting all discussion posts into one document to skim through them and compose one facilitation response message that addresses the whole group (Haavind, 2008). Oosterhof's (2000) method of individualizing e-mail allowed for consolidating messages and providing some automatic answering options when working with large classes. Replies to students can be brief but need to be meaningful. Both large and small classes can benefit from the use of e-communication when the technology is geared to meet specific teaching-learning objectives.

■ Future Directions

The present context offers a wealth of options—sometimes it can even feel like there are too many possibilities. But it is also important to stay abreast of new developments, as well as to anticipate technologies that are fading from use. The New Media Consortium's Horizon Project, an annual report, is a relatively easy way to keep current. Looking beyond 2013, as mobile devices make it possible for people to access e-mail, text messages, the Web, podcasts, social media, and a host of other apps from a pocket-sized device, we can expect that e-communication will become simultaneously ubiquitous and infinitesimally smaller. At first glance, these tiny devices may raise as many problems as they solve. But as educators open themselves up to considering the wealth of possibilities, to rethinking assumptions about where, when, and learning takes place, opportunities will be vast even though the mechanism for communication is small.

TEACHING EXAMPLE:

Discussion Boards, Wikis, and E-Portfolios

This example describes how three e-communication tools are used in conjunction within a fully online course to achieve synergistic learning. The tools serve the following three different pedagogical purposes: wikis for collaborative authoring (cocommunication), threaded discussions for interpersonal dialogue and collaborative meaning making, and e-portfolios for intrapersonal reflection and metacognitive integration.

Emerging Trends in Education is a fully online, core course within the Master of Education program at Northeastern University. The Master of Education program also includes an e-portfolio requirement, for which students are expected to place at least one reflection and a work sample in their e-portfolios during or after every course that they complete.

In online courses, students typically begin by introducing themselves within a threaded discussion, an exercise that is repeated for each course. This practice can become tedious for students pursuing an entire degree online, particularly for those who have already "met" each other in previous courses. Students in Emerging Trends link to their e-portfolios. As opposed to perfunctory introductions, e-portfolios have the capacity to depict many facets of the author's identity, including experience, interests, goals, and dreams. Students claim that they get to know their peers better when they browse each other's e-portfolios. People who do not already know each other can click through to read about their peers, but old friends can forgo that process. This makes it possible to focus introductory threaded discussions on what students hope to gain from the course, launching a dialogue about connections between the topic, students' relevant prior experiences, and their goals for learning.

The e-portfolio and threaded discussions work in tandem. Sometimes the e-portfolios provide peer background information that helps students begin threaded discussions at a deeper level; sometimes threaded discussions serve as a prewrite and sounding board for

(continued)

entries that students later make in their individual e-portfolios. For example, at the beginning of the course, students use a course-based threaded discussion to assert and discuss their vision for education, using the following writing prompt to guide the conversation:

> If you could reinvent our system for education starting from scratch today, how would it be different? From your vantage point as an educator (and/or as a student) . . . What should be kept? What could we survive without? How would this approach to education be different from, or similar to, current model(s)? Please also include information about the educational setting in which you work so that we can get a better picture of your perspective.

> Don't worry about being right because we are just getting started with our conversation on this topic. Your first message is a snapshot of your thinking at the beginning of the course. You'll have a chance to revisit it later to see how your thinking has changed and grown.

Students attach this preliminary vision for education to their e-portfolios at the end of the first week so that they can revisit it at the end of the course.

At the end of the first week of class, students are assigned to one of five wiki study groups, using the wiki tool that is available within the learning management system. Each week, each group is given a different set of resource materials (readings, websites, and videos) that pertain to the week's topic and related models for education. Sample wiki study group topics include open education, digital citizenship and media literacy, and global education. Within their respective wikis, group members pool notes and thoughts on the week's resource materials and then coauthor a starter message that includes a central question for discussion. A representative from each group posts the group's starter message to the threaded discussion board for the whole class to read. In the second half of each week, all students read the five starter messages and select one discussion thread to participate in during a follow-through discussion.

In the last week of the course, students revisit the vision statements that they composed during the first week. In a threaded discussion, they consider the following questions:

- How has your thinking changed or matured? Which aspects of your vision remain constant?
- Which opportunities do you see for bringing your vision to life? Thinking about your vision, identify one thing that you intend to do differently in your life and work. It doesn't have to be a big change, just something that is doable now, with the resources, social, and professional networks you already have in place.

After the discussion, students post revised vision statements and final reflections in their individual e-portfolios. The following prompt helps students "zoom out," looking at their e-portfolio as a whole, to reflect on the ways that their course-based learning relates to their entire academic program, and to the bigger picture of their personal goals and growth.

> Take a step back and look at the work you did for this course, reflecting on what it demonstrates. As you examine this work, ask yourself the following: What does it tell you about how your thinking has changed or expanded? Which evidence does it provide about your growth in this course?

Now consider your e-portfolio as a whole. What do you want to say about your evolving goals, recent insights, and the next steps you plan to take in your development? Based on where you are now, what's next for you in your learning journey? Are there resources from this and other courses that you want to save for future reference?

This assignment is the final piece of work each student completes for the course. It is designed to close the loop between course-based work and the larger learning arc that each student experiences within the program.

REFERENCES

Bates, A. W., & Poole, G. (2003). *Effective teaching with technology in higher education*. San Francisco, CA: Jossey-Bass.

Batson, T. (2008). Machines are dumb. *Campus Technology*. Retrieved from http://campustechnology.com/Articles/2008/11/Machines-are-Dumb.aspx

Burgstahler, S., & Cory, R. (Eds.). (2008). *Universal design in higher education*. Cambridge, MA: Harvard University Publishing Group.

Carnevale, D. (2006). Email is for old people. *Chronicle of Higher Education*. Retrieved from http://chronicle.com/article/E-Mail-is-for-Old-People/4169

Clark, R. C., & Mayer, R. E. (2003). *E-learning and the science of instruction: Proven guidelines for consumers and designers of multimedia learning*. San Francisco, CA: Jossey-Bass/Pfeiffer Edition.

Collision, G., Elbaum, B., Haavind, S., & Tinker, R. (2000). *Facilitating online learning: Effective strategies for moderators*. Madison, WI: Atwood.

Effink, V. L., Davis, L. S., Fitzwater, E., Castleman, J., Burley, J., Gorney-Moreno, M. J., .. Martin, A. (2000). The Nightingale Tracker Clinical Field Test Nurse Team: A comparison of teaching strategies for integrating information technology into clinical nursing education. *Nurse Educator, 25*(3), 136–144.

Green, T. D., Brown, A., & Robinson, L. (2008). *Making the most of the Web in your classroom: A teacher's guide to blogs, podcasts, wikis, pages, and sites*. Thousand Oaks, CA: Corwin Press.

Haavind, S. (2008). Facilitating online discussions. Retrieved from http://at.simmons.edu/blendedlearning/learnhow/casestudies/haavind

Lane, C. (2006). UW podcasting: Evaluation of year one. *Catalyst Papers*. Seattle, WA: University of Washington Office of Learning Technologies. Retrieved from http://catalyst.washington.edu/research_development/papers/2006/podcasting_year1.pdf

Littlejohn, S. (2002). *Theories of human communication*. Belmont, CA: Wadsworth.

Matthews-DeNatale, G. (2013). Northeastern University Master of Education Program ePortfolio resources. Retrieved from https://northeastern.digication.com/master_of_education_eportfolio_resources

Michaels, S., & O'Connor, S. (2011). *Talk science primer*. Cambridge, MA: TERC. Retrieved from http://inquiryproject.terc.edu/shared/pd/TalkScience_Primer.pdf

Mitra, A., & Steffensmeier, T. (2000). Changes in student attitudes and student computer use in a computer-enriched environment. *Journal of Research on Computing in Education, 32*(3), 417–432.

Oosterhof, A. (2000). Efficiently creating individualized e-mail to students. *Journal of Computing in Higher Education, 11*(2), 75–90.

Read, B. (2005). Duke U. assesses iPod experiment and finds it worked—in some courses. *Chronicle of Higher Education, 51*(43), A26. Retrieved from http://chronicle.com/article/Duke-U-Assesses-iPod/27063

Reid, S. (2009, March 2). Online courses and how they change the nature of class. *First Monday, 14*(3). Retrieved from http://firstmonday.org/htbin/cgiwrap/bin/ojs/index.php/fm/article/viewArticle/2167/2114

Reynard, R. (2008). 6 ways not to become rote using instructional technology. *Campus Technology*. Retrieved from http://campustechnology.com/Articles/2008/11/6-Ways-Not-To-Become-Rote-Using -Instructional-Technology.aspx

Shannon, C. E., & Weaver, W. (1949). *A mathematical model of communication*. Urbana, IL: University of Illinois Press.

TERC. (2011). The Inquiry Project: Library of resources. Retrieved from http://inquiryproject.terc.edu /prof_dev/library.cfm

Weerts, S. E., Miller, D., & Altice, A. (2009). "Clicker" technology promotes interactivity in an undergraduate nutrition course. *Journal of Nutrition Education & Behavior, 41*(3), 227–228.

CHAPTER 20

Synchronous Distance Education: Bringing Everyone Together

■ SHARON M. COSPER AND LYNN JAFFE ■

Today distance education is offered using a variety of media-based technology. The debate over the merits of distance education used to vary from blind adoration with assertions that teaching with technology resolved weaknesses in traditional teaching methods to opposition insisting that distance teaching was not capable of producing the same learning outcomes as traditional teaching methods (Allen & Seaman, 2011). However, sufficient research has been completed, particularly in medical and healthcare education, to allow for meta-analysis that suggests that online and blended learning are at least equal to, if not better than, face-to-face learning (U.S. Department of Education, 2010).

The purpose of this chapter is to describe synchronous distance education learning methods used in teaching in the healthcare professions. Technological advances have increased the ability to provide quality health-related professional education across distance. However, the merit of this strategy comes down to the teaching and accurate use of the methods themselves.

■ Definitions and Purpose

Distance education, as opposed to correspondence education/courses, refers to a substantially interactive instructional delivery method occurring when learners and educators are separated by time and/or distance (Higher Learning Commission, 2010). The term *technology* is broadly used in the literature to describe hardware and software including computers, videoconferencing, Internet, and other resources to provide instruction (Higher Learning Commission, 2010). Technology has become integral to the learning experience for the new generations of learners but is still a challenge to some faculty and students (Oblinger & Hawkins, 2006). The use of technology allows teacher–learner interaction in two formats: synchronous and asynchronous. The main focus of asynchronous educational theory is to use instructional technology to effectively transmit learning content to individuals at another site, while enabling real-time interaction between faculty and students as well as among students (Ely, 2000; Higher Learning Commission, 2010). Asynchronous technology is available to be accessed any time. The use of distance education provides alternative educational opportunities that might not otherwise be available due to learners' constraints. Students enrolled in healthcare professional curricula benefit from a maximal level of interaction to facilitate the mastery needed for complex knowledge, skills, and behaviors expected by the professions (Gallagher, Dobrosielski-Vergona, Wingard, & Williams, 2005).

■ Theoretical Foundations

The theoretical foundation of distance education had its roots in correspondence courses and was based on the concept that education could be further equalized and accessible if learners were not constrained to a time and place for educational experiences (Garrison, 2000). Theories of distance education have evolved as the technology has advanced. Early theories focused on the independence of the learners and their responsibility to make the most of the educational process. Distance methodology was evaluated under theories of traditional education, but then came to be deemed unique, and a theory of equivalency was proposed (Pyari, 2011). This theory called for all educational experiences to be equal between on-campus cohorts and their distance education peers (Simonson, Schlosser, & Hanson, 1999). Current federal funding for distance education requires the interactions now made possible by synchronous technology, differentiating it from correspondence courses (e-CFR §600.2; Poulin, 2012). The advances in technology that have enabled real-time conversation between groups over distance refocused theory on communication and the learning experiences (Garrison, 2000; Roushanzamir, 2004), which aligns the theoretical foundations closer to traditional educational beliefs. (For a concise review of distance education theory, see Roushanzamir, 2004.)

Studies involving a variety of health professionals have examined the pros and cons of educating future health professionals using distance education and have described successful learning outcomes (Condon, 2013; Wells & Dellinger, 2011). One study in a clinical laboratory science program examined academic performance between distance students and on-campus students. The analysis revealed there was no significant difference in the mean final grade-point averages and certification scores between the two groups. The findings document the success of the clinical lab science distance program for educating entry-level scientists (Russell, Leibach, Pretlow, & Kraj, 2007).

■ Types of Learners

Programs that use distance education allow for a broader, more diverse student audience. More specifically, healthcare professionals are generally upper-division or graduate-level students and may include many nontraditional students. Students enrolled in distance education tend to be a bit older than traditional students, are often working full time, may have served in the military, and may have a disability (EducationCounsel, 2012). An important touchstone of distance education has been the ability to contribute to the development of individual learners regardless of life circumstances. Nontraditional students tend to select distance education courses due to conflicting life priorities. Distance education programs allow these individuals expanded opportunities to pursue a healthcare career.

Studies examining the success of distance education and student profiles indicate learner and instructor familiarity with technology is beneficial to the overall learning outcomes. Also, learner motivation and a sense of interactivity are highly predictable of learner success (Gallagher et al., 2005). The level of motivation to succeed among these learners is helpful for attaining learning outcomes. Synchronous distance education is appropriate for all types of healthcare learners if attention is paid to the learners' access to the technology, adjustment to the new learning environment, and the importance of understanding the learners' perspectives of distance education (White, 2005). Even though younger learners are considered digital natives, they may not be familiar with either the specific learning management system in use or the etiquette of a formal online educational experience. As for mature students, they are sometimes at more of a disadvantage since they may have been digitally naïve prior to enrollment, although this gap in abilities is narrowing as technology use continues to become more and more prevalent.

■ Conditions for Learning

Three crucial conditions for effective distance education are the quality of the instructional process (Moser, 2007), the technology, and sufficient support for the students and faculty. The most common quality indicator in distance education is student–teacher interaction (Chaney et al., 2009). Another critical condition for success is the quality of the technology and immediate technology support (Hilgenberg & Tolone, 2000; Moser, 2007). Training on using the technology is of major importance, as is the ready support of information technology staff. The importance of the quality of faculty preparation has been emphasized, as has early communication with students to ensure learner motivation and success. The methods include additional or flexible scheduling if confronted with technology downtime. It should be expected that technological problems must be addressed immediately to allow for learning to occur (Zapantis & Maniscalco-Feichtl, 2008).

The investment of preparation is essential for effectiveness in distance education; unlike face-to-face classes, spontaneity faces challenges of ensuring that the distance students have all the materials they may need in sufficient time. While few students depend on dial-up connections, there may be some who will not be able to immediately access and print materials that are posted just as an instructor is beginning the class. The types of learning activities used in distance education require thought and awareness—they cannot simply consist of content posted onto a website if effective learning is to take place. Projects, case studies, peer interaction, and other interactive experiences must be employed (Oblinger & Hawkins, 2006).

Studies examining learning characteristics have identified a positive relationship between self-motivation and distance learning success. Five central distance education themes have been described: (1) the learner's access to education; (2) the learner's access to the learning materials and understanding of the technology; (3) clear instructions; (4) time to adjust to the new learning environment; and (5) the time it takes the instructor to identify the learners' needs, characteristics, and perspective of distance education (Zapantis & Maniscalco-Feichtl, 2008). This matches recommendations from the NEA (2000), which published a multisite study establishing the following benchmarks as necessary for successful distance education strategic planning: (1) institutional support; (2) course development; (3) teaching/learning; (4) course structure; (5) student support; (6) faculty support; and (7) evaluation and assessment.

Faculty support and commitment, as well as student support and commitment, are development areas needed to enhance the knowledge, skills, and buy-in for learning within a technological learning environment. For distance education to effectively meet the needs of the students, the institution must support the faculty (Moser, 2007). Published literature examining motivators and inhibitors for faculty with regard to distance education have identified intrinsic motivators as a more common driving force behind faculty desire for involvement than extrinsic motivators. Some of the top intrinsic motivators identified in the literature include ability to reach new audiences, intellectual challenge, and personal motivation to use technology. The most prevalent trends in concerns related to inhibitors of faculty involvement included a concern with the lack of technical support available and increased time necessary to prepare for distance education curriculum. These areas of concern must be addressed by the institutional administration to ensure successful implementation of distance education; otherwise, the success and quality of the program will be at risk (Cook, Ley, Crawford, & Warner, 2009).

Initial faculty skills in using the selected instructional technologies will be varied. Faculty will need technological assistance, and the institution should plan to provide this support. Some faculty members will require support to successfully transition from traditional teaching methods to using the technology. Peer mentoring may be helpful to faculty members who are new to distance education. Faculty should be aware of institutional resources to assist the learners' use of distance education and how to troubleshoot or access resources if the technology is problematic. One recommendation for successful learning is to have courses developed and delivered by teams since the skill sets and time commitment can be overly challenging for an individual (Oblinger & Hawkins, 2006).

Many institutions embark on distance education without first analyzing the impact on the teaching, the faculty, and the learners. The financial impact on the administration and the control of intellectual property are also serious synchronous learning issues. The development of new higher learning administration strategic plans and policies that embrace distance education and change is needed. The process should create an organizational plan that anticipates consequences and develops trouble-shooting resources. The level of administration, faculty, and student commitment is a good predictor of distance education success. The technology selection should be guided by sound instructional design choices that optimally facilitate the desired knowledge, skills, values, and interaction needed for competency and satisfaction of the lifelong learning needs of the targeted group. Technology selection must include a faculty voice in the decision-making process. The models proposed in this chapter require an interactive relationship between curriculum design, instructional design, technology selection, and the financial implications (Boettcher, 2000).

Healthcare educators must carefully address the aforementioned identified needs and suggested strategies. Valuing the use of technology and synchronous distance education will be critical to successful applications. Faculty should identify any potential barriers and plan professional development and alternative solutions to resolve impending issues (Boaz, Foshee, Hardy, Jarmon, & Olcott, 1999; Dupin-Bryant, 2004).

■ Using the Method

Once decisions have been made about the learning management system and synchronous interaction options, the business of using distance education is similar to regular instruction. Ground rules for students include all the standard education criteria, such as reading the details offered in the course syllabus, the use of the syllabus as a critical source of information, and respectful treatment of peers and instructors. Faculty need to include clear instructions regarding response time to e-mail and messages, often including hours of availability. Today's learners, who are used to instant messaging and frequent access to Twitter and Facebook, tend to expect immediate responses to questions. It is beneficial to include both faculty and student response time in the syllabus and occasionally reinforce the times of office hours though announcements in the courseware. Additional guidance regarding etiquette over distance is useful. Faculty should caution students that in a live videoconference situation their every move or comment may be broadcast to more than one location at any given moment.

Faculty need to set aside time, or a survey structure, for gaining an understanding of the learning needs of the distance learners and their individual learning contexts. The spontaneity of conversation in a classroom becomes a bit cumbersome in a distance situation due to time lag in the communication and the potential loss of attention because of the virtual environment. In face-to-face classes, there are often students who stop paying attention; this penchant is magnified when students believe no one is watching what they do. One method of combatting this drift of attention is to use frequent interaction techniques, such as polling, sharing desktops among the class, or employing novel bits of technology such as Wordle, a web-based software

■ **Figure 20-1** Wordles of conditions for learning section, two layouts (any which way and mostly horizontal)

that generates word clouds based upon frequency of response (http://www.wordle .net/) to prompt immediate responses from the students (see **Figure 20-1**). Some studies have investigated the use of Twitter for encouraging student engagement, one of which had positive results on both engagement and grades related to a highly structured use of Twitter with active faculty engagement (Junco, Elavsky, & Heiberger, 2012).

In synchronous distance education courses, using technology easily, with adequate time and support, enables the instructor to approach the teaching–learning relationship through multiple methods. These methods can be quite effective, no matter the size of the class, as evidenced by the work of Curtis Bonk, who is a master of the massively open online class (MOOC). His continuing education classes have enrollment upward of 500 people (issues of time related to grading do not come into play). Bonk uses elements that affect student motivation, such as feedback, engagement, meaningfulness, and peer interaction, and he implements a variety of activities to tap each of these elements and more, including the use of ice breakers, cases, surveys and polling, and debates (Dennen & Bonk, 2007; for complete information see *The World Is Open,* by Curtis Bonk, 2009). The use of creative, focused tasks shows the students you care about their participation and learning.

Because the learners are participating in the learning process from a computer or an electronic classroom, the need for nontraditional interaction with the content, the professor, and other students is critical to the learning process. The sound and video transmission must have good quality. Poor learning outcomes have been noted with poor sound and video transmission (Mills, Bates, Pendleton, Lese, & Tatarko, 2001; Saba, 2005). Currently, there are many platforms for effective synchronous distance learning technology. These platforms vary from individual contact, such as through Skype, to whole-classroom connectivity via Wimba Collaborate, Adobe Connect, WebEx, or other commercial platforms that can be incorporated into the major learning management systems that form the basis of distance learning at higher education entities, such as Blackboard, Desire2Learn, Moodle, Pearson Learning, and Sakai. Whole-classroom connectivity can be incorporated into most of these platforms, although some will require an additional cost to the institution. These systems can employ chat functions where the learner types a question or comment to the professor or class and receives answers as well as two-way audio/video. The best examples of employing two-way interactivity usually have an assistant helping the professor monitor the chat function. The assistant could be a hired work-study or technology person, or he or she could be a class member who takes on the role for a given class period. Having such an assistant allows the professor to keep focus without losing the interactions in a stream of comments that scroll through the chat window.

The common feature of all these platforms is of communication being interactive between the sites, preferably with audio as well as written comments. When working with groups of people, each site needs to be equipped with videoconferencing equipment, cameras, and microphones. Educators may need a personal wireless microphone. Instructors view students on monitors on the multiple campuses. The remote site views a video image of the instructor and other students at the transmission site. The instructor may use traditional educational supports such as PowerPoint slides or a Smart Board, or he or she may use features built into the platforms, such as whiteboards or polling features to gather information from the students. A document camera may be used to project documents or demonstrations of practice techniques—for example, the correct methods for management of a hand contracture. The process is effective with facilitated faculty-to-student and student-to-student interactions with supportive experiential and flexible presentations (Anderson et al., 2003).

■ Resources

These days, there are a variety of books (such as *The World Is Open*, mentioned previously), articles (see references list), and websites on effective use of distance learning technology. Some of the more useful websites include:

> Educause, an organization dedicated to improving higher education through technology, with a focus on teaching and learning: http://www.educause.edu/eli

> Florida Center for Instructional Technology: A teacher's guide to distance learning, Chapter 10, Implementing distance learning: http://fcit.usf.edu /distance/chap10.htm

> State University of West Georgia: How interactive are YOUR distance courses? A rubric for assessing interaction in distance learning: http://www.westga .edu/~distance/roblyer32.html.

■ Potential Problems

There are negative impacts on learning outcomes when the audio or video transmission is poor. The potential disruption needs to be anticipated with backup instructional plans to ensure student learning. Clear interaction and communication are required for effective professional learning. The literature clearly states technology problems directly contribute to poor learning outcomes (Hilgenberg & Tolone, 2000). Because of the potential for disruptions in signal transmission, which may compromise the quality of sound or video production, it is necessary for the educator to schedule for technology downtime and disturbances (Anderson et al., 2003; Zapantis & Maniscalco-Feichtl, 2008).

Distance education may put learners at a greater risk for taking in the factual information but not gleaning experientially the functional application of knowledge. This transition from knowledge to skill is imperative for future healthcare providers to experience. Ways of optimizing available resources to provide this transition must be considered when offering a distance program (Billings, 2007). Some of this can be more readily addressed in the synchronous two-way interactive environment but does require considerable attention from the instructor.

Another challenge to a distance model is the amount of time required by the faculty member to prepare quality web-based content and implement one-on-one instruction. Evidence suggests that the teacher–student ratio be 1:15 to ensure optimal delivery of quality instruction to the students (Boettcher, 1999), despite the current examples of MOOCs (which are frequently not for credit and involve no grading, so they are quite different from degree offerings). This is in contrast to a traditional class ratio of 1:25–30. It is imperative that time be arranged when the faculty is available to provide direct assistance and meet the individual needs of students. This can be challenging in a distance model, due to varying schedules limiting availability of both the faculty and students, yet it can be accommodated.

The interaction between instructor and learners should be positive, collaborative, and interactive. Faculty should role model the needed level of support and connection between the various learning sites. It is important that the faculty member ensure equal interaction time for all learning sites. Student expectations and faculty support should also be equal. It is important to avoid any tendency to respond to questions that are not open to all learners and all campuses. All learners should be included in course discussions, directions, and communication of any changes, and all students need to feel valued. One major concern is whether the students are contributing to the class. This particular concern is more easily met in asynchronous methods unless the class size is small.

A tangential, but tangible concern with distance education is the belief held by many faculty that the efforts expended on distance education are not fully credited in tenure and promotion decisions (Allen, Seaman, Lederman, & Jaschik, 2012). Working through faculty governance to ensure proper career credit for time spent with distance education classes is necessary. Preparing well and implementing distance learning are time consuming and can be invasive if faculty do not set specific response time parameters. Remember—it is best practice to state formally in a syllabus what the expectations are for both faculty and student communications.

■ Conclusion

Distance education has become a fact of higher educational life. If done well, it has been shown to be as effective as traditional education. If the instructor meets the expected learning considerations such as organization, interactivity, effective communication, and experiential learning, the outcomes are comparable. Distance students require organization, experiential learning, and interaction with the instructor. Selection of the appropriate technology methods must consider the needed program competencies and learner characteristics. The quality of the technology support from the institution is critical to the students' learning and the overall success of the distance education program (Anderson et al., 2003; Zapantis & Maniscalco-Feichtl, 2008).

REFERENCES

Allen, I. A., & Seaman, J. (2011). *Going the distance: Online education in the United States.* Babson Park, MA: Babson Survey Research Group and Quahog Research Group.

Allen, I. E., Seaman, J., Lederman, D., & Jaschik, S. (2012). Conflicted: Faculty and online education, 2012.. Babson Park, MA: Babson Survey Research Group and Quahog Research Group.

Billings, D. (2007, June). Optimizing distance education in nursing: Editorial. *Journal of Nursing Education, 46,* 247–248.

Boaz, M., Foshee, B., Hardy, D., Jarmon, C., & Olcott, D., Jr. (1999). *Teaching at a distance: A handbook for instructors.* Monterey, CA: Archipelago Productions.

Boettcher, J. V. (1999). Designing for learning: How many students are just right in a web course? Retrieved from http://www.designingforlearning.info/services/writing/number.htm

Boettcher, J. V. (2000). The state of distance education in the United States: Surprising realities. *Syllabus: New Directions in Educational Technology, 13*(7), 36–40.

Chaney, B. H., Eddy, J. M., Dorman, S. M., Glessner, L. L., Green, B. L., & Lara-Alecio, R. (2009). A primer on quality indicators of distance education. *Health Promotion Practice, 10,* 222–231.

Condon, B. (2013). The present state of presence in technology. *Nursing Science Quarterly, 26,* 24–28.

Cook, R. G., Ley, K., Crawford, C., & Warner, A. (2009). *Motivators and inhibitors for university faculty in distance and e-learning.*

Dennen, V. P., & Bonk, C. J. (2007). We'll leave the light on for you: Keeping learners motivated in online courses. In B. H. Khan (Ed.), *Flexible learning in an information society* (pp. 64–76). Hershey, PA: The Idea Group.

Dupin-Bryant, P. A. (2004). Teaching styles of interactive television instructors: A descriptive study. *American Journal of Distance Education, 18*(1), 39–50.

e-CFR Electronic Code of Federal Regulations, Title 34: Education. §600.2. Definitions. Retrieved from http://www.ecfr.gov/cgi-bin/text-idx?c=ecfr&sid=0900b7322acc5a5a10c558b8fe15ad7b&rgn=div8&view=text&node=34:3.1.3.1.1.1.23.2&idno=34

EducationCounsel. (2012). Commission on Regulation of Postsecondary Distance Education: A call to action in light of federal and state legal and policy issues and trends. Retrieved from http://ide.sreb.org/fedregs/Commission%20White%20Paper%20Final-Updated%20post%20June%20meeting%20Final%20II%20.pdf

Ely, D. (2000). Looking before we leap: Prior questions for distance education planners. *Syllabus: New Directions in Educational Technology, 13*(10), 26–28.

Gallagher, J. E., Dobrosielski-Vergona, K. A., Wingard, R. G., & Williams, T. M. (2005). Web-based vs. traditional classroom instruction in gerontology: A pilot study. *Journal of Dental Hygiene, 79*(3), 1–10.

Garrison, R. (2000). Theoretical challenges for distance education in the 21st century: A shift from structural to transactional issues. *International Review of Research in Open and Distance Learning, 1*(1), 1–17.

Higher Learning Commission. (2010). Approval of distance and correspondence education. Retrieved from http://www.dmi.illinois.edu/nca/DistanceEdApproval2010.pdf

Hilgenberg, C., & Tolone, W. (2000). Student perceptions of satisfaction and opportunities for critical thinking in distance education by interactive video. *American Journal of Distance Education, 14*(3), 59–73.

Junco, R., Elavsky, C. M., & Heiberger, G. (2012). Putting Twitter to the test: Assessing outcomes for student collaboration, engagement and success. *British Journal of Educational Technology.* doi: 10.1111/j.1467-8535.2012.01284x

Mills, O. F., Bates, J. F., Pendleton, V., Lese, K., & Tatarko, M. (2001). Distance education interactive videoconferencing in a family practice residency center. *Distance Education Online Symposium News, II.* Retrieved from http://www.ed/psy.edu/acsde/deros/deosnews/deosnews11_7.asp

Moser, F. Z. (2007). Faculty adoption of educational technology. *Educause Quarterly, 1,* 66–69.

National Education Association (NEA). (2000, June 13). Quality online: Maintaining standards in the distance education course. *Syllabus: New Directions in Educational Technology, 10,* 10.

Oblinger, D. G., & Hawkins, B. L. (2006, January/February). The myth about online course development: A faculty member can individually develop and deliver an effective online course. *Educause Review,* 14–15.

Poulin, R. (2012, April 20). Is your distance education course actually a correspondence course? [Web log post]. Retrieved from http://wcetblog.wordpress.com/2012/04/20/correspondence-definition/

Pyari, D. (2011). Theory and distance education: At a glance. *5th International Conference on Distance Learning and Education IPCSIT, 12.* Retrieved from http://www.ipcsit.com/vol12/18-ICDLE2011E10011.pdf

Roushanzamir, S. (2004). *Theories of distance education meet theories of mediated (mass) communication.* Distance learning roundtable presented at Association for Educational Communications & Technology Conference, Chicago, IL. Retrieved from http://roushan.myweb.uga.edu/EDIT7000/aect2004.pdf

Russell, B. L., Leibach, E. K., Pretlow, L., & Kraj, B. (2007, Summer). Evaluating distance education in clinical laboratory science. *Clinical Laboratory Science, 20*(3), 137–138.

Saba, F. (2005, October). Critical issues in distance education: A report from the United States. *Distance Education, 26*(2), 255–272.

Simonson, M., Schlosser, C., & Hanson, D. (1999). Theory and distance education: A new discussion. *American Journal of Distance Education, 13*(1). Retrieved from http://www.c3l.uni-oldenburg.de/cde/found/simons99.htm

Tucker, S. (2001). Distance education: Better, worse, or as good as traditional education? *Online Journal of Distance Education Administration, 4*(4), 1–13. Retrieved from http://www.westga.edu/~distance/ojda/winter44/tucker44.html

U.S. Department of Education, Office of Planning, Evaluation, and Policy Development. (2010). *Evaluation of evidence-based practices in online learning: A meta-analysis and review of online learning studies.* Washington, DC: Author.

Wells, M., & Dellinger, A. (2011). The effect of type of learning environment on perceived learning among graduate nursing students. *Nursing Education Perspectives, 32*(6), 406–410.

White, C. (2005, October). Contribution of distance education to the development of individual learners. *Distance Education, 26*(2), 165–181.

Zapantis, A., & Maniscalco-Feichtl, M. (2008, May 15). Teaching in a distance education program. *American Journal of Health-System Pharmacy, 65*, 912–920.

ONLINE RESOURCES

Listing of journals and magazines: http://depd.wisc.edu/html/mags3.htm
Education and technology resource listing: http://mason.gmu.edu/~montecin/disedresource.htm
Distance Education Clearinghouse: http://www.uwex.edu/disted/index_new.htm

CHAPTER 21

Social Media as a Context for Connected Learning

■ GAIL MATTHEWS-DeNATALE ■

It was only a few years ago that the now shopworn term *21st-century learning* seemed fresh and exciting. With the turn of the century, we looked forward to the dawn of a new era in education with an optimism that seems naïve in hindsight. More recently, Harvard School of Management's Clayton Christensen has described higher education as an environment in peril. He posits that bigger, better, and more sophisticated incremental improvement results in a behemoth that crumbles under its own weight, and he predicts that many colleges and universities will succumb to that fate. In contrast, institutions that embrace disruptive change and fundamentally "change their DNA" by becoming more nimble and responsive will survive and thrive (Christensen & Eyring, 2011).

While technology features prominently in Christensen and Eyring's work as an agent of disruption, it does not inevitably lead to positive change. For example, digital projection systems are no more revolutionary than the acetate overhead projectors that preceded them, and very few of us have achieved the paperless office that was forecast with the advent of personal computers. Corporations often solicit Christensen's opinion on strategic directions for development, hoping to gain cutting-edge advantage through disruption instead of incremental change. Christensen demurs, saying that he "doesn't have an opinion," but that his theory of disruptive change "has an opinion". If we understand the theory, we will be able to make prescient decisions about change within our own practice. As we incorporate the newest technologies into our teaching, how can we know if we are making a significant difference that improves learning instead of simply swapping a digital teaching tool for its analog predecessor?

Past is prologue, even in the midst of disruption. Revisiting the history of technology in higher education can provide insight into the larger patterns and motivating factors at play—the DNA that Christensen says we need to

The author wishes to thank Doug DeNatale for his review and contributions to this piece.

change. If we understand the larger narrative arc associated with history, we will be better equipped to apply the theory of disruption and to make wise decisions about what's worth disrupting in our teaching.

Educators who have used technology for more than a decade will remember the early days when e-mail and electronic mailing lists were considered cutting-edge technology. E-mail was useful for one-on-one communication, while electronic mailing lists supported one-to-many discussion. The first iterations of these tools were clunky and unforgiving; command-line interfaces made it difficult to correct even simple typos without having to start over. But over time, these technologies improved. Electronic mailing lists still serve a purpose, and e-mail is central to our daily work in higher education.

In the early 1990s, the increasing popularity of the World Wide Web gave rise to learning management systems (LMSs). Web Course in a Box, one of the first LMSs to be used widely in higher education, provided faculty and students with a suite of password-protected tools especially designed for learning contexts—syllabus builder, threaded discussions, web-based quizzes, and a class roster that could include student-written biographies with photos. The invention of the LMS was important because it signaled a shift from technology as a discrete tool (i.e., software, hardware) to technology as an online *place* where learning could happen. The LMS provided us with a virtual classroom that could accommodate many modes of learning and the development of coherent learning communities, including asynchronous and live, self-paced and group based, text based, and audio/video. The first learning management systems were inexpensive or free to use, but commercial products such as WebCT and Blackboard soon followed, along with a series of mergers and acquisitions. Today, only a few commercial LMS products dominate the field.

We have come a long way from the early days of blinking cursors, glowing iridescent green on tiny black screens, and our expectations have become increasingly sophisticated as well. Even though faculty and students assume that their institutions will provide some form of LMS for coursework, many wish that these online educational environments were more visually appealing and easier to use. In addition, LMS costs skyrocketed when a few major vendors acquired competitors and captured the market, reducing competition. Open source products such as Moodle are promising but require in-house technical expertise, and they are often not robust enough for large-scale implementation. The LMSs have gotten bigger, better, more sophisticated, and more expensive. Educational technology, LMSs in particular, has become the behemoth that Christensen's theory describes as ripe for disruption.

We find ourselves longing, simultaneously, for more *and* less—more flexibility to accommodate a wider range of learning preferences and scenarios, and less complexity to shorten the learning curve and lower barriers to entry. This is the near-recent context in which Web 2.0 arrived on the scene in 2004–2005, bringing with it an explosion of social media tools that were visually engaging, elegantly designed, and easy to use. Unlike the LMS, a cumbersome Swiss Army knife of tools, these light-weight apps could be used separately or in conjunction with one another as mashups. They exemplified the best of the Web because they were, in the words of David Weinberger, "small pieces loosely joined" (2003).

The rise of social media tools represented a radical departure because they did not try to be the best or most sophisticated. They embodied Web 2.0's read-write ethos that made Internet multimedia authoring possible for the rest of us. Web 1.0 tools helped online authors connect things (hyperlinked documents, embedded images and videos within documents). Web 2.0's social media tools helped people connect with people. These technologies felt, and continue to feel, like a breath of fresh air in the increasingly stodgy context of technology in higher education. They open up possibilities for learning that engage all types of students in active and collaborative work.

First, social media have a strong visual component, making it possible for students to represent their developing understanding through a combination of text and images (and often audio/video). They help learners make their thinking visible to their peers and teachers (Ritchhart, Church, & Morrison, 2011). These multisensory artifacts of learning can also be used to assess progress and set goals for improvement, and they can be revised to reflect the current state of understanding.

Second, these tools are designed to support networking between users, a process that can be leveraged to achieve what Randy Bass calls "social pedagogy" (Bass, 2012). Learning management systems are designed to support teacher-directed, course-centric learning. Students submit assignments and post messages, embedding their work within a course that disappears after the semester's close or graduation. Social media tools allow students to create work within personal accounts that can be networked, tagged, and commented upon, supporting a process of connected learning during which students pool originally produced media, compare differing perspectives, look for commonalities, analyze observations to discern meaning, and create an enduring record of learning. Learners both own and share their understanding.

By way of example, students enrolled in Michael Wesch's fall 2007 cultural anthropology course at Kansas State University conducted primary research, created a polished 5-minute video about their findings, and posted the video, entitled *A Vision of Students Today*, for public viewing on YouTube. This is not necessarily a novel assignment; students have been making digital stories for years (Lambert, n.d.). What is striking is that by September 2009, the video had been viewed more than 3,340,000 times, and as of March 2013 it had been viewed 4,800,245 times (Wesch, 2007). In the words of social media, the video went viral. The work of these students has extended beyond the duration of the class, beyond the KSU campus, and even after 5 years, it continues to serve as a catalyst for intellectual discussion that spans continents. As of March 2013, over 9,676 people had used YouTube's commenting tool to post their thoughts about the video in the discussion area located directly below the piece.

Imagine the sense of accomplishment that Wesch's students must feel. No LMS-based assignment could claim this level of engagement and impact on society as a whole. According to Diana Oblinger, president of Educause:

> When many of us started in this field we were excited about the possibilities of e-learning, and we still are, but e-learning may be a term and a concept that's limited by history and perception ... Initially e-learning was about the digital dissemination of information. We were in the *information* age, and e-learning allowed us to get more information faster and more conveniently. However, we've moved beyond the information age; we are in the *connected* age. Everyone and everything is connected. Anyone can participate, and it isn't just about being face-to-face *or* online, it's a continuum ... What does e-learning look like when it shifts from being about information to being about connections? The next step in next generation learning is connected learning. (Oblinger, 2013)

When used appropriately, with thoughtful guidance, social media can be a powerful conduit for helping students connect life and learning.

■ Theoretical Foundations

Given that technological options grow exponentially over time, how can educators avail themselves of emerging technologies without sacrificing precious learning time with their students? All too often, teachers who want to experiment with technology begin by selecting the tool and then determining its educational use. This strategy is both *inefficient*, because it forces educators to learn about all technologies regardless of their relevance to a particular learning scenario, and pedagogically *ineffective*, because it takes the focus off the most important drivers: learning goals, desired outcomes, and evidence of learning.

Lee Shulman, president emeritus of the Carnegie Foundation for the Advancement of Teaching, describes the following five dimensions that are central to effective teaching: vision, design, interactions, outcomes, and analysis (1998). A good course functions as a coherent whole; discrete assignments are engaging and often creative in design, yet the pieces are interconnected and create a synergistic learning experience. Likewise, good teaching is responsive to learners, differentiated to address a variety of capabilities while also tailored to meet the needs of specific populations enrolled in the course. Georgetown University's Randy Bass describes this process of learning design as identifying the problem:

> I realized I didn't know really if the better students in a course who demonstrated a real understanding of the material by the end of the semester were actually acquiring that understanding in my course, or were merely the percentage of students who entered the course with a high level of background and aptitude. Similarly, I realized I didn't really know if the students who I watched "improve" from their early work to later work were really understanding the material and the paradigm from which I was operating, or merely learning to perform their knowledge in ways that had adapted to my expectations. (Bass, 1999, para 9)

In response to these uncertainties, Bass and other proponents of the "scholarship of teaching and learning" advocate focusing on "the relationship between student prior understanding and their capacity to acquire new understanding" to investigate how students' "self-awareness of learning might help them develop a deeper understanding of certain disciplinary principles more quickly and meaningfully" (Bass, 1999, para 11). With this approach, courses and assignments are developed in response to and as an investigation of students' learning needs and developing abilities.

In the article "Disrupting Ourselves: The Problem of Learning in Higher Education," Bass describes this approach to teaching and learning as a "porous" blurring of boundaries, a process that creates "not only promising changes in learning but also disruptive moments in teaching" (2012, p. 1). He goes on to explain:

> By "disruptive moments," I'm not referring to students on Facebook in classrooms. I mean "disruption" in the way Clayton Christensen uses the term. Christensen coined the phrase *disruptive innovation* to refer to a process "by which a product or service takes root initially in simple applications at the bottom of a market and then relentlessly moves up market, eventually displacing established competitors." ... I am asserting that one key source of disruption in higher education is coming not from the outside but from our own practices, from the growing body of experiential modes of learning, moving from margin to center, and proving to be critical and powerful in the overall quality and meaning of the undergraduate experience. (Bass, 2012, p. 1)

This problem-based approach helps faculty select emerging technologies that disrupt or transcend the confines of course-based learning in a way that is both meaningful and productive, realizing the full potential that technology holds for transforming higher education. The disruptive use of emerging technology in education is grounded in a vision for learning that:

- *Is responsive* to learners' intellectual and social needs.
- *Fosters connections* between the course at hand and students' life experiences (e.g., friends, family, regional, ethnic, and cultural affinity groups).
- *Creates a bridge* between the course and students' larger learning contexts (e.g., other courses, internships, service learning, and co-ops).
- *Taps into diverse preferences and perspectives,* allowing students to play to their strengths as they grapple with course concepts.
- *Helps students achieve deeper conceptual understanding* and *develop core capabilities* in relationship to the course topic or discipline.

Expanded Approaches to Learning

Historically, higher education has best served students who learned best through reading, listening to lectures, note taking, and sequential problem solving such as mathematical calculation. In 1983, with the publication of his seminal work on multiple intelligences, Howard Gardner challenged the very notion of intelligence itself, and since then the concept of multiple intelligences has crossed over from academic educational circles into popular thought and understanding (Gardner, 1983). This new taxonomy of intelligence has far-reaching pedagogical implications. Logic dictates that if there is more than one way to be smart, there should also be more than one way to learn and be taught. In the intervening years, educational researchers have developed a host of theoretical models designed to help teachers leverage the strengths and preferences found among learners in a heterogeneous classroom (Butler, 1986; Felder & Soloman, n.d.; Kolb, 1984). The following four-part model put forth by Felder and Soloman is particularly useful in exploring the relevance of social media for higher education:

1. Reflective and active
   - Reflective involves learning by thinking.
   - Active involves learning by doing.
2. Sensing and intuitive
   - Sensing involves learning by facts and verifiable experience.
   - Intuitive involves learning through innovation and possibility thinking.
3. Verbal and visual
   - Verbal involves learning through the written and spoken word.
   - Visual involves learning through images, diagrams, and timelines.
4. Sequential and global
   - Sequential involves drawing on details and facts to construct larger understanding.
   - Global involves starting with the big picture and then analyzing the whole to understand the sum of its parts.

Note that these pairs are continuums of learning preference, not dichotomies. All learners exhibit these eight styles in greater or lesser degrees. Yet social media are particularly adept at supporting active, intuitive, visual, and global learning. **Table 21-1** maps selected social media tools to Felder and Soloman's framework of learning preferences.

Table 21-1 Learning Preferences and Emerging Technologies

Preference	Social Media Example
Active (learning by doing)	Students pool lab work or field-gathered data into a wiki, authoring a collaborative analysis of their primary data.
Intuitive (innovation and possibility thinking)	Students browse the TED Talks video site and identify thought leaders who can provide a big-picture analysis of a given topic (e.g., epidemiology students access a talk on pandemics given by Larry Brilliant).
Visual (images, diagrams, time lines)	Students identify stories of previous experiences that relate to a given topic, then create and share digital stories using VoiceThread (3- to 5-minute videos that combine images and words). Classmates use VoiceThread's annotation tool to comment on each other's stories.
Global (big-picture thinking)	Students use Gliffy to create mind maps that provide a holistic picture of a topic or concept, then use a blog or Twitter aggregator to compile an overview of all recent posts written about that topic.

▪ Using the Method

When technology developers set out to create a new product, they begin by surveying the needs of their users. The next step is to develop a spec—a specification document that describes all the things that the product will need to be able to do. In integrating emerging technologies into teaching, a similar process is useful. Begin with the questions:

1. What should my students know and understand by the end of the course (or assignment or module)?
2. Which skills or capabilities, academic or disciplinary, are essential to achieving the goals for learning?
3. What is the problem (à la Randy Bass) that I am trying to solve—which of the goals for learning have been difficult for learners to achieve when I taught this course in the past?
4. What do I want for myself and for my students? For example, you may want to obtain a clearer picture of students' thought processes, or you may want your students to connect course concepts to everyday life.
5. By the end of the learning sequence, which evidence will I and my students need to be confident that learning goals have been achieved? Along the way, which evidence would help me and my students identify trouble spots to address areas of concern and make adjustments as necessary?
6. Which modes of learning are particularly relevant to the topic or leaning goals? For example, epidemiology may lend itself to mapping, clinical decision making to visual and other data analysis, and cultural competence or medical ethics to multimedia storytelling (Matthews-DeNatale, 2008).

The answers to these question provide a spec that can be used in seeking out emerging technologies that best align with the learning scenario. This preliminary work, often called "learning design," also saves time because the faculty member needs to investigate only technologies that will meet specific criteria for learning.

In evaluating emerging technologies, faculty need not be alone. Educause, the national organization dedicated to technology in higher education, publishes a series entitled 7 *Things You Should Know About* ... (Educause Learning Initiative, n.d.). Each brief focuses on a single technology or practice, describing what it is, how it works, and why it matters to teaching and learning. As of March 2013, there were 94 briefs in the series, with approximately 12 publications added to the collection each year. The Educause Learning Initiative, in collaboration with the New Media Consortium, also produces the *Horizon Report* (New Media Consortium, n.d.), an annual digest of technologies that are likely to have a significant impact on teaching and learning in the near future, along with examples of those technologies at use in higher education. An online self-paced workshop called 23 *Things* (n.d.), developed by the Public Library of Charlotte and Mecklenberg County as part of its Learn 2.0 initiative, also provides a guided introduction to social media.

In addition, most colleges and universities have instructional designers who are current with recent developments in technology, eager to share their knowledge, and equipped to provide consultation on the use of technology for learning. These professionals are usually located within centers for teaching and learning or centers for teaching and learning with technology. Whether consulting with an instructional designer or browsing 7 *Things* briefs, the result will be more satisfactory and efficient if the faculty member first uses the method to create a spec that identifies desired learning goals, processes, and outcomes.

■ Potential Problems

Despite social networking's capacity to increase student engagement, metacognition, and connected learning, educators have also found that these tools can be confusing, somewhat intimidating, and even scary. The associated terminology can sound like something penned by Lewis Carroll—*Twas Pinterest and the slithy blogs did tweet and wiki in the wabe!*

Sometimes social media are *too* easy to use, with the consequence that embarrassing and inappropriate youthful dalliances are posted online for enduring public scrutiny. These horror stories might make some educators leery of incorporating social media into their work with students.

The accelerated pace of change is also dizzying—each week dozens of new resources arrive on the scene while others are either acquired or go out of business altogether. As soon as the public became accustomed to the term *Web* 2.0, technologists began speaking about a Web 3.0 that featured mobile technologies (e.g., GPS-enabled smartphones, tablet computers, e-readers, and Android devices) that are location aware and context tailored (e.g., tracking interests and settings to offer only pertinent resources and information). The use of version numbers (e.g., 2.0, 3.0, and beyond) quickly became as problematic as the hackneyed phrase *21st-century learning*. Instead of focusing on the generation of a given technology and its specifics, perhaps we should focus our attention on the learning theories that, Christensen believes, have an opinion about the aspects of education that need to be disrupted (Christensen & Eyring, 2011).

Emerging technologies are a grand adventure that can add a new dimension to learning, but there is a price for teaching outside the box of institution-supported learning management systems. Educational institutions are careful to make regular backups of courses in their LMSs—they cannot risk losing credit-bearing discussion posts or test results. In contrast, emerging technologies come with no guarantee of backups, security, or even ongoing existence. An assignment that previously worked well using a given technology may need to be adapted in response to new versions, acquisition by another company, or even the disappearance of a much-loved tool.

Unlike learning management systems, social media tools come unbundled, are rarely supported at the institutional level, and therefore place the onus for technical orientation and support on the teacher. Because the tools are selected à la carte, it is the educator's responsibility to weave technologies together into a coherent learning environment. Students can become frustrated when a course includes too many different technologies. When using an LMS, the student experiences it as *one* software application, even though the learning system can do many things. When using emerging technologies, students experience each one as a different tool—a different "place" to go to do coursework, a different interface to learn, a different login, and a unique application that has its own technology troubleshooting challenges. One strategy is to use the LMS as a portal or door through which students can access all other tools used in the class. This is can be accomplished by inserting links to all technologies on a course page or as needed within course modules. Another strategy is to integrate emerging technologies thoughtfully and sparingly—no more than two or three tools unless the course is about technology itself.

When taking the leap into emerging technologies, it is important to realize that this is uncharted territory. Students take their cues from their teachers, and these technologies require a pioneering spirit—so plan accordingly and encourage your students to take an adventurous approach as well.

■ Conclusion

Higher education is in a period of disruption, creating new opportunities for learning with social media that are visually rich and socially connected, and that extend formal learning beyond the confines of school into everyday life. Emerging technologies provide educators with a rich palette of opportunities for enhancing learning, but technology should not lead the decision making. Newer, unbundled technologies are intuitive, are particularly well suited to active and global learning, and accommodate diverse learning preferences and differentiated perspectives. Even though emerging technologies can breathe new life into coursework, enrich communication, increase student engagement, and promote social learning, these technologies often evolve, and therefore it is wise to have a contingency plan in place. Rather than selecting a tool and then deciding what to do with it in an assignment, those who want to incorporate emerging technologies into their teaching are cautioned to focus on pedagogy first, to identify the problem of practice or change that they wish to see in students' development, and then select tools that best meet these learning needs.

TEACHING EXAMPLE

Gail Matthews-DeNatale and Ellen Lust

In 2011, Yale University launched an initiative to offer undergraduate core courses over the summer in two formats, with face-to-face and fully online sections of the same course running in parallel. As part of this initiative, Professor Ellen Lust worked with the author to develop the following exercise for a class entitled "Introduction to Middle East Politics."

On the first day of class, prior to any instruction or review of the syllabus, both the online and face-to-face students were asked to do the following exercise.

(continued)

WHERE IS THE MIDDLE EAST?

This exercise is designed to be completed *before* you go through the syllabus, do Session One readings, and view the Session One videos—you are on your honor to not peek!

When you look at a map, the boundaries of nations and continents are clear. But regions such as the Middle East are open for interpretation. The regional boundaries that we draw can tell us a great deal about our underlying assumptions.

As we will discuss in more detail during the semester, one of the major goals of the course is to understand which factors unite the Middle East, which important distinctions exist across the region, and how these influence domestic and regional politics.

Before reading through the syllabus in detail, use Scribble Maps to draw a map of the Middle East. Session One's materials, located in the course website, include a Scribble Maps quick start guide that provides set-by-step directions for signing up for and using this online mapping tool. After you've completed your map, consider the following questions and capture your thoughts in writing.

1. Which factors tie together the countries you identified as a region?
2. What are your reasons for excluding other, neighboring countries?
3. Which important differences exist across countries that you, nevertheless, see as part of the Middle East?

When you have finished, post the link to your map and your responses online in the Session One drop box. Your responses will serve as the basis for our discussion during the first session. Please note that we will view and refer to your maps during the discussion on Thursday, so it is very important for you to post your maps before the specified deadline.

Rudimentary Scribble Map created on the first day of class.
Used with permission from Ellen Lust.

In the face-to-face section of the class, students used the computer projector to navigate to their maps, discuss their decision-making process, and compare perspectives. In the online section, Lust held a "live classroom" synchronous webinar, during which students used a similar process to share and discuss their maps.

In subsequent weeks, students granted advanced map access permission to each of their peers. This allowed them to use Scribble Maps' online commenting and tagging features to engage in dialogue within each other's maps, developing a differentiated yet shared understanding of the complexities of the region. Each person's map continued to look different from the others, but every week students did a common set of exercises to refine and annotate their maps.

Sample Scribble Map annotations that can include embedded images and links
to other websites.

For example, during one week they posted markers on their maps to record the history of colonialism and independence in the countries they considered to be part of the Middle East region. In other weeks they underwent a similar process to note the presence of Islam, fossil fuels, women's rights, and other dimensions that factor into the politics of the region.

(continued)

Sometimes students decided to change the boundaries of the Middle East in their maps in response to the rich patterns they identified during this annotation process; others kept the same construct but deepened their understanding of the decisions they had made. The map made their developing thinking visible to others and also visible to themselves.

Scribble Map that conveys refined perspective on the region.
Used by permission from Ellen Lust.

By the end of the course, each student had created an individualized, layered, and multimedia-rich map that represented his or her growth in understanding. By comparing the initial maps with those submitted for the culminating assignment, both the students and their teacher could see how far they had come.

As of this writing in 2013, Lust still uses Scribble Maps in her teaching. When asked to reflect on the assignment and its pedagogical impact, she provided the following explanation:

The exercise serves two purposes. First, it provides a great discussion tool for the initial meetings of class. It engages students directly, as each makes active decisions about which countries are and aren't included in the region and, more importantly, why that's the case. These are easily put onto the screen for class discussion, and it's really the engagement of students and a discussion about what "makes the Middle East" that I aim for at that first meeting. Second, the map becomes a resource and sort of "diary" of the learning journey the students experience in the class. The students update the maps throughout the course, adding the dates of independence, colonial experience, resource wealth (especially oil), and other features into the map. At the end, they have an easy reference for many of the basic distinguishing features of the region, and also a way to look back at all that they have learned through the course.

Much of this could be done with a physical paper map, but the exercise would be much more cumbersome. Sharing the maps for discussion would be more difficult, and near impossible for distance learning. It's also more desirable than simply having a group discussion about boundaries based on a large, classroom map (which is what I'd done previously), since this engages *all* of the students in making their own map, and not simply the more vocal students who are willing to describe boundaries. Updating the map is also technically feasible with a paper map, but often those maps get mangled over the course of a semester—a problem that doesn't exist with the electronic option.

In retrospect, Lust commented that the experience "really changed not just the course, but how I think about teaching" (personal communication).

Middle East Scribble Maps created for the class in 2011 are still functional in 2013, despite the vagaries of social media. While the Middle East mapping assignment is designed for a course in political science, it is generalizable because it illustrates social media's capacity to engage students in the development of visible knowledge that persists for the duration of a course and long after the class has been completed. For example, within the field of nursing and health sciences, this exercise could be adapted for use in a community health windshield survey assignment, an epidemiological analysis, or any other experience in which health professionals need to be aware of, and sensitive to, their surrounding context.

REFERENCES

23 Things. (n.d.). Self-paced online workshop developed by the Public Library of Charlotte and Mecklenberg County. Retrieved from http://plcmcl2-things.blogspot.com

Bass, R. (1999). The scholarship of teaching: What's the problem? *Inventio: Creative Thinking About Learning and Teaching, 1*(1), 1–10. Retrieved from http://wiki.biologyscholars.org/@api/deki/files/820/%3D11RR_Assignment_2_Readings.pdf

Bass, R. (2012). Disrupting ourselves: The problem of learning in higher education. *Educause Review Online*. Retrieved from http://www.educause.edu/ero/article/disrupting-ourselves-problem-learning-higher-education

Butler, K. (1986). *Learning and teaching style: In theory and practice*. Columbia, CT: Learners' Dimension.

Christensen, C., & Eyring, H. (2011). *The innovative university*. San Francisco, CA: Jossey-Bass.

Educause Learning Initiative. (n.d.). 7 things series. Retrieved from http://www.educause.edu/ELI/ELI Resources/7ThingsYouShouldKnowAbout/7495

Felder, R. M., & Soloman, B. A. (n.d.). Learning styles and strategies. Retrieved from http://www4.ncsu.edu/unity/lockers/users/f/felder/public/ILSdir/styles.htm

Gardner, H. (1983). *Frames of mind: the theory of multiple intelligences*. New York, NY: Basic Books.

Kolb, D. A. (1984). *Experiential learning: Experience as the source of learning and development*. Englewood Cliffs, NJ: Prentice-Hall.

Lambert, J. (n.d.). *Digital storytelling: History*. Berkeley, CA: Center for Digital Storytelling. Retrieved from http://www.storycenter.org/history

Matthews-DeNatale, G. (2008, January). *Digital story-making: Understanding the learner's perspective*. Paper presented at Educause Learning Initiative Annual Conference, San Antonio, TX. Retrieved from http://www.educause.edu/Resources/DigitalStoryMakingUnderstandin/162538

New Media Consortium. (n.d.). The Horizon Project. Retrieved from http://www.nmc.org/horizon

Oblinger, D. (2013, February). *Student success does not arrive by chance*. Opening remarks given at the Educause Learning Initiative 2013 Annual Conference, Denver, CO. Retrieved from http://www.educause.edu/eli/events/eli-annual-meeting/public-webcasts

Ritchhart, R., Church, M., & Morrison, K. (2011). *Making thinking visible: How to promote engagement, understanding, and independence for all learners.* San Francisco, CA: Jossey-Bass.

Shulman, L. (1998). Course anatomy: The dissection & analysis of knowledge through teaching. In P. Hutchings (Ed.), *The course portfolio: How faculty can improve their teaching to advance practice and improve student learning* (pp. 1–15). Washington, DC: American Association of Higher Education.

Weinberger, D. (2003). *Small pieces loosely joined.* Jackson, TN: Basic Books.

Wesch, M. (2007). A vision of students today. Retrieved from http://www.youtube.com/watch?v=dGCJ46vyR9o

CHAPTER 22

Blended Learning

■ ARLENE J. LOWENSTEIN ■

To an experienced educator who was also a digital immigrant, the first entry into online teaching was a challenge but has now become a love affair.

—*Arlene*

■ Definition and Purposes

Garrison and Vaughan (2008) define blended learning as "a coherent design approach that openly assesses and integrates the strengths of face-to-face and online learning to address worthwhile educational goals" (p. x). They note that it is a *thoughtful* fusion of classroom teaching and online learning experiences. *Thoughtful* is the key word here, because the learning opportunities and experiences are crucial, and the course needs to be specifically designed to allow students to discover and work with those opportunities. Blended learning requires a restructuring of class contact hours with the goals of engagement of the student in the learning process and extending access to learning opportunities that may be found on the Internet (Garrison & Vaughan, 2008).

Online teaching can be *synchronous*, where students will be online at the same time (e.g., chat rooms, teleconferences, and online synchronous class sessions with programs such as Adobe Connect), or *asynchronous*, where students can access the course and post responses at any time, day or night, in different time zones. Blended learning, also known as *hybrid* or *mixed mode*, is a combination of online plus face-to-face (f2f) classroom sessions. Blended learning may utilize less face-to-face class time but adds asynchronous learning time and could even include some synchronous class sessions, but that is not required. A blended course may be designed to have 50% on-site classroom and 50% online time, or 70% and 30%, or other percentages. The ratio will vary depending on the course and needed content. The method chosen and class design depends on the learning objectives and the technology available.

Understanding the Blended Course Environment

A learning management system (LMS) is used to allow students to access course information. Popular systems include Blackboard, Moodle, and Sakai, among others. Depending on the school's procedures, students can log in with the user name and password anytime, beginning a few days before the first day of class. Access to class materials after the course ends is determined by school policy. The course syllabus and other posted classroom materials, including PowerPoint or other forms of presentation tools, videos, or other lecture materials, such as podcasts/audio lectures and interactive teaching modules, allow students to review materials and refresh their memory if they so choose to do so. Announcements and communication methods, such as e-mailing the students, group discussion boards, blogs, social media, and wikis may also be available. Social media are becoming more common in use in the classroom and can be used with blended learning as appropriate (McEwan, 2012; Moran, Seaman, & Tinit-Kane, 2011; Steer, 2012).

The instructor can post materials anytime during the course, so that lecture materials may be posted before the class during which the lecture is given, to encourage preparation, or after the lecture has taken place, to allow the students to review for exams or assignments. However, a blended learning environment can enable the "flipping" of the classroom—a new term that describes having learners ingest the course materials for a lesson (readings, video lectures, podcasts) *outside* the classroom before a session (Berrett, 2012; Brunsell & Horejsi, 2011; Sams & Bergmann, 2013). That allows the valuable class time to be used for the digesting and discussion of the material, rather than listening passively to a lecture.

Discussion Posts

Discussion posts may be assigned at varying times during the blended course, or weekly, again depending on class design. Students need clear instructions as to what is expected in the posts, the length of the post for assigned discussions, and what is expected for responses to classmates. A good discussion among students develops a learning community, where students learn from each other, as well as from the instructor (and especially when students are encouraged to use the literature to develop their discussions, the instructor can also learn from the students). One example may be for the instructor to develop specific discussion questions based on course objectives, materials that have been presented online, and readings, but that ask for more evidence than was given, such as finding a new reading on the question or a broader question. This type of question can help the student develop a higher level of critical thinking (Palloff & Pratt, 2005). Along with scholarly work, students can be asked to discuss appropriate experiences they have had or know about that illustrate some of the issues within the questions. Student responses to their classmates' threaded discussion postings and faculty comments help set up the learning community dialogue to the benefit of all.

Assignments

Papers and group and individual projects can be assigned along with specific assignments, such as searching for additional resources and websites to share through the postings. Assignments may be posted and graded online or turned in on class days, depending on teacher preference. Antiplagiarism software (like TurnItIn and Safe-Assign) may be used to help cut down on cheating or plagiarism. Quizzes and exams may be given online or in class.

▪ Theoretical Foundations

In the 1990s, Badrul H. Kahn (2005) was concerned with what it takes "to provide the best and most meaningful flexible learning environments for learners worldwide." His answer to this question was developed into a framework for online learning, and this model is used internationally (Kahn, 2007). Kahn understood that e-learning did not include just teaching, but rather required a combination of factors to be effective. His framework (**Figure 22-1**) consisted of eight elements. The first is *institutional*, which discusses administrative elements and the need for administration understanding and support. *Pedagogical* refers to the learning goals and design and the need for adaptation to the expansion of opportunities available through online

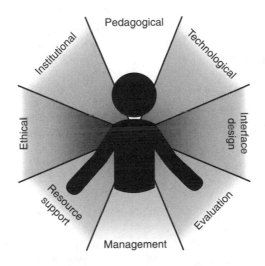

▪ **Figure 22-1**   A framework for e-learning.

Source: Badrul, H. (2009). E-learning framework. http:badrulkhan.com learning. The ***technological*** section refers to the infrastructure available to produce effective online teaching, avoiding the frustration that can occur with poor technology; this goes along with the ***interface***, which discusses how the user interfaces through the technology with those learning opportunities. ***Evaluation*** is critical for both learners and content to understand the problems and seek solutions to improve the learning. The ***management*** section is the management of the learning environment, including who is responsible and how is it done, and the ***resource support*** refers to required resources other than the nontutorial components. The ***ethical*** portion is related to diversity issues and ethical concerns in the learning.

Harvey Singh (2003) adapted Kahn's framework to blended learning programs to serve as a guide to planning, developing, delivering, managing, and evaluating blended learning programs. He noted that blended learning includes several forms of learning tools and mixes various event-based activities, including face-to-face and e-learning that can include both synchronous and asynchronous learning activities along with self-paced learning.

Singh's (2003) studies have found that blending provides various benefits over using any single learning delivery medium alone. He recognizes that learning is not a one-time event, but rather a continuous process. The concepts in the Kahn framework demonstrate the need for a broad base of support, as well as the instructional or pedagogical issues to implement and carry out blended learning offerings. Singh has looked at each piece of Kahn's framework in relation to how it can be developed to establish effective blended learning.

Ausbum (2004) explored instructional features most important to adult learners in blended classes. She found that most adults in her study valued course designs that contained options, personalization, self-direction, variety, and a learning community. They enjoyed and highly valued two-way communication with their classmates and instructor, and felt they benefited from frequent announcements and reminders from their instructors. However, she also found that in online instruction, as in more traditional environments, learners with different learning styles and characteristics do prefer and benefit from various instructional features and goals, depending on their previous experiences or learning style. Their preferences were not all the same.

Means, Toyama, Murphy, and Baki (2013) carried out a meta-analysis of 45 studies contrasting fully or partially online (blended) with fully face-to-face instructional conditions. Most courses lasted more than 1 month. Results showed that on average, students in online learning conditions performed modestly better than those receiving all face-to-face instruction, but there was a significant advantage over face-to-face instruction for students in blended learning conditions. Active and self-paced learning established in blended learning can relate effectively to different learning styles and student preferences. Studies designed with blended learning tend to involve additional learning time, instructional resources, and course elements that encourage interactions among learners (Means et al., 2013).

Faculty development is key to a successful blended program (Myers, Mixer, Wyatt, Paulus, & Lee, 2011). Faculty need to become comfortable with the technology and the transition between classroom and online. When attending a faculty development program about blended learning, faculty are required to shift their roles from teachers to students. That shift can enrich their learning about teaching (Myers et al., 2011).

▪ Types of Learners

Blended learning designs can be used for undergraduate- and graduate-level students. In today's world, technology is commonplace. Digital natives are usually younger students who grew up with and are familiar with computers and are facile in using them, but there still may be younger students who require assistance. Digital immigrants are those of us who did not grow up with computers (Prensky, 2001). Some of the student immigrants have been able to adapt well, while others take longer and may require assistance. However, there are older students who are very competent with technology, and younger students who may have difficulty with it.

It may take time for some students to understand this format and how to work with it, especially when they have not previously worked in online coursework. Some students will have had blended or fully online courses previously, but ordinarily there will be learners who will be in their first blended course. It is important for the instructor to be able to explore with students their level of comfort with this technology and to make sure that students understand how and where they can get assistance if needed. Students need access to the Web and the learning management system and must be oriented to accessing and using the online posts and materials.

A blended learning course requires students to be self-directed and take responsibility for their learning. It is active learning, and it may take time for them to learn that their behavior needs to be different from attending a totally in-class lecture course—and changing behaviors is not easy. Faculty need to assist students with learning new organizational ways to manage their course responsibilities and reduce confusion. All students need to know where to go for help with technical problems. Technical glitches cause frustration for both students and instructors.

▪ Conditions for Learning

Know Your Learners

It is important to understand who your learners are. What is the size of the class? Small classes will be treated differently from larger classes and will need to use different teaching methodologies. What background do students have prior to entering this course? Have they taken courses that provide the background material for the current course? Can you assess or can students tell you what their preferred learning style is? Today's students may be very diverse. What are the forms of diversity in the class? Do you have students who have specific learning disabilities, and how can they be supported in their learning activities? Cultural and ethnic diversities can enrich all students by fostering cultural understanding and learning, but also may need to be monitored to avoid stereotyping and negative feelings and communications. Students with English as a second language may need assistance or specific programs to assist them in writing assignments. Some of these questions can be answered in the introduction to the course, either in class with an introductory exercise or online where students introduce themselves to faculty and classmates.

Working with Technology

Faculty need to work with instructional technology to learn to work with the LMS and keep up-to-date with changing technology. It is critically important for you to have a good understanding of what the LMS offers and how to work with it prior to designing your course. It is very helpful to have a connection with the technology resources in your institution so you know who you can contact to provide support when technology glitches occur, but also to help you avoid those glitches. Success in online teaching requires close collaboration with the school's instructional technology department. Understand how to contact them, and make them your best friend if possible. It is very helpful to have a specific person to work with. Technology changes rapidly, with some older technological teaching strategies being outdated and new ones coming in. Technology personnel can help keep you up-to-date on new technological teaching strategies that have been developed and can let you know if there are financial obligations for the use of some of those technologies.

Technologies such as wikis (excellent for group projects because students can access and edit a group paper, rather than using e-mail), blogs, voiceover PowerPoint presentations, podcasts, and other technologies can be incorporated within the course, but too many different technologies can be overwhelming to students. It is critical to meet technology deadlines in preparing your classes so the course template can be set up on time.

Check whether there are faculty technology orientation programs or workshops that you can take advantage of. Encourage students to attend technology orientations and to contact the student technology support system with computer issues. Orientation to a course may include a scavenger hunt for students within the e-learning environment, which may allow students to download certain files, take practice quizzes, send an e-mail, and enter the results, information from the documents, or a special word from an e-mail message to guarantee that they can access all e-learning tools and successfully access the tools required for the course.

▪ Using the Method

Planning and Modifying

In online and blended learning courses, good planning is critical to a successful course. Planning out and posting the course prior to implementation makes teaching easier. Adjustments can be made as needed, but the course will be well organized and the instructor is freed up to focus on the discussions and other online activities, rather than taking time to prepare a weekly class. A schedule of in-class and online or out-of-class activities should be set up for each week. That allows the students to know what is required in class (readings or other assignments to bring to class) and what will be required out of class (such as discussion posts, podcasts, quizzes, or other online teaching methodologies).

Planning is also very important to develop a coherent course that stays within the expectations for a student workload that is necessary, but not excessive for the topic. It is very important that you do not overload students with work for the course and that students feel that the work is doable, which can encourage student motivation in self-directed learning (Keller, 2008). The Simmons College Academic Technology Department presented a workshop for instructors interested in establishing a blended learning course, and participants were asked specific questions to think about as they worked on their course plans (**Table 22-1**). Planning takes time and needs to be carried out well before the classes begin. The online portion must be completely developed and posted prior to the beginning of the course. Last-minute preparation that may occur with traditional classroom lectures must be avoided, although modifications, such as adding more information and resources or correcting information, can be made during the course with appropriate notification to students.

Begin planning a blended course by defining course objectives (**Table 22-2**). Meeting objectives is a prime responsibility in designing a course lesson plan. The next step is to carry out a literature review of articles and websites that will be used for course readings and can be assigned to students to supplement the textbook and used for discussion post assignments. During the course, asking students to research and post appropriate articles and websites expands their learning opportunities.

Develop a detailed lesson plan for each class, which includes each area of the f2f and online course environments, and quizzes, exams, and other learning assessment strategies as appropriate (**Box 22-1**). This is the thoughtful portion of the class, designing the course around the objectives and determining appropriate learning activities. Objectives and learning activities should be determined for each week of the course. This is also where the instructor decides the content needed for the course, how it will be presented, which technology can be used, and what students will be asked to present or develop using other methods. The purpose is to provide the best learning opportunities in the classroom and online for students to be sure the needed content can be learned. Based on the objectives, it is important to develop a grading rubric and clear expectations for discussions and other assignments (**Box 22-2**). Writing discussion questions and assignments for each week of the course comes next.

Discussion questions should relate to the weekly class objectives and the overall course objectives. Students can also be asked to research articles or other materials and present them in the discussion board for that week, so that the other students

Table 22-1   Questions to Think About for Blended Course Design

1. What do you want students to know when they have finished taking your blended course?

2. As you think about learning objectives, which would be better achieved online and which would be best achieved face to face?

3. Blended teaching is not just a matter of transferring a portion of your traditional course to the Web. Instead, it involves developing challenging and engaging online learning activities that complement your face-to-face activities. Which types of learning activities do you think you will be using for the online portion of your course?

4. Online asynchronous discussion is often an important part of blended courses. Which new learning opportunities will arise as a result of using asynchronous discussion? Which challenges do you anticipate in using online discussions? How would you address these?

5. Can synchronous online sessions be incorporated into the course? Is a synchronous program available, and what would the purpose of using it be? How much time can be allotted to those sessions? Would students have access to a synchronous online class from a technology and time perspective?

6. How will the face-to-face and time-out-of-class components be integrated into a single course? In other words, how will the work done in each component feed back into and support the other component?

7. When working online, students frequently have problems scheduling their work and managing their time, as well as understanding the implications of the blended course module as related to learning. What do you plan to do to help your students address these issues?

8. How will you divide the percentage of time between the face-to-face portion and the online portion of your course? How will you schedule the percentage of time between the face-to-face and online portions of your course (e.g., one 2-hour face-to-face session followed by one 2-hour online session each week)?

9. How will you divide the course grading scheme between face-to-face and online activities? Which means will you use to assess student work in each of these two components?

10. Students sometimes have difficulty acclimating to the course website and to other instructional technologies you may be using for face-to-face and online activities. Which specific technologies will you use for the online and face-to-face portions of your course? Which proactive steps can you take to assist students to become familiar with your course's e-learning and those instructional technologies? If students need help with technology later in the course, how will you provide support?

11. There is a tendency for faculty to require students to do more work in a blended course than they normally would complete in a purely traditional course. What are you going to do to ensure that you have not created a course and a half? How will you evaluate the student workload as compared to that of a traditional class?

Source: Blended Learning Institute, School for Health Studies. (2008). *Academic technology.* Boston, MA: Simmons College.

can see and develop a conversation about them. The next step is to prepare quizzes, exams, and guidelines for assignments. Exams may be offered in class or online. The instructional technologist should be able to help faculty with learning how to utilize and post online quizzes. Once the instructor has compiled the information and learning activities that will go into the course, it is time to prepare the course syllabus,

Table 22-2 Blended Learning Preparation

- Define course objectives.
- Carry out a literature review of articles and websites.
- Develop a detailed lesson plan for each class that includes each area of the f2f and online course environments, noting quizzes, exams, and other learning assessment strategies as appropriate.
- Write discussion questions and assignments for each week of the course.
- Prepare quizzes and exams.
- Develop a grading rubric and clear expectations for discussions and other assignments.
- Prepare the course syllabus to be posted on the Internet platform.
- Prepare a welcoming letter.
- Materials for student access should be posted prior to the first day of class, although access dates may be controlled.

which puts the lesson plan information into a document explaining what will be expected from students for the course, includes the grading rubric, and contains a schedule of the dates and times students are expected to be in class or posting on the discussion board, with deadlines for the posting process. Instructors can provide individual feedback by e-mail to students when needed instead of using the discussion board, but students need to know that, and when they should, or should not, utilize e-mail rather than the discussion board. E-mail is typically used for personal or grading issues that allow for student privacy. Materials for student access should be posted prior to the first day of class, although access dates may be controlled.

Developing the Learning Community

As part of the planning process, it is important to consider and develop a discussion learning community where students feel safe to talk to each other with little interference, except for guidance and nurturing from the instructor. Trust takes time to build, and the instructor needs to support students in this, so they do not keep quiet or hold back in the discussion because of fear of criticism. Students need to be given guidelines for discussion posts. Students need to be instructed about *netiquette*; for example, derogatory personal comments or attacks must be avoided. Instructor responses must demonstrate that mistakes are expected in a learning environment, and students do not need to be embarrassed, punished, or ashamed of those mistakes because they will learn from them. Instructors can provide constructive critiques via e-mail to ensure privacy and avoid embarrassment for individual students as needed. Discussion boards can be more informal than required papers; however, students using traditional Internet-speak may need to define those abbreviations for new computer uses, and a smiling face can be used to provide emotion :-).

Encouraging students to ask questions when unsure of the lecture or e-learning environment is valuable, and instructors should be sure students know not to hold

Box 22-1 Lesson Plan Template

Course Title: NUR 390 Theory and Research, Integration and Synthesis for Professional Nursing Practice
Course Developer: Arlene Lowenstein

Course Objectives:
Upon completion of the course the student will:

1. Address the historical influences in health care, nursing research, and in the nursing profession and their influences on the nursing profession today.
2. Explore the application of theories within the discipline of nursing and other disciplines and consider their use in practice and research.
3. Identify and explore the various research methods utilized to advance nursing science.
4. Recognize the responsibilities of the professional nurse to advance nursing through research critique and utilization.
5. Consider the role of the nurse in formulating research questions and contributing to conduct and dissemination of research findings.
6. Apply principles of evidence-based practice and research utilization as related to clinical practice issues.

Goals for Learning (what graduates will know, understand, be able to do)	As Evidenced by (products of student work that correlate with the goal)	Experiences (course experiences that will generate this evidence)	Online (experiences most suited to online)	Face-to-Face (experiences most suited to f2f)	Blend (integration/ synergy between online and f2f)
Become aware of historical influences in the areas of health care, nursing research, and the nursing profession that have influenced the current-day nursing profession.	Discussion posts relate readings that discuss historical issues to their nursing practice.	Viewing movie *Sentimental Nurses Need Not Apply* Lecture/discussion on historical issues—timeline.		Week 1: Viewing movie. Classroom lecture/ discussion.	

Explore the application of a theory from nursing and one other discipline and explain how they can be used in nursing practice and research.	Following guidance from the instructor, select one nursing theorist and one theory from another discipline and search the literature for two to three articles and an appropriate website for each theory that include use in practice and research. Post the resources to the discussion with a short explanation of key points and how they have been used.	Theory and theorist lecture will introduce them to basic areas to explore.		Part 2 of Week 1: Lecture introducing nursing theory and theories from other disciplines. Classroom discussion.	Week 2: Online assignment to find website from one nursing theorist and one additional theorist.
Understand basic elements of quantitative and qualitative research design.	Submit two 6- to 8-page papers, one critiquing a qualitative research article and one critiquing a quantitative research article. Papers will follow guidelines that include analyzing the basic elements of the research design.	Textbook readings. Research examples.	Discussion posts.	Week 3, Session 1: Quantitative research concepts. Week 3, Session 2: Qualitative research concepts. Classroom discussion.	Discussion posts.
Recognize the responsibilities of the professional nurse to advance nursing through research critique and utilization.	Critiques of quantitative and qualitative research studies. Select two articles and disseminate to the class.	Textbook readings and lecture re: critiquing.	Exploring Web and articles online.	Week 3: Concepts of critiquing. Classroom discussion.	Posting resources online. Week 4: Quantitative paper due. Week 5: Qualitative paper due.

(continued)

Box 22-1 (continued)

Goals for Learning (what graduates will know, understand, be able to do)	As Evidenced by (products of student work that correlate with the goal)	Experiences (course experiences that will generate this evidence)	Online (experiences most suited to online)	Face-to-Face (experiences most suited to f2f)	Blend (integration/ synergy between online and f2f)
Consider the role of the nurse in formulating research questions and contributing to conduct and dissemination of research findings.	Discussion posts show evidence of dissemination of research findings.	Textbook readings. Evidence-based practice examples.	Online literature search.	Weeks 4 and 5: None.	Discussion posts.
Apply principles of evidence-based practice and research utilization as related to clinical practice issues.	Presentation identifying evidence-based practice with references and recommendations for practice.	Textbook examples and literature review. Course wrap-up.	Online literature search. Develop PowerPoint presentation.	Student presentations and discussion. Course wrap-up and evaluation.	None.

Note: This 6-week course was taught in the summer for 13 undergraduate RN to BSN students. Because of the accelerated nature of the course, a discussion board was used each week.

BOX 22-2 GRADING RUBRIC FOR DISCUSSIONS

A Grade	B Grade	C Grade
Utilizes knowledge of adult learning theory in discussions and responses—meets objectives most of the time with minimal guidance and/or shows growth in learning from guidance and other student responses. Usually keeps up-to-date in responses.	Utilizes knowledge of adult learning theory in discussions and responses most of the time with consistent guidance. Responds late some of the time.	Content is usually satisfactory, but the student is late in responding much of the time.
Discussion submissions meet course objectives with minimal guidance and/or student demonstrates growth in learning from guidance and other student responses. Usually keeps up-to-date in responses.	Discussion submissions meet course objectives in discussions and responses most of the time with consistent guidance. Responds late some of the time.	Content is usually minimally satisfactory but may lack thoroughness much of the time. The student is often late in responding.

back because they may feel the question was a silly one. There are no silly questions! One student's question may also be in the mind of other students who were afraid to ask because they may feel it was dumb, or they should have known and did not want to receive criticism from the instructor and/or classmates or be embarrassed. It can be helpful to have a separate discussion board where students can ask the instructor questions, and the instructor's response is then available to all students. Depending on the technology available, it may be possible to allow a student to post a question anonymously. Students should be instructed that personal questions or comments should be handled by e-mail.

Discussions should promote evidence-based practice and encourage students to apply the research they are reading to their clinical environments. Asking students to apply the readings to case studies, to their clinical practice, and to personal experiences promotes critical thinking and spurs interest by making the material come alive and become relevant, thereby enhancing the lecture material. While classroom discussions are limited in the numbers of students who can be active, online discussions involve everyone. In large classes, small discussion groups can be established, and it can be exciting to see the different impressions and experiences that students talk about among themselves.

Instructors need to stay in the background during the discussions, allowing the students to create a dialogue among themselves—acting as the guide on the side, rather than the sage on the stage (Collison, Elbaum, Haavind, & Tinker, 2000). However, it is important that students recognize the instructor's contacts and presence in the online portion of the course. Instructors can correct or add information to the discussions when specific points need attention, but the discussion needs to be student centered. Avoid a constant student-to-instructor and back again conversation, but encourage students to discuss with each other instead. The student who provides a main post should be instructed to return to that thread and answer classmates' response posts, challenges, and questions. Students should also be instructed to avoid cheerleading—posting a one-line post that says nothing more than "that was a good post" or "great post." Students need to be told to say why it was a great post, but also to constructively challenge and ask questions, and to express their own experiences that relate to the thread under discussions and to add resources that will add to the learning for all. As you monitor the discussions, you will get to know your students well and learn from them as they learn from you.

Implementing Blended Learning

It is helpful to prepare and post a welcoming letter that clearly explains your teaching methodology, expectations for student participation, and who students should contact for technical issues and help. That welcoming post by the instructor can introduce the blended learning concept, help orient students to the syllabus, and provide a road map for students to understand what will be done in the classroom and what is expected outside of class. A discussion post can be set up and used for students to introduce themselves to their classmates and to the instructor, and it can be helpful for the students to have introductory information about the instructor(s) as well. That introductory post can ask students for their previous experience with online and blended learning.

The outline of the course and the discussion questions should have been posted on the LMS, so it is important to check that everything posted is accurate. Once the course begins, it is the responsibility of the instructor to monitor the discussions and assignments. In any course, things rarely go as planned, and corrections to the course may be carried out as needed and appropriate.

Course evaluations may be carried out in class on the last day of class or online if the last class is a scheduled online class. As with quizzes and exams, evaluations can be developed in an online format. Online capabilities also allow for keeping statistics, such as how often students access the course online, to assist in course evaluation (Ginns & Ellis, 2009). A caution to be considered is that steps need to be taken to see that course instructors do not have access to the evaluations posted online that includes identifying information from the students. Students need to be sure that their online posting is anonymous from their instructor, and this may be a technical issue to be resolved.

■ Potential Problems

Student Self-Direction

Successful students are self-disciplined in completing assignments and discussion posts on time. Patterns of late or missed discussions need to be recognized and challenged using a positive and nonpunishment-oriented approach, especially early in the course as students are getting used to the process. Avoid criticizing students on the discussion board for everyone to see, but use e-mail or conferences to discuss the problems individually with students. There will be some students who are exceptional in their postings, and others who will barely meet the minimum requirement. It is helpful to provide feedback to both types of students. It is important to remember that life can interfere with a student's ability to participate at times. Illness, family celebrations, or a death of someone close needs to be recognized and students supported as much as possible. Students need to understand that they need to notify the instructor of such occurrences as soon as possible and make arrangements for missed work if possible.

Plagiarism

Plagiarism policies need to be clearly spelled out. Many online platforms use or provide programs to examine papers for evidence of plagiarism. Instructors need to emphasize the importance of citing references.

Technology Issues

As mentioned earlier, technology problems can occur in the online portion or classroom portion. Faculty need to know who to contact and how to reach them, and it can be helpful to have a help discussion board in the class that is monitored by an instructional technologist who can respond to students' questions. Systems do slow down or go offline at times, and it is important that students have an understanding of how to work with the specific LMS in use in their facility.

▪ Conclusion

Overall, the author has found that students in online and blended courses learned better and faster and retained more information that they were able to apply, than students in f2f classes.

Comparison of Blended and f2f Courses

Blended Course Advantages

- Blended courses encourage active learning and student responsibility for their own learning. Increased student participation can increase retention of learning.
- Students learn from each other as well as the instructor, as experiences and resources are shared among them.
- Required on-site classroom time may be reduced, and students can work on their own time and be able to avoid conflicts with family and work schedules.
- The online and in-class interactions allow faculty to get to know their students well, if not better than in the straight classroom, through constant individual communications via the discussion board.

Blended Course Disadvantages

- Students require knowledge of working with computers. This can be more difficult for digital immigrants, usually older students, than for digital natives, younger students who have grown up with computers, although both groups may need strong support.
- Technical glitches can be frustrating and time consuming.
- Some students have difficulty with being self-directed and taking responsibility for their learning. This approach may be new to them if they have been used to lectures where all they had to do was sit in class. Change can be difficult. Patience, encouragement, and support may be needed until they become accustomed to the process.

The author also learned an inordinate amount of new information from those students, which is a great benefit to her, and it has added to her reference and resource lists. The author found that she was able to have students learn as much or more in a shorter period of time than the traditional 12- or 14-week semester. The teaching example following this discussion demonstrated that idea, as it discusses a summer, 6-week session while the usual fall semester was 14 weeks in length. The author found she was able to include all the information from the longer semester, and students were able to retain the material. However, adjusting to a new format definitely took some getting used to for both students and faculty. Faculty may need to experiment to see which teaching strategies work best at which time. All in all, the author has found the rewards much greater than any problems that have surfaced, and so have her students.

TEACHING EXAMPLE:

The following example is from a nursing research course the author taught for RN to BSN students. The course was held in the hospital in which the students were working. This was a summer course for 13 students, taught in a 6-week time frame, rather than the traditional 12- to 14-week format used in the fall and spring courses. The traditional format for this four-credit summer course would have had two lecture sessions each week, but that would be difficult for the students, who were all working as RNs, and for the hospital in which they were employed. Although the author had taught fully online courses prior to this course, she had no experience with a blended format, but knew about that possibility. She decided to try that for this semester. She spoke with her academic technology department for advice and was invited to a blended learning workshop for other faculty members who were interested in blended learning, and she attended and began to develop and plan the course. That workshop was extremely valuable as she looked at the differences between a strictly online course and a strictly classroom course and worked on the blended model of including both modalities. The course description and objectives were based on the traditional course description and objectives as follows.

COURSE DESCRIPTION

This upper-level course is designed to assist the senior-level student in the continued integration and application of research and theory in nursing practice. Theoretical and historical perspectives will be discussed as integrated within the research process. A spirit of inquiry will also be fostered as many clinical questions that require a nursing perspective for future study remain. Principles of nursing research, critique, and utilization in clinical practice will be highlighted, and students will be given the opportunity to develop a research-based project. Independent learning, self-direction, and understanding of group interaction in the teaching–learning process will be stressed. Intellectual integrity, creativity, and open communication will be fostered in an environment of cooperative learning.

COURSE OBJECTIVES

Upon completion of the course the student will:

1. Address the historical influences in health care, in nursing research, and in the nursing profession, along with their influences on the nursing profession today.
2. Explore the application of theories within the discipline of nursing and other disciplines and consider their use in practice and research.
3. Identify and explore the various research methods utilized to advance nursing science.
4. Recognize the responsibilities of the professional nurse to advance nursing through research critique and utilization.
5. Consider the role of the nurse in formulating research questions and contributing to conduct and dissemination of research findings.
6. Apply principles of evidence-based practice and research utilization as related to clinical practice issues.

Based on the course objectives, developing the course lesson plan (Box 22-1) was the first step, followed by the discussion board rubrics (Box 22-2). The rubrics were developed on the basis of achieving the course objectives, and each rubric dealt with one or more of those objectives. However, in some instances, the author found the rubric to be too subjective, and it may need some revision in future classes, but it serves as an example of the process. The course was implemented very successfully.

REFERENCES

Ausbum, L. J. (2004). Course design elements most valued by adult learners in blended online education environments: An American perspective. *Educational Media International*, 42(4), 327–337.

Berrett, D. (2012). How "flipping" the classroom can improve the traditional lecture. *Education Digest*, 78(1), 36–41.

Brunsell, E., & Horejsi, M. (2011). Flipping your classroom. *Science Teacher*, 78(2), 1.

Collison, G., Elbaum, B., Haavind, S., & Tinker, R. (2000). *Facilitating online learning: Effective strategies for moderators*. Madison, WI: Atwood Publishing.

Garrison, D. R., & Vaughan, N. D. (2008). *Blended learning in higher education: Framework, principles, and guidelines*. San Francisco, CA: Jossey-Bass.

Ginns, P., & Ellis, R. (2009). Evaluating the quality of e-learning at the degree level in the student experience of blended learning. *British Journal of Educational Technology, 40*(4), 652–663.

Kahn, B. H. (2005). *Managing e-learning strategies: Design, delivery, implementation and evaluation.* Hershey, PA: Information Science Publishing.

Kahn, B. H. (2007). *Flexible learning in an information society.* Englewood Cliffs, NJ: Idea Group.

Keller, J. M. (2008). First principles of motivation to learn and e3-learning. *Distance Education, 29*(2), 175–185.

McEwan, B. (2012). Managing boundaries in the Web 2.0 classroom. *New Directions for Teaching & Learning, 131,* 15–28.

Means, B., Toyama, Y., Murphy, R., & Baki, M. (2013). The effectiveness of online and blended learning: A meta-analysis of the empirical literature. *Teachers College Record, 115*(3, special section), 1–47.

Moran, M., Seaman, J., & Tinit-Kane, H. (2011). *Teaching, learning, and sharing: How today's higher education faculty use social media.* Babson Survey Research Group. Retrieved from ERIC database (ED 535130).

Myers, C. R., Mixer, S. J., Wyatt, T. H., Paulus, T. M., & Lee, D. S. (2011). Making the move to blended learning: Reflections on a faculty development program. *International Journal of Nursing Education Scholarship, 8*(1), Article 20.

Palloff, R. M., & Pratt, K. (2005). *Collaborating online: Learning together in community.* San Francisco, CA: Jossey Bass.

Prensky, M. (2001). Digital natives, digital immigrants. *On the Horizon, 9*(5), 1– 6. Retrieved from http://www.marcprensky.com/writing/prensky%20-%20digital%20natives,%20digital%20immigrants%20-%20part1.pdf

Sams, A., & Bergmann, J. (2013). Flip your students' learning. *Educational Leadership, 70*(6), 16–20.

Singh, H. (2003). Building effective blended learning programs. *Educational Technology, 43*(6), 51–54.

Steer, D. (2012). Improve formal learning with social media. *T + D, 66*(12), 31–33.

Teaching in Unstructured Settings

This section addresses teaching and learning in the most unstructured settings, such as that of the clinical care environment. Clinical teaching is one of the most significant features of a health professions education. Chapters in this section are introduced by philosophical underpinnings that should guide each instructor when planning and carrying out clinical instruction. This edition presents a how-to chapter for instructors who conduct a very structured clinical experience, such as in nursing. The clinical teaching chapters evolve from an introductory skills lab to addressing complex situations, such as student preceptor issues and service learning, including study abroad. Critical thinking and the development of higher order thinking are key components of the chapter on concept mapping. To meet the challenges of finding diverse clinical experiences, chapters on faculty practice clinics and study abroad present creative ideas for enhancing clinical learning. With these opportunities, students can achieve a higher degree of independence, self-awareness of personal strengths and weaknesses, and enhanced critical-thinking skills.

CHAPTER 23

Philosophical Approaches to Clinical Instruction

■ MARTHA J. BRADSHAW ■

The purpose of clinical instruction is to give the student opportunities to bridge didactic information with the realities of practice. Clinical learning within the realm of health professions education is best achieved when there is consistent and meaningful interaction between the students and the clinical instructor who is part of an educational institution. In guided situations, students blend theoretical knowledge with experiential learning, in order to effect a synthesis and understanding of those endeavors known collectively as *good clinical practice*. Clinical learning is directed by an educator who operationalizes his or her practical knowledge about teaching. Through use of this practical knowledge, the instructor translates the didactic content into application for use in health care. Clinical instruction in all health professions has become more challenging because of changes in the healthcare environment and the need for health professionals to fulfill increasingly diverse roles. Instructors need to examine their personal philosophy (underlying beliefs) about teaching, especially considering the changes in traditional models of clinical learning. The need for clinical judgment or clinical reasoning, especially in complex patient settings, calls for dual competence—content-specific knowledge and an ability to use the information for clinical practice and decision making. However, constant changes in the practice settings make competence elusive and demanding (Little & Miliken, 2007).

■ Role of the Clinical Instructor

The goal of the clinical learning experience is for the instructor to guide the novice in what constitutes safe practice and to develop clinical reasoning abilities. In the clinical setting, planning and selection of clinical learning activities tends to be instructor driven. Depending upon the amount of experience and sense of self-efficacy held by the instructor, the nature of clinical learning may become more student centered. In either case, the teacher guides the students in applying theory to patient care. Faculty roles in clinical instruction are as diverse and demanding as are the settings. The instructor is expected to be competent, experienced, knowledgeable, flexible, patient, and energetic. The instructor should be capable of balancing structure with sponta-neity. Clinical learning is aimed at knowledge application, skill acquisition, and pro-fessional role development. The instructor must be aware of the didactic information the students are studying in order to provide parallel opportunities for application. In nursing, students are led in practicing and improving patient care skills, and they need guidance in valuing the skills (Clark, Owen, & Tholcken, 2004). By recognizing the importance of a skill and performing it safely and efficiently, students will increase confidence in their abilities to provide direct patient care. Clinical instructors also help students understand and respect the uniqueness of each client and family in order to individualize holistic care (Northington, Wilkerson, Fisher, & Schenk, 2005). Nursing students have indicated that their most successful clinical experiences (over time, such as a semester or rotation) are ones in which the instructor uses strategies to improve self-confidence, foster responsibility, and encourage them to think criti-cally (Etheridge, 2007). In summary, the role of the clinical instructor is to direct the student to think like a physical therapist, nurse, or dentist.

Typically, the following two approaches to clinical instruction exist: technical or task focus and outcomes focus (Forbes, 2010). Task mastery instruction is based on the instructor's decisions about which behaviors and ways of thinking are important for care providers and, therefore, need to be reproduced in students. In essence, clinical instructors are gatekeepers, allowing students to enter the profession once they have demonstrated their ability. With the outcomes approach, the instructor serves as a mentor, guiding students in patient-centered decision making, actions, and evaluation that serve as the framework for comprehensive care. The technical approach may be suitable with novice students or in technical programs, but the outcomes-focused approach has a more far-reaching effect on students as they progress in their educa-tional program.

The successful student clinical experience—measured in terms of learning out-comes and an internalized sense of fulfillment—is largely influenced by the planning and selection of learning activities available to the students. Selection of activities, as well as actual teaching, is value laden and reflects the faculty member's philosophical approach to clinical learning and the role or roles the instructor chooses to fulfill. The functions in which individual instructors see themselves may include interaction with students, serving as a role model, and being an expert reference. Qualities that students see as important for clinical instructors to hold have been identified as being knowledgeable and professionally competent, being encouraging and supportive, being providers of helpful feedback, having organizational skills, and showing respect for others, especially students (Cook, 2005; Hanson & Stenvig, 2008). Once this self-image is determined, teachers consciously or subconsciously shape situations that enable them to enact their various roles. This action enhances teacher effective-ness because the instructor is most comfortable in fulfilling preselected roles.

There is some indication that background knowledge and preferences for ori-entation to practice strongly influence planning and decision making by teachers

(Yaakobi & Sharan, 1985). Therefore, an instructor with a concrete, structured practice background (such as surgical nursing) may select or plan patient assignments that are more structured than those selected by an instructor from a less structured background (such as psychiatric nursing). The potential for conflict exists between teacher and student regarding learning and practice preferences. Consequently, an effective clinical instructor is one who has the knowledge and practice experience plus understands students learning preferences and educational needs. Furthermore, new graduates report that their best learning opportunities in clinical experiences were when they had a variety of patient care experiences (Etheridge, 2007).

▪ Foundations for Selection of Clinical Activities

Another philosophical perspective that governs clinical learning is the instructor's view of the *purpose* of the clinical learning experience. The three most common purposes are for students to (1) apply theoretical concepts, (2) experience actual patient situations, and (3) see and implement professional roles. Based on the chosen perspective, the instructor selects the agency or unit and plans the type of clinical assignment that is best suited for the identified purpose. The realism of clinical activities brings added benefit to any of the three types of experiences.

The planning and supervising of clinical learning call for the instructor's own philosophical stance to be blended with the selected goal(s) of the clinical experience. Student assignments may have one of the following goals:

- Learn the **patient**: provide one-to-one total care
- Learn the **content area**: practice a variety of care activities in one setting
- Learn the **role(s)**: function as a staff or team member, practitioner, administrator, or other selected role

The instructor who selects a student focus for clinical assignments may value empowerment as part of his or her philosophical approach to teaching. The aims of this approach are the cultivation of responsibility, authority, and accountability in novice practitioners (Manthey, 1992). Selected clinical activities directed toward empowerment could include:

- *Analytic nursing*: Use of actual experiences (instructor or student based) to define and solve problems
- *Change activities*: Develop planned change and identify resources to effect this change
- *Collegiality*: Professional interactions (instructor–student, student–student, student–staff) to solve problems and promote optimal care
- *Sponsorship*: Collaboration and interaction with preceptors or administration; analysis of the bureaucratic system (Carlson-Catalano, 1992)

Within the framework of the assignment, the instructor then makes decisions about which activities will enhance learning outcomes. This process again reflects the teacher's values, beliefs about how learning should take place, and beliefs about how teacher role fulfillment should influence this learning. For example, the instructor who values participatory learning and role modeling will be actively involved in many aspects of the students' activities, and his or her presence will be felt by the students—at the bedside or interacting with staff members. Role modeling, an encouraging attitude, and serving as a resource person are attributes that decrease student anxiety about the clinical experience and strengthen the instructor–student relationship (Cook, 2005; Hanson & Stenvig, 2008). The instructor who wishes to foster independence in students may take on the role of resource person and become centrally available to students as needed. The instructor who places emphasis on organization and task accomplishment will oversee numerous student activities and facilitate completion of the assignments within a designated period. Many instructors value all of these activities as a part of student learning. Accomplishing all of these activities calls for a great deal of diversity and planning by the teacher. There are clear advantages for students who become engaged in more than one type of learning experience from one clinical day or week to the next. This broadens the possibilities for learning plus strengthens understanding of multiple roles and diversity of settings. Students who experience multiple clinical placements describe themselves as more adaptable in new environments (Adams, 2002).

Some philosophical approaches to teaching and role assumption by educators are more subtle, yet promote more complex, higher-order learning. More specifically, the teacher who values empowerment and accountability in students will take on a less directive role and assume one that is more enabling for each student. Bradbury-Jones, Sambrook, and Irvine (2007) point out that the concept of empowerment is associated with decision making, ability to express one's own needs, and negotiation. Personal empowerment is closely aligned with self-esteem, a much-needed characteristic for self-confidence. Sense of self-confidence and empowerment develop through positive experiences and reflection of self during the experience. A student who has the freedom and opportunity to advocate for the patient, volunteer a plan of care, and give an opinion about decisions of care will feel more empowered. The instructor who wishes to promote independence in students must be willing to release a certain amount of control, in order to give freedom for students to learn and grow.

Periodic, timely feedback is essential. Students can recognize strengths and areas for improvement only when they are given objective, constructive feedback. Feedback should be not only evaluative but also encouraging in order to bolster confidence and independence. Augustine (1992) investigated feedback by clinical instructors and discovered that, in addition to group feedback, such as in conferences or orientation, students felt the need for personal feedback from the instructor until they were certain what the instructor wanted from them. This need indicates not only the value of the instructor as a guide but also the emphasis students place on feedback for clinical success or failure. Furthermore, feedback is an opportunity for the student to refine his or her practices by gaining insight from an experienced clinician (the instructor). The topic of feedback and clinical evaluation is addressed in depth elsewhere in this text.

■ Clinical Activities and Clinical Reasoning

The instructor who promotes clinical reasoning in students fashions learning activities to meet this goal. Discovery learning is one way in which student autonomy, problem solving, and clinical reasoning can be enhanced. Students can have experiences where they can realize, or discover, patient responses to certain aspects of care, or how structuring an activity differently is more time saving. These discoveries boost self-esteem when students see what they have learned on their own or that they have the ability to resolve certain problematic situations. The instructor then is rewarded by seeing growth take place in the students.

According to a meta-analytic review conducted by Alfieri, Brooks, Aldrich, and Tenenbaum (2011), a discovery learning task can range from implicit pattern detection, to the elicitation of explanations and working through manuals, to conducting simulations. Discovery learning can occur whenever students are not provided with an exact answer but rather the resources to find the answer themselves. Detecting implicit patterns can occur with beginning students by having them assume an observational role. By watching the practitioner conduct routine responsibilities, learners develop an "aha!" about the role. The next step is seeking explanations for actions and a description of decision making. This especially can be accomplished in a student–preceptor relationship. These observations and thought processes can be applied in simulated, then actual, patient situations as students continue to grow in knowledge and expertise.

Another approach to promoting problem-solving abilities is placing emphasis on the clinical, or patient, problem, rather than on the clinical setting. Student assignments that take place in a familiar, repetitive setting enable students to deal with patients *in that setting*. In addition to learning how to deal with clinical problems, students in new or unexpected settings experience professional socialization through role discontinuity. In making the transition from instructor-directed, structured, familiar assignments to empowering, unstructured, undefined patient problems, students experience new ways of defining their own roles and responsibilities as practitioners. The chapter on clinical pathways describes how to structure and evaluate students in a one-time clinical setting.

■ Student-Centered Learning

The strategy of reciprocal learning not only meets clinical learning needs but also promotes collegiality. Reciprocal learning usually takes the form of peer teaching, or student-to-student instruction. This learning informally occurs within most clinical groups and can become more purposeful and goal directed through instructor planning. Through pairing of students for specific learning activities, the student learner gains information, experience, and insight in new ways. Learners receive individualized, empathetic instruction and may feel more relaxed with a peer than with a faculty teacher. The student teacher also learns about instruction, helping, and working with others. Peer support is useful for building student self-confidence, for providing a mechanism for feedback from someone other than the clinical instructor, and as a means to initiate the students into the collaborative role (Morarity, 2009).

From the viewpoint of the instructor, student-centered learning increases student accountability and independence. This is especially beneficial for students who are closer to graduation and need to break ties to the instructor. As students increase independence, the instructor can receive satisfaction from this new level of student performance. Students appreciate the trust that the instructor conveys to them. In fact, the promotion of cooperative learning, active involvement, and recognition of diverse ways of learning are attributes that students rank highly in effective teachers (Wolf, Bender, Beitz, Wieland, & Vito, 2004).

■ Faculty Development

The powerful influence of the instructor as a person should not be overlooked. Development of an effective clinical instructor and the evolution of a meaningful, positive, clinical learning experience are based on insight, planning, and implementation by the faculty member. Therefore, individual teachers need to cultivate an appropriate self-image as a teacher. In addition, the clinical instructor should indulge in periodic self-reflection, asking the following questions: Is my own clinical competence being maintained? Are my own views on the profession and the teaching–learning process congruent with student perspectives and needs? Should teaching strategies, types of assignments, or communication skills be revised? Just as encouraging self-reflection in students guides them in viewing their clinical experience as a success (Hanson & Stenvig, 2008), self-reflection by the instructor will also bring about synthesis of the experience and evaluation of successes and failures. The effective faculty member then may need to reshape his or her own teaching perspectives to better blend with those perspectives held by the clinical students.

■ Conclusion

The philosophical approach to teaching is the foundation by which the instructor operationalizes his or her own practical knowledge. The responsibilities for the instructor are great, calling for clinical expertise, role modeling, and understanding of teaching and learning principles for a variety of students, settings, and clinical experiences.

Carlson-Catalano (1992) pointed out that much of the instruction that takes place is related to how the instructor has internalized professional values and developed a self-image as a practitioner and role model. The instructor who wishes to promote empowerment in students must see himself or herself as empowered to do so. Only then can needed socialization and empowerment take place. The empowered instructor is able to visualize the potential learning opportunities in the clinical environment (Chally, 1992). The nature of clinical practice has been redefined, and so must the nature of clinical learning experiences.

Effective clinical instruction emerges from conscious efforts by the instructor. These efforts should be based on background knowledge, strongly formed values, and a well-defined self-image as a nurse teacher. Applying these personal resources enables the teacher to bring about effective clinical instruction. Formal and personal learning outcomes then are achieved.

REFERENCES

Adams, V. (2002). Consistent clinical assignment for nursing students compared to multiple placements. *Journal of Nursing Education, 41*, 80–82.

Alfieri, L., Brooks, P. J., Aldrich, N. J., & Tenenbaum, H. R. (2011). Does discovery-based instruction enhance learning? *Journal of Educational Psychology, 103*(1), 1–18. doi: 10.1037/a0021017

Augustine, C. J. (1992). *Dimensions of feedback in clinical nursing education* (Doctoral dissertation). Available from ProQuest Dissertations and Theses database (UMI No. PUZ9318414).

Bradbury-Jones, C., Sambrook S., & Irvine, F. (2007). The meaning of empowerment for nursing students: A critical incident study. *Journal of Advanced Nursing 59*(4), 342–351.

Carlson-Catalano, J. (1992). Empowering nurses for professional practice. *Nursing Outlook, 40*, 139–142.

Chally, P. S. (1992). Empowerment through teaching. *Journal of Nursing Education 31*, 117–120.

Clark, M. C., Owen, S. V., & Tholcken, M. A. (2004). Measuring student perceptions of clinical competence. *Journal of Nursing Education, 43*, 548–554.

Cook, L. J. (2005). Inviting teaching behaviors of clinical faculty and nursing students' anxiety. *Journal of Nursing Education, 44*, 156–161.

Etheridge, S. A. (2007). Learning how to think like a nurse: Stories from new nursing graduates. *Journal of Continuing Education in Nursing, 38*(1), 24–30.

Forbes, H. (2010). Clinical teachers' approaches to nursing. *Journal of Clinical Nursing, 19*, 785–793.

Hanson, K. J., & Stenvig, T. F. (2008). The good clinical nursing educator and the baccalaureate nursing clinical experience: Attributes and praxis. *Journal of Nursing Education, 47*, 38–42.

Little, M. A., & Miliken, P. J. (2007). Practicing what we preach: Balancing teaching and clinical practice competencies. *International Journal of Nursing Education Scholarship, 4*, 1–14.

Manthey, M. (1992). Empowerment for teachers and students. *Nurse Educator, 17*, 6–7.

Morarity, B. (2009). Implementation of a peer-support system in the clinical setting. *Nursing Standard, 23*(27), 35–39.

Northington, L., Wilkerson, R., Fisher, W., & Schenk, W. (2005). Enhancing nursing students' clinical experience using aesthetics. *Journal of Professional Nursing, 21*, 66–71.

Wolf, Z. R., Bender, P. J., Beitz, J. M., Wieland, D. M., & Vito, K. O. (2004). Strengths and weaknesses of faculty teaching performance reported by undergraduate and graduate nursing students: A descriptive study. *Journal of Professional Nursing, 20*, 118–128.

Yaakobi, D., & Sharan, S. (1985). Teacher beliefs and practices: The discipline carries the message. *Journal of Education for Teaching 11*, 187–199.

CHAPTER 24

Crafting the Clinical Experience: A Toolbox for Healthcare Professionals

■ STEPHANIE S. ALLEN AND LYN S. PRATER ■

Clinical teaching is where it happens, and the clinical teacher needs to be able to know what to do and make it happen. Healthcare education historically has been based upon the expert–novice or mentor–protégé model. Optimal learning outcomes are not achieved when the teacher is just an authority figure and content expert. Rather, optimal clinical learning is best achieved when the teacher is a true educator. In order for expert clinicians to become effective teachers in their professional programs, an additional knowledge base and skill set is required. The clinical experience is a time in which the student applies theory to practice. It is the role of the clinical instructor to facilitate this application and evaluate learner outcomes. Establishing and maintaining professional boundaries with students, remaining current in practice, teaching, and implementing evidence-based practice are both an art and a science. It is the purpose of this chapter to provide a framework for how to implement the use of best teaching practices in the areas of clinical teaching and evaluation.

■ Role Preparation

Role preparation for health professions faculty typically came from graduates completing educational preparation in order to practice in their chosen professions, clinical experience, and an interest in teaching. So although the educator may be an expert clinician in his or her field, as a novice educator he or she may not have the foundation necessary to be a successful clinical teacher (Bartels, 2007). It is thus incumbent upon the educational institution to provide the necessary mentoring for new faculty so that not only the scholarship of discovery can be implemented, but also the scholarship of integration, application, and teaching can be developed. These roles identified by Boyer (1990) provide a pathway for faculty to develop and flourish in the structure of higher education.

The scholarship of *discovery*, as noted by Boyer (1990), is the need for scientific inquiry into the discipline of healthcare professions, and this faculty research role is imperative in higher education. "The degree to which faculty engage in the role of scholarly discovery, as well as the approach taken to actualize the role, will depend on the rewards and structure of the academic environment" (Bartels, 2007, p. 156). The scholarship of *integration* is that part of the faculty role where meaning, perspective, making connections across disciplines, and placing the specialties in a broader context can be explored and applied. Bartels reminds us that "nursing faculty must be prepared to assume this role of interdisciplinary integration, finding ways to connect not only with evidence discovered within the profession, but also with evidence generated across professions" (p. 156). The scholarship of *teaching* is the heart of health professions education but is often not a part of the basic education for entry into practice. For example, Beitz and Wieland (2005), when analyzing teaching effectiveness of nursing faculty, determined that 70% said their educational program did not prepare them to teach clinically. This is unfortunate because formal preparation for the educator role has been best addressed in nursing and less so in other professional fields.

The scholarship of *application* is relevant in the healthcare professions because it calls for the educator to maintain competency in the clinical field. Remaining current in practice heightens the ability for the educator to blend academic and practice roles. The scholarship of application "requires that faculty come to their academic role with an advanced understanding and preparation in the profession and applies clinical experience in their area of practice expertise" (Bartels, 2007, p. 156). Teaching will likely be the primary activity of most nursing faculty, so it is imperative that this role be articulated and developed in new faculty. Clinical teaching is especially challenging, as the situation/clinical sites can vary greatly from institution to institution and faculty must help students assimilate into their role of caregiver in an increasingly acute setting. Ongoing changes in technology along with a generation of students who must learn to conform to an intense and highly standardized system for healthcare delivery make the clinical teaching event both challenging and rewarding. Clear objectives, professional boundaries, and collegial relationships with healthcare staff are all important components for clinical faculty to realize a successful clinical experience for students. This area of scholarship is especially pertinent for nursing faculty, as nursing is an applied practice. The scholarship of application is invaluable as faculty prepare and guide their students for the practice arena of the future. An ongoing process for evaluating the effectiveness of the clinical instructor is an important aspect for performance assessment and feedback for professional development. Input from a variety of evaluators, including students, agency personnel, and the academic clinical coordinator, will provide for comprehensive feedback (Buccieri, Brown, & Malta, 2011).

In addition to incorporating Boyer's model into a personal teaching style, the clinical educator must be aware of and able to implement effective clinical teaching behaviors. Kelly's (2007) case report related to physical therapy education describes five exemplary clinical instructor teaching strategies: (1) creating and maintaining an open, collegial relationship; (2) adapting the experience to the student; (3) facilitating clinical reasoning; (4) making time for the student; and (5) receiving environmental support. For instance, once the collegial relationship has been established, the ability to provide direct feedback, both positive and corrective, is achieved. The open collegial relationship is maintained by providing clear and consistent expectations. Adapting the experience to the student requires student participation in determining learning goals and needs. Kelly (2007) refers to this as "meeting them where they are" (p. 65). An important category of facilitating clinical reasoning is utilizing thinking out loud with the student. The benefit of receiving environmental support lies in feeling valued. According to Beitz and Wieland (2005), respectful and caring interpersonal relationships between the instructor and the student result in supportive and approachable communication. Also, students view faculty as positive role models if they are current in their specialty. An additional aspect of role preparation according to Wetherbee, Peatman, Kenney, Cusson, and Applebaum (2010) is for the clinical and academic stakeholders to mutually agree on standards and outcomes to work toward a common goal.

Role preparation is critical to the success of the healthcare professional as an educator. Utilizing resources available and garnering support from seasoned faculty will make the implementation of the educator role easier. Bartels (2007) reminds us that "critically important to supporting and retaining faculty in their multiple roles is the creation of an environment that allows for flexibility, encourages creativity and sustains faculty energy" (p. 157).

■ Implementing the Role

Students recognize and respond to clinical instructors who exhibit passion and enthusiasm for their work. Passion is contagious and promotes the development of a positive learning environment. According to Spurr, Bally, and Ferguson (2010), there are five dimensions of passion that can provide a framework for clinical teaching:

1. Commitment
2. Achievement
3. Trust
4. Caring
5. Collaboration

As clinical faculty define and develop their teaching approaches, these passions may be used as a framework for building their philosophy of teaching and support their values.

Clinical Orientation: How to Get off to a Good Start

It is the responsibility of the clinical instructor to complete all required agency orientation and be knowledgeable of agency policies and procedures. Good rapport will be maintained between the instructor and clinical site when students and faculty follow agency guidelines. This both shows respect for the agency and allows an opportunity for professional development in the students. Instructors cannot just drop off students on a unit or at a clinical agency and expect the staff to provide all of the teaching. Staff nurses appreciate an instructor who is present, acts as a team member, has experience, is relaxed, and is organized. According to Matsumara, Callister, Palmer, Cox, and Larson (2004), instructors who dropped their students off and expected staff to do the teaching were resented by the staff nurses, which ultimately affected the quality of the student experience. A component of orientation will be identifying for the staff what their responsibilities will be. Frequently, the clinical staff as agency employees are called upon to participate in the educational experience. Clinical staff are familiar with their role as patient care providers and in teaching patients and family members, but they may not have been provided any formal instruction on the teaching or serving as preceptor of students. Consequently, clinical instructors need to communicate clear expectations for each clinical experience. Unless the educational institution provides a structured orientation for this process, the clinical instructor will be responsible for this process as well. If this formal process does not take place, each student's clinical experience will differ due to the varying quality of instruction provided by the instructor/preceptor within each clinical setting. Establishing rapport with the clinical management and staff takes time and dedication. Refer to **Figure 24-1**, which is a typical schedule for new faculty orientation. An additional consideration for ensuring a positive experience for faculty and students related to clinical placement is to ensure the faculty members have consistent placement on clinical units from semester to semester. This provides organizational familiarity, continuity, and a positive sense of belonging for students (Newton, Cross, White, Ockerby, & Billett, 2011).

Crafting the Clinical Experience

Once faculty have oriented themselves and the students to the clinical site, it is critical to craft the clinical experience so that the assignments match the course objectives and are congruent with the theoretical concepts. For example, the instructor would assign patients who have fluid and electrolyte deficits during the time frame the students are learning about this concept in their theory course. Additional practice with calculating maintenance fluids and analyzing lab values will help the students make the connections between theory and practice. More background on the selection of clinical activities can be found elsewhere in this text.

In clinical settings in which the patient care activity is very specific, the clinical instructor might want to use an assignment sheet or form. This communication tool provides an easy reference for the unit staff to know which students will be caring for which patients. Because this assignment sheet contains sensitive information, it must be posted away from public access. Outlining clearly on the assignment sheet which student is doing what/when helps the staff know which experiences to save for a student and which ones they themselves are responsible for. At the beginning of the clinical day, the instructor will review the student's preclinical preparation and determine whether there are any gaps or inconsistencies for care. The student will receive report from the primary caregiver assigned to his or her patient and assume care within

New Faculty Orientation

Room 407

Lyn Prater, PhD, RN, Undergraduate Clinical Coordinator

1. Welcome and introductions

2. Baylor mission, philosophy, and curriculum

3. Human needs framework

4. Intranet

5. Care plans

6. Learning contract

7. Midterm evaluations

8. Final evaluations

9. Clinical evaluation tool

10. Schedule

11. Workroom, secretary, and communications

12. Clinical expectations

13. Dress code

14. Questions and answers

■ Figure 24-1 Orientation for New Clinical Faculty

the context of the agency guidelines and clinical assignment. "Oral shift reporting can stimulate learning if it includes consultation and discussion between nursing students and the nursing staff" (Skaalvik, Normann, & Henriksen, 2010, p. 2300). In order for the clinical instructor to organize a number of students within a clinical setting, he or she must negotiate and communicate the student's responsibility. As an example, even if a student has read the procedure for lab blood draws, he or she will benefit from watching it done at least once before attempting it on the patient.

It is imperative to follow agency policies regarding the procedures in which students may and may not participate. Please refer to **Figure 24-2**, which is an example of an agency schedule for student orientation. Credibility as a clinical instructor may be initially tested by staff members as well as by students. This is not unusual and should not threaten the instructor's sense of clinical competence. Once trust is established, the clinical instructor will find that this testing dissipates. Purposeful assignments should, in addition, be congruent with the evaluation tool. Keeping detailed anecdotal notes and documenting the student's progress or lack thereof in meeting the course objectives makes the final evaluation process less subjective. Providing students with specific, positive examples as well as examples of omissions or errors helps guide them in reflective practice. An important question that is worth discussing is, "What would you do differently next time?"

Guidelines and Expectations for Students: Presbyterian Hospital Dallas Nursing Clinical Experience/Rotation

Presbyterian Hospital Dallas Nursing Staff/ Support	Nursing Institution/Instructor	Students
• RNs/all patient care staff will ultimately maintain responsibility for patients. • Nursing staff will show a positive attitude and willingness to mentor students and be role models. • Nursing staff will share objective observations regarding students' clinical performance with faculty. • Provide cooperation to promote the success of the student clinical rotation. • Designate an individual on unit as a student contact. • RNs may observe students do procedures with patients *only* after instructors have checked off students. • NPD is the department responsible for coordinating all student affiliation educational rotations; *any changes* of rotation *must be approved* by NPD. • Maintain professional and courteous behavior with instructors and students. • Maintain standards of patient care. • NPD provides orientation for faculty and students to hospital and assigned units. • Nursing staff provides orientation on the assigned unit. • Recommend a maximum faculty-to-student ratio of 1:10.	• Faculty must always be on assigned units and be available for students' learning experience. • Faculty must be proficient and qualified in the area of teaching experience/clinical assignment. • Disseminate and post clinical assignments (length, dates, hours of clinical experience) and phone/pager numbers as appropriate for each service area/unit and NPD (include student/faculty names and numbers). • Arrange own conference space as needed. • Supervise students' *first* time using clinical skills with patients on units. • Notify unit personnel and NPD of student objectives for the learning experiences in writing. • Clinical assignment changes must be approved by NPD. • Seek information from RNs about student performance. • Provide NPD with proof of malpractice/liability insurance and CPR certification of both faculty and students prior to the beginning of the semester (day of orientation). • Provide NPD with Texas Nursing Registration number of each faculty member assigned to PHD. • Maintain professionalism and courtesy with both staff and students.	• Responsible for action with patients. • Responsible for reporting to the nursing staff information concerning patients. • Be prepared for clinical assignments; show initiative in learning and work as a partner with the staff nurse. • Exhibit professional and courteous behavior with patients and staff. • Notify the unit if unable to be onsite for the assigned day. • Always report/check out with the RN assigned to patients before leaving the unit either for a break or for the conclusion of the clinical day. • Complete end-of-semester PHD evaluation regarding the learning experience at PHD. • Be vaccinated for HBV; the series of injections must begin prior to the beginning of the semester and proof must be provided to NPD. • Maintain confidentiality of patient information.

■ **Figure 24-2** Agency Orientation Schedule

- NPD provides an evaluation tool for completion by students and gives results to staff.
- PHD requires faculty and nursing students to be vaccinated for HBV.

- Obtain approval from NPD for any faculty/substitute on the clinical schedule throughout the rotation.
- Conduct end-of-semester PHD evaluation with students regarding the learning experience at PHD and return to NPD.
  - Be vaccinated for HBV; the series of injections must begin prior to the beginning of the semester and proof must be provided to NPD.
  - Maintain confidentiality of patient information.

■ **Figure 24-2** *(continued)*

CPR, cardiopulmonary resuscitation; HBV, hepatitis B virus; NPD, nursing professional development; PHD, Presbyterian Hospital Dallas; RN, registered nurse.

Source: Used with permission from Texas Health Resources, Presbyterian Hospital Dallas.

Clinical Rounds

Clinical rounds provide an opportunity to observe students interacting with their patients and family members. Introductions by either the student or the instructor are important to facilitate ongoing rapport. Rounds also provide the opportunity for spontaneous learning by using the teachable moment. An astute clinical instructor will use these teachable moments as she or he encounters the student engaged in the delivery of real-time care. Guidance and/or gentle prompting regarding additional resources for the teaching/learning event can be given, and role modeling by the instructor can be provided at the bedside. According to Close and Casteldine (2005), "It is felt that the rounds are particularly useful in developing clinical practice, evidence-based care, [and] understanding [of] patients and the conditions they experience, while linking theory and practice" (p. 982).

The clinical instructor may observe students assuming responsibility in their role or having difficulty and becoming an onlooker. The onlooker may describe himself or herself as being excluded from delivering care, unable to overcome obstacles, and feeling insecure in his or her role. In this situation, the clinical instructor must recognize and intervene for the patient's safety and well-being and must provide timely feedback to promote independence and increase confidence (Hellstrom-Hyson, Martensson, & Kristofferzon, 2012). Timely feedback may prevent students from making incorrect assumptions about clinical competence and allows for the improvement in future performance (Hauer & Kogan, 2012; Nottingham & Henning, 2010). Melo, Williams, and Ross (2010) stated:

To best support students in a rigorous and demanding program of study faculty development should include strategies and tools to assist clinical tutors with assessing students for signs of psychological distress. Early intervention through psychological counseling may provide much needed support for students who are highly anxious. (p. 773)

Ongoing care and teachable moments are excellent occasions for challenging students to grow by using directed questioning. An example of this type of questioning would be when the instructor asks the student to discuss the rationale for a medication's use as a treatment modality that differs from the drug's primary action (e.g., nifedipine in the preterm labor patient). According to Hoffman (2008), clinical instructors should be utilizing higher-level questions to facilitate critical thinking skills in the clinical setting. "These questions require the student to correlate clinical findings with textbook descriptions and apply this content to the care of their patients" (p. 234). It is important to avoid spoon feeding the answers. Make the student look up policies and procedures and medical terminology. This provides an opportunity to utilize resources and to become self-directed in their pursuit of knowledge in the profession.

One of the goals of the clinical teaching experience is to provide the students with an experience that keeps them engaged and places them in the role of a total patient care provider. By eliciting feedback from both the student and the staff members, the instructor will be able to determine whether the assignment is too challenging or is not keeping the student engaged and will be able to adjust accordingly. Developing self-awareness in students is a professional priority. It is important to share observations made by the staff and instructor that promote a positive professional demeanor as well as those that detract from a student's professional demeanor. When a student is overly focused on programming an IV pump and not making eye contact with a family member who is asking a serious question, the establishment of a therapeutic relationship is affected. Actions by students such as washing hands in the patient's room and then running those hands through their hair before putting on sterile gloves for a central line dressing change may diminish trust when observed by patients and family members. At these times, the instructor must redirect the student to ensure safety using a professional approach.

Clinical Decision Making

Baxter and Boblin (2008) have provided insight into the types of clinical decisions students make depending upon the level of placement within their program. Students progress from assessment decision making to interventional decision making with the capability of appraisal with risk to themselves as well as to the patients. It is important, then, for the clinical instructor to monitor and support the student throughout the clinical day and semester by being present and providing feedback for the decisions the student makes.

In addition to clinical rounds, preclinical and postclinical conferences provide a rich opportunity for clarification and teaching. There are advantages and disadvantages to preplanned conference activities. An instructor should have a planned conference activity but should be able to be flexible and spontaneous when the need arises. Utilizing student–nurse dyads or group activities are proven strategies designed to create a supportive learning environment enabling students to meet the clinical learning objectives (MacGowan, 2010; Ruth-Sahd, 2011). Some examples of activities to use in postclinical conferences are discussed next.

Postclinical Conferences

Example One: Taking Action Based on Analysis of Patient Information

Analyzing patient information guides the students in cultivating analytical abilities and assuming accountability for action.

Step 1. Each student identifies abnormal assessment findings.

Step 2. Each student analyzes which nursing implications those abnormalities have for patient care.

Step 3. Each student shares with the group how patient care was altered and the team process for implementation.

Example 2: Applying Evidence-Based Research to Practice

Applying evidence-based research to practice prompts students to examine current evidence regarding practices in which they have participated in during the clinical day. Exercises such as this will enable the professional in practice to remain current in practice.

Examples of these activities include using current clinical situations from the day's experiences and pulling the current theory content threads out to interact with away from the bedside. This provides a nonthreatening atmosphere that is not time dependent and allows for exploration in greater detail. For example, the week that fluid and electrolyte content is covered in class, the instructor could use the following steps.

Step 1. Assign each student to look up abnormal lab values for every patient cared for.

Step 2. Print the lab data and remove all patient identifiers.

Step 3. Lay the lab data out on the table and ask each student identify which are their patient's data.

Step 4. Provide 10 minutes to research before asking the students to report back to the group the necessary implications the abnormalities have for the care they provided.

It will be instantly clear who included lab preparation within their preclinical preparation.

Example 3: Incorporating Evidence-Based Practice

Another example for postclinical conference learning and discussion would be incorporating evidence-based practice into students' care for the day.

Step 1. The students are instructed to bring an evidence-based research article that is related to some aspect of their patient's care.

Step 2. Students present the research findings along with an example of how they incorporated the findings into their patient care with the clinical group.

Example 4: Peer-to-Peer Feedback

A fourth example for postclinical conference is peer-to-peer feedback. Guiding students through the process of critiquing each other's documentation emphasizes the significance of attention to detail and provides a model for future communication with professional peers. The ability to give and receive peer-to-peer feedback as students is a rehearsal for future practice as we prepare students for entry into peer interaction within their practice.

Lundberg (2008) states:

> Relating clinical experiences to others helps students develop realistic expectations of their clinical skills and allows for immediate feedback from others, thus reinforcing their perceived abilities to function as a nurse. Shared stories are another form of peer modeling where other students can witness how their peers work through difficult situations. (p. 88)

Step 1. Have students sit next to one another in pairs.

Step 2. Provide each pair with a tool to analyze the written documentation they have completed during that clinical experience.

Step 3. The students hand over their documentation to their peer; the peer evaluates it using the standardized tool.

Step 4. Once the evaluation is complete, the peers share their findings and make suggestions for additions and corrections to the documentation.

Closure at the end of the clinical experience is an important last step for both students and clinical instructors. One last question might be, "Which lessons did you learn that you would take up in your future practice?" (McAllister, Tower, & Walker, 2007, p. 311). This question prompts the students to reflect on their experiences and charges them to take a more autonomous role in their professional practice.

FIDeLity

Constructive feedback regarding the students' performance is an important part of the clinical educator's role. Fink (2003) provides an acronym, *FIDeLity*, to guide educators in providing this much-needed feedback.

FIDeLity:

> *F*requent
> *I*mmediate
> *D*iscriminating (based on criteria and standards)
> Done *L*ovingly (or supportively) (Fink, 2003)

F—Frequent

Fink (2003) describes the widespread practice of giving feedback only in the form of a midterm and a final grade as being insufficient. No matter how often feedback is provided, the students may request more. It is worth the instructor's time to elicit whether the feedback provided is meeting the students' needs or whether they require additional information.

I—Immediate

Utilizing a broad, open-ended question upon exiting the patient's room such as "How do you think that went?" will allow the student the opportunity to reflect on his or her clinical performance. If the instructor has observed a break in sterile technique and the student did not self-correct, the instructor has to intervene at the bedside. If the student required excessive prompting during a procedure, the instructor needs to clearly articulate that the student is not performing up to speed. At this point it is the instructor's responsibility to design remediation activities away from the clinical site to provide additional opportunities for instruction and practice.

The problem with delayed feedback is that students cease to care about why their answer or activity was good or not. When the feedback comes a week or more after the learning activity, they just want to know, "Wha'd I get?" (Fink, 2003, p. 96).

D—Discriminating

Discriminating and distinguishing features of good and poor performance in ways that are clear to students are imperative. One way to accomplish this is in postclinical conference with the instructor asking the question, "What was the best part of your day and what was the worst part of your day?" This will give the students the opportunity to hear about their peers' issues and will provide a milieu for open sharing and debriefing. It is not uncommon for some experiences among students to be similar, and this provides opportunity for peer-to-peer feedback and support. This situation may result in confidence building in the growing professional. Anderson and Kiger (2008) point out about students, "their experiences of managing in different situations [serve] to enhance their belief in themselves and their abilities" (p. 445). In addition, when giving feedback regarding written assignments, the instructor must provide detail as described by Fink (2003): "Knowing that their organization was good but their use of evidence and reasoning was poor provides more discriminating and useful feedback than either 'OK' or a 'B'" (p. 96).

L—Lovingly

Feedback delivered lovingly, with empathy and personal understanding, is an essential component in providing the feedback. Providing feedback by acknowledging the students' feelings in their attempts to be successful communicates the instructors' personal empathy and understanding. There are times when the consequences of the students' unsafe actions will result in their removal from the clinical setting. This may be one of the most challenging aspects of the clinical instructor role. An example of this type of feedback provided by the instructor to the student is, "I know you are trying, but you performed three unsafe actions in 3 hours, and I am dismissing you from clinical practice for the day." As the instructor of record provides feedback to clinical students, she or he may wish to integrate the FIDeLity acronym as a communication tool.

Conducting the Clinical Day

Every instructor should develop a purposeful, organized method for conducting the clinical day. Typically, the structure is based on a plan for both instructor and students. Patient care assignments for each clinical experience must be tied to course objectives. The instructor will map his or her day by using a master sheet for jotting notes. This tool, which includes all aspects of patient care, helps the clinical instructor track and plan times for specific interventions such as medications and treatments. To ensure that interventions and medications are administered in a timely manner, restrictions will need to be placed on the number of students participating in direct patient care activities at one time. For instance, during a 12-hour shift, all eight students will have a medication administration experience; however, four students will give medications at the beginning of the shift while the remaining students will administer medications during the last 6 hours of the shift. During this process it is the responsibility of the student to keep the instructor and staff informed of the outcome(s) of the interventions implemented. Documentation is an important aspect of the learning activity and may be regulated by the clinical institution. Regardless of whether the student or the staff actually document in the medical record, it is the responsibility of the student to provide accurate and timely patient status reports. An additional responsibility of the instructor is to keep accurate anecdotal notes during the clinical day for use in formative and summative evaluations.

Anecdotal notes are an important tool for the clinical educator as they can be used to evaluate the student's progress and are a critical component in the documentation process of formative and summative evaluation. A word of caution regarding written notes was described by Indar-Maraj (2007): "Teachers must carefully examine their value systems, philosophies and beliefs and not allow these to influence their evaluation of students" (p. 8). Record keeping of clinical student behaviors over time is captured in the form of instructor-generated anecdotal notes. Instructors may wish to develop a tool to be used during each clinical experience and that is directly related to the institution's formal clinical evaluation tool. (Please refer to **Figures 24-3** and **24-4**, which are formats for anecdotal notes.)

Pediatric Clinical Anecdotal Notes Form

Absences _____   Makeup work _____   Name _____

	Family Assessment	DDST	Physiological	Psych	Social	Spiritual
WEEK 1						
WEEK 2						
WEEK 3						
WEEK 4						
WEEK 5						

■ **Figure 24-3** Anecdotal Notes Form

DDST, Denver Developmental Screening Test.

N4435 Level III Nursing Practicum

Student _____

Clinical Evaluation: Daily Data Form

Date _____ Unit _____

Assessment: Interaction(s) _____ Use of time _____ Activities _____

Use of standardized clinical tools _____ Thoroughness and depth in assessment _____

Evidence of preclinical prep _____ Level of thrp. comm. tech. _____

Adapts comm. to Pts state _____ Presentation of data at post conference _____

Meds: Name _____ Action _____ Dosage _____ S/E _____ S/E Obs _____ Nsg. Implic _____ **Lab** _____

Analysis: Level of clinical decision making _____ ID of Nsg. Dx/interventions/priorities _____

Planning: Realistic and measureable goals _____ Can formulate an in depth plan of care _____

Takes initiative in planning pt/family education based on specific needs _____

Implementation: Ability to thrp. comm. _____ Awareness of specialty standards of practice _____

Communicates accurately verbally and in writing _____ Collaborates _____

Nursing actions evident today _____

Evaluation: Evaluates care provided and client outcomes _____

Evaluates all interventions for client and family response _____

Develops alternative interventions and goals when needs not/partially met _____

Professional Behaviors: Arrived on time _____ Compliance with dress code _____ Self-initiative/self-direction _____

Shows interest in learning _____ Seeks out learning experiences _____

Asks pertinent questions _____ Supportive/respectful of peers _____

Respects client confidentiality _____ Assumes responsibility for actions _____

Comments:

■ **Figure 24-4** Anecdotal Note Format

Source: Judy Howden, RN, PhD

■ Student Issues

A hallmark of a good clinical educator is knowledge of the student's background and learning needs (Hanson & Stenvig, 2008). Emerging workforce generation characteristics were discussed elsewhere in this text. In addition, instructional strategies need to be tailored to the cognitive style of the student. This requires the educator to be flexible and adapt his or her teaching style to the needs of each student in the clinical setting (Noble, Miller, & Heckman, 2008). Cognitive styles were discussed previously in this text.

Hopkins (2008) found that early identification of at-risk nursing students is related to success and retention in their academic program. This early identification begins with the admissions process, where academic and nonacademic predictors can be utilized for student selection. Stinson (2009) recommends early intervention with students who are not doing well in clinical practice to improve their performance. It is prudent to have a clinical faculty member serve on the admissions committee, as the admission criteria can make or break the clinical experience for students. "Admission policies can either promote success or facilitate failure in a baccalaureate nursing program" (Newton, Smith, & Moore, 2007, p. 440). Once the program identifies which predictors of success are valid, the next step is to develop a model of student support. Academic institutions may have this additional support in the form of a success center or additional student services.

At times the clinical instructor may be called upon to manage a challenging student situation. The purpose of the next few pages is to address some issues that may challenge the clinical instructor. Setting and enforcing boundaries is a key element in establishing the instructor–student relationship. Although codes of ethics may be initially introduced in a theory course, it is in the clinical setting where students are bound to practice by these codes of ethics. Having students describe their ethical responsibilities during a certain clinical situation or having them discuss how they protected their patients' confidentiality are examples of integrating this concept into the clinical experience (Numminen, Leino-Kilpi, van der Arend, & Katajisto, 2010). By defining and maintaining clear boundaries, the instructor is role-modeling behavior that will be expected in future practice. Setting emotional boundaries with the student will facilitate the educator's role in managing the clinical experience. Maintaining this professional boundary prevents the clinical instructor from usurping his or her power and getting off track with the student. To maintain this balance will require focus, vigilance, and self-awareness.

Unprofessional Behavior

One challenging student situation involves unprofessional behavior on the part of the student. This may be something that the clinical instructor observes while it is occurring or it may be reported by someone else. This could range from a minor infraction such as nontherapeutic communication to a major issue such as a HIPAA violation. "Students should be engaged early-on in the significance of professional accountability for security and confidentiality related to information technology" (Day & Smith, 2007, p. 141). It is within the instructor's role to enforce compliance with professional issues such as tardiness, absence, and dress codes. Consistency among faculty related to enforcing policies such as these provides the student with a standardized approach and allows for integration of these professional behaviors over time. Infractions involving unprofessional behavior must be dealt with immediately, and the student must be confronted with the issue and given the opportunity to problem-solve future prevention strategies. This is an appropriate time to explore with the student the question, "What would you do differently next time?" Many evaluation tools include professional behavior as a grading criterion, and any infraction may cause the lowering of the final clinical grade.

Incivility

Incivility is a form of unprofessional behavior. Entry into professional practice requires individuals to conduct themselves with a professional demeanor. The instructor must role-model these professional behaviors at all times. Defining clear guidelines and setting boundaries should begin on the first day of the clinical experience as this will set the tone for the entire instructor–student interaction. Regardless of the instructor's clear expectations for professional behavior, there may be a student who is unable to conform. Uncivil acts such as challenges to faculty knowledge or credibility, general taunts or disrespect to faculty or other students, inappropriate e-mails, or telephone conversations, vulgarity, harassing comments, and threats of physical harm are issues that require addressing and reporting through appropriate institutional channels. If the clinical instructor's interventions with the student are unsatisfactory, seeking the guidance of a more seasoned faculty member is a prudent strategy. One should never feel as though one is faced with decisions in isolation. According to Clark and Springer (2007), "Evidence suggests that incivility on American college campuses, ranging from insulting remarks and verbal abuse to violence, is a serious and growing concern" (p. 7). The effect of uncivil behavior on faculty members may include lower productivity, lower self-esteem, loss of confidence in their teaching abilities, and overall job dissatisfaction that may result in the instructor leaving the teaching profession (Luparell, 2007a). Uncivil encounters disrupt the teaching–learning environment; therefore it is incumbent upon clinical faculty members to help students learn to cope with conflict in healthy and constructive ways. Additionally, Clark (2010) points out that incivility can be inflicted upon a student by his or her instructor, which may result in long-term consequences such as fractured self-esteem. In her paper "Why Civility Matters," Clark (2010) states:

> Civility is an authentic respect for others that requires time, presence, willingness to engage in genuine discourse and intention to seek common ground. Civility matters

because treating one another with respect is requisite to communicating effectively, building community and creating high-functioning teams. (para 1)

Academic Dishonesty and Unethical Behavior (Honor Code)

Most institutions have an honor code. It is the responsibility of the clinical instructor to be familiar with and comply with the policy as well as to report violations in a timely manner. Baxter and Boblin (2007) found in their study that students may view unethical clinical behaviors differently from unethical classroom behaviors. Altering charts or failing to report a mistake may result in patients experiencing negative outcomes. At times these aberrant behaviors may be a symptom of a more serious problem such as chemical dependence, which may contribute to unsafe patient care. Reporting guidelines and testing of students for chemical usage may be covered by both agency and educational institution policies. For healthcare professionals, it is crucial that this moral development be examined for entry-level practice. "As nurse educators, we have the responsibility to ensure that we are preparing competent, autonomous, ethical practitioners who can provide quality nursing care" (Baxter & Boblin, 2007, p. 26).

Safety

Safety in the clinical setting is imperative and is receiving unprecedented attention on several fronts. Due to the ethical imperative of "first, do no harm," the integration of quality and safety content into the clinical curriculum is paramount. Safety issues related to patient care center on near misses and adverse events and require healthcare professionals to comply with a code of ethics. Reporting, investigating causal systems failures, and revealing the primary error to the physician and possibly the patient is a primary role of the healthcare professional (Lachman, 2007). It is the instructor's responsibility to assess each student's preparation for delivering safe patient care prior to the beginning of the clinical experience. If the instructor determines that the student is inadequately prepared, he or she may choose to dismiss the student from the clinical setting in order to prevent a breach in patient safety. A breach in patient safety is commonly a critical point for failure in the clinical course. An example of this breach of safety is a student coming inadequately prepared for medication administration. As Harding and Petrick (2008) remind us, "The practice of purposefully incorporating medication safety knowledge throughout connected theory and practice courses" is beneficial to student learning (p. 47). Medication administration is an opportunity for the student to incorporate theory into practice. It is incumbent upon the clinical instructor to document and provide feedback to the student who has had a breach of patient safety. The clinical instructor must also follow agency guidelines for reporting such incidents. "Educators should monitor student errors and incidents over time (i.e., quality assurance determinants) to identify how education structures and processes are contributing to potential and actual student error" (Gregory, Guse, Davidson, & Russell, 2007, p. 81).

■ Evaluation of Clinical Learning

The purpose of evaluation is to help the student grow in his or her profession. Traditionally, evaluation has been looked upon as a negative or punitive act and can be viewed as adversarial between the student and faculty member. This, however, is not the case because evaluation is an opportunity for growth. The evaluation of clinical performance should not be subjective, because it is based on a standardized evaluation tool, and the instructor must collect data sufficient to weigh the evaluation against the behavioral outcomes over time.

Even though the instructor should have given oral and written feedback during the clinical day, a formal midterm and final evaluation of the student's performance is necessary to provide formative feedback and as a mechanism for grade assignment. The purpose of formative evaluation is to provide specific and detailed feedback to the student and observe his or her ability or inability to integrate this feedback into his or her clinical practice. One of the goals of this formative evaluation is to allow the students the opportunity to internalize the processes of self-reflection and self-discovery in their personal practice. It is the hope that this ongoing communication between the students and instructor will promote insight into the strengths and weaknesses of the students' professional practice. Susan Luparell (2007a) makes a good point when she encourages clinical instructors to "Say what you mean and mean what you say" (p. 105).

Luparell states:

> I have come to realize that, although there is some good to be found in the sandwich approach to providing feedback, this may contribute to the meat of the message being lost. When the student does not hear the true message, he or she cannot make the necessary adjustments for success. It is not caring to inhibit student progression toward the goals. I now realize that sugar coating the message is not equivalent to caring for my students. Rather, caring is demonstrated when a respectful tone within the context of trust is used to deliver a sometimes tough message. (p. 105)

Sample formats for midterm evaluations, as shown in **Figures 24-5** and **24-6**, can be utilized as a means to provide specific formative feedback on clinical performance. Figure 24-5 is a narrative response tool where the instructor provides areas of strengths and weaknesses to this point in the clinical experience. Figure 24-6 is an example of a tool that describes specific behavioral outcomes that the student must display in order to be a safe and effective care provider. Often, once they see a letter grade, students ask, "What can I do to improve my grade?" By receiving a list of outcome behaviors, the student has the opportunity to incorporate them into his or her practice. "Be specific" was a common phrase used by a colleague during midterm evaluations. She often wrote "increase specificity" on assignments, and the students would question what that meant. By providing specific examples the instructor helped students understand what to do differently before repeating the assignment.

Anecdotal notes are an important means by which the clinical instructor can provide specific details regarding the student's performance that will require remediation as well as documenting areas of superior performance. Hall, Daly, and Madigan (2010) reported that the majority of clinical nursing faculty use anecdotal notes on a weekly basis as a means for collecting data for summative evaluation. Cooke, Mitchell, Moyle, Henderson, and Murfield (2010) suggest the use of a clinical progression portfolio format to capture students' progress in clinical practice.

BAYLOR UNIVERSITY, LOUISE HERRINGTON SCHOOL OF NURSING

Nursing 3425 Level II Clinical

Faculty:

Student Midterm Progress Report

Student: [Student Name]

Preparation for clinical experiences:

Assessment skills

Analysis *(application of physiologic and pathophysiologic concepts to clinical practice)*

Planning for care

Implementation of nursing interventions

Medications/IVs knowledge and administration

Patient/family education

Communication skills

Evaluation of care

Professionalism

Student signature: **Date:**

■ **Figure 24-5**   Student Midterm Progress Report

Expected Clinical Performance Behaviors

The following behaviors are examples of the expectations of students in Practicum III, are based on the Baylor University Louise Herrington School of Nursing (BULHSON) Clinical Performance Evaluation tool.

Assessment

1. **Collects data through appropriate physical assessment techniques**
   a. Assessment data is collected independently by student and reflects consistent application of principles taught in NUR 3314.
   b. Techniques and equipment are used correctly throughout collection of assessment data.
   c. Student demonstrates awareness of any deficiencies he or she may have in physical assessment skills and seeks opportunities/assistance to remedy these deficiencies.
   d. Physical assessment skills reflect an in-depth knowledge of anatomy and physiology.
   e. Physical assessment data collections are adapted correctly/appropriately for the client in the pediatric and psych settings.

2. **Collects data (subjective and objective) from available resources**
   a. All references/resources utilized for practicum experiences/written work are from appropriate, practice-specific professional nursing texts, journal articles, or resources recommended by faculty. References are recent (within past 5 years) and reflect current research.
   b. All references/resources used for practicum experiences/written work are specific to needs of assigned clients/families.
   c. Student uses agency policies and procedures as guidelines for data collection.
   d. Advanced interviewing skills are used to collect in-depth data from the client/family.
   e. Before utilizing data of staff, student will validate those findings in assessment of the client/family.
   f. Data collection from the chart reflects in-depth understanding of information recorded.
   g. All pertinent diagnostic/lab/screening values are noted and analyzed. Results not on chart are obtained from computer or lab via phone.
   h. The student is aware of all current medical and nursing orders for the patient.
   i. The student continuously assesses the patient/family environment.
   j. The student demonstrates an awareness of the nursing unit environment in terms of where supplies, equipment, and resources are located.

3. **Documents assessment data in a clear and organized manner**
   a. All documentation of data is obtained from student's own assessment.
   b. Documentation of assessment data is thorough and is entered in the chart in a timely/correct manner using charting standards for agency.
   c. The student takes the initiative to chart data on all unit-specific and client-specific flow sheets.

4. **Shows evidence of pre-clinical preparation**
   a. Student consistently has required data base/worksheet completed prior to the beginning of each clinical day.
   b. Student can verbalize to instructor an appropriate plan of nursing care specific to the patient/family at the beginning of the clinical day.
   c. Student demonstrates in-depth knowledge of physiologic and pathophysiologic concepts applicable to assigned client.
   d. Student demonstrates knowledge of all medications (routine, one time, as needed) ordered for the client or that the client has recently received at the beginning of the

■ **Figure 24-6** Expected Clinical Performance Behaviors

clinical day. Student only has to look up newly ordered medications during the practicum day.
   e. Student demonstrates preparedness for nursing procedures that he/she may perform for the patient.
   f. Student has reviewed appropriate resources; that is, information from Baylor School of Nursing skills lab (NUR 3414), Medical City procedure manuals, skills discussed in required or reserved materials specific to this course, or other resources as designated by the instructor.
   g. Student takes the initiative to obtain information from staff nurse (during report) needed to care for client/family.
   h. Student comes prepared for clinical day with needed equipment.

Analysis

1. **Clinical decision making reflects an understanding of the relationships of assessment data to the client's problem/diagnosis**
   a. Student can verbalize or describe in written work an in-depth understanding of client/family condition/status based on accurate synthesis of data collected in relation to nursing theory base.
   b. Student takes initiative during the clinical day to discuss with instructor the meaning of assessment findings and implications for clinical decisions. Student can analyze situation with minimal cues from instructor.

2. **Identifies priorities requiring nursing actions based on assessment and determines reassessment is indicated**
   a. Student consistently verbalizes in clinical setting or documents in written work the most important client/family needs that require nursing action. This is based on sound nursing theory, nursing assessment/reassessment data, and incorporates collaboration with client/family.

3. **Formulates nursing diagnosis based on assessment data**
   a. All nursing diagnoses are based on active client/family problems that are pertinent while student is present in the clinical setting.
   b. Student utilizes appropriate format for writing nursing diagnoses as taught in NUR 3310.
   c. Etiology portion of the nursing diagnoses are always based on problems that can be alleviated with nursing interventions.
   d. Student's written work or verbalization demonstrates accurate assessment data to support the diagnoses.
   e. Student comes prepared for the clinical day with appropriate nursing diagnoses as required.

Planning

1. **Formulates appropriate and measurable goals for self and client**
   a. Student verbalizes at the beginning or during of the clinical day (or includes in written work) measurable client/family goals based on data analysis. As data analysis fluctuates or changes, student can revise patient/family goals. Goals formulated by the student are realistic and achievable during the time period the student cares for the family.

▪ **Figure 24-6** (*continued*)

   b. Student can consistently verbalize or document in written work personal goals that will enhance nursing care and contribute to own professional growth. Student takes initiative to actively achieve these goals.

2. **Plans care in a systematic, logical, organized manner**

   a. The student is able to articulate an in-depth plan of holistic nursing care to the instructor at any time during the clinical day. This is also consistently reflected in written work.

   b. The plan of care is flexible enough to meet patient/family needs in a timely manner and coincides with plans/activities of other healthcare personnel.

   c. The student is able to consistently verbalize rationale for each nursing activity within the plan of care.

   d. All plans of care are consistent with procedural guidelines for specific nursing units at the agency.

3. **Plans health teaching based on identified learning needs and readiness of client**

   a. The student can independently interview client/family to determine/assess actual learning needs and plan to meet those needs.

   b. Patients/families under the student's care are consistently evaluated for readiness and understanding before nursing care activities are performed.

   c. The student demonstrates the ability to develop in-depth teaching plans for specific client/family learning needs based on concepts taught in NUR 3222.

   d. Patient/family health teaching is an ongoing process during the care provided by the student.

   e. The student demonstrates preparation for anticipated client/family learning needs.

   f. All health teaching is based on current nursing theory and is planned at an appropriate developmental stage/knowledge base of the client/family.

   g. The student keeps the instructor informed of planned or incidental health teaching the instructor can observe.

   h. Student uses agency resources (computer programs, videotapes, teaching manuals) with clients and families.

4. **Communicates clearly regarding nursing care plan (NCP) with all appropriate individuals**

   a. The family is informed by the student of his/her plan of care at the beginning of the shift and on an ongoing basis. The client and/or family is informed of the student's scope of responsibility.

   b. The student informs the staff nurse of all assessment and care he/she will provide at the beginning of and throughout the clinical day.

   c. The student takes initiative on the unit to enhance learning experiences without compromising assigned patient care.

   d. The student consistently takes initiative to keep the staff and instructor informed of the plan of nursing care and changes in that plan.

Implementation

1. **Utilizes effective and appropriate verbal/nonverbal communication skills**

   a. Student communication with clients/families is consistently goal-oriented.

   b. Student demonstrates advanced skill in establishing rapport and effective communication with client/families who have complex/complicated interactive behaviors.

■ **Figure 24-6** *(continued)*

    c. Student is aware of and able to modify personal barriers/behaviors that can interfere with therapeutic communication.

    d. Student is able to maintain a level of objectivity while establishing rapport and trust with client/family.

    e. Student demonstrates behavior that promotes confidence of the patient/family in the student's skills.

    f. Student is able to continue therapeutic communication as appropriate with client/family in the presence of nurse, instructor, physician, or other health team members.

2. **Provides direct patient care in a safe, accurate, organized manner**

    a. Student's care consistently provides for client safety. The student demonstrates anticipation of patient behaviors that could compromise health/safety and plans care accordingly.

    b. All care provided reflects the nursing diagnosis and patient/family needs and is based on appropriate nursing theory.

    c. The student demonstrates an ability to anticipate supplies/equipment, etc., needed for care and has items needed readily available.

    d. The student demonstrates critical thinking skills in carrying out nursing care in a logical, patient-centered manner.

    e. The student consistently calculates medication and intravenous (IV) fluid dosages correctly without assistance and in a timely manner. The student can determine safe dosage ranges without assistance.

    f. The student notifies the instructor of all procedures for which the instructor needs to be present.

    g. The student assumes responsibility for keeping the patient's environment orderly, safe, equipped with needed supplies, and esthetically appropriate.

3. **Administers medications safely according to established procedure**

    a. Student consistently observes "5 rights" in administering all medications, IV solutions, etc.

    b. Student notifies instructor of all medications to be administered.

    c. Student verbalizes to instructor, without prompting, the following information regarding medications the patient has recently received, medications the student is administering, or those the patient has ordered:

        i. Classification of drug

        ii. Purpose of medication for patient

        iii. Safe and correct dose

        iv. How drug acts/pharmacology of drug

        v. Potential drug interactions

        vi. Pertinent side effects the patient may experience and how the student will manage potential side effects

        vii. How the drug will be administered; that is, drip rate, type of syringe to be used, how client currently takes medication, etc.

        viii. Client/family teaching that will be needed regarding medication

        ix. Nursing implications for administration of drug

        x. Student's plan for monitoring drug effectiveness and side effects

        xi. Developmental considerations of medication

    d. Student demonstrates proficiency in all aspects of medication administration and documentation.

■ **Figure 24-6** (*continued*)

4. **Communicates accurately verbally and in writing (charting and reporting)**
   a. Student's charting provides thorough documentation of nursing care provided. The charting consistently reflects action taken when assessment is abnormal.
   b. All health teaching is consistently documented on appropriate forms.
   c. All charting reflects appropriate medical/nursing abbreviations, correct grammar and spelling.
   d. Student consistently takes initiative to keep staff nurse informed of nursing interventions, patient/family status, etc. Student reviews his/her charting with staff nurse when reporting off.
   e. Student consistently reports off to appropriate staff nurse without being reminded.
   f. Student immediately reports to new nurse if there is a change in the patient's primary nurse assignment during the clinical day.
   g. The student's documentation follows agencies charting procedures.

5. **Collaborates with client/family/health team and other appropriate individuals**
   a. Student consistently informs nurse and instructor at outset and throughout shift of his/her plan for care, medication administration, charting, and referral needs.
   b. The student takes the initiative to discuss clarification of medical orders with the appropriate nurse and physician.
   c. The student takes the initiative as appropriate to consult with other health team members (e.g., physician, social worker, child life specialist, dietitian, etc.) to validate his/her plan of care.
   d. The student provides nursing care in which the client and family are active participants.
   e. Care provided by the student consistently reflects an integration of individual family member needs to promote family growth.

Evaluation

1. **Uses evaluation appropriately in the nursing process (utilizes data to validate if identified goals are met)**
   a. Student consistently evaluates the results of the care provided in relation to the outcome criteria established for the patient/family goals. Student documents all data regarding outcomes.
   b. Student demonstrates objectivity in evaluation process.

2. **Evaluates effectiveness of specific interventions**
   a. Student consistently observes for side effects and patient response of all medications and therapies the patient is receiving.
   b. Individual nursing actions are evaluated and documented on a consistent basis.
   c. Client/family response to care provided is observed and documented.
   d. Evaluation and documentation of client/family education is in measurable terms.

3. **Develops alternate interventions and goals when appropriate**
   a. The student demonstrates awareness of and planning for differing outcomes. The student can verbalize in advance alternate nursing interventions for these outcomes.
   b. Student demonstrates the proper course of action that should be taken if the client experiences ineffective response or adverse reaction to (1) specific therapies (e.g., medications, IV therapy, blood products, etc.); or (2) normal process of adaptation.
   c. The student can implement alternate interventions while demonstrating flexibility, objectivity, timely organization, and professionalism.

■ **Figure 24-6** *(continued)*

Professional Behaviors

1. The student demonstrates promptness in attendance at all clinical experiences, post-conferences, and seminars.
2. The student consistently demonstrates honesty and integrity in the provision of care and his/her clinical performance.
3. The student will adhere to professional behaviors as listed in the NUR 4435 syllabus.
4. The student's behavior in the clinical setting consistently reflects maturity; responsibility for own actions; and respect for patients, staff, instructors, and peers.
5. The student assumes responsibility for adherence to verbal and written guidelines set forth by individual faculty members in the pediatric, psych, and community settings.
6. The student consistently demonstrates professional behavior and a pleasant demeanor despite personal problems/concerns/issues.

■ **Figure 24-6** (*continued*)

The final clinical evaluation allows the instructor to analyze and deliver to students the progress of their clinical performance over time. This summative event prepares students to move forward in their program with guided input regarding their current state of practice. Assigning a grade plays an important role in determining whether competencies have been met during directly supervised clinical experiences (Amicucci, 2012). Although the tools are standardized, it is important for the clinical instructor to individualize his or her evaluation comments.

Edgecombe and Bowden (2009) remind us that "Learning outcomes [are] expressed as both intrinsic and extrinsic" (p. 97). The summative evaluation will examine the students' ability to meet the course objectives that were imposed by the program curriculum. The intrinsic objectives of each student's personal need to learn upon exposure to nursing practice in the clinical environment should also be documented and discussed. To prepare for final clinical evaluations, an appointment time should be scheduled, which is agreed upon with both the faculty member and each student. The meeting place should provide privacy because the evaluation content and conversation should remain confidential. When a student arrives for the evaluation, a copy of the completed tool is provided for the student to read and sign, following any discussion of reflective practice, clarification of evaluative comments, and an opportunity for self-appraisal on the part of the student. When meeting with students to give midterm and final evaluations, it is a good practice to have two clinically based faculty members present. This could be two faculty members who have simultaneously taught the student during the evaluation period or two faculty members from the same content domain. This practice validates for the student the significance of the evaluation comments and provides for physical and emotional safety of the primary instructor in situations in which the evaluation becomes emotionally charged. Learning contracts or clinical practice warning forms are documents used by clinical instructors to delineate unsafe clinical practice or a breach in professional practice. These contracts become a part of the evaluation process and typically include a remediation plan. The purpose of these learning contracts is to provide additional structure and clear communication as to what the student must do to be successful in the clinical course. Orientation for clinical faculty assists in their providing effective clinical instruction.

> For example, use of a clinical warning form to document inadequate, unsafe student performance may help with optimal formative and summative evaluation of a struggling student in that it creates a paper trail for legal purposes and an educational wake-up call for the student. (Beitz & Wieland, 2005, p. 44)

As Barrington and Street (2009) found in their research regarding learner contracts, these tools improved learner–faculty communication and reflection on learning. For a sample document regarding safety in the clinical setting, refer to **Figure 24-7**. For an example of how to record a breach in professional behavior, refer to **Figure 24-8**. Writing and delivering the learning contract to the student who is not performing at an acceptable level should not be a contentious process, but it should be presented in a clear and compassionate manner. The clinical instructor cannot ensure success solely through the use of the contract but is responsible for designing the plan for success. The learning contract outlines the roles both instructor and student play in any additional remediation sessions that may take place outside the clinical setting. Part of the process for implementing the learning contract is to provide the student with feedback during each clinical experience. This may be referred to as meeting or not meeting the terms of the contract. If safety issues are not remediated, the student may not be allowed to continue in the clinical setting, which may result in a course failure.

> Nurse educators need to be fully present with students who are at risk of failing clinical courses in ways that foster personal and professional growth, rather than distance themselves. This is not easy work. As educators we are inclined to disconnect from students to protect our own vulnerability, particularly when performance issues arise. (McGregor, 2007, p. 509)

Ultimately the student must display the outcome behaviors necessary for success in the course, which are directly related to the standardized final clinical evaluation tool. The learning contract is signed by both clinical instructor and student and a copy is placed in the student's academic file.

Clinical Practice Failure

Clinical practice failure is the lack of clinical competence and the inability of the student to meet the course objectives. Issues such as unsafe clinical practice, unprofessional behaviors, attendance, inability to implement appropriate interventions, falsification of patient records, omissions in documentation, nontherapeutic

BAYLOR UNIVERSITY LOUISE HERRINGTON SCHOOL OF NURSING STANDARDS OF SAFE CLINICAL PRACTICE

In all clinical situations students are expected to demonstrate responsibility and accountability as professional nurses with the ultimate goal being safe patient care. The Baylor University Louise Herrington School of Nursing (LHSON) believes that this goal will be attained if each student's daily clinical practice is guided by the Standards of Safe Clinical Practice that always includes, but is not limited to, the following behaviors.

The student will:
1. Know and conform to the Texas Nursing Practice Act and Texas Board of Nursing rules and regulations as well as all federal, state, or local laws, rules, or regulations.
2. Adhere to the American Nurses Association (ANA) Code of Ethics.
3. Adhere to Health Information Portability and Accountability Act (HIPAA) and institutional privacy practices.
4. Prepare for clinical learning assignments according to course requirements and as determined for the specific clinical setting.
5. Practice within the boundaries of the nursing student role as established by the LHSON and the assigned agencies.
6. Provide nursing care required to promote health and prevent illness or further complications.
7. Demonstrate the application of previously learned skills and principles in a safe manner while providing nursing care.
8. Administer medications and/or treatments in a safe manner according to guidelines provided by LHSON and the assigned clinical agency.
9. Promptly report significant client information in a clear, accurate, and complete oral or written manner to the appropriate person(s).
10. Comply with institutional policies and procedures when implementing nursing care.
11. Meet the clinical expectations as outlined in the course syllabus and the LHSON Clinical Performance Evaluation Tool.

I have read the Baylor University Louise Herrington School of Nursing Standards of Safe Clinical Practice, Texas Nursing Practice Act Rules 217.11 and 217.12, ANA Code of Ethics, HIPAA, and clinical course syllabus. I understand that these standards are expectations that guide my clinical practice and will be incorporated into the evaluation of my clinical performance in all clinical courses. Failure to meet these standards may result in my removal from the clinical area, which may result in clinical and course failure.

Student signature and date: _____

Student printed name: _____

■ **Figure 24-7** Clinical Safety Contract

communication, and errors in medication administration are all examples of critical elements of practice that may result in clinical practice failure. "Not all nursing students can be successful, yet when failure is the outcome, students' dignity, self-worth and future possibilities must be preserved" (McGregor, 2007, p. 504). Some clinical practice failures indicate that the student needs more exposure or time in the clinical setting to be successful.

Baylor University Louise Herrington School of Nursing Professional Behaviors Student Counseling Record

Student: **Instructor:**
Date: **Course:**

Data Record and Statement of the Problem
Noncompliance with course expectations and performance standards for NXXXX, level XX related to professional behaviors

   Date and time of occurrence: [Faculty comments added here.]

   Description of occurrence: [Faculty comments added here.]

Course Expectations and Performance Standards
As professionals, students are expected to demonstrate professional behaviors as listed in the course syllabus.

* Project a positive image through the use of language, accountability, behavior, and appearance.
* Demonstrate professional behaviors at all times during the clinical experience (arrives on time, respects client confidentiality, assumes responsibility for own actions, is in appropriate uniform with pertinent equipment, etc.).
* Demonstrate an active role in own learning process (shows interest in learning experience, seeks out learning opportunities, and asks pertinent questions).

Student Goals
The student will adhere to professional behaviors. [Faculty comments added here.]

Student Responsibilities
1. The student will review professional behaviors in the NUR XXXX syllabus, Level XXX Clinical Evaluation Tool, LHSON Student Information Guide, and Baylor University Student Policies and Procedures found at http://www.baylor.edu/student_policies.
2. The student will implement chain of command as necessary.

Faculty/Instructor Responsibilities
The instructor will continue to be available during clinical and business hours to answer any questions concerning the clinical experience which includes, but is not limited to, professional behaviors.

Evaluation
Failure to demonstrate any of the clinical professional behaviors outlined in the NUR XXXX syllabus, Level XXX Clinical Performance Evaluation Tool, LHSON Student Information Guide, Baylor University Student Policies and Procedures, and/or this Student Counseling Record may result in the lowering of the numerical grade and/or a failure of the course.

Instructor Comments

Student Signature: _____ Date: _____
Instructor Signature: _____ Date: _____

THE ORIGINAL COPY OF THIS FORM MUST BE GIVEN TO THE UNDERGRADUATE PROGRAM DIRECTOR WITHIN 24 HOURS OF COMPLETION.

▪ **Figure 24-8** Student Counseling Record

There are implications for clinical instructors as well as their students when clinical practice failures occur. From the student's perspective, the failure may result in a wake-up call that leads to revising his or her strategies for success throughout the remainder of the clinical experiences. A second outcome for the student may be the revelation that the health profession chosen is not for him or her, at which time he or she may choose to revise his or her degree plan. At other times, the student may become angry and blame his or her failure on the clinical instructor. This reaction of the student will have implications for the clinical instructor as he or she may become a part of an appeals process. Rutkowski (2007) reminds us that assessing nursing students' competence during practice placements may result in a clinical practice failure. Safeguarding the public is the goal of safe clinical practice. Each healthcare professional's code of conduct must be the standard against which competency is measured. McGregor (2007) summarizes the picture of clinical practice failure by stating:

> In the face of a clinical failure, what really matters is how the student and the teacher interact. When tensions about clinical performance arise, teachers need to become partners who stand with, rather than against, vulnerable students who are struggling to become competent nurses. (p. 510)

Clinical Practice Success

The ultimate goal of clinical teaching is clinical practice success for the student. This means the student has met the objectives of the course and is ready to progress in the program or into the workforce. Creating supportive clinical learning environments, utilizing interprofessional mentoring, infusing evidence-based practice at the bedside, honing interpersonal skills with patients and families, and incorporating reflective practice on a daily basis are all pillars that provide the foundation for the clinical professional to focus on and overcome challenges that are constantly present in the ever-changing healthcare environment. Students who have inherited a passion for lifelong learning from their clinical instructors will be well equipped and resilient to meet the demands as they grow in their professional roles.

Conclusion: Light at the End of the Tunnel

The outcomes of our teaching experience directly advance our chosen healthcare profession. It is continually rewarding to write letters of recommendation for students as they enter the clinical practice arena and prepare for graduate school. The ebb and flow of the academic calendar can provide a predictable schedule for those who like a beginning and ending point to their work. The clinical practice day may be unpredictable and the generation of learners may change but clinical teaching still provides a stimulating and rewarding practice field.

REFERENCES

Amicucci, B. (2012). What nurse faculty have to say about clinical grading. *Teaching and Learning in Nursing, 7,* 51–55. doi: doi.org/10.1016/j.teln.2011.09.002

Anderson, E., & Kiger, A. M. (2008). "I felt like a real nurse": Student nurses out on their own. *Nurse Education Today, 28*(4), 443–449.

Barrington, K., & Street, K. (2009). Learner contracts in nurse education: Interaction within the practice context. *Nurse Education and Practice, 9,* 109–118.

Bartels, J. (2007). Preparing nursing faculty for baccalaureate-level and graduate-level nursing programs: Role preparation for the academy. *Journal of Nursing Education, 46*(4), 154–158.

Baxter, P. E., & Boblin, S. L. (2007). The moral development of baccalaureate nursing students: Understanding unethical behavior in classroom and clinical settings. *Journal of Nursing Education, 46*(1), 20–27.

Beitz, J. M., & Wieland, D. (2005). Analyzing the teaching effectiveness of clinical nursing faculty of full- and part-time generic, BSN, LPN-BSN, and RN-BSN nursing students. *Journal of Professional Nursing, 21*(1), 32–45.

Boyer, E. L. (1990). *Scholarship reconsidered: Priorities of the professoriate.* New York, NY: Carnegie Foundation for the Advancement of Teaching.

Buccieri, K. M., Brown, R., & Malta, S. (2011). Evaluating the performance of the academic coordinator/director of clinical education: Developing tools to solicit input from program directors, academic faculty, and students. *Journal of Physical Therapy Education, 25*(2), 26–35.

Clark, C. (2010). Why civility matters. *Reflections on Nursing Leadership, 36*(1), 4.

Clark, C., & Springer, P. J. (2007). Incivility in nursing education: A descriptive study of definitions and prevalence. *Journal of Nursing Education, 46*(1), 7–14.

Close, A., & Casteldine, G. (2005). Clinical nursing rounds, Part 4: Teaching rounds for nurses. *British Journal of Nursing, 14*(18), 982–983.

Cooke, M., Mitchell, M., Moyle, W., Henderson, A., & Murfield, J. (2010). Application and student evaluation of a clinical progression portfolio: A pilot. *Nurse Education in Practice, 10,* 227–232.

Day, L., & Smith, L. (2007). Integrating quality and safety content into clinical teaching in the acute care setting. *Nursing Outlook, 55*(3), 138–143.

Edgecombe, K., & Bowden, M. (2009). The ongoing search for best practice in clinical teaching and learning: A model of nursing students' evolution to proficient novice registered nurses. *Nurse Education and Practice, 9,* 91–101.

Fink, L. (2003). *Creating significant learning experiences.* San Francisco, CA: Jossey-Bass.

Gregory, D. M., Guse, L. W., Davidson, D., & Russell, C. K. (2007). Patient safety: Where is nursing education? *Journal of Nursing Education, 46*(2), 79–82.

Hall, M. A., Daly, B. J., & Madigan, E. A. (2010). Use of anecdotal notes by clinical nursing faculty: A descriptive study. *Journal of Nursing Education, 49*(3), 156–59. doi: 10.3928/01484834-20090915-03

Hanson, K. J., & Stenvig, T. E. (2008). The good clinical nursing educator and the baccalaureate nursing clinical experience: Attributes and praxis. *Journal of Nursing Education, 47*(1), 38–42.

Harding, L., & Petrick, T. (2008). Nursing student medication errors: A retrospective review. *Journal of Nursing Education, 47*(1), 43–47.

Hauer, M., & Kogan, J. R. (2012). Realizing the potential value of feedback. *Medical Education, 46*(2), 140-142. doi: 10.1111/j.1365-2923.2011.04180.x

Hellstrom-Hyson, E., Martensson, G., & Kristofferzon, M. (2012). To take responsibility or to be an onlooker. Nursing students' experiences of two models of supervision. *Nurse Education Today, 32*(1), 105–110.

Hoffman, J. (2008). Teaching strategies to facilitate nursing students' critical thinking. In M. Oermann (Ed.), *Annual review of nursing education* (6th ed., pp. 225–236). New York, NY: Springer.

Hopkins, T. H. (2008). Early identification of at-risk nursing students: A student support model. *Journal of Nursing Education, 47*(6), 254–259.

Indar-Maraj, M. (2007). Clinical evaluation of nursing students: Challenges and solutions. *MedSurg Matters, 16*(4), 6–8.

Kelly, S. P. (2007). The exemplary clinical instructor: A qualitative case study. *Journal of Physical Therapy Education, 21*(1), 63–69.

Lachman, V. (2007). Patient safety: The ethical imperative. *Medsurg Nursing, 16*(6), 401–403.

Lundberg, K. (2008). Promoting self-confidence in clinical nursing students. *Nurse Educator, 33*(2), 86–89.

Luparell, S. (2007a). The effects of student incivility on nursing faculty. *Journal of Nursing Education, 46*(1), 15–19.

Luparell, S. (2007b). Managing difficult student situations: Lessons learned. In M. Oermann & K. Heinrich (Eds.), *Annual review of nursing education* (pp. 101–110). New York, NY: Springer.

MacGowan, M. (2010). Finding and integrating the best available evidence into the group work field practicum: Examples and experiences from MSW students. *Social Work with Groups, 33*(2–3), 210–228.

Matsumara, G., Callister, C., Palmer, S., Cox, A., & Larson, L. (2004). Staff nurse perceptions of the contributions of students to clinical agencies. *Nursing Education Perspectives, 25*(6), 297–303.

McAllister, M., Tower, M., & Walker, R. (2007). Gentle interruptions: Transformative approaches to clinical teaching. *Journal of Nursing Education, 46*(7), 304–312.

McGregor, A. (2007). Academic success, clinical failure: Struggling practices of a failing student. *Journal of Nursing Education, 46*(11), 504–511.

Melo, K., Williams, B., & Ross, C. (2010). The impact of nursing curricula on clinical practice today. *Nurse Education Today, 30*(8), 773–778.

Newton, J. M., Cross, W., White, K., Ockerby, C., & Billett, S. (2011). Outcomes of a clinical partnership model for undergraduate nursing students. *Contemporary Nurse: A Journal for the Australian Nursing Profession, 39*(1), 119–127.

Newton, S., Smith, L., & Moore, G. (2007). Baccalaureate nursing program admission policies: Promoting success or facilitating failure? *Journal of Nursing Education, 46*(10), 439–511.

Noble, K. A., Miller, S. M., & Heckman, J. (2008). The cognitive style of nursing students: Educational implications for teaching and learning. *Journal of Nursing Education, 47*(6), 245–253.

Nottingham, S., & Henning, J. (2010). Provision of feedback to students, Part 1: Overview of strategies. *Athletic Therapy Today, 15*(5), 19–21.

Numminen, O. H., Leino-Kilpi, H., van der Arend, A., & Katajisto, J. (2010). Nurse educators' teaching of codes of ethics. *Nurse Education Today, 30*(2), 124–131. doi: doi.org/10.1016/j.nedt.2009.06.011

Ruth-Sahd, L. A. (2011). Student nurse dyads create a community of learning: Proposing a holistic clinical education theory. *Journal of Advanced Nursing, 67*(11), 2445–2454.

Rutkowski, K. (2007). Failure to fail: Assessing nursing students' competence during practice placements. *Nursing Standard, 22*(13), 35–40.

Skaalvik, M. W., Norman, H. K., & Henriksen, N. (2010). To what extent does the oral shift report stimulate learning among nursing students? A qualitative study. *Journal of Clinical Nursing, 19*(15–16), 2300–2308.

Spurr, S., Bally, J., & Ferguson, L. (2010). A framework for clinical teaching: A passion-centered philosophy. *Nurse Education in Practice 10*, 349–354. doi: 10.1016/j.nepr.2010.05.002

Stinson, S. (2009, Spring). Maximizing minority students' success in clinical. *Minority Nurse*, pp. 1–5. Retrieved from CINAHL with Full Text database.

Wetherbee, E., Peatman, N., Kenney, D., Cusson, M., & Applebaum, D. (2010). Standards for clinical education: A qualitative study. *Journal of Physical Therapy Education*. Retrieved from http://www.highbeam.com/doc/1P3-2279669081.html

CHAPTER 25

Concept Mapping: A Meaningful Learning Tool to Promote Conceptual Understanding and Clinical Reasoning

■ GREGORY PASSMORE ■

Instruction can be described as existing on a continuum from teacher-centered/content-oriented to student-centered/learner-oriented actions (Ertmer & Newby, 1993; Passmore, Owen, & Prabakaran, 2011). Various models of this continuum exist in health professions instruction, bringing forth reactive to proactive student behavior and participation and passive to active involvement of the instructor in learning. Traditionally, curricula for health professions instruction have been developed to meet the behavioral learning outcomes desired by national accrediting and credentialing bodies. These traditional curricula are often content centered to meet these desired outcomes. However, the current healthcare environment is demanding graduates who can think critically and problem solve in a variety of clinical practice areas (Daley & Torre, 2010; Edmondson, 1994; Novak & Cañas, 2008; Passmore et al., 2011; Pinto & Zeitz, 1997; Regan-Smith et al., 1994; Rendas, Fonseca, & Rosado-Pinto, 2006; Wheeler & Collins, 2003). Critical thinking, problem solving, and clinical reasoning are poorly served by most content-centered instruction. Educational theorists such as Novak and Gowin (1984) believe that the key to successful critical thinking and problem solving is the cognitivist/constructivist-based meaningful learning–centered methods of instruction to promote active processing of concepts leading to problem-solving skills.

The key to meaningful learning is that learning is an individual, cognitive process, where each learner must construct his or her own understanding of concepts, relationships, and procedures. For a student to accomplish this style of learning, a learner would have to mentally integrate the new information acquired during learning activities into what the learner already knows or differentiate what the learner knows to accommodate the new information (Ausubel, 1963; Ausubel, Novak, & Hanesian, 1978; Heinze-Fry & Novak,

1990; Novak, 1990, 2003; Novak & Cañas, 2008; Novak & Gowin, 1984; Passmore, 1995; West, Park, Pomeroy, & Sandoval, 2002).

Meaningful learning, then, is how the student organizes, saves, and retrieves information or knowledge in a relational fashion. Meaningful learning is based on the premise that knowledge is bundled in packets called concepts (defined as recognized regularities in events or objects), and recalled from memory based on how the concepts are attached to one another. New information is nonarbitrarily attached to concepts already familiar to the learner through linkages that the learner identifies as meaningful. In contrast to rote learning, the outcome of meaningful learning is that the new information is transferred into long-term memory through a meaningful linkage, thus enabling retrieval needed for critical thinking and problem solving (Novak, 1990; Novak & Cañas, 2008; Pinto & Zeitz, 1997).

The purpose of instruction is for the student to develop a knowledge base within the discipline, but also to be able to acquire new knowledge as the discipline changes with advancements in technology and practice. Students who are taught how to learn meaningfully by the nonarbitrary assimilation of new concepts and procedures into the learner's knowledge structure or accommodate their knowledge structures to accept the new information should be able to meet the discipline's needs today and tomorrow. One learning intervention that helps identify an individual's unique knowledge structure of a topic or process is a graphic organizer of topical concepts commonly known as a concept map. Concept maps provide both teacher and student a guide from which to base further learning (Ausubel, 1963; Novak, 1990; Novak & Gowin, 1984; Passmore, 1996; Pinto & Zeitz, 1997).

■ Definition and Purposes

A concept map is a concise, two-dimensional, schematic representation of the collection of concepts and linking relationships in a student's knowledge set of a topic or process. Two or more concepts and their linking relationships become meaningful statements about some object or event one is trying to define, classify, or purpose. It is the identification of the linking relationship between concepts in a concept map that makes this graphic organizer unique and separates the concept map from other less communicative organizing techniques, such as outlines, nursing process care plans, or flow charts. Concept maps can be used by individual students and groups as tools for learning, by teachers and students for remediation, and by teachers for assessment (Adler, Wilson, & Coulter, 2008; Dansereau & Cross, 1990; Edmondson, 1994; Hsu & Hsieh, 2005; Novak, 1990; Novak & Gowin, 1984; Novak & Wandersee, 1990; Passmore, 1995, 1996; West et al., 2002).

Concept maps have been used as a learning intervention for individuals and groups in traditional didactic and distance courses, in laboratories, in clinical courses, and in critical thinking and problem-solving courses, with the emphasis in the health-care literature on clinic, critical thinking, and problem solving (Daley & Torre, 2010;

Pinto & Zeitz, 1997). By creating concept maps, students learn that the conceptual understanding they gain in their didactic coursework has a procedural counterpart in their laboratory and/or clinical application courses and clerkships (Hunter-Revell, 2012; Passmore, 1996, 1998). In essence, using concept maps as a meaningful learning intervention helps students to develop a more complete and meaningful understanding of the theoretical knowledge they gain didactically and to bridge the gap between the theoretical knowledge and the procedural knowledge they gain in the laboratory and the clinic (Hicks-Moore, 2005; Novak & Gowin, 1984; Passmore, 1998). Further, the concept map's visual interpretation of an individual's knowledge structure can simplify discussion and lead to enhanced understanding between individuals, either in groups or in providing an opportunity between teacher and student for misconception remediation (Dansereau & Cross, 1990; Novak & Cañas, 2008; Novak & Gowin, 1984; Passmore, 1995, 1996, 1998). Additionally, the concept map lends itself to quantitative and qualitative assessment using rubrics such as the one developed by Novak and Gowin (1984), allowing a teacher and the student to measure the extent of the knowledge represented by the concept map.

■ Theoretical Rationale

The continuum of learning theories begins with the behaviorist theory, where learning is confirmed by specific behavioral responses to specific stimuli; passes through the cognitivist theory, where learning is confirmed by the behavioral and mental solutions to specific stimuli; and ends with the constructivist theory, where learning is individualized and based on the stimuli as they are presented. More simply, this continuum might be described as moving from rote learning or memorization through meaningful learning and problem solving to autonomous learning and invention (Novak & Cañas, 2008; Passmore et al., 2011).

The shortcomings of behaviorist learning theory applied to students in the health professions can be seen in the example of the student who correctly performs a healthcare protocol in clinical practice, but who fails when he or she is exposed to variations in the protocol or patients. If the student has been conditioned to respond to certain stimuli in the protocol, when the learning stimuli are different, the learner may not be able to respond appropriately until he or she has memorized all possible variations of the protocol.

Further, the student taught using cognitivist learning theories and given the same set of variations in clinical protocols as previously mentioned understands the need or existence of the variations. This student does not see the required variations as an impediment to accomplishing the task, since he or she has developed a mental schema that allows for processing of critical thinking and problem-solving strategies that come with meaningful learning.

Students taught in the constructivist learning environment may or may not be able to accomplish a health professions–associated task. Constructivist learning theory supports creativity in problem solving because it asks the student to approach the problem from different perspectives where knowledge of previous protocols may be advantageous, but not necessary. However, by its definition, a protocol establishes a set of procedures used to carry out a task. Reinventing that set of procedures every time the task is required would be inefficient and time consuming, and it is a weakness with constructivist learning in situations where conformity is essential and divergent thinking may cause problems.

The cognitive psychologist David Ausubel (1968) summed up the purpose of learning interventions as actions designed to "ascertain this [what the student already knows] and teach him accordingly" (p. vi). The fundamental idea in Ausubel's cognitive psychology is that learning takes place either by the assimilation of new concepts into existing conceptual or cognitive structures held by the learner or by accommodation of the learner's cognitive structure to the new concept. Thus, personal knowledge is typically constructed like a house or a car, and not usually discovered like oil or a new planet (Novak & Gowin, 1984).

The learning theory that is to be utilized in instruction should be the one that best meets the outcomes of the learning objectives, the type of learning task, and the student's level of competence. In the health professions, this leads to instruction that both meets the predicated curricular objectives of its accrediting agencies and promotes meaningful learning to best meet the needs of the student. Instruction is provided for the student to develop a knowledge base within the discipline. However, the student has to be able to learn new knowledge as the discipline changes with advancements in technology and practice. Rote learning will provide most students with a body of facts, such as lab values, anatomy and physiology, and even some clinical protocols. However, students who are taught how to learn meaningfully by the nonarbitrary assimilation of new information or new concepts and procedures into the learner's knowledge structure have been shown to be better critical thinkers/problem solvers, and thus should be able to more completely meet their discipline's needs and challenges (Daley & Torre, 2010; Edmondson, 1994; Ertmer & Newby, 1993; Passmore et al., 2011; Wheeler & Collins, 2003).

How the student organizes and recalls knowledge is the key to meaningful learning. Meaningful learning is based on the premise that knowledge is bundled in concept packets and recalled from memory based on how the concepts are attached or linked to one another when stored in long-term memory. Concept maps are two-dimensional graphic representations or organizers of multiple concepts designed to help students recall and structure their knowledge in relational maps. It is this process of identifying or naming the linking relationships between concepts in the map that makes this graphic organizer an effective learning intervention (Novak & Cañas, 2008; Passmore, 1995).

Well-developed concept maps also display cross-links. These are linking relationships between concepts in different levels or conceptual clusters of the concept map and are an important characteristic of concept maps. Cross-links help us see how a concept or process in one domain of knowledge represented on the map is related to a concept in another domain shown on the map, indicating a deeper level of understanding (Angelo & Cross, 1993; Dansereau & Cross, 1990; Novak, 1990; Novak & Cañas, 2008; Novak & Gowin, 1984; Passmore, 1995, 1996, 1998).

Meaningful learning requires the learner to become an active participant in the learning process. The process of creating a concept map by identifying relevant concepts and their relationships between them is an active learning process. Meaningful learning strategies, such as concept mapping, allow learners to actively organize their knowledge structures into powerful, integrated patterns. A concept map becomes a concise, visual interpretation of an individual's knowledge structure (Angelo & Cross, 1993; Dansereau & Cross, 1990; Heinze-Fry & Novak, 1990; Novak, 1990; Novak & Cañas, 2008; Novak & Gowin, 1984; Passmore, 1995, 1996, 1998). Whereas rote memorization is typically static, concept mapping allows for the growth of the individual's knowledge structure. **Figure 25-1** represents a student concept map depicting understanding of fundamental radiation safety concepts before (a) and after (b) multiple teacher–student remediation activities. Note that a relational linking term exists between concepts, and the postremediations map has several levels of hierarchies and clusters of understanding. This pair of maps shows how a student's understanding can grow following instruction, laboratory, or remediation.

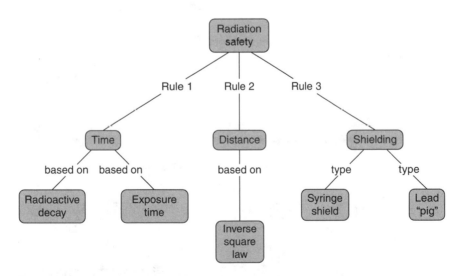

■ **Figure 25-1a** Student concept map depicting understanding of fundamental radiation safety concepts prior to remediation

■ Conditions

Concept maps have been used as guides to instruction, meaningful learning organizers, misconception remediation facilitators, and assessment tools across all levels of education. Construction of concept maps requires reflection on the part of the individual constructing the map, whether student or teacher (Novak & Gowin, 1984). Individuals with a penchant for rote learning activities and assessments should be given the opportunity to familiarize themselves with the processes of map construction. Teachers and students who focus more on memorization rather than deep understanding have expressed state anxiety in using mapping activities. This is exemplified in Roth and

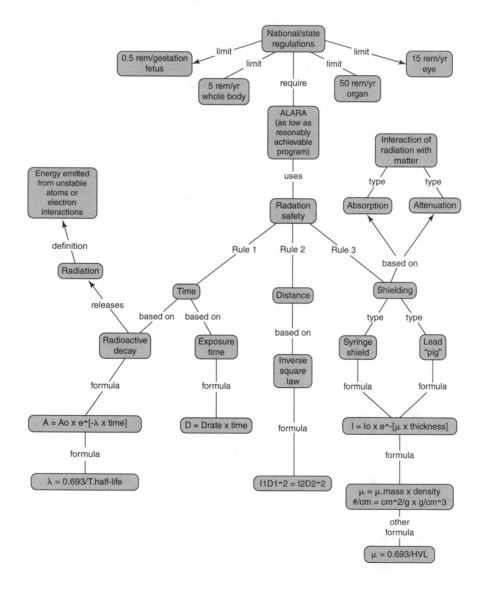

Roychoudhoury's 1993 study of elementary education majors taking a physical science course for their specialty certification. These researchers found that the concept mapping activity was attitudinally accepted by 81% of the student teachers in the program, leaving 19% to declare themselves attitudinally resistant as they were being moved from rote learning to meaningful learning practices. Similarly, Passmore (1996) found some attitudinal resistance in his longitudinal study of radiologic science students; however, these feelings of resistance seem to be abated with long-term use (Feldsine, 1987; Passmore, 1998). Concept maps have been used successfully in the academic environment, the business environment, and the military environment (Novak & Cañas, 2008).

Implementation

Concept mapping needs to be taught to students, researchers, or clinicians when the method is intended to be utilized in the classroom, laboratory, or clinic (Adler et al., 2008; Novak & Cañas, 2008; Novak & Gowin, 1984; Passmore, 2008; Pinto & Zeitz, 1997). This is a process activity, and it should be treated just as any other process with stepwise instruction and practice (Gagne, 1985). Passmore (2008) uses a 2- to 4-hour workshop to introduce the mapping process to health professions students and teachers. Since the audience for this workshop is discipline diverse, the workshop is initiated by having participants identify concepts and relationships from a general list of biologic and sociology concepts and relationships (Dansereau & Cross, 1990). The workshop concludes with participants (in small-group units) developing a concept map from a two-paragraph description of the information processing model of memory using long-term and short-term memory, using a skeleton map as a starting point. In this instructional process, it is important to begin with a limited domain of knowledge that is familiar to the student. This creates a context that will help determine the structure of the concept map. While experienced map makers may employ topical, broad-scope maps, novice map makers should be provided with a

---

■ **Figure 25-1b** Post remediation: Student concept map depicting understanding of fundamental radiation safety concepts

Terminology Key: rem = unit of dose equivalent (J/kg); HVL = half-value layer measure of attenuation in linear dimension units (e.g., mm); D = dose or amount of energy deposited in matter (J/kg); Drate = rate of energy deposited in matter (J/kg/unit time); μ = linear attenuation coefficient derived from the ratio of the ln2/HVL; T = half-life, the time required for a radioactive sample to decay to one-half the sample's original activity; λ = radioactive decay constant derived from the ratio of the ln2/T; inverse square law = I = radiation intensity, D = distance from source from which radiation intensity was measured or for which is to be calculated.

clear, specific domain, root concepts or skeleton map, and/or focus question around which they can develop their maps (Cañas, Novak, & Reiska, 2012; Novak & Cañas, 2008; Passmore, 2008). The next step is for the map maker to list the key concepts in the domain. From this list the map is developed with the most general concepts at the top and the most specific concepts at the bottom. One technique for identifying subordinate concepts from the superordinate, general concept is to ask descriptive questions about the general concept (Dansereau & Cross, 1990), such as questions of types, characteristics, and parts that pertain to the general concept, or questions of process such as what leads to the general concept, or what follows.

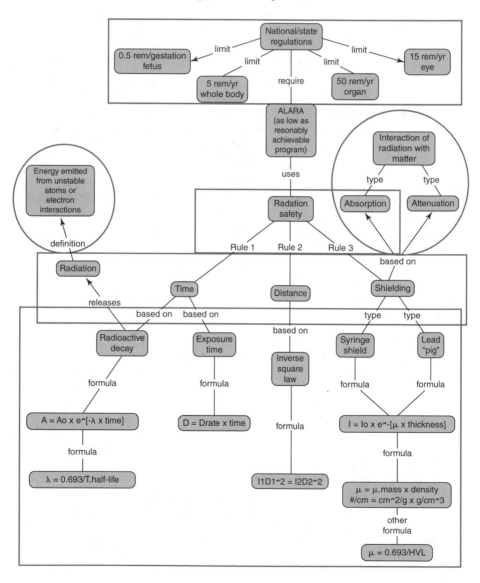

Once this list is generated, map construction can begin, typically with a preliminary map. In the preliminary map, the concepts can be positioned in a fashion that is unique for the map maker. Lines are drawn between concepts and labeled with a few relational words that describe the relationship between the concepts. As this map develops, the maker usually sees that the most organized fashion for the map is with the most general, superordinate concept at the top with the subordinate concepts clustered beneath. However, whereas these hierarchical maps seem intuitive in science-based fields, this may not be the case in all disciplines. Many maps start with the most general concept as a central node, and the subordinate concepts radiate out and beneath the central concept (Dansereau & Cross, 1990; Passmore, 2004). Dynamic or cyclic maps can also be generated as the discipline requires to indicate temporal distributions in the conceptual structures, such as the assessment, evaluation, and follow-up process involved in many patient care activities (Dansereau & Cross, 1990; Safayeni, Derbentseva, & Cañas, 2005).

■ **Figure 25-2** The scoring process applied to Figure 25-1b. Note that a relational linking term exists between concepts, and the postremediation map has several levels of hierarchies and clusters of understanding. Each map was scored based on the rubric described above. This map shows how a student's increased understanding following instruction, laboratory, or remediation can be quantified in place of other formal or summative assessments.

Score:
28 conceptual links $\times$ 1 point each
1 definition $\times$ 1 point
4 levels of hierarchy $\times$ 10 points each
1 supporting cluster $\times$ 10 points
= 79 points

Terminology Key: rem = unit of dose equivalent (J/kg); HVL = half-value layer measure of attenuation in linear dimension units (e.g. mm); D = dose or amount of energy deposited in matter (J/kg); Drate = rate of energy deposited in matter (J/kg/unit time); μ-linear attenuation coefficient derived from the ratio of the ln2/HVL; T = half-life, the time required for a radioactive sample to decay to one-half the sample's original activity; λ-radioactive decay constant derived from the ratio of the ln2/T; Inverse Square Law = I = radiation intensity, D = distance from source from which radiation intensity was measured or for which is to be calculated.

One notable aspect of concept maps that makes the intervention such a powerful, meaningful learning tool is that cross-links between subordinate concepts or clusters of concepts should be sought and labeled, since these indicate a deeper understanding of the relationships in any domain. Another feature that may be added to concept maps is specific examples of events or objects that help to clarify the meaning of a given concept. These early drafts are followed by subsequent drafts until the final draft that the map maker feels explains his or her understanding of the response to the initial question or domain. Revisions using pencil and paper can be somewhat cumbersome and time consuming. However, there are software packages available that allow for frequent revisions, but may be a little restrictive compared to pencil-and-paper mapping activities (Novak & Cañas, 2008). The revisions also provide an orderly sequence of iterations between working memory and long-term memory, using the map as the scaffold or template to build knowledge frameworks (Novak, 1990). The concept maps can now be used as an individual study guide, as a collaborative group discussion format, as a basis from which misconceptions can be identified and remediated a priori to testing (Figure **25-1**), and as a form of assessment themselves (**Figure 25-2**) (Abel & Freeze, 2006; Adler et al., 2008; All & Huycke, 2007; Daley & Torre, 2010; Gonzalez, Palencia, Umana, Galindo, & Villafrade, 2008; Hinck et al., 2006; Hsu & Hsieh, 2005; Mahler, Hoz, Fischl, Tov-Ly, & Lernau, 1991; Novak & Gowin, 1984; Passmore, 1996; 2011; West et al., 2002; West, Pomeroy, Park, Gerstenberger, & Sandoval, 2000).

▪ Types of Learners

The physical construction of concept maps as a learning intervention has been shown to facilitate meaningful learning by enabling students from elementary school through college and graduate school to actively seek and develop conceptual relationships. Researchers have shown the utility of concept mapping as a learning and evaluation tool in multiple educational environments, to include expository lecture, laboratory, critical thinking, problem solving, cooperative group learning, clinical, case study analysis, patient care planning, and distance learning (Daley & Torre, 2010; Novak & Cañas, 2008; Passmore, 1996; Passmore et al., 2011; Preszler, 2004).

Research in multiple intelligences (Gardner, 1983) and learning styles (Felder, 1993; Kolb & Kolb, 2005) has been well accepted and draws attention to the wide range of differences in student abilities for various types of learning and performances. Concept mapping, being a form of graphic organizer, would seem to fit well with those individuals who rely on visual/spatial techniques for learning. Other forms of learning preferences, such as verbal/auditory and tactile, can also benefit from generating concept maps. If learning style preferences are long-term learner adaptations to facilitate learning, then activities that enhance meaningful learning should be adapted to just as readily given time and practice, irrespective of the learning style (Laight, 2004; Novak & Cañas, 2008).

■ Using the Method

Concept maps can be used for a variety of educational processes from the perspective of the teacher and the student, in the form of knowledge acquisition/structuring template, critical-thinking/problem-solving intervention, misconception remediation guide, meaningful-learning/authentic-assessment template, research/project-planning guide, and curriculum-planning guide. These tasks are applied in several different curriculum models to include lecture/laboratory, critical thinking/problem solving, cooperative learning, clinical processes, case study analysis, case/care planning, distance learning environments, and postprofessional continuing education (Cañas et al., 2003; Daley & Torre, 2010).

Student Uses of Concept Maps

Meaningful Learning from Lecture/Laboratory Curriculum

Concept maps can be used as meaningful learning tools within a lecture-based course. Students can map lectures and textbook passages to gain a meaningful understanding of the presented material. Concept mapping can be used by students to organize and integrate multiple concepts and as a template for growing their conceptual understanding. As a meaningful learning activity, students can document their existing knowledge, gain new understandings, and then relate the new information to what they already know. In addition, students can detect areas where there are misconceptions, expressed as dissatisfaction with their own cognitive structures in trying to connect concepts in a meaningful and organized way. Whether self-determined or discovered through study group or teacher–student interaction, misconceptions provide an opportunity for remediation, a process where student misconceptions are replaced with more scientifically valid concepts and relationships, which is discussed more fully in the *Teacher Uses of Concept Maps* section later in this chapter (Daley & Torre, 2010; Novak & Cañas, 2008; Novak & Gowin, 1984; Passmore, 1995, 1996, 1998; Pinto & Zeitz, 1997; Roth & Roychoudhury, 1993).

Concept maps also can be used in other study methods, such as distance learning and laboratory. Distance learning demands communication between students and teachers, as well as between students. Concept maps make excellent vehicles for long-distance discussion between individuals, to include misconception remediation activities (Coffey & Canas, 2000; Novak & Cañas, 2008; Passmore et al., 2011; Pinto & Zeitz, 1997).

Additionally, concept maps used in laboratory will help the student understand the relationships between the concepts that are driving the procedures the student is following. Many laboratory study guides provide the conceptual understanding required for purposeful learning in a laboratory protocol. However, unless the student is acting on the information in a meaningful fashion, the student may miss the understanding and simply follow the procedure. Having students construct a relational concept map can help them identify how the laboratory procedures are derived from the theoretical and conceptual basis. Concept maps used this way will tend to have a descriptive component as well as a dynamic, procedural component, thus giving them access to the "Why is the procedure done this way?" instead of "It is done this way" encountered so often in laboratory and clinical practice (Dansereau & Cross, 1990; Hicks-Moore, 2005; Novak & Gowin, 1984; Passmore, 1998; Safayeni et al., 2005).

One goal of radiologic science physics teaching has traditionally been to help students become proficient problem solvers. Several studies point out that traditional methods of applying formulas to sets of problems at the end of a chapter fail to encourage concept development; thus, the student has no knowledge base (appropriate memory) from which to draw the needed information and procedures to develop a solution set (Champagne & Klopfer, 1981; Glynn, Yeany, & Britton, 1991; Novak, Gowin, & Johansen, 1983; Passmore, 1998; Prankratius, 1990; Roth & Roychoudhury, 1994). Prankratius (1990) compared concept mapping groups to nonconcept mapping groups in physics instruction and concluded that the groups that often performed concept mapping scored significantly higher on a problem-solving assessment than the traditionally instructed groups that relied on practice alone.

Meaningful Learning from Critical Thinking/ Problem-Based Learning Curriculum

Students in a problem-based learning (PBL) program use their concept maps to identify the student-generated informational learning opportunities that emerge during case study. Additionally, each PBL group can concept map out a model specific to the case study. A case-specific concept map would have the students incorporate basic science concepts, clinical science concepts, procedural concepts, and student-generated hypotheses into a case-specific model of the case study that would potentially include multiple cross-linkages and layers (Dansereau & Cross, 1990; Pinto & Zeitz, 1997). Giddens (2006) based a curriculum development activity for graduate student nurses on using concept maps as a guide to critical thinking and deeper understanding. Attitudinal outcomes were positive, as participants felt that the mapping activity led to discussions of content and theory. These were possible after organizing, analyzing, and communicating interrelationships among concepts identified in the mapping process. Hicks-Moore and Pastirik (2006) quantified critical thinking in a study to assess the level of critical thinking with concept maps. Their results indicate that critical thinking was enhanced by developing concept maps.

Meaningful Learning from Clinical Curriculum

Students in clinical courses, to include community medicine, preventive medicine, and healthcare delivery, can use concept mapping when learning important concepts and procedures that are the basis for their clinical rotations or clerkships. As described previously in the *Meaningful Learning from Lecture/Laboratory Curriculum* section, the concept map processes used for meaningful learning of basic science knowledge can also be used for meaningful learning of clinical procedures, ensuring that students understand the science behind the procedures they are learning, giving the student understanding in both declarative and procedural knowledge bases. One example of this process applied clinically is in clinical care plans that incorporate concept maps as part of the critical-thinking, problem-solving process. Concept mapping encourages a patient-centered focus in a comprehensive care environment (Abel & Freeze, 2006; Atay & Karabacak, 2012; Hinck et al., 2006; Novak & Gowin, 1984; Passmore, 1998; Pinto & Zcitz, 1997; Weiss & Levison, 2000; Wheeler & Collins, 2003).

Meaningful Learning from Medical Residency Curriculum

Medical school programs consist of medical program education followed by a long period of residency training. A longitudinal use of concept maps is seen in medical residents' use of maps made during early clinical experiences as a basis for meaningful learning of new concepts encountered during residency training. These individually unique concept maps can serve as a means for integrating the new knowledge acquired during residency training with the knowledge achieved and meaningfully learned during medical school (Mahler et al., 1991; Pinto & Zeitz, 1997; West et al., 2002; West et al., 2000).

Meaningful Learning from Postprofessional Curriculum

For healthcare professionals, learning does not stop upon completion of professional training. New knowledge emerges with increasing frequency, a fact not lost on the certification/registry boards that require either recertification every few years or continuous education every year. Thus, healthcare professionals are obligated to gain a meaningful understanding of the new science and care concepts developed in their discipline, and to integrate these new concepts with prior concepts retained in long-term memory. Concept mapping can be used as a meaningful learning strategy for knowledge identification in this lifelong, often self-directed, postprofessional learning environment (Cañas et al., 2003; Pinto & Zeitz, 1997).

Teacher Uses of Concept Maps

Concept Maps as Planning Tools

Teachers can make a concept map to use as a teaching guide to help organize a lecture. This helps the teacher identify what he or she feels is important for students to understand. Also, this strategy provides for a conceptual flow in the lecture. Programmatic curriculum and lesson planning through the use of concept mapping have been suggested by Novak and Gowin (1984) and documented by Starr and Krajcik (1990), who studied the development of a curriculum by elementary teachers using the concept map technique. These group concept maps were analyzed for levels of hierarchical structure, topical differentiation, and integrative reconciliation. As each curriculum map revision took place, the curricular concepts to be learned and the relationships between them were clarified until a conceptually cohesive, integrated, and hierarchically arranged curriculum guide was produced. This process can enhance authentication of teacher evaluation. Teachers who use concept maps to guide their lectures and curricula will be in a better position to evaluate their teaching performance when they consider how well their knowledge set describes the hierarchical relationships and complexity of the material to be taught (Dansereau & Cross, 1990; Glynn et al., 1991; Trowbride & Wandersee, 1994).

Giddens (2006) used concept mapping in a group activity to promote critical thinking about curriculum design. Graduate student nurses were asked to develop nursing curricula while working in groups. The activity generated much discussion and problem solving within the groups, and positive affective outcomes were noted. Additionally, participants claimed that the concept mapping activity provided a guide that led to group discussions concerning related reading assignments. A deeper understanding was the most cited outcome of these discussions.

Daley and Torre (2010) report on a research effort where teacher-generated concept maps were used to augment didactic learning materials. However, caution suggests that complete teacher maps should not be shared with students. Recall that concept maps are individually unique, and expert maps have been shown to either be so complex that the learning objectives and concepts are difficult for the viewer to identify or too simplistic because much of what the expert knows is subsumed in more general concepts, which are not elaborated upon in the expert's map (Bogden, 1977). Also, the action of a teacher handing out a teacher-prepared concept map sets up the condition for students to memorize the map by rote, which does little in helping them to cognitively understand or integrate the material (Cañas, Novak, & Reiska, 2012; Novak, personal communication, September 3, 2012). It has been shown that a skeleton map of a few main concepts and initial relationships may be given as a guide to help students see the organization and integration of the important concepts, allowing the students to build or expand on these maps, which will negate rote memorization and encourage meaningful learning (Novak & Cañas, 2008).

Concept Maps as Misconception Remediation Tools

Having students concept map a lecture can give the teacher feedback information on student misconceptions, thus prompting mentoring and/or misconception remediation. Misconceptions that have occurred as a result of the interaction of the student and the instruction from lecture, laboratory, or clinic need to be successfully identified and remediated (Griffiths, Thomey, Cooke, & Normore, 1988; Renner, Abraham, Grzybowski, & Marek, 1990; Roth, 1990; Wandersee, Mintzes, & Novak, 1994). Misconceptions are identified in concept maps as a linkage between two concepts that is false or as a linkage that fails to address the main idea relating the two or more concepts (Novak & Gowin, 1984). One method of examining the student's concepts and relationships is through a preinstruction and postinstruction interview. Since concept maps are a concise representation of the concepts and relationships in a learner's knowledge set, they allow teachers to quickly recognize invalid or underdeveloped knowledge claims, which would suggest a need for remediation (Novak, 1990; Novak & Gowin, 1984; Roth, 1990; Wandersee et al., 1994).

Passmore (1995, 1996) used concept maps as a postinstruction format for misconception remediation prior to formal assessment with radiologic science students (Figure 25-1), finding concept maps to be both an efficient and effective form of communication between the student and the teacher. Learning gains were evident in the concept mapping group, as evidenced by the ability of the concept mapping intervention to alter the predictive ability of SAT scores in the concept mapping group. Student attitudes toward having remediation before the assessment instead of traditionally after the assessment were positive. Wallace and Mintzes (1990) used concept maps to document conceptual change in biology for elementary education majors. The authors note that a teacher can observe how the student's individual cognitive structures grow and mature by comparing successive student concept maps as the student gains mastery of the domain.

Correcting long-held misconceptions of basic science or social science phenomena requires conceptual change. Students' dissatisfaction with their own cognitive structures in trying to connect concepts in a meaningful and organized way is a requirement in cognitive/constructivist philosophy as a first step in conceptual change, a process where student misconceptions are replaced with more scientifically valid concepts and relationships, ideally through meaningful learning activities (Roth & Roychoudhury, 1993).

Concept Maps as Assessment Tools

Concept maps are a tool for teachers wanting a more authentic or meaningful evaluation than standardized achievement tests. Meaningful learning activities such as concept mapping should be followed by meaningful evaluation, and using the student-generated concept map as the evaluation tool is one method for achieving this goal. Scoring concept maps for the validity or completeness of conceptual or procedural relationships, for what the teacher or discipline determines to be correct conceptions, for multiple levels of hierarchical structure, and for complexity described by concept differentiation and integration is a more authentic assessment than end-of-course achievement tests, which are often rote memorization oriented (Abel & Freeze, 2006; Daley & Torre, 2010; Markham, Mintzes, & Jones, 1994; Novak, 1990; Novak & Gowin, 1984; Passmore, 1995, 1996, 1998; Roth & Roychoudhury, 1993; West et al., 2002).

To use the concept map as an assessment tool, the teacher must construct a domain-specific expert concept map and compare each student's map to the expert map. A scoring scheme based on Novak and Gowin's (1984) suggestion follows:

- 1 point for each correct conceptual relationship and concept example or definition
- 5 points for cross-linking relationships
- 10 points for conceptual clusters and hierarchical structure

This process can be used as a prelesson and/or postlesson formative or summative assessment or in assistance to the remediation process discussed previously, as the change in quantitative values attached to a student's concept map can serve as an extrinsic motivator to reinforce the learning process (Abel & Freeze, 2006; Daley & Torre, 2010; Novak & Gowin, 1984; Passmore, 1995, 1996, 1998; West et al., 2002). Figure 25-2 has a score associated with a student's concept map following several remediation efforts. A change in map complexity preinstruction–postinstruction activity or remediation activity reflects the increase in the student's increase in learning and can be quantified by scoring the preinstruction–postinstruction activity concept maps.

The teacher should be aware that assessment of concept maps may well indicate differences in success for students who typically score well on standardized assessments. Novak and colleagues' (1983) analysis suggested that students who best understood the science concepts were not necessarily the students who received the best grades on standardized tests. Additionally, Passmore's (1995) study outcomes using concept map assessment showed that concept mapping altered the predictive ability of SAT scores. West and others (2000) compared preinstruction–postinstruction concept map scores, noting improvement. However, the improvement in map scores did not correlate with course outcomes or standardized test scores. These observations support the differences in assessment and achievement for rote and meaningful learning.

■ Conclusion

Meaningful learning for health professions students and practitioners is an important, cognitive individual skill that can be enhanced through the use of concept mapping. Concept maps can be used by teachers, students, and postgraduate professionals to enable meaningful learning for themselves, their students, and their colleagues. Educationally oriented research using these two-dimensional graphic organizers has shown that students can benefit from drawing how they are integrating new knowledge, as well as identifying misconceptions, for use as a guide for discussion and understanding in group work, critical thinking/problem solving, and relating conceptual knowledge to the procedural knowledge needed for clinical reasoning and performance. Teachers can use concept maps as meaningful assessments, as enablers for misconception remediation, as guides in group work, and as devices that allow for a complete lesson and/or curriculum-planning process. Professionals, too, can gain from the process of concept mapping by integrating new concepts required for current practice with previously learned concepts in a format that allows for information to be recalled in a usable manner. The multiplicity of researched uses of this graphic organizer show the extent of the utility of this meaningful learning tool in helping students and professionals shift from rote learners to meaningful learners.

REFERENCES

Abel, W., & Freeze, M. (2006). Evaluation of concept mapping in an associate degree nursing program. *Journal of Nursing Education, 45*(9), 356–364.

Adler, S. R., Wilson E., & Coulter, Y. Z. (2008). Assessing students' socio-cultural knowledge frameworks through concept mapping. *Medical Education, 42,* 1125.

All, A. C., & Huycke, L. I. (2007). Serial concept maps: Tools for concept analysis. *Journal of Nursing Education, 46*(5), 217–224.

Angelo, T. A., & Cross, K. P. (1993). *Classroom assessment techniques: A handbook for college teachers* (2nd ed.). San Francisco, CA: Jossey-Bass.

Atay, S., & Karabacak, U. (2012). Care plans using concept maps and their effects on the critical thinking dispositions of nursing students. *International Journal of Nursing Practice, 18,* 233–239.

Ausubel, D. P. (1968). *Educational psychology: A cognitive view.* New York, NY: Holt, Rinehart, and Winston.

Ausubel, D. P., Novak, J. D., & Hanesian, H. (1978). *Educational psychology: A cognitive view.* New York, NY: Holt, Rinehart & Winston.

Bogden, C. A. (1977). *The use of concept mapping as a possible strategy for instructional design and evaluation in college genetics.* Master's thesis, Cornell University, Ithaca, NY

Cañas, A. J., Coffey, J. W., Carnot, M. J., Feltovich, P., Hoffman, R. R., & Novak, J. D. (2003). *A summary of literature pertaining to the use of concept mapping techniques and technologies for education and performance support.* Prepared for the chief of naval education and training, Pensacola FL. Pensacola FL.: Institute for Human and Machine Cognition. Retrieved from http://www.docstoc.com/docs /DownloadDoc.aspx?doc_id=3753282

Cañas, A. J., Novak, J. D., & Reiska, P. (2012). Freedom vs restriction of content and structure during concept mapping: Possibilities and limitations for construction and assessment. In A. J. Cañas, J. D. Novak, & Vanhear (Eds.), *Concept maps: Theory, Methodology, Technology: Proceedings of the Fifth International Conference on Concept Mapping.* Valletta, Malta. www.ihmc.us

Champagne, A. B., & Klopfer, L. E. (1984). Research in science education: The cognitive psychology perspective. In Holdzkom, D. & Lutz, P. (Eds.), *Research within reach: Science education* (pp. 171–189). Washington, DC: National Science Teachers Association.

Coffey, J. W., & Cañas, A. J. (2000). A learning environment organizer for asynchronous distance learning systems. *In Proceedings of the Twelfth IASTED International Conference on Parallel and Distributed Computing and Systems, Las Vegas, NV. www.ihmc.us*

Daley, B. J., & Torre, D. M. (2010). Concept maps in medical education: An analytical literature review. *Medical Education, 44*(5), 440–448.

Dansereau, D. F., & Cross, D. R. (1990). *Knowledge mapping: Cognitive software for thinking, learning, and communicating.* Ft. Worth, TX: Department of Psychology, Texas Christian University.

Edmondson, K. M. (1994). *Concept mapping for the development of medical curricula.* Paper presented at the Annual Conference of the American Educational Research Association, Atlanta, GA. Retrieved from ERIC database (ED 360 322).

Ertmer, P. A., & Newby, T. J. (1993). Behaviorism, cognitivism, constructivism: Comparing critical features from an instructional design perspective. *Performance Improvement Quarterly, 6*(4), 50–72.

Felder, R. M. (1993). Reaching the second tier: Learning and teaching styles in college science education. *Journal of College Science Teaching, 23,* 286–290.

Feldsine, J.E. (1987). *The construction of concept maps facilitates the learning of general college chemistry: A case study.* PhD dissertation, Cornell University. Dissertation Information Service, Ann Arbor, MI.

Gagne, R. (1985). *The conditions of learning and theory of instruction* (4th ed.). New York, NY: Holt, Rinehart and Winston.

Gardner, H. (1983). *Frames of mind: The theory of multiple intelligences.* New York, NY: Basic Books.

Giddens, J. (2006). Concept mapping as a group learning activity in graduate nursing education. *Journal of Nursing Education, 45*(1), 45–46.

Glynn, S. M., Yeany, R. H., & Britton, B. K. (1991). A constructive view of learning science. In S. M. Glynn, R. H. Yeany, & B. K. Britton (Eds.), *The psychology of learning science* (pp. 3–20). Hillsdale, NJ: Lawrence Erlbaum Assoc.

Gonzalez, H. L., Palencia, A. P., Umana, L. A., Galindo, L., & Villafrade, M. L. A. (2008). Mediated learning experience and concept maps: A pedagogical tool for achieving meaningful learning in medical physiology students. *Advances in Physiology and Education, 32*(4), 312–316.

Griffiths, A. K., Thomey, K., Cooke, B., & Normore, G. (1988). Remediation of student-specific misconceptions relating to three science concepts. *Journal of Research in Science Teaching, 25*(9), 709–719.

Heinze-Fry, J. A., & Novak, J. D. (1990). Concept mapping brings long-term movement toward meaningful learning. *Science Education, 74*(4), 461–472.

Hicks-Moore, S. L. (2005). Clinical concept maps in nursing education: An effective way to link theory and practice. *Nurse Education Practice, 5*, 348–352.

Hicks-Moore, S. L., & Pastirik, P. J. (2006). Evaluating critical thinking in clinical concept maps: A pilot study. *International Journal of Nursing Education Scholarship, 3*, Article 27.

Hinck, S. M., Webb, P., Sims-Giddens, S., Helton, C., Hope, K. L., Utley, R., ... Yarbrough, S. (2006). Student learning with concept mapping of care plans in community-based education. *Journal of Professional Nursing, 22*(1), 23–29.

Hsu, L., & Hsieh, S. I. (2005). Concept maps as an assessment tool in a nursing course. *Journal of Professional Nursing, 21*(3), 141–149.

Hunter-Revell, S. M. (2012). Concept maps and nursing theory: A pedagogical approach. *Nurse Educator, 37*(3), 131–135.

Kolb, A. Y., & Kolb, D. A. (2005). Learning styles and learning spaces: Enhancing experiential learning in higher education. *Academy of Management Learning & Education, 4*(2), 193–212.

Laight, D. W. (2004). Attitudes to concept maps as a teaching/learning activity in undergraduate health professional education: Influence of preferred learning style. *Medical Teacher, 26*(3), 229–233.

Mahler, S., Hoz, R., Fischl, D., Tov-Ly, E., & Lernau, O. Z. (1991). Didactic use of concept mapping in higher education: Applications in medical education. *International Sciences, 20*, 25–47.

Markham, K. M., Mintzes, J. J., & Jones, M. G. (1994). The concept map as a research and evaluation tool: Further evidence of validity. *Journal of Research in Science Teaching, 31*(1). 91–101.

Novak, J. D. (1990). Concept mapping: A useful tool for science education. *Journal of Research in Science Teaching, 27*, 937–949.

Novak, J. D. (2003, Summer). The promise of new ideas and new technology for improving teaching and learning. *Cell Biology Education, 2*, 122–132.

Novak, J. D., & Cañas, A. J. (2008). *The theory underlying concept maps and how to construct them.* Technical report. IHMC CmapTools 2008-01, Florida Institute for Human and Machine Cognition. Retrieved from http://cmap.ihmc.us/Publications/ResearchPapers/TheoryUnderlyingConceptMaps.pdf

Novak, J. D., & Gowin, D. B. (1984). *Learning how to learn.* New York, NY: Cambridge University Press.

Novak J. D., Gowin D. B., & Johansen, G. T. (1983). The use of concept mapping and knowledge vee mapping with junior high school science students. *Science Education, 67*(5), 625–645.

Novak, J. D., & Wandersee, J. H. (1990). Perspectives on concept mapping. *Journal of Research in Science Teaching, 27*(10), 921–1075.

Passmore, G. G. (1995). Constructing concept maps facilitates learning in radiologic technologies education. *Radiologic Science and Education, 2*(2), 50–59.

Passmore, G. G. (1996). *The effects of Gowin's vee heuristic diagramming and concept mapping on meaningful learning in the radiation science classroom and laboratory.* Doctoral dissertation, University of Missouri, Columbia, MO.

Passmore, G. G. (1998). Using vee diagrams to facilitate meaningful learning and misconception remediation in radiologic technologies laboratory education. *Radiologic Science and Education, 4*(1), 11–28.

Passmore, G. J. (2004). Extending the power of the concept map. *Alberta Journal of Educational Research, 50*(4), 370–390.

Passmore, G. G. (2008). *Concept mapping construction: Meaningful learning activity and assessment tool. A report on the empirical evidence.* Multimedia Educational Resource for Learning and Online Teaching—MERLOT Tegrity presentation, learning materials category. Retrieved from http://www.merlot.org/merlot/viewMaterial.htm?id=317905

Passmore, G. G., Owen, M. A., & Prabakaran, K. (2011). Empirical evidence of the effectiveness of concept mapping as a learning intervention for nuclear medicine technology students in a distance learning radiation protection and biology course. *Journal of Nuclear Medicine Technology, 39*, 284–289.

Pinto, A. J., & Zeitz, H. J. (1997). Concept mapping. A strategy for promoting meaningful learning in medical education. *Medical Teacher, 19*(2), 114–122.

Prankratius, W. J. (1990). Building an organized knowledge base: Concept mapping and achievement in secondary school physics. *Journal of Research inScience Teaching, 27*(4). 315-333.

Preszler, R. W. (2004) Cooperative concept mapping improves performance in biology. *Journal of College Science Teaching, 33*, 30–35

Regan-Smith, M. G., Obenshain, S. S., Woodward, C., Richards, B., Zeitz, H. J., & Small, P. A. Jr. (1994). Rote learning in medical school. *Journal of the American Medical Association, 272*, 1380– 1381.

Rendas, A. B., Fonseca, M., & Rosado-Pinto, P. (2006). Toward meaningful learning in undergraduate medical education using concept maps in a PBL pathophysiology course. *Advances in Physiology Education, 30*, 23–29.

Renner, J. W., Abraham, M. R., Grzybowski, E. B., & Marek, E. A. (1990). Understandings and misunderstandings of eighth graders of four physics concepts fund in textbooks. *Journal of Research in Science Teaching, 27*(1), 35–54.

Roth, W. M. (1990). Map your way to a better lab. *The Science Teacher, 57*(4), 31–34.

Roth, W. M., & Roychoudhury, A. (1993). Using vee and concept maps in collaborative settings: Elementary education majors construct meaning in physical science courses. *School Science and Mathematics, 93*(5), 237–244.

Safayeni, F., Derbentseva, N., & Cañas, A. J. (2005). A theoretical note on concepts and the need for cyclic concept maps. *Journal of Research in Science Teaching, 42*(7), 741–766.

Starr, M. L., & Krajcik, J. S. (1990). Concept maps as a heuristic for science curriculum development: Toward improvement in process and product. *Journal of Research in Science Teaching, 27*(10), 987–1000.

Trowbride, J. E., & Wandersee, J. H. (1994). Identifying critical junctures in learning a college course on evolution. *Journal of Research in Science Teaching, 31*(5), 459–473.

Wallace, J. D., & Mintzes, J. J. (1990). The concept map as a research tool: Exploring conceptual change in biology. *Journal of Research in Science Teaching, 27*(10), 1033–1052.

Wandersee, J. H., Mintzes, J. J., & Novak, J. D. (1994). Research on alternative conceptions in science. In D. Gabel (Ed.), *Handbook of research on science teaching and learning* (pp. 177–203). Washington, DC: National Science Teachers Association.

Weiss, L. B., & Levison, S. P. (2000). Tools for integrating women's health into medical education: Clinical cases and concept mapping. *Academic Medicine, 75*(1), 1081–1086.

West, D. C., Park, J. K., Pomeroy, J. R., & Sandoval, J. (2002). Concept mapping assessment in medical education: A comparison of two scoring systems. *Medical Education, 36*, 820–826.

West, D. C., Pomeroy, J. R., Park, J. K., Gerstenberger, E. A., & Sandoval, J. (2000). Critical thinking in graduate medical education: A role for concept mapping assessment? *Journal of the American Medical Association, 284*, 1105–1110.

Wheeler, L. A., & Collins, S. K. R. (2003). The influence of concept mapping on critical thinking in baccalaureate nursing students. *Journal of Professional Nursing, 19*(6), 339–346.

CHAPTER 26

The Preceptored Clinical Experience

■ BRIAN M. FRENCH AND MIRIAM GREENSPAN ■

The preceptored clinical experience provides an opportunity for students, new graduate clinicians, experienced clinicians new to a work setting or practice area, or others to work with an experienced staff member to begin socialization and role transition, as well as gain exposure to the healthcare arena. This experiential teaching and learning methodology provides clear benefits to the learner, preceptor, school, and healthcare setting.

■ Definition and Purposes

In 15th-century England, the word *preceptor* was first used to identify a tutor or instructor. The term first appeared in the nursing literature in the mid-1970s (Peirce, 1991). The more recent use of the term *preceptorship* denotes an experience lasting a designated period of time, during which an experienced clinician or preceptor enters into a one-on-one relationship with a novice clinician learner (the student, preceptee, or orientee) to assist the novice in the transition from learner to practitioner (Baggot, Hensinger, Parry, Valdes, & Zaim, 2005; Benner, Tanner, & Chesla, 1996; Marcum & West, 2004; O'Malley, Cunliffe, Hunter, & Breeze, 2000). The preceptorship is a process during which the preceptor, through role modeling, information sharing, coaching, and direction, teaches the preceptee the art of professional practice. The precepted clinical experience is a planned and organized instructional program with specific objectives and goals. It can be useful in supporting the learning process of students at all levels during a clinical, management, education, or research practicum. Other uses include orienting new graduate clinicians or experienced clinicians transferring between clinical areas. Visitors to the clinical area, such as clinicians from another country seeking exposure to the U.S. healthcare system and roles, can also benefit from being precepted.

Student precepted experiences typically take place within a capstone clinical course during the later part of the curriculum. Such a course might be designed to promote synthesis of theoretical knowledge, allow for more in-depth study of a specific patient population, and apply evidenced-based research to the clinical practice area. In addition, preceptors can assist students to demonstrate leadership and collaborative skills and provide experiences to enhance understanding of organizational behavior as well as ethical, legal, economic, and political issues.

Preceptorship is often used as a way of facilitating the role transition of novice clinicians. Preceptorship can also be used as a methodology for orienting experienced clinicians who are new to a particular patient population or institutional setting. This offers the clinician learner the opportunity to apply previously acquired knowledge in an experiential manner while safely accumulating new knowledge and experiences for future reference (Benner et al., 1996). During the preceptorship, a partnership in which both the preceptor and the preceptee contribute to the outcome is formed (Godinez, Schweiger, Gruver, & Ryan, 1999; O'Malley et al., 2000). The partnership becomes an ongoing mutual exchange between the preceptor and the learner, in a mutually trusting, supportive environment. The preceptor offers information, direction, and feedback, and the preceptee offers insight about personal goals, learning needs, and learning styles. During the preceptorship both the student and the graduate clinician learn the rules, language, and behaviors of the work environment (Godinez et al., 1999; Horsburgh, 1989; O'Malley et al., 2000; Tradewell, 1996).

The preceptored experience differs from spend-the-day shadowing experiences or informal pairing relationships that are typically geared toward providing a broad exposure to the healthcare environment or toward promoting individual career awareness or understanding of the clinician role. It also differs from the mentor–mentee experience, which is generally a long-term relationship designed to promote career growth and development and may be mutually supportive and collaborative in nature (Alspach, 2000).

The preceptorship is the opportune time for the novice to be socialized into the new work setting. In the case of students, it may be the first exposure to the roles, responsibilities, and accountabilities of the clinician role. For the graduate clinician, the preceptorship serves as a period of transition from the role of student to that of professional. The experienced clinician moving into a new work setting also requires assistance with socialization and must adjust previous experiences to fit into the new work setting with new rules, new languages, and new patient populations.

■ Theoretical Foundations

Socialization has been defined as the passing of a role from one person to the next, the process by which a person acquires and internalizes new knowledge and skills (Horsburgh, 1989; Santucci, 2004; Tradewell, 1996). Socialization enables the transition from previous roles to new roles and from familiar to unfamiliar work environments. Tradewell also states that socialization occurs through observing the preceptor role model behaviors and language as well as by exposure to incumbent staff as they reflect on their practice through stories of their own work experiences.

Santucci states that the socialization period involves the learning of work systems, staff roles, and employer expectations for students and new employees alike. The preceptor informs, guides, and supports the clinician in navigating the social mores of the workplace and applying knowledge gained from past clinical and classroom experiences to the technologic and physiologic aspects of patient care in the new setting.

During this period, preceptees may experience a loss of confidence in their abilities to perform skills and think critically. For experienced clinicians entering a new practice arena, the loss of their self-confidence is particularly difficult. In their previous work setting, they have been capable, experienced practitioners, relying on past experiences and intuition to function effectively. They were comfortable in their practice and felt knowledgeable about the expectations of the work environment, resources, and sources of support. In the new work environment, their self-image has changed as they find themselves unsure of how to behave or practice and lacking in knowledge regarding resources and support systems. This unfamiliarity engenders a self-image or vision that is difficult to accept, even if the period is transient.

During the transition, the preceptee begins to leave behind previously learned beliefs and behaviors and integrates new standards and expectations into his or her practice. Kramer (1974) described this difficult process as reality shock, a period in which the learner begins to recognize differences and inconsistencies in the new environment in comparison to the old environment. Students transitioning to the professional role are exposed to the realities and contradictions of the real world, as compared to the known and ordered world of academia. The preceptee may question the value of what was learned as well as the ethics of what is observed in the workplace. Finding a balance and learning to mesh the academic and work environments in a way that is acceptable for the learner may be difficult and emotionally stressful as familiar support and social systems are left behind. The work of learning, performing in a new role, balancing new and old roles, and making meaning of new work is an exhausting process that requires high-energy consumption by the learner and significant support from the preceptor.

Communication and feedback are the backbone of the preceptor–preceptee relationship. Open, honest, compassionate, and timely feedback is valued by the preceptee. Such communication requires mutual trust and respect. While it takes time to develop this trust, the reality of the preceptorship experience is that it is of the moment, existing only within a limited time frame. It is critical that an initial meeting between the learner and the preceptor include a discussion of their past experiences, expectations, and goals for the relationship, and personal, work, learning, teaching, and communication styles. This conversation sets the stage for a successful, sharing relationship.

The preceptor is called on to be teacher, counselor, and clinician to guide the preceptee through this complex transition (O'Malley et al., 2000). A safe, supportive, and informative environment is vital during this period (Goh & Watt, 2003). While the key relationships are between preceptor and preceptee, supportive faculty and unit staff are critical. Faculty, managers, and clinical specialists must meet with preceptors to describe the course or orientation program objectives and enlist the assistance of other staff as necessary to assist in designing the preceptorship. In this way, there is an investment and support for the program from the beginning. Consideration should be given to the kind of support that will be provided to the preceptors throughout the experience. Support can be in the form of public acknowledgment of their work, scheduled meetings with the preceptor to ascertain whether assistance is needed or with the preceptor and preceptee to discuss progress, support for the types of assignments the preceptor selects, and possible schedule adjustments for the preceptor to enhance the learning experience.

■ Types of Learners

Whether the individual involved in the precepted experience is a student, new graduate, experienced clinician, or a temporary visitor, he or she is an adult learner who actively participates on some level in the identification of individual learning needs and designing or choosing learning experiences intended to meet those needs. The precepted experience takes place in a complex and dynamic clinical environment with the preceptor facilitating the learning. The experience is enhanced by learners who exhibit well-developed adult learning characteristics. This includes an independent self-concept, willingness to freely share their life experiences with others, active engagement in the process to meet learning goals, an openness to learning opportunities regardless of when they occur in the experience, and a problem-centered approach to learning.

■ Conditions for Learning

The two most commonly named goals for the preceptored learning experience reported in the literature include the facilitation of socialization into the work setting and role transition from student to graduate clinician or from newly hired orientee to staff member (Gaberson & Oermann, 1999; Guhde, 2005; Smith & Chalker 2005). Gaberson and Oermann also reported benefits for students in terms of the ability to integrate classroom theoretical knowledge with actual clinical practice within a healthcare organization. In addition, the preceptor has the ability to provide individualized attention and guidance to the learner and improve the learner's clinical competence and confidence. The schools also benefit from preceptored experiences because students have less dependence on faculty because preceptors serve in the educator role. In this way, a faculty member can more effectively manage a group of students through collaborative relationships with preceptors.

From the organizational perspective, student-preceptored clinical rotations may assist in meeting mission statement goals, such as a commitment to educating future clinicians. In addition, preceptorships may facilitate recruitment of employees because the learner has a relationship within the organization and is exposed to the workplace and staff. The supportive relationship between an orientee and a preceptor may also impact new employee recruitment, job satisfaction, and retention rates (Casey, Fink, Krugman, & Propst, 2004; Gaberson & Oermann, 1999).

■ Resources

Although the preceptored experience may take place in any organization that delivers health care, it is important to ensure that the clinical environment matches the goals of the experience from either the course and student or the program and orientee perspective. The length of the experience is dependent on the goals to be achieved. In short, the experience can be of any length but must be long enough to provide the varied clinical exposure and experiences to ensure achievement of course or orientation objectives.

Whether it is a student or orientee experience, the preceptor and learner will benefit from contact and guidance from a faculty member or organization-based educator, clinical specialist, or manager. Preceptors should have access to a student's goals and objectives or an orientee's competency checklist to facilitate planning, track achievements, and evaluate performance.

Organizations that provide clinical placements to student clinicians require qualified staff to precept. In addition, they require qualified staff to precept new or transferring employees. Depending on the staff mix in a given clinical area, there may not be an adequate supply of interested, committed, and educationally prepared staff to serve in the preceptor role, and this could be a limiting factor for the number of students or new hires a unit or department is able to absorb. This is particularly true if the unit or department also welcomes groups of students and a clinical instructor at the same time, thus creating competition for patient assignments. Staff may view the role of preceptor and the teaching and evaluation responsibilities as added work, and this may also limit the number of students or orientees for a given clinical area. All of these scenarios require commitment on the part of the unit or department manager, clinical specialists, educators, and faculty to create a learning environment that supports staff throughout the process so that they are prepared to serve and feel valued in their role as preceptor.

Recognition for clinicians who are preceptors can take many forms. Schools may appoint preceptors to adjunct faculty status, provide access to continuing education programs, provide certificates of appreciation or recognition receptions, and, in some cases, offer vouchers for free or reduced tuition for selected courses. Although these recognition and reward efforts may have a budgetary impact on the academic institution, benefits may also be realized through recruitment of preceptors to enroll in academic programs. Healthcare organizations may or may not provide similar incentives for staff who are preceptors, including certificates of appreciation, preceptor awards, luncheons, less off-shift or weekend scheduling, lighter than usual patient assignments, or pay differentials. Again, these methods of recognizing staff for their role as preceptor may have a budget impact but may also encourage staff to participate in this key role and contribute to job satisfaction and retention through recognition of their hard work. Speers, Strzyzewski, and Ziolkowski (2004) report that nonmaterial benefits had greater relative importance for staff in their decision to serve in the preceptor role.

■ Using the Method

Under the guidance of an experienced clinician preceptor, the student or novice clinician begins to apply the knowledge and theory learned in the classroom to the reality of patient care and begins to transition from learner to professional. It is equally important that the environment is one in which the novice feels safe enough to ask questions and take risks. Having clear expectations for the precepting experience for both the preceptor and the novice further contributes to a successful experience. Faculty should review the goals prior to the experience if the novice is a student. If the novice is a new graduate clinician or an experienced clinician new to a particular work setting, he or she should come with expectations for the precepting experience and be prepared to discuss them with the preceptor. The preceptor, working with unit-based leadership, should also develop a set of goals and expectations for the precepting experience. During the initial meeting between the preceptor and the preceptee, goals and expectations for the experience should be shared and reworked into a mutually agreed-upon plan with time frames for achievement.

The preceptor is the key to the success of this experience. When designing the precepting experience, time and attention should be paid to the selection, preparation, and ongoing support of the preceptor. Attention should also be given to the roles and responsibilities of the learner, the clinical faculty, and the unit leadership in this learning experience.

The Preceptor

Precepting requires an individual who is committed to nurturing and teaching the next generation of professionals, someone who is both caring and clinically competent. On occasion, preceptors are selected based on their availability, convenience, and clinical abilities, but an outstanding clinician does not always translate into a skillful preceptor. There are four criteria for selecting a qualified preceptor. The first criterion in selecting a preceptor should be the clinician's interest in and willingness to assume the role in addition to his or her patient care responsibilities.

The second criterion is ensuring a positive relationship between the preceptor and the preceptee. The relationship must include trust and understanding if learning is to take place. Factors that can facilitate this trusting relationship include ensuring that the preceptor reviews written goals and objectives for the experience to facilitate upfront planning; reviewing preceptor and preceptee expectations for communication, behavior, and timelines for goal achievement; and providing time for meetings for discussion, reflection, and feedback throughout the experience. Other factors that may influence the relationship include involving the potential preceptor in the interview process for a new staff member and having a manager or clinical specialist choose a preceptor who matches the perceptions of the preceptee based on his or her knowledge of both individuals, including such factors as communication, learning, and teaching styles.

Clinical knowledge, skill, and ability are the components of the third criterion for choosing an ideal preceptor. A practitioner with a depth of understanding of the patient population and a high level of technical skill is necessary when selecting a preceptor. Benner and colleagues (1996) state that the competent practitioner often provides the best guidance for the new clinician. The competent practitioner is adept at assessing and diagnosing patient needs in a step-by-step fashion. This attention to detail and use of a logical and orderly process is useful when teaching the student or novice practitioner. Proficient, expert clinicians have a breadth of knowledge and intuition not possessed by the competent practitioner, but their skill often proves to be too abstract for the novice and therefore may not be the best choice to serve as a preceptor. As a task-focused learner, the novice is comfortable with the concrete precepts of the competent practitioner.

The ability to listen and communicate with respect describes the fourth criterion for the preceptor. During the transition from student or orientee to practitioner, the amount of new information, new experiences, and new responsibilities may be overwhelming. Students and orientees may experience a range of emotions from excitement and eagerness to anger and frustration during the transition period. The preceptor will need to be attuned to these reactions and adapt the learning experience accordingly. To manage this, the preceptor will need to be able to listen closely and assess the needs of the preceptee, much as the preceptor assesses the needs of the patient.

The preceptor's role will be multifaceted. As teacher and guide, the preceptor will be introducing the novice to clinical practice (Godinez et al., 1999). In the first meeting between preceptor and preceptee, the preceptor will discuss the goals for the precepting experience. The preceptor will also determine the preceptee's learning needs and learning style. This can be done by simply asking how the preceptee learns best (e.g., visual, auditory, audiovisual, verbal, or kinesthetic) or through a more formal assessment process using any of a number of standardized tools such as Kolb's learning style inventory (Kolb, 2005; Kolb & Kolb, 2005).

Role modeling patient care skills from interpersonal interactions to assessment and diagnosis, and finally to intervention and evaluation, will be the initial primary method of teaching. Ongoing explanations for each action will inform the learner of the reasons for the choices the preceptor makes. In addition to modeling practice at the bedside, the preceptor will model skills in communication with the interdisciplinary team involved in patient care, as well as with the patient and family.

In the early phase of the precepted experience, the novice will observe and listen to the preceptor role model. As the experience progresses, the role of the preceptor will move to teacher, as the preceptor instructs the learner in providing direct patient care, using technology, interacting with the multidisciplinary team, and accessing the resources available within the work environment.

The preceptor will spend time coaching the preceptee by role playing interactions before they occur. For instance, the preceptor may have the preceptee practice reviewing the plan for participating in patient care rounds before they occur or giving a clinician-to-clinician report before the shift ends. The skill of the preceptor will be called into action, including knowing when to hover close by the preceptee as he or she provides direct care and knowing when to allow the learner to practice independently. As the patient dynamic changes, so will the choices the preceptor makes relative to the autonomy of the novice. When the patient's condition is acute or changes unexpectedly, the preceptor will work closely with the learner as he or she provides care, makes assessments, and plans with other members of the healthcare team. When the patient is well known to the preceptor and learner, with a stable or improved condition, the preceptor may choose to review the care plan with the learner and then observe and evaluate the learner's ability to implement the plan.

Along with the responsibility for teaching at the bedside, the preceptor must introduce and socialize the preceptee to the work environment to assist in the transition from student or orientee to professional clinician. It is incumbent upon the preceptor to introduce the preceptee to the culture of the unit, the values of the staff, the formal and informal roles occupied by members of the staff, and the formal and informal rules by which the unit functions. Preceptors will need to explain basics such as how the schedule works and how to manage the hospital's communication system, as well as how to cope with the realities of the healthcare environment. The preceptor becomes a guide to the learner who has left behind familiar environments and support systems and must form a new and stable base on which to grow as a clinician.

When working with new clinicians, the preceptor, with support from unit leadership, should attempt to carve out some time for reflection. While this is challenging in today's fast-paced clinical environment, it does serve several important purposes. Time away from the clamor of the unit allows the preceptor and learner to review the patient experience and to discuss in greater depth how and why specific patient care decisions were made. Perhaps most importantly, this time provides a safe space for the learner to reflect on his or her own thoughts and feelings about what has occurred with the patient and how he or she has performed. Through these discussions, the relationship between preceptor and preceptee is built, trust is developed, and communication is enhanced. This is vital for later discussions as the pair evaluate the success of the practicum or process of orientation and each person's behavior in the process. Most likely, students will be familiar with this time for reflection, as this is common practice in an instructor-led clinical practicum.

The Preceptee

The preceptee is an active participant in the precepting experience and must assume a leadership role in ensuring the success of the experience. In addition to the initial sharing of goals for the experience, the learner is responsible for informing the preceptor when the goals are not being met, when new lessons are not clear, or when he or she is uncomfortable performing a new skill. Feedback from the learner helps the preceptor adapt and adjust the experience in a meaningful way that leads to a successful outcome. Without feedback, the preceptor will only be making assumptions that may not always be correct. The learner is also accountable for following through on the suggestions and recommendations made by the preceptor. This may include practicing a skill, researching an unfamiliar aspect of clinical care, or reading a suggested article or chapter about a particular patient condition.

The Faculty and Unit Leadership

A strong collaborative partnership between academic faculty and service providers, including both unit leadership and staff, is a critical factor in ensuring a successful experience for students (Corlett, Palfreyman, Staines, & Marr, 2003). The role played by faculty and unit leadership will vary depending on the level of experience of both the preceptor and the preceptee. If the preceptor is new to the role, then the faculty or unit leadership will play a mentoring role in the process and may need to provide more guidance to ensure success. As the preceptor gains experience in the role, faculty and unit leadership may need to meet with the preceptor and preceptee only occasionally to monitor the process or consult on more complex issues that the preceptor is unable to solve independently. Regardless of the experience level of the preceptor, faculty or unit leadership must maintain open communication and monitor the experience on some level to ensure objectives are met and intervene if there are issues that arise in the preceptor–preceptee relationship. Such support can be offered in direct discussions that occur periodically throughout the preceptorship or by phone or e-mail when specific questions or concerns arise.

Evaluating the Preceptored Clinical Experience

Ideally, evaluation should be a formative and ongoing process, part of the daily communication between preceptor and preceptee. Discussion and feedback about skill performance, assessment and diagnosis, and bedside interactions should be part of the regular communication of each day. By incorporating this process into the routine of the day, it becomes a respectful, helpful activity and one that moves the precepting experience continuously forward. Competency-based tools, timelines, or lists of objectives can serve as valuable guidelines for such discussions. If goals have been set at the beginning of the precepting experience, discussion can be based on how closely the experience has come to meeting those goals. Asking simple questions such as "How do you think you performed today?" "Is there anything you would do differently?" and "How close are we to reaching each goal?" provide a basis for self-reflection and allow the preceptor to evaluate the learner's understanding of his or her performance. The preceptor can then compare his or her assessment of the preceptee's performance with the learner's self-assessment and provide constructive feedback to support or improve the preceptee's performance. If only summative evaluation is used to evaluate the precepting experience, the learner will not benefit from the preceptor's suggestions and recommendations since it has not been provided in a time-sensitive or event-sensitive manner. As the orientation is nearing the end of its prescribed timeline, the burden of evaluating the orientee becomes more acute. Many schools and clinical units have created evaluation tools that consider the preceptor's actions, the preceptee's actions, or both. In addition, both the American Association for Critical-Care Nurses (AACN) and the Center for Nurse Executives have used survey data and focus groups to determine lists of core competencies (Berkow, Virksis, Stewart, & Conway, 2009; Hickey, 2009). Important generic competencies identified in these documents include basic knowledge application, assessment, technical skill attainment, time management, critical thinking, and communication. For the new clinician, such tools most often follow a competency-based format that covers the various aspects of caring for a particular patient population, including skill acquisition, problem solving, and decision making. For the student, tools generally focus on goal attainment and the overall clinical experience, including the effectiveness of the preceptor. Preceptors may use a self-evaluation model focusing on the various aspects of the preceptor role or they may receive feedback from the preceptee, faculty, or unit leadership using a more inclusive method.

Faculty or unit leaders should participate in the evaluation process periodically during the precepting experience. They can offer objective insight into the progress being made and recommendations gleaned from their expertise in patient care and teaching. They can also serve as role models and support the preceptor in handling more complex feedback issues that might occur during the precepting experience. Preceptors take their role very seriously and may feel they are solely responsible for the outcome of the experience. Indicators for lack of readiness for independent practice have been identified through focus groups and individual interviews. Preceptors have listed a lack of basic knowledge, followed by the inability to perform frequently taught and demonstrated skills, as the most concerning general indicators of a preceptee's lack of readiness for practice; specific behaviors that raise red flags include an inability to develop organizational skills, an apparent lack of interest in engaging with patients, and an unwillingness to participate in self-reflection or critical self-assessment (Luhanga, Yonge, & Myrick, 2008; Modic & Harris, 2007). Active and timely faculty or unit leadership involvement will help the preceptor manage some of the perceived burden of the preceptor's sense of responsibility for the outcome of the experience.

▪ Potential Problems

For a successful partnership to develop, consistent, interested, capable preceptors are necessary (Boychuck-Duchsher, 2001; Boyle, Popkess-Vawter, & Taunton, 1996; Casey et al., 2004; Oermann & Moffitt-Wolfe, 1997). On the other side of the equation, there must be an engaged, participative preceptee (O'Malley et al., 2000).

The challenges described by students and new graduates during this transition include being able to set priorities and organize patient care needs, acquiring time management skills, fearing communication with physicians, lacking confidence in their performance, and struggling with dependence and independence in the preceptor–preceptee relationship (Casey et al., 2004; Oermann & Moffitt-Wolfe, 1997). The issue of independent practice is a dilemma for preceptors as well as preceptees. Knowing when to allow the preceptee to practice more independently or when to step in and actively guide and participate in the patient care is subjective and varies from moment to moment. An event that can be handled by a preceptee in one instance may require the direct involvement of the preceptor in another case because of the impact of individual patient characteristics. This seeming inconsistency in preceptor behavior may contribute to the preceptee's issues of confidence and highlights the need for open, honest communication between preceptor and preceptee.

Potential problems can arise in the preceptorial experience because of factors related to the preceptor, the learner, or the process. The importance of formal training in preparing a staff member to function effectively as a preceptor is well documented in the literature (Alspach, 2000; Neumann et al., 2004; Speers et al., 2004). Although clinicians chosen to be preceptors are typically well prepared to care for their patients, to be effective as staff preceptors they must also be knowledgeable regarding the principles of adult education and adult learning, learning styles, planning and implementing learning experiences, reality shock, and the principles of evaluation and providing constructive feedback. Faculty, managers, clinical specialists, and staff educators must provide opportunities for advanced education in these areas to adequately prepare clinicians to serve in their assigned role and to maximize the potential success of the preceptor–preceptee relationship and achieve a positive outcome. In addition, staff preceptors should have periodic contact with faculty and their managers, clinical specialists, and educators throughout the preceptorship to enhance communication, problem solve, and continue their development as preceptors through evaluative feedback of their performance. For preceptors, the sense of responsibility they feel for the experience extends beyond the clinical teaching that occurs. They often feel responsible for diagnosing and resolving all problems that occur, even those that are beyond their scope to manage. Frequent involvement of faculty or unit leadership helps to establish a relationship in which the preceptor feels comfortable sharing concerns and seeking an expert's advice.

Learners must receive clear, upfront communication regarding their responsibility for the learning process, achievement of outcomes, preceptor expectations, and what they can expect of their preceptor as well as practical issues such as adhering to assigned schedules and completion of assignments. This helps avoid misunderstandings about their role as learner and the goals of the experience. It also removes the primary responsibility for the success of the experience from the preceptor and ensures that the preceptee is aware of his or her accountability for successful outcomes.

Beyond preparation of both preceptor and learner, other issues internal to the individual must be considered as affecting the relationship. There are many potential causes for perceived or real personality conflicts between a preceptor and a preceptee, but many can arise when there is a clash of values and beliefs that can occur between different age groups. The need to manage generational issues in the workplace is well documented in the literature (Gerke, 2001; Weston, 2001). Differing worldviews, personal motivating factors, preferred work environments, perceptions of work–life balance, and individual strengths and differences can create conflicts between a preceptor of one generation and a preceptee of another. Awareness and understanding of these different generational values, behaviors, and expectations is the first step in working toward a successful preceptor–preceptee relationship. Integration of this information into preceptor preparation programs is key to assisting with the teaching and learning challenges created by a multigenerational workforce.

Preparation of preceptors and preceptees requires a structure to support expected outcomes. Educational preparation of preceptors to serve in their role, orientation of learners as to what to expect in the clinical setting, written course or orientation program objectives, competency or skill checklists, articulated time frames for outcome achievement, appropriate matching of preceptor and learner, and appropriate scheduling and identification of resources to assist in the process are all aspects of a well-planned and organized preceptorship. Effective planning and creation of tools to support the process allow the preceptor and learner to focus on the learning process within the context of the busy clinical environment.

The acuity and pace of the current clinical environment provide unique challenges for the preceptor and the student or orientee. The preceptor is no longer serving in one role, that of caregiver and coordinator of care, but also fills the role of teacher of caregiving and care coordination (Alspach, 2000). The challenge of teaching while providing high-quality care requires the preceptor to balance these roles. Most often, the student or new orientee has less clinical knowledge and skill than the more experienced preceptor. The preceptor must consider the rights of the patients and adhere to the ethical standard of beneficence, the duty to help, to produce beneficial outcomes, or at least to do no harm within the context of the teaching and learning process (Gaberson & Oermann, 1999). Patients must be aware that a learner is involved in their care as part of informed consent, and preceptors should ensure that the learner has demonstrated the knowledge and skill to provide care safely prior to doing so independently. The challenge for the preceptor is to achieve not only the desired patient clinical outcomes but also the desired educational outcomes for the student or orientee. The preceptor's judgment must be used exquisitely to determine when a learner can provide care safely and learn safely to achieve both goals.

■ Conclusion

The preceptored clinical experience is a valuable teaching and learning methodology with clear benefits for academic institutions and healthcare organizations alike. Students and orientees who are in the preceptee role benefit from the real-world experience of seasoned clinical staff preceptors. Preceptors benefit by adding this credential to their experience and learning new and valuable teaching, communication, and evaluation skills. Planning and communication are the keys to ensuring a successful period of socialization and role transition for the preceptee.

TEACHING EXAMPLE:

New Graduate Critical Care Program

The new graduate critical care program (Mylott & Ciesielski, 2003; Mylott & Greenspan, 2005) is a 6-month orientation and continuing education program designed to develop and support baccalaureate-prepared new graduate registered nurses (RNs) in the acquisition of experiential nursing knowledge and the application of theory and research in the care of critically ill patients. The program takes place at Massachusetts General Hospital. Using Benner's (1984) and Benner and colleagues' (1996) concepts explicating the development of novice nursing practice, the program combines participative and reflective didactic sessions with a preceptored clinical practicum in the intensive care unit of hire. Preceptor development is facilitated through group workshops and individual consultation as requested. Eight intensive care units participate in the program, including medical, surgical/trauma, cardiac surgery, neurological, pediatric, burn, postanesthesia, and coronary care. A team of central and unit-based critical care nurse directors, clinical nurse specialists, educators, and human resources staff meet regularly to provide program oversight and development.

The majority of participants complete the program within the allotted time. Formal didactic instruction is completed within 5 months, and the last month is class free to allow for immersion in practice. This approach serves as a transition period to full professional responsibility. This time frame is consistent with the literature on similar programs, and the nursing leadership believes that a 6-month orientation is needed for the new graduate to acquire the experiential knowledge and clinical skills to practice safely and independently. Preceptors and leadership believe that much of the variation in readiness to practice occurs in the last 2 months, when the work is largely about becoming an independent clinician.

PARTICIPANT CHARACTERISTICS

Through experience, the leadership group has identified several attributes that are associated with success. These attributes include experience working as a nursing assistant in critical care, passing the NCLEX RN licensing exam on the first attempt, and a committed desire to practice in critical care.

The average age of the program's new graduate nurse participants is 24.5 years, as compared with an average age of over 46.8 years for the general nursing population in the United States (U.S. Department of Health and Human Services [HHS], 2004). Implications for a growing proportion of younger nurses in the practice environment are described within the literature (Nursing Executive Center, 2002). In response, the program planners implemented a workshop on generational differences as an intervention to facilitate communication and the development of positive relationships between preceptors and new graduates that is delivered as needed (Tyrrell, 2005). Program evaluations of this workshop have been positive to date.

(continued)

To evaluate the professional development of the new graduate participants, e-mail surveys with questions targeted toward their achievements were sent to participants in the first four classes ($n = 24$) who were employed at the institution. An 88% response rate ($n = 21$) was achieved, and collated responses indicated that respondents had accomplished much professionally and were highly involved in professional development activities. In addition to the items cited in **Table 26-1**, five respondents had served as preceptors to subsequent new graduate program participants.

Table 26-1 Professional Development Survey Responses

Professional Development Indicators	*Affirmative Response (%)*	*Number*
Enrolled in graduate school	37	8
CVVH competent	94	20
Serves as unit resource nurse	59	12
Has passed CCRN exam or completed review course with intent to take exam	37	8
Clinical advancement program participation	10	2
Project Hope humanitarian effort participation	6	1

CCRN, critical care registered nurse; CVVH, continuous veno-venous hemofiltration.

CURRICULUM

The curriculum addresses the learning needs of both the new graduate preceptees and the experienced nurse preceptors. For the preceptees, a variety of learning options and supports are offered throughout the 6-month experience. The style of teaching is case based, including simulation, narrative, and discussion sessions. Topic areas cover pathophysiology encountered in critically ill children and adults and interventions for each illness discussed. Content focuses on managing the patient requiring mechanical ventilation as well as patients requiring close cardiac monitoring, invasive hemodynamic monitoring, and neurologic monitoring. Simulation sessions include respiratory distress and failure, shock, dysrhythmias with hemodynamic consequences, and cardiopulmonary arrests. These sessions require participants to work as a team to assess the patient, identify actual and potential problems, communicate and collaborate with various members of the healthcare team to identify and initiate interventions, and evaluate outcomes.

The preceptors are offered a workshop prior to participating in the program. The content includes new graduate behavior as described by Benner and colleagues (1996), teaching strategies, learning styles, communication and feedback skills, and interventions for precepting challenges. Techniques include simulation, case-based discussions, reflection, and role modeling. There is a panel discussion with experienced preceptors. Throughout the course of the 6-month program, preceptors are offered the opportunity to meet and discuss challenges with their peers.

The program's effectiveness is evaluated using a variety of measures. A focus group of preceptors and orientees is held in the fifth month to review the effectiveness from the participants' perspective. An evaluation tool is given to both preceptors and orientees to determine program effectiveness and areas in need of change. The tool's elements require both preceptors and orientees to evaluate the orientees' readiness to practice independently. In addition, both preceptors and orientees complete self-evaluations of how they fulfilled their program roles, as well as evaluate their partner's effectiveness in fulfilling program roles. Finally, a postprogram review of each orientee's capabilities is done using standards agreed to by the intensive care unit leadership. The standards include participants' ability to:

- Manage patients requiring invasive, closely monitored treatments such as continuous venous-to-venous hemodialysis.
- Serve as a resource nurse responsible for managing the flow of patients and staff during a work shift.
- Function as a program preceptor within 2 years of program completion.

NEW GRADUATE IN CRITICAL CARE PRECEPTOR NARRATIVE

The following is an adaptation of a narrative written by an experienced staff nurse preceptor (Albert, 2004). It describes the events of a typical day spent orienting a new graduate nurse participating in Massachusetts General Hospital's new graduate critical care program. The narrative was submitted as part of a portfolio in support of the preceptor's nomination as the first Norman Knight Preceptor of Distinction award. Nominees are asked to submit a narrative that illustrates their abilities as a preceptor. The author of the narrative, Jennifer Albert, RN, BSN, a staff nurse in the surgical/trauma intensive care unit, received the award. Awardees receive funds to attend a graduate course of their choice or protected paid time to complete a course of study with a clinical nurse specialist in their area of interest. An annual ceremony is held to announce the award and is followed by a reception for the hospital community and invited guests. A plaque that describes the award's purpose and lists the names of awardees is prominently displayed on the first floor of the hospital. The names of the patient and preceptee used in the narrative have been changed to ensure anonymity.

I am a staff nurse in the surgical intensive care unit, where I have practiced for the past 7 years. My nursing career began in 1989, 6 months before graduating from nursing school. As part of my senior practicum, I spent 20 hours per week working one-on-one with an experienced nurse on the surgical/trauma floor. I was blessed with a preceptor who was warm and welcoming, patient and professional, and who, above all, had the desire to share her knowledge and expertise with me, the neophyte nurse. I credit this positive experience with my willingness to take the challenge of reciprocating 2 years later when I was approached about precepting a student nurse from my alma mater. I was a bit apprehensive, as I had no previous teaching experience. What I did have, however, was the desire to share my newly acquired knowledge and to make this a fulfilling experience for this student, just as had been done for me 2 years previously.

(continued)

Since my first experience in 1991, I have had the opportunity and privilege to serve as a preceptor for over a dozen nurses, all with varied levels of experience. My intent here is not to sound boastful, but rather grateful. For it is I who have truly been enriched both professionally and personally by each of these individuals whom I've had the opportunity to precept over the years.

Presently, I am nearing the halfway mark in a 6-month orientation process with my preceptee, Sue, a new graduate nurse enrolled in the critical care program. The narrative that follows is a glimpse into one of our days together.

Andy is a 39-year-old with a history of psoriasis who had presented to an outside hospital with diffuse erythema extending from his thigh to his ankle, fever, and worsening renal failure and mental status, despite having received a dose of IV antibiotics in that hospital the previous night. His symptoms were most likely the result of either renal failure or profound sepsis. He was transferred to our hospital for further evaluation, and his admitting diagnosis was necrotizing fasciitis. Andy would most likely be the most challenging and complex patient Sue had cared for thus far. Yet, as a preceptor, I knew the circumstances couldn't be more ideal because Sue had already had some exposure to this patient, as she had had the opportunity to observe his surgery, as well as participate in admitting him to our unit.

We assembled outside of Andy's room at 7:00 AM with the flow sheet to get report from the night nurse. I made the calculated, but hopefully inconspicuous decision to move my seat, so that I was sitting next to Sue so that she was sandwiched between the night nurse and me. A few years ago, it never would have occurred to me that where I sat during report had any relevance. Yet, one of my former orientees commented to me one day, "Have you ever noticed that during report they (the nurses giving report) tend to always address you?" Frankly, I had never made this observation, but as I watched over the next few months, it became apparent that this was indeed true. My colleagues had the tendency to talk directly to me, almost turning their backs toward my orientee at times. To prevent this, I began to position myself directly next to my orientee, so that there was no confusion and we were both being addressed during report.

We were told that Andy was started on drotrecogin alfa. Other critical pieces of data we received during report were that his platelet level had fallen to 40,000, his hematocrit was trending down, and his leg dressing, which had not been bloody during the night, was saturated with blood, only 1 hour after the surgeons had changed it.

We entered the room together and Sue began the morning routine of zeroing and leveling transducers, setting alarms, and checking drug doses and infusion rates. I noted, but chose to not yet verbalize my own observation, that there was heparin in all of the transducer bags. I quietly wondered if Sue had made the same observation, and if she had, would she make the connection that even this small amount of heparin could be contributing to Andy's thrombocytopenia and therefore needed to be removed from the transducers? Sue began a thorough physical assessment. Andy's neurological status was difficult to assess since he was heavily sedated.

Recalling that with previous patients we had shut off the propofol drip to get a more thorough exam, Sue questioned whether we should do this with Andy. Sue's ability to incorporate previous experiences was becoming evident and I supported her plan but cautiously reminded her about what had been relayed to us in report—that Andy became dyssynchronous with the ventilator and tended to drop his oxygen saturation when awake or undersedated. My role as preceptor was to help Sue anticipate this potential instability and I did so by questioning her about how she planned to react and which interventions she planned to employ if Andy became unstable. With an action plan in place, Sue moved ahead.

Having completed her physical exam, Sue discussed her findings and observations. She was particularly concerned and focused on the continued bleeding from Andy's leg. His dressing was saturated with blood. At that point in her orientation, Sue had no previous experience to draw on that would allow her to differentiate normal from excessive bleeding. I attempted to coax from her what she might expect to see in a patient who had lost significant blood volume by asking, "How might the patient's hemodynamic profile change?" "Which lab values would be of particular concern?" and "Which medications might be contributing to this ongoing bleeding?" Together we explored the answers, examining the most recent vital signs, interpreting the reading from the Swan Ganz catheter, and discussing the signs of hypovolemia. Lastly, I prompted Sue about the medication that might have been contributing to the patient's condition. She reviewed Andy's medication list but was unable to identify the two drugs that I found concerning. I suggested that she take a close look at the transducer bags. I immediately saw the smile go across her face as she identified her earlier oversight, even before actually looking at the bags. Sue removed the heparin from the transducers and I recommended that she take a 10-minute break to read about drotrecogin alfa, knowing that once she did, she would be able to identify my second concern—that this medication increases the risk of bleeding and is contraindicated with acute bleeding.

Sue was far enough along in her orientation that she had begun to take an active and participatory role in rounds. That day I took a backseat role and allowed her the primary role of interacting with the physicians during rounds. In preparation for this, I assisted her in generating a list of questions in regard to the bleeding that she might want to have answered or addressed. Rounds began and I stepped back into the patient's room, far enough away so that I could hear the discussion, yet not be directly involved in it. This allowed Sue the opportunity to independently interact with the physicians, while providing her with the security of knowing I was close by should she need my assistance. Following rounds, I had Sue reiterate the plan for the day, which she might have thought was redundant, but I needed to know she had extrapolated the correct information from rounds and that she was clear on how we were to proceed.

(continued)

UNBUNDLING THE NARRATIVE

Ms. Albert's narrative provides an insightful view into the thinking and practice of an expert preceptor. She chose to become a preceptor based on her own positive experience working with a caring and skilled preceptor, her wish to continue that experience for others, and finally her realization of the rewards of precepting through her own personal and professional sense of enrichment. Ms. Albert's passion for the role came through clearly in the course of the narrative.

The expertise of precepting is apparent from the way Ms. Albert introduced the patient she selected for the shift. She was thoughtful and goal directed in the choice of patient assignment and gave specific reasons for her selection. She also displayed her awareness of the level of acuity this patient presented and the challenge this would be for Sue, her preceptee. Ms. Albert's clinical expertise is woven throughout the narrative, as she was able to guide her preceptee while anticipating potential patient problems and possible interventions.

Ms. Albert described the importance of having a sharing, respectful relationship with a preceptee. When a preceptee she had worked with previously presented her with a critical observation regarding staff behavior toward preceptees during report, Ms. Albert felt compelled to followed up to confirm. This resulted in a decisive change in her personal placement during report, underscoring her openness as a preceptor. She mirrored this behavior later in the narrative when she described her placement in the background during rounds with the physician staff. Ms. Albert never left Sue completely alone but choreographed her presence such that it would not prevent other healthcare team members from treating the preceptee as the patient's nurse.

Ms. Albert's awareness of the new graduate's need for routine was clear as she described the daily regimen Sue must follow when starting the shift. She was constantly aware of the patient and his needs and was thinking many steps ahead of the preceptee, but allowed the preceptee time to think through and problem solve for herself. Rather than specifically telling Sue directly what to look for, she coached, provided clues, and asked thoughtful questions to guide her. In so doing, Ms. Albert taught and informed the preceptee while preparing her to begin her own critical thinking process. Ms. Albert used this process several times during the shift to help Sue identify actual and potential clinical issues and also to help her devise a plan for intervention. The tactic was also utilized to prepare Sue to participate in rounds with the healthcare team. Prepping the preceptee is another example of how an expert preceptor teaches and helps build the new graduate's self-confidence and self-esteem.

Finally, Ms. Albert was tuned into her preceptee's own needs. When she provided time for Sue to review drotrecogin alfa, she was aware of her preceptee's informational needs and also her need to step back and consider all that had occurred to that point in the day. The same held true when Ms. Albert reviewed the discussion from rounds that created an opportunity for Sue to not only review the care plan, but also to ask questions or clarify the points discussed. Finally, Ms. Albert was aware of how Sue might have felt about this process and was prepared to explain her reasons for engaging in such a manner.

Ms. Albert's narrative exemplifies the characteristics of an expert preceptor, starting with her commitment to precepting, extending through her own clinical expertise, and concluding with her ability to teach, coach, and guide her preceptee in a compassionate, respectful, yet structured manner.

REFERENCES

Albert, J. (2004). Preceptor narrative. *Caring Headlines, 1*, 4–5.

Alspach, J. G. (2000). *From staff nurse to preceptor: A preceptor development program. Instructor's manual* (2nd ed., pp. 11–13). Aliso Viejo, CA: American Association of Critical Care Nurses.

Baggot, D., Hensinger, B., Parry, J., Valdes, M. S., & Zaim, S. (2005). The new hire/preceptor experience: Cost-benefit analysis of one retention strategy. *Journal of Nursing Administration, 35*(3), 138–145.

Benner, P. (1984). *From novice to expert: Excellence and power in clinical nursing practice.* Upper Saddle River, NJ: Prentice Hall.

Benner, P., Tanner, C., & Chesla, C. (1996). Entering the field: Advanced beginner practice. In P. Benner, C. Tanner, & C. Chesla (Eds.), *Expertise in nursing practice: Caring, clinical judgment, and ethics* (pp. 48–77). New York, NY: Springer.

Berkow, S., Virkstis, K., Stewart, J., & Conway, L. (2009). Assessing new graduate nurse performance. *Nurse Educator, 34*(1), 17–22.

Boychuck-Duchsher, J. (2001). Out in the real world: Newly graduated nurses in acute-care speak out. *Journal of Nursing Administration, 31*(9), 426–439.

Boyle, D. K., Popkess-Vawter, S., & Taunton, R. L. (1996). Socialization of new graduate nurses in critical care. *Heart and Lung, 25*(2), 141–154.

Casey, K., Fink, R., Krugman, M., & Propst, J. (2004). The graduate nurse experience. *Journal of Nursing Administration, 34*(6), 303–311.

Corlett, J., Palfreyman, J. W., Staines, H. J., & Marr, H. (2003). Factors influencing theoretical knowledge and practice skill acquisition in student nurses: An empirical experiment. *Nurse Education Today, 23*(3), 183–190.

Gaberson, K., & Oermann, M. H. (1999). *Clinical teaching strategies in nursing.* New York, NY: Springer.

Gerke, M. L. (2001). Understanding and leading the quad matrix: Four generations in the workplace: The traditional generation, boomers, Gen X, nexters. *Seminars for Nurse Managers, 9*(3), 173–181.

Godinez, G., Schweiger, J., Gruver, J., & Ryan, P. (1999). Role transition from graduate to staff nurse: A qualitative analysis. *Journal for Nurses in Staff Development, 15*(3), 97–110.

Goh, K., & Watt, E. (2003). From "dependent on" to "depended on": The experience of transition from student to registered nurse in a private hospital graduate program. *Australian Journal of Advanced Nursing, 21*(1), 14–20.

Guhde, J. (2005). When orientation ends . . . Supporting the new nurse who is struggling to succeed. *Journal for Nurses in Staff Development, 21*(4), 145–149.

Hickey, M. (2009). Preceptor perceptions of new graduate nurse readiness for practice. *Journal for Nurses in Staff Development, 25*(1), 35–41.

Horsburgh, M. (1989). Graduate nurses' adjustment to initial employment: Natural field work. *Journal of Advanced Nursing, 14*(8), 610–617.

Kolb, A. Y., & Kolb, D. A. (2005). *The Kolb learning style inventory-version 3.1: 2005 technical specifications.* Boston, MA: Hay Resources Direct.

Kolb, D. A. (2005). *The Kolb learning style inventory-version 3.1: Self scoring and interpretation booklet.* Boston, MA: Hay Resources Direct.

Kramer, M. (1974). *Reality shock: Why nurses leave nursing.* St. Louis, MO: C. V. Mosby.

Luhanga, F., Yonge, O., & Myrick, F. (2008). Hallmarks of unsafe practice. *Journal for Nurses in Staff Development, 24*(6), 257–264.

Marcum, E. H., & West, R. D. (2004). Structured orientation for new graduates: A retention strategy. *Journal for Nurses in Staff Development, 20*(3), 118–124.

Modic, M. B., & Harris, R. (2007). Masterful precepting: Using the BECOME method to enhance clinical teaching. *Journal for Nurses in Staff Development, 23*(1), 1–8.

Mylott, L., & Ciesielski, S. (2003). It takes a village: New graduate nurses enter critical care at Massachusetts General Hospital. *Advance for Nurses, 29*–30, 32.

Mylott, L., & Greenspan, M. (2005). *MGH-IHP new graduate in critical care program annual report.* Executive summary presented to the vice president for patient care and chief nurse, Massachusetts General Hospital, and the director, graduate program in nursing, MGH Institute for Health Professions, Boston, MA.

Neumann, J. A., Brady-Schluttner, K. A., McKay, A. K., Roslien, J. J., Twedell, D. M., & James, K. M. G. (2004). Centralizing a registered nurse preceptor program at the institutional level. *Journal for Nurses in Staff Development, 20*(1), 17–24.

Nursing Executive Center. (2002). *Nursing's next generation: Best practices for attracting, training, and retraining new graduates.* Washington, DC: Advisory Board Company.

Oermann, M. H., & Moffitt-Wolfe, A. (1997). New graduates' perceptions of clinical practice. *Journal of Continuing Education in Nursing, 28*(1), 20–25.

O'Malley, C., Cunliffe, E., Hunter, S., & Breeze, J. (2000). Preceptorship in practice. *Nursing Standard, 14*(28), 45–49.

Peirce, A. G. (1991). Preceptorial students' view of their clinical experience. *Journal of Nursing Education, 30*(6), 244–249.

Santucci, J. (2004). Facilitating the transition into nursing practice: Concepts and strategies for mentoring new graduates. *Journal for Nurses in Staff Development, 20*(6), 274–284.

Smith, A., & Chalker, N. (2005). Preceptor continuity in a nurse internship program: The nurse intern's perception. *Journal for Nurses in Staff Development, 21*(2), 47–52.

Speers, A. T., Strzyzewski, N., & Ziolkowski, L. D. (2004). Preceptor preparation: An investment in the future. *Journal for Nurses in Staff Development, 20*(3), 127–133.

Tradewell, G. (1996). Rites of passage: Adaptation of nursing graduates to a hospital setting. *Journal of Nursing Staff Development, 12*(4), 183–189.

Tyrrell, R. (2005). *Understanding and leading a multigenerational workforce.* Boston, MA: Massachusetts General Hospital.

U.S. Department of Health and Human Services. (2004). The registered nurse population: Findings from the March 2004 national sample survey of registered nurses. Retrieved from http://bhpr.hrsa .gov/healthworkforce/rnsurvey04/ http://bhpr.hrsa.gov/healthworkforce/rnsurveys/rnsurvey2004.pdf

Weston, M. (2001). Coaching generations in the workplace. *Nursing Administration Quarterly, 25*(2), 11–21.

RECOMMENDED READING

Baltimore, J. (2004). The hospital clinical preceptor: Essential preparation for success. *Journal of Continuing Education in Nursing, 35*(3), 133–140.

Flynn, J. P., & Stack, M. C. (Eds.). (2006). *The role of the preceptor: A guide for nurse educators, clinicians, and managers* (2nd ed.). New York, NY: Springer.

Johnson, S. A., & Romanello, M. L. (2005). Generational diversity: Teaching and learning approaches. *Nurse Educator, 30*(5), 212–216.

Yonge, O., & Myrick, F. (2004). Preceptorship and the preparatory process for undergraduate nursing students and their preceptors. *Journal for Nurses in Staff Development, 20*(6), 294–297.

CHAPTER 27

Student Learning in a Faculty– Student Practice Clinic

■ JENNIFER E. MACKEY, MARJORIE NICHOLAS, AND LESLEY MAXWELL ■

If we are to pursue excellence in any field, we must go beyond knowledge and skills in our education of graduate students. We need to identify the qualities of mind that underlie excellence and leadership potential in our disciplines, and we need to build those qualities into the foundations of our educational programs.

What does it mean to have a critical spirit? Experts in the field of critical thinking use this metaphorical phrase to mean "a probing inquisitiveness, a keenness of mind, a zealous dedication to reason, and a hunger or eagerness for reliable information" (Facione, 2009, p. 10.). The faculty of the graduate program in communication sciences and disorders at the MGH Institute of Health Professions asked itself this question: What are the foundational qualities of mind that excellence and leadership in the field are built upon and how can they be identified and nurtured in our graduate students? The result has been the development of an enhanced clinical curriculum that emphasizes excellence and systematically develops critical thinking, innovation, collaboration, social perception, risk taking, and self-knowledge and reflection in our students.

Professional licensure and program accreditation standards form the basis of the academic and clinical curriculum of clinical education programs. The American Speech-Language-Hearing Association (ASHA) requires that the education of graduate students who are seeking to become speech-language pathologists includes the acquisition of both *knowledge* and *skills* in a variety of content and disorder areas (ASHA, 2005). The breadth and depth of knowledge and skill that are required for recent healthcare graduates to practice effectively in current times are immense. Programs of all types are struggling to develop the sophisticated knowledge and skills in their graduates needed to meet an ever-expanding scope of practice. So why expand the demands on students and faculty by developing an extra set of requirements related to the esoteric ideas of excellence or leadership?

The reason is simple. In a world where knowledge is exploding and skill sets must keep pace, the most valuable education is one that teaches one to think critically, to be innovative, to collaborate effectively, to take the perspectives of others and modify one's behavior accordingly, to understand the value of taking thoughtful risks, and to practice in a manner that is self-reflective. Education should teach students how to unlock their personal potential to spend a lifetime pursuing excellence and becoming leaders in their chosen field.

As in most healthcare programs, ensuring that students gain the requisite knowledge base required by the accrediting body is accomplished primarily via academic coursework. Furthermore, like education models in many healthcare professions, most programs in speech-language pathology in the United States utilize a series of clinical externships in which students work in different healthcare and educational settings to acquire the clinical skills they will need to become professional practicing clinicians. Most also have on-site clinics in which students learn the preliminary clinical skills they need before venturing out to their externships. In this chapter, we describe the MGH Institute of Health Professions' faculty–student practice clinic, known as the Speech, Language and Literacy Center. The center operates as both an entry-level and an advanced practice clinic. While the examples we provide will necessarily be related to speech-language pathology, we believe the lessons learned from this clinical educational model are pertinent to a broad range of healthcare professionals.

The model of clinical education we will describe in this chapter is known as the *teacher-practitioner model* (Meyer, McCarthy, Klodd, & Gaseor, 1995; Montgomery, Enzbrenner, & Lerner, 1991; Peach & Meyer, 1996). One of the important features of the implementation of this model that we will highlight is the integration of academic (knowledge based) with clinical (practical and excellence skills based) education. We describe both entry-level and advanced-practice clinics and then discuss the positive outcomes and challenges of using this model.

▪ Definition and Purpose of the Teacher-Practitioner Model

The essential principle of the teacher-practitioner model is that students learn best from individuals who have dual roles as teachers and practicing clinicians. In this model, the supervising faculty member teaches the student in the classroom and also directs the clinical interaction with clients in the clinic through modeling and guided practice. In one of the most well-known models of supervision in speech-language pathology (Anderson, 1981; McCrea & Brasseur, 2003), a continuum of skill development is emphasized for both the student and the supervisor. Interaction between the two parties is also a key feature of the continuum model. This interaction and the continuum of skill development are also fundamental features of the teacher-practitioner model. This model is used by many academic institutions and seeks to create a strong link between scholarly and professional roles of the supervisor. Students have opportunities to see firsthand how theory relates to their clinical work with individuals with communication disorders. This model is the foundation for the faculty–student practice clinic, which serves the following two primary purposes: (1) it operates as a site for the education of students, and (2) it provides communication therapy services to the community.

In its main role as a setting focused on student learning, the clinic provides an atmosphere for the integration of academic knowledge and research-based practice in a clinical environment. As a place where supervisors mentor beginning clinicians, an on-site clinic is an ideal environment for linking clinical practice with theory and academic coursework. This setting encourages the development of excellence skills as well as the development of students' self-evaluation and self-reflection skills and the establishment of personal goals for clinical and professional growth. Superficially, it might appear that the best learning atmosphere is a real-world setting, such as a hospital, rehabilitation center, or specialty clinic. While these settings offer diverse, rich, and important experiences, the pressures of productivity, insurance issues, and medically complex patients make these environments exceptionally challenging for beginning clinicians (ASHA, n.d.). Like many healthcare professionals, speech-language pathologists face personnel shortages and increased requirements for documentation. External supervisors, or preceptors, often struggle with the demands of high caseloads and not enough time to teach and support students with limited knowledge and experience. Therefore, these settings are often best suited to advanced students who have already developed a solid basis for the understanding of intervention planning, diagnosis, and professional interaction.

The design of the teacher-practitioner model at the MGH Institute is uncommon across graduate programs in speech-language pathology nationally. Because of institutional requirements related to tenure and financial pressures at many colleges, academic faculty rarely participate in clinical work, and clinicians involved in supervising students within graduate school clinics are often not faculty and are frequently unfamiliar with the academic curriculum. Thus, the split between researcher/academic and clinician begins immediately in the educational process itself. Beginning students need clear paths drawn from the classroom to clinical application if they are to learn to think critically while developing a scholarly approach to practice based on evidence from research. A teacher-practitioner setting provides this bridge from the classroom to the clinic. It is a bridge that is crossed in both directions, because research in applied fields should be guided by questions that arise in the real world of practice.

A secondary purpose of the faculty–student practice clinic is to provide diagnostic and therapeutic services to community members with communication disorders. Since the faculty–student practice clinic is an integral part of the educational program, the hosting educational institution financially supports the clinic as a place for student learning. Therefore, the clinic is not dependent on outside sources such as state or governmental funding or payments from insurance or private-pay individuals. Clients are requested to pay a nominal user fee to support purchase of materials used in the clinic such as books, diagnostic tests, treatment materials, and software. This fee can be waived or reduced depending on individual circumstances. No client is ever denied services because of the inability to pay this fee. Having a free clinic is possible because of the nature of the integration of academic and clinical resources, including teachers and supervisors. Furthermore, because the clinic is not dependent on outside funding, it is able to provide services to underserved and underprivileged populations.

■ Use of the Teacher-Practitioner Model

The Entry-Level Clinic

The Speech, Language and Literacy Center was designed as a space for beginning graduate students to work with children and adults with various speech and language disorders, as well as for experienced graduate students to work in a simulated outpatient setting with adults who have acquired language disabilities. The physical layout of the center includes 14 individual treatment rooms and one large group/conference room. A digital observation system allows parents, caregivers, students, and supervisors to observe and record sessions. All treatment rooms have video cameras that project to a third observation room equipped with television monitors. Supervisors can observe sessions in this room and also have the ability to operate the camera remotely from the computer on their office desks. This gives student clinicians independence in the therapy room while they are carefully observed by a supervisor.

Students are supervised by licensed speech-language pathology faculty members with advanced expertise in their field. These supervisors, often called instructors, mentors, or preceptors, are faculty members in the communication sciences and disorders department. The majority of the supervisors also teach academic and clinical courses. This integration of academic and clinical information and experience allows for a unique learning atmosphere for the students and a rich collegial environment for faculty. This model of blending academic with clinical instruction is the basis of the teacher-practitioner model and allows students to fully assimilate information from classes into direct therapy with clients.

Students in their first year of the graduate program will have two semesters of clinical experience in the center. During one of these semesters, students work with children with spoken language disorders, such as toddlers, preschoolers, or early school-aged children who demonstrate difficulties in the areas of expressive or receptive language, articulation or phonology, or social communication. These children might also present with a specific diagnosis such as autism, cerebral palsy, or Down syndrome, but most often they do not have a specific diagnosis. Students also spend one semester with school-aged children and adults with reading and writing disorders. Some of these clients have a diagnosis of dyslexia.

These two semesters of clinical experience occur during the first and second semesters of the students' graduate program. In the first semester (fall), the entire class is divided in half and students are assigned randomly to one section—either spoken language or written language. Students move to the alternate section during the second semester (spring) to give them experience with another population.

Within each section, each student is paired with another student as a dyad partner. Dyad partners share two clients who are each seen twice a week for individual sessions. Each partner is responsible for the creation of weekly lesson plans as well as participating in diagnostic and therapeutic activities. This experience of working with a partner was designed to explicitly facilitate the development of professional collaboration skills.

Beginning clinical work is often highly stressful for novice clinicians. Some students have experienced some type of clinical environment during their undergraduate education, but many see the clinical world as foreign and daunting. Pairing students with another beginning graduate student fosters a feeling of companionship and collegiality. Since speech-language pathologists rarely work independently in the healthcare and educational fields, learning how to function as part of a collaborative team is a crucial skill. In addition, working in a partnership provides students with direct experiences with more than one client. This diversity of clients leads students to a greater understanding of a variety of disorders and fosters clinical growth in a manner that working independently with only one client would not allow.

In addition to the dyad partnership, students participate in a weekly case discussion (CD) group. Students are provided written documentation of CD group expectations and responsibilities. These include examples of behaviors demonstrating the core clinical excellence skills as well as process requirements for case presentation. For example, students are expected to actively participate in group discussions by asking questions that demonstrate critical thinking, giving examples of innovative approaches that they have developed, taking the risk to discuss and analyze errors, reflecting on and assessing their performance, thinking from the perspective of their client, and communicating in a professional manner. Each week, students spend 2 hours with a small group of students in a discussion format, facilitated by a faculty member. Therapy sessions are videotaped so that students can then select a digital segment to present to the group. For example, students might select a clip of a therapy activity that yielded unexpected results, had a positive outcome, or perhaps led them toward a question about the client and the therapeutic process. Each student is given time to discuss issues pertaining to his or her client and is also required to participate in discussions regarding other clients. This forum engages each student in a learning process that expands his or her knowledge base beyond a single client. Since multiple clients are represented, students learn about therapy techniques and treatment planning for a variety of disorders. This type of peer group supervision allows students to expand their perspectives to include different viewpoints and to learn from their peers as well as their supervisor (Williams, 1995).

A clinical discussion group syllabus guides the faculty member in facilitating the group. The syllabus includes the core excellence skills to be targeted that week and the knowledge and skill objectives and activities for the week. A questioning hierarchy based on Bloom's Taxonomy of Educational Objectives (Anderson & Krathwohl, 2001; Bloom & Krathwohl, 1956) is used by faculty to facilitate growth in critical thinking.

Students are provided with the hierarchy and Bloom's Taxonomy, which are also used to guide written feedback in planning documentation. Students are given explicit information about how to advance through the hierarchy of critical thinking toward advanced skills and self-supervision (Anderson, 1988) and how that progress is facilitated by supervisory scaffolding and the use of facilitative questions (Facione, 2009).

Encouraging active engagement in the learning process as a group facilitates critical thinking and self-evaluation in all members. The goal of supervision should be to assist students in their own development of self-analysis and evaluation as well as problem-solving skills so that the students will become independent (Anderson, 1988). Active engagement in their own learning encourages students to maintain an inquisitive nature and nurtures the development of critical thinking (Facione, 2009). These critical thinking concepts and self-evaluation measures are outlined for students in a tool that the authors developed (**Table 27-1**), which states the expectations for participation in case discussions as well as guidelines to help students consider their own development of communication skills and application of theory to practice within the group setting. The tool was based on the descriptive work of Peter A. Facione (2009) in the area of critical thinking.

This self-evaluation tool uses a directional arrow to illustrate a continuum of development of skills. One would expect a beginning student to be toward the left-hand side of the continuum (or the beginning) with such critical thinking skills as analysis or inference. Similarly, one might also expect to see a beginning student at a less developed level in his or her ability to self-reflect or demonstrate innovation and creativity. This continuum allows students to see their own growth as clinicians as a developmental process. Few, if any, students in their first term in graduate school would be at a well-developed level for all of these skills.

The concept of a continuum utilizes a mastery approach to clinical learning and gives the students a feeling of acceptance of current skills, with appropriate vision for areas of needed growth. Students are asked to self-evaluate and identify strengths and areas of growth in the beginning of the first term. Students then return to this form to reevaluate their own progress periodically throughout the first and second terms of clinical practice. Supervisors also look at the student's self-assessment of skills and progress and use this information as a point of discussion during mid-term and final evaluations. It is common, for example, for students to either overestimate or underestimate their skill level in a particular area. Discussions between supervisors and students about perceived skills allow for the self-evaluation process to become a part of the supervision process. Supervisors can then guide students in determining appropriate goals and objectives for growth. Students are encouraged to take this self-assessment tool into external practicum experiences and share it with supervisors in these environments to continue the learning process with new populations and professional communication situations.

Communication skills are of great importance to anyone practicing in the health professions, yet they do not always come naturally to beginning clinicians.

Table 27-1   Student Self-Assessment Form for Clinical Excellence and Critical Thinking Skills

Clinical Excellence Skills		
Skill	*Ranking of Performance*	
	Not Yet Present	*Well Developed*
Facilitates discussions Comes prepared, summarizes information, poses questions, analyzes strengths and weaknesses of session	├————————————————————▶	
Uses professional communication style Uses appropriate vocabulary, grammar, voice, speech rate, and articulation	├————————————————————▶	
Demonstrates self-reflection • Fair-minded in appraising reasoning • Honest in facing one's own biases, prejudices, stereotypes, or egocentric tendencies • Prudent in suspending, making, or altering judgments • Willing to reconsider and revise views where honest reflection suggests that change is warranted • Accurate in identifying strengths and weaknesses • Able to self-correct	├————————————▶ ├————————————▶ ├————————————▶ ├————————————▶ ├————————————▶ ├————————————▶	
Demonstrates innovation and creativity	├————————————▶	
Collaborates effectively	├————————————▶	
Analysis Identifies the intended and actual inferential relationships between concepts, facts, questions, descriptions, judgments, experiences, reasons, information, or opinions	├————————————————————▶	
Inference Identifies and secures elements needed to draw reasonable conclusion; forms conjectures and hypotheses; consider relevant information and induces consequences	├————————————————————▶	
Explanation States the result of one's reasoning; justifies that reasoning in terms of the evidential, conceptual, methodological, and contextual considerations; presents one's reasoning in the cogent arguments	├————————————————————▶	
Evaluation Assesses the credibility of statements or other representations; assesses the logical strength of the actual or intended inferential relationships among statements, descriptions, or questions	├————————————————————▶	

Supervisors seek to encourage students to use both a high-level vocabulary and clear definitions when defining diagnostic terms as well as when discussing specific therapeutic strategies and techniques. Within the case discussion group, students have weekly opportunities to orally present information to their peers and supervisor. This develops oral skills of summarization of information, use of clear terminology, and improved professional interaction with colleagues, clients, and caregivers.

Application of theory to practice is not only part of the beginning student's self-assessment process, but also a journey for everyone throughout his or her career. Application involves taking information learned from an academic class, a journal article, or a professional presentation and applying it to clinical practice in a meaningful way. This is a skill that all professionals should strive for and is a major component of both the clinical and academic experiences in the MGH program. The authors believe that the teaching of this skill begins with the individuals who are instructing their students.

Faculty members are often engaged in both the teaching process and the supervision of students in the MGH clinic. Most faculty continue to practice within their field of expertise, which allows individuals to keep in close contact with their populations of interest. Some examples include serving as a consultant in early intervention agencies or schools and working in area hospitals or clinics. This also allows a faculty member to remain clinically active, which in turn provides an immediate experience to share with students who are beginning to understand the clinical process. All too often, clinical skills are taught by individuals who have not had an opportunity to practice clinically for many years. The teacher-practitioner model, in contrast, allows students to benefit not only from an instructor's past experience, but also from recent interactions in the clinical field.

The model encourages faculty to perform in dual roles as clinical supervisors and academic teachers. First of all, new clinical supervisors attend weekly clinical seminars and courses on the theory of speech and language development along with beginning students. This allows new supervisors to understand the perspective and philosophy of the program and to experience firsthand the coursework required of students. The supervisor can then refer students to readings from class, specifics of class lectures, or comments made by the course professor. Often, the professor of the class will engage the new supervisor in a discussion within the class. Perhaps a particular therapeutic approach is the class topic and the professor might have the supervisor discuss a personal experience or clinical opinion on the use of such an approach. If questions about a particular theory or clinical application arise in a subsequent clinical supervisory session, the professor of the related course can be consulted.

This integration of academic and clinical practice is beneficial to all involved. Students gain a deeper appreciation for course material when it can be applied to clinical experiences. They view the link between information taught in a course and planning for a therapy session as an integration of ideas. Academic information fuels intervention planning, and vice versa. Clinical supervisors gain an understanding of the students' academic experience and its relation to current clinical issues. Academic professors find opportunities to link what is taught in the classroom with what happens in the clinical world. This regular interaction among faculty fosters a rich learning environment for students, as well as a rewarding intellectual atmosphere for everyone. The idea that all professionals should continue to explore and grow is an important lesson for students to learn.

The participation of supervisors in academic courses is extended into direct teaching experiences. For example, supervisors might teach a class on a particular topic within a course, or they could teach an entire course in their field of expertise. When clinical faculty teach in academic courses, students benefit from the overt integration of academic information with its practical application to the clinic.

Another way the program uses the teacher-practitioner model is to have primarily academic faculty supervise in the clinic. Professors teaching academic courses also offer professional opinions regarding challenging cases in the clinic. Thus, the program purposely chooses not to draw a clear distinction between faculty who are primarily academic instructors and those who are primarily clinical supervisors.

The Advanced Practice Clinic

The advanced practice clinic specializes in providing diagnostic and treatment services to adults with acquired neurogenic speech and language disorders such as aphasia, dysarthria, alexia, agraphia, and other cognitive-linguistic disorders resulting from brain damage. The clinic was started to provide a site for a subset of the second-year graduate students to gain clinical experience working with adults.

It is modeled on a typical outpatient rehabilitation clinic that provides speech-language pathology services to people who have had strokes and other adults with acquired communication disorders. The advanced practice clinic operates simultaneously with the entry-level clinic, so that both first- and second-year students are seeing clients in the clinic at the same time. Many other speech-pathology graduate programs throughout the country operate on a similar model.

The clinical excellence curriculum and the teacher-practitioner model provide the base for clinical education across terms. In keeping with the philosophy of the entry-level clinic, clinical supervision is provided in the advanced practice clinic by faculty members who also teach the acquired communication disorders courses. This allows for a meaningful integration of the academic knowledge students gain in their courses with the mentored clinical experiences they have with actual clients. As stated previously, the authors believe that this aspect of the clinical education model is perhaps the most important and novel feature of the program. Students in the advanced practice clinic are expected to develop their clinical excellence and critical thinking skills identified in the curriculum (Table 27-1) to a more advanced level than is expected for the students in the entry-level clinic. In addition, because they have already taken the academic coursework relevant to their clientele, they are expected to be more independent in developing evidence-based treatment plans for their clients.

In addition to providing a clinical practicum experience, the advanced practice clinic allows the students to learn several important realities of the larger healthcare arena. With the high costs of health care in the United States and the limited availability of funds to pay for services, many adults with communication disorders no longer qualify for services. The reasons for this are varied but generally arise from severe limitations in funds for chronic conditions such as aphasia. While a variety of therapies are generally covered by insurance plans in the first few months post stroke or injury, many insurance plans will no longer cover treatments for communication disorders in the chronic phase. As they enter the postacute period, many people with brain injuries from stroke or head trauma are denied further treatment. This is particularly true for individuals with limited means or those without family members to advocate for extended coverage beyond the acute period.

Settings such as the advanced practice clinics in universities and other healthcare education institutions can serve as bridges across this gap in service. Patients can receive the treatments they require, and students gain valuable insights into both the nature of chronic impairments and how variably people respond to their chronic conditions.

Individuals in need of services are referred to the advanced practice clinic usually by speech-language pathologists at local hospitals and rehabilitation centers. In addition, many clients are self-referred. Like clients at the entry-level clinic, clients at the advanced practice clinic are requested to pay the nominal clinic user fee. In the advanced practice clinic, because the majority of clients are middle-aged or elderly adults who were forced to retire from working because of their strokes or other injuries, most have requested waivers of the fee.

The clinical supervisors in the advanced practice clinic manage all new referrals and discharges of clients. Clients may continue to receive services in the clinic for as long as they are benefiting from the intervention provided. Both impairment-based and life participation–based treatments are incorporated into the clinical practice model. Impairment-based therapies are those that would be considered standard treatments to improve a specific speech or language deficit that is interfering with communication to some extent. For example, direct treatment targeting impairments in syntax (the rules for combining words in language) would be a type of impairment-based therapy that could be provided. Life participation–based treatment approaches are attempts to take another step to address the effects the communication impairment has on an individual's quality of life.

In their academic coursework covering acquired adult language disorders, students learn about the life participation approach to aphasia (LPAA; Chapey et al., 2001). A group of practitioners adhering to the LPAA has published a set of core values that stress that services should be provided to people with aphasia as long as they are needed, that the explicit goal of intervention should be the enhancement of life participation, and that both personal and environmental factors should be the targets of intervention. Similarly, the National Aphasia Association has recently published its aphasia bill of rights, which stresses similar values (National Aphasia

Association, n.d.). Students learn about this approach and other recent advances in their academic coursework, but experiencing them firsthand in the advanced practice clinic makes them come alive for the students.

Students have experiences providing both impairment-based therapies in individual treatment sessions and life participation enhancements with each client. For example, there is a cafe adjacent to the clinic where many clients meet to have lunch prior to the weekly aphasia support group meeting. Within the model of the LPAA, an appropriate intervention target would be to work with the staff at the cafe to educate them about aphasia and to teach them strategies to maximize communication interactions with people who may have communication impairments. Another target might be to work with the cafe to encourage it to have aphasia-friendly menus and signs that have pictures in addition to words. These actions would result in an improved quality of life for the clients, even though the clients would not receive the interventions directly.

Each semester, in addition to developing and carrying out individualized treatment plans, the students are required to assist with the aphasia support group and help plan group outings into the community. These outings have included events such as lunch at a nearby restaurant, seeing an IMAX movie at the local science museum, and attending a major league baseball game. Making the arrangements for these events has forced the students to think about how their clients must cope with physical, cognitive, and language disabilities in everyday life situations. As a result of their participation in these events, every student in the advanced practice clinic has commented on how inspired they have been by these experiences.

Students may also gain research experience in either the entry-level or advanced practice clinic. They have an option to complete a master's thesis during their 2-year program, and many have completed projects either fully or partially within the on-site clinic. Individual case studies, small-group assessment studies, and short-term treatment studies are possible types of projects that can be conducted within the clinic. In planning and conducting their research, students become familiar with the process necessary to complete a research project, from the initial step of getting approval from an institutional review board (IRB) to the final stages of data analysis and interpretation. While students are not required to do their research projects in the clinic, the availability of subjects of all ages with a variety of communication disorders on-site makes the process easier to accomplish for many students.

Students who elect not to do a master's thesis have been able to gain research experience by participating in various faculty members' projects. For example, one of the clinical supervisors had an ongoing project investigating the efficacy of an alternative communication treatment software program. Students assisted in the project by delivering the treatments according to the research protocol and conducting the periodic assessment sessions.

Having the advanced practice clinic on-site at the institute operating year-round also provides opportunities for first-year students to observe second-year students, as well as opportunities for students from other programs (e.g., nursing, physical therapy) to watch sessions. In addition, students are assigned projects in their academic coursework that require them to observe a treatment session and carefully document what they observed, and to determine what they think the treatment goals were in that session. Individual clients with aphasia and other neurogenic communication disorders have also been invited to be guest speakers in the class on aphasia. While students have many opportunities to watch videotaped examples of people with aphasia, they find that live interactions with people are even more valuable.

Finally, the mix of clients in the waiting areas who are attending either the entry-level or the advanced practice clinic has resulted in some interesting learning experiences pertaining to living with disabilities among students, faculty, clients, and their families. For example, the authors observed children attending the clinic reading books with an adult with aphasia in the waiting room. Young children have direct observation of individuals with disabilities, and adult clients have opportunities to interact with young people in a social communication situation that might not otherwise be available to them. Similarly, students, faculty, and staff members benefit from the environment. For example, students in the entry-level clinic have the opportunity to interact with adults who have aphasia in the social environment of the waiting room before they have the course on aphasia. This gives the students initial exposure to a population that they will learn about later in their education.

■ Types of Learners

A faculty–student practice clinic can support a wide range of student learning styles and needs, including students who have little experience with clinical application as well as those who are moving toward independence. Using the teacher-practitioner model, supervisors can often be matched to students with specific needs. For example, an instructor who is an expert writer might supervise a student who needs assistance with the development of clinical writing skills. This model also facilitates the learning styles of students who lack confidence as well as those who may be considered overconfident.

It is common for students facing their first clinical encounter to feel unprepared, anxious, and frightened. Although many of these students find they are able to move beyond this fear and quickly become acclimated to the clinical environment, some students continue to lack confidence in their clinical and interpersonal skills. The teacher-practitioner model allows the instructor to approach this type of student in a positive, supportive manner. Supervisors might spend time in the therapy room with the student clinician to model techniques and strategies before moving outside of the room to observe via camera. Students are encouraged to use self-evaluation and peer discussion as a means of improving self-confidence and awareness of areas of strength.

Likewise, students who have exaggerated perceptions of their knowledge and clinical skills (Brasseur, McCrea, & Mendel, 2005; Dowling, 2001) can be supported in a faculty–student practice clinic. It is for these students that the development of self-evaluation skills is most critical prior to sending a student into an external placement. Analysis of a video after the session can be useful so that the student can have an objective view of what occurred in the session. For example, a supervisor might assist a student in analyzing a video clip of a session where a client's desired behavioral objective was not met. The supervisor can then help the student identify clinical and personal skills that need to be further developed.

■ Conclusion

Many positive outcomes have emerged as a result of this clinical training model. First, the teacher-practitioner model has allowed students to be highly prepared when entering external practicum experiences. In fact, many external supervisors report that students are good critical thinkers and adopt professional roles easily. As a result, the authors' students receive multiple job offers upon graduation and have become highly successful professionals in the field. The emphasis on excellence throughout the program allows students to become lifelong learners who see their professional growth as a continuum of development. Many alumni currently volunteer to precept the authors' students in their clinical settings, and several former students have returned to the MGH program to teach courses and supervise students in the on-site clinic.

The on-site clinic is a student learning environment that enhances the integration of academic and clinical experiences and provides a rich atmosphere for the sharing of knowledge and expertise among faculty and students. The use of peers as dyads during the students' first year fosters personal growth in a collegial, supportive environment. Students learn to work as team members and to interact with a variety of clients as they learn to apply academic knowledge to clinical practice.

Some challenges of this model are common to many clinical education settings. These include logistical matters such as coordinating academic and clinical schedules with students, faculty, and clients; space management; parking; and maintenance of clinical materials. Another challenge is ensuring the right mix of clients each semester for student clinicians. Clients with complex communication disorders who require expert therapeutic intervention may not be appropriate for a clinic geared toward the education of beginning clinicians. Similarly, clients with mild disorders are often challenging for novice clinicians because mild disorders are sometimes difficult to perceive. Therefore, finding clients who will benefit from working with graduate students is an important consideration when planning a faculty–student practice clinic.

It is crucial that faculty have time built into their schedules to meet and discuss student issues, for academic planning, and for coordination of course topics with clinical needs. For example, conducting a class about how to use diagnostic materials is especially helpful if this class comes before a student needs to test a client in the clinic. This is one example of how the teacher-practitioner model can function at its highest level.

This model in a faculty–student practice clinic allows for the integration of academic knowledge, the development of clinical skills, and the beginning preparation for a lifetime of excellence. The on-site practice clinic is a well-traveled bridge between the classroom and the clinic.

Leadership and the pursuit of excellence are not something that universities train into students. Students sit before us with the potential for a lifetime of excellence in service; it is our job to facilitate the unfolding of that potential.

References

American Speech-Language-Hearing Association (ASHA). (2005). 2005 standards and implementation procedures for the certificate of clinical competence. Retrieved from http://www.asha.org/certification/slp_standards.htm

American Speech-Language-Hearing Association (ASHA). (n.d.). Responding to the changing needs of speech-language pathology and audiology students in the 21st century. Retrieved from http://www.asha.org/academic/reports/changing

Anderson, J. (1981). Training of supervisors in speech-language pathology and audiology. *ASHA, 23,* 77–82.

Anderson, J. L. (1988). *The supervisory process in speech-language pathology and audiology.* Boston, MA: College-Hill Press.

Anderson, L., & Krathwohl, D. (2001). *A taxonomy for learning, teaching and assessing: A revision of Bloom's taxonomy of educational objectives.* New York, NY: Longman.

Bloom, B. S., & Krathwohl, D. (1956). *Taxonomy of educational objectives: The classification of educational goals, by a committee of college and university examiners. Handbook I: Cognitive domain.* New York, NY: Longmans, Green.

Brasseur, J. A., McCrea, E. S., & Mendel, L. L. (2005). Remediating poorly performing students in clinical programs. *Perspectives on Issues in Higher Education, 9*(2), 20–26.

Chapey, R., Duchan, J. F., Elman, R. J., Garcia, L. J., Kagan, A., Lyon, J.G., ... Simmons-Mackie, N. (2008). Life participation approach to aphasia: A statement of values for the future. In R. Chapey (Ed.), *Language intervention strategies in aphasia and related neurogenic communication disorders* (5th ed.). Philadelphia, PA: Lippincott Williams & Wilkins.

Dowling, S. (2001). *Supervision: Strategies for successful outcomes and productivity.* Boston, MA: Allyn & Bacon.

Facione, P. A. (2009). *Critical thinking: What it is and why it counts.* Millbrae: California Academic Press, Insight Assessment. Retrieved from http://www.insightassessment.com/pdf_files/what&why2004.pdf

McCrea, E. S., & Brasseur, J. A. (2003). *The supervisory process in speech-language pathology and audiology.* Boston, MA: Allyn & Bacon.

Meyer, D. H., McCarthy, P. A., Klodd, D. A., & Gaseor, C. L. (1995). The teacher-practitioner model at Rush-Presbyterian-St. Luke's Medical Center. *American Journal of Audiology, 4,* 32–35.

Montgomery, L., Enzbrenner, L., & Lerner, W. (1991). The practitioner-teacher model revisited. *Journal of Health Administration Education, 9,* 9–24.

National Aphasia Association. (n.d.). Aphasia bill of rights. Retrieved from http://www.aphasia.org

Peach, R. K., & Meyer, D. H. (1996, April). The teacher-practitioner model at Rush University. *Administration and Supervision Newsletter,* pp. 9–13.

Williams, A. L. (1995). Modified teaching clinic: Peer group supervision in clinical training and professional development. *American Journal of Speech-Language Pathology, 4,* 29–38.

CHAPTER 28

Service Learning

■ HENDRIKA MALTBY ■

Students in clinical placements are expected to acquire skills, problem solve, and prepare for future employment in professional fields. Many courses also require students to reflect on their practice—what went well, what did not, and how practice could be improved for the future. Experiential learning and reflection are two of the components of service learning. The involvement of the agency as a true partner in the meeting of agency needs and student learning adds the third component. The focus needs to be on both the students and the recipients of care in partnership (Bailey, Carpenter, & Harrington, 2002). That is, meeting community needs, students' learning objectives, and formal reflection of the experience are the components of service learning. This chapter describes the use of service learning in the health professions.

■ Definition and Purpose

The Community-Campus Partnerships for Health (CCPH) organization has defined service learning as:

> A structured learning experience that combines community service with preparation and reflection. Students engaged in service-learning provide community service in response to community-identified concerns and learn about the context in which service is provided, the connection between their service and their academic coursework, and their roles as citizens. (CCPH 2013)

Using this definition, healthcare professionals have discovered that there are many opportunities to work with communities in enhancing health, as well as work with each other. "Service-learning not only connects theory with application and practice but also creates an environment where both the provider of service and the recipient learn from each other" (Norbeck, Connolly, & Koerner, 1998, p. 2). This ties in with the philosophy of a liberal education, common in North American universities:

> Liberal education has always been concerned with cultivating intellectual and ethical judgment, helping students comprehend and negotiate their

relationships with the larger world, and preparing them for lives of civic responsibility and leadership. It helps students, both in their general-education courses and in their major fields of study, analyze important contemporary issues like the social, cultural, and ethical dimensions of the AIDS crisis or meeting the needs of an aging population. (Schneider & Humphreys, 2005, p. B20)

Service learning operationalizes liberal education. Its purpose is to involve students in the community to provide a service that is determined by the community and connected to learning objectives in a course. Students begin to "understand that the people of a community are the true experts in knowledge of their community, because both the problems and the assets belong to them" (Mayne & Glascoff, 2002, p. 194).

■ Theoretical Foundations

Service as a concept in the community has been implemented since ancient times when people provided support and care to families (Cohen, Johnson, Nelson, & Peterson, 1998). Dewey was one of the first champions of service learning in the early 1900s when service and educational goals were connected (Bailey et al., 2002). Over the years, various American presidents have established a variety of organizations that provided service to communities, such as the Peace Corps, VISTA volunteers, the Foster Grandparents program, and the Office of National Service.

Increasingly, community partnerships and interdisciplinary education are coming to the forefront of health professional education. In the Pew Health Commission's 1998 final report, a number of recommendations were made, and a set of 21 competencies for the 21st-century health professional were outlined that transcend disciplinary differences (Bellack & O'Neil, 2000). A main recommendation of this report was the requirement that all health professionals have interdisciplinary competence. This incorporates the competencies of partnering with communities to make healthcare decisions and working in interdisciplinary teams. More recently, the Institute of Medicine (IOM) has made recommendations for education of public health professionals for the 21st century, noting that "effective interventions to improve the health of communities will increasingly require community understanding, involvement, and collaboration" (IOM, 2003, p. 15). Service learning is part of this education.

CCPH is a nonprofit organization founded in 1996 that assists in fostering health-promoting partnerships between communities and health professional schools (Seifer & Vaughn, 2002). It is a "network of over 1000 communities and campuses throughout the United States and increasingly the world that are collaborating to promote health through service-learning partnerships for improving health professional education, civic engagement and the overall health of communities" (CCPH, 2009). Seifer (1998) also clarifies the differences between service learning, traditional clinical education, and volunteerism. In service learning, there is a balance between service and learning objectives and an emphasis on reciprocal learning, developing citizenship skills and achieving social change, reflective practice, addressing community-identified needs, and the integral involvement of community partners. Seifer emphasizes that service learning is not required volunteerism, which lacks reciprocity and reflection and may not be connected to course objectives.

Using service learning in nursing and other health professions enables the development of perceptions and insight as described in cognitive learning theories in the opening chapter. Developing a variety of teaching strategies to complement student learning styles is necessary to enhance this development. Students in health professions are usually practice oriented and want to do something, which relates to the adult learning principles of Knowles (1975) of recognizing the meaning or usefulness of the information learned. Cultural understanding can be a key element of this learning as students work with a variety of populations. Service learning allows the student to implement classroom learning objectives while providing a wanted service to a community.

■ Types of Learners

Service learning is suitable for any level of student in any health education program. One resource, Campus Compact, a national coalition, is "committed to fulfilling the civic purposes of higher education" (Campus Compact, 2013b, first para.) by assisting faculty to integrate service learning into the classroom with institutional commitment to community engagement. To date, almost 600 colleges and universities have become signatories to the Presidents' Declaration on the Civic Responsibility of Higher Education (Campus Compact, 2013a), which challenges higher education to become engaged with the community so that the knowledge gained by the students can benefit society. Service learning has been added to courses and programs outside of health care as well such as geography, political science, education, environment, and mathematics. At the University of Vermont, for example, 75 courses now have the SL designation so that students can easily find a course in which they can engage with the community (University of Vermont, 2013). These are at all levels and include undergraduate and graduate courses.

Examples in health care include a variety of professions in multiple settings. Cashman, Hale, Candib, Nimiroski, and Brookings (2004) had medical and nurse practitioner students provide depression screening at a community clinic through the application of service learning, providing a mutually beneficial opportunity. Chabot and Holben (2003) integrated service learning into dietetics and nutrition education. Health law students travel from the University of Maryland to Mississippi to partner with the Mississippi Center for Justice to examine hospital charity policies and debt collection practices (Rowthorn, 2012). Graduate rehabilitation students worked with inner-city seniors to provide primary prevention through service learning and also learned about interdisciplinary roles and advocacy for those in need (Hamel, 2001). Occupational and physical therapy students provided service at a child care facility (Hoppes, Bender, & DeGrace, 2005).

The nursing profession uses service learning in partnership with many community agencies. Much of the recent literature involved community/public health nursing clinical rotations focusing on the Veterans Administration Medical Center (Hudson, Gaillard, & Duffy, 2011), homeless individuals and families (Loewenson & Hunt, 2011), a sheriff's department (Fuller, Alexander, & Hardeman, 2006), a tuberculosis screening clinic (Schoener & Hopkins, 2004), an adult day care center (Ross, 2012), a Community Health Improvement Center (Carter & Dunn, 2002), and a variety of community health agencies (Mallette, Loury, Engelke, & Andrews, 2005; Redman & Clark, 2002; Riedford, 2011). Additionally, service learning has been used as a tool for developing research skills (Janke, Pesut, & Erbacker, 2012), facilitating leadership and management skills (DeDonder, Adams-Wendling, & Pimple, 2011; Groh, Stallwood, & Daniels, 2011), learning about health policy (O'Brien-Larivée, 2011), and increasing cultural awareness with prenursing students in a first-year experience course (Worrell-Carlisle, 2005).

All of the examples cited here use service learning; students provided a necessary service that was tied into the coursework they were undertaking. Reflection on the service and the process was a key element. Students were able to examine issues such as homelessness in the elderly (Hamel, 2001), disabled children (Hoppes et al., 2005), social justice (Groh et al., 2011; Redman & Clark, 2002), mental health in the community (Riedford, 2011), the financially disadvantaged (Scott, Harrison, Baker, & Wills, 2005), and culture (Worrell-Carlisle, 2005). Moreover, students had their worldview challenged and often changed their view in the process.

▪ Conditions for Learning

Service learning courses can be placed anywhere in the curriculum, and students can be partnered in groups or as individuals working with homeless people, working with those with diabetes, in residential living centers, in health departments—in fact, almost anywhere and with anyone. The learning environment becomes very broad, especially when not bound by classroom walls. The first step is to build partnerships with community agencies that match course goals and objectives. Dunlap, Marver, Morrow, Green, and Elam (2010) discuss some of the variables that can affect campus/community partnerships that must be considered, such as leadership, the academic calendar, and changing student cohorts. The CCPH website has a tool that can be used to inventory current partnerships to make decisions about the future partnership work.

Prerequisites include teaching students what service learning is and how it differs from volunteerism. Outlining reflection requirements and how to incorporate this component is essential because reflection helps students to connect the service to course objectives and to understand why service is important. Reflection can be done in a variety of ways, such as in-class writing assignments, final papers, presentations, and journals.

■ Resources

Resources can be as much or as little as needed depending on partnerships. Many placements are able to provide necessary supplies for projects, whereas others may rely on students providing the materials they need. For example, the agency may be able to fund clinics (e.g., screening for tuberculosis, influenza immunizations, cholesterol); other funding may be found through other sources such as area health education centers (AHECs) or the college/university. AHECs were begun by the U.S. government in the late 1970s "to address health staffing distribution and the quality of primary care through community-based initiatives designed to encourage universities and educators to look beyond institutions to partnerships that promote solutions which meet community health needs" (University of Vermont, College of Medicine, 2013). Research grants can also be applied for to incorporate service learning into the curriculum and to evaluate partnerships.

One of the major requirements is time, particularly when developing partnerships. Partners can be found anywhere. This may be through a partnership-type office at the educational institution (such as the Community-University Partnerships and Service-Learning office at the University of Vermont) that keeps a list of partners and their needs (e.g., a town planning office looking for geography students). The faculty member may have contacts via other courses, clinical experiences, service, or research in which they are involved.

Students also need time to provide the service. For example, a 3-credit-hour course takes about 9 hours of preparation time for students outside of class; therefore, the service can be a part of the 9 hours. Time can range from 10 to 15 hours over a semester to a concentrated 90 to 135 hours. The revision of assignments for the course can also incorporate the service learning projects. Suggested websites that may serve as a resource for faculty are listed at the end of this chapter.

■ Using the Method

Health seldom takes place in a vacuum. It requires the efforts of the individual, family, group, university, and community working in partnership. Service learning works to address the needs identified by a partner. Therefore, one of the first essential steps is to identify a partner. This can be done over a summer, during the semester prior to the service learning, or at the beginning of the course. Maurana, Beck, and Newton (1998) have outlined some principles of good partnerships, including common goals, mutual trust and respect, building on strengths, clear communication, and continuous feedback. They list three key themes in building successful partnerships: "1. Always remember that community members are experts in their community; 2. Promise less and deliver more; and 3. Be committed for the long haul" (p. 51). Once the partner has been identified, the contract can be as informal as a verbal agreement ("students will help ...") or can be a formal written agreement outlining the roles and responsibilities of faculty, students, and partners. Websites identified in the *Notes* section at the end of the chapter provide examples of different types of contracts. Partnerships can become one of the strengths of the course and can be utilized each time the course is offered.

The course syllabus needs to incorporate service as part of the course and not as a "mere sidebar" (Heffernan, 2001, p. 1). Heffernan goes on to describe six models of service learning (**Table 28-1**). The model of service learning chosen for the course will depend on the goals and objectives that students need to meet.

Decisions on the partners and model of service learning lead to the other required components that should be included in the syllabus. How are the students going to engage with the partner? Will students work individually or in groups? Will the partner be a guest speaker in the class? Will students meet partners on their own or will the faculty arrange formal meetings? Will projects be outlined in the syllabus or will the partner and student(s) decide on this together? Will the projects be presented?

The reflection on service in conjunction with course objectives needs to be clear. How are these reflections going to be done (e.g., in-class writing assignments that are announced or unannounced, final paper)? How will they be graded? Are there specific criteria to be used? Will students have a grading rubric? Ash and Clayton (2004) provide an articulated learning structure for reflection through four questions: What did I learn? How did I learn it? Why does this learning matter? In what ways will I use this learning? Similarly, Kuiper (2005) suggests prompts for reflection such as "The problems I encountered ... ; I think I solved them by ... ; When I had difficulty I ..." (p. 353). Using prompts guides students to critically reflect on the experience and how it affects both the partner and themselves. **Table 28-2** provides two examples of grading rubrics. More tools are available at http://www.ccph.info/.

Table 28-1 Models of Service Learning

1. Pure service learning where the service is the course content.

2. Discipline-based service learning that makes the link between content and experience explicit.

3. Problem-based service learning in which students may act as consultants.

4. Capstone courses usually offered to students in their final year.

5. Service internships—intense experiences with regular and ongoing reflection.

6. Community-based action research (or community-based participatory research) using research to act as an advocate for the community.

Source: Heffernan, K. (2001). *Fundamentals of service-learning course construction.* Providence, RI: Campus Compact.

Table 28-2 Grading Rubrics

Health Promotion Across the Life Span: In-Class Reflections

There will be four in-class writing assignments based on the readings and your work to date. A question will be posed during the class. You will need to tie in your reading and other work in the response. These will be assessed by how well you link the readings to your work and your thoughts about the two. They will be short and unannounced ahead of time (five marks each).

Community/Public Health Nursing

Journal

Students will complete a journal every 2 weeks (for a total of 6) throughout the semester. The journals will be submitted electronically to the clinical faculty with whom you are working.

Due dates: Journal entries are due Monday mornings.

You will need to address the following items:

1. Summary and reflection of practice: This is a general overview of activities over the past 2 weeks including your thoughts, feelings, judgments, and an evaluation of your experience to this point. It should consist of no more than two pages (typed, double-spaced).

2. Describe how you used previous knowledge and experience during the past 2 weeks. Link experiences to specific course objectives. For example, if you are teaching children about asthma, you would incorporate child development, teaching, and learning strategies, coping skills, respiratory diseases, chronic illness, environmental issues, and so on. By the end of the semester you need to have addressed all course objectives. Be sure to include the ethical standards.

3. Which research and/or practice questions can you generate based on your 2 weeks' experience? Which additional knowledge do you require for your practice in the next 2 weeks? How will answering these questions improve your practice?

4. Discuss one research-, practice-, or theory-based article that relates to each question in number 3 and reflects evidenced-based practice. How does what you learned from the article relate to your practice?

5. Describe the value of activities to your individual learning and meeting personal objectives.

6. Discuss the impact on your personal beliefs about nursing, health care, the nurse in community and public health, and community partnerships.

Topic (Possible Points)	Your Grade
Summary (5)	
Previous knowledge/course objectives (5)	
Question/additional knowledge improvement for practice (10)	
Article and relation to practice (10)	
Value of activities (5)	
Impact on personal beliefs (5)	
Total (40)	

Finally, how will reciprocity be accomplished? Usually evaluations by and of all partners (the community, the students, the faculty) are necessary. These can be formal or informal. Shinnamon, Gelmon, and Holland (1999) have developed evaluation of service learning tools for students, faculty, and community partners and asked questions about attitude, experiences, and influence on future work using a Likert scale. Evaluations help to create better relationships and a stronger experience. Other evaluation tools for student, partner, and faculty assessments are available on the CCPH website. Showcasing service learning projects during class presentations or a campus-wide poster presentation contributes to reciprocity by recognizing the work of the students and the partners.

■ International Service Learning

Another option for service learning is study abroad—immersion experiences of living and learning in another culture. This has several advantages, including increased student awareness of their own beliefs, values, practices, and behaviors and how that affects care; ability to learn from clients and provide culturally appropriate care; and ability to cope with factors affecting health and living conditions (Lipson & Desantis, 2007). A number of authors have described study abroad experiences, including preparation of students and faculty (Doyle, 2004; Robinson, Sportsman, Eschiti, Bradshaw, & Bol, 2006), descriptions of the study abroad opportunities (Anders, 2001; Bentley & Ellison, 2007; Harrison & Malone, 2004; Johanson, 2006; Tabi & Mukherjee, 2003), and learning cultural competence through these types of experiences (Caffrey, Neander, Markle, & Stewart, 2005; Koskinen & Tossavainen, 2004; Walsh & DeJoseph, 2003; Warner, 2002). Readers are encouraged to explore the literature concerning these experiences.

Service learning during study abroad experiences requires a long-term commitment (at least five years) for both learning and service with a partner outside of the country. Chisholm (2003) outlines the following three principles for international partnerships: trust, mutuality of benefit, and open communication. Trust entails being clear about goals, budgets, and limitations and includes being sure promises made can be kept. There must be a benefit for both partners (inherent in service learning). Open and complete communication is essential, ranging from the formal evaluation plans to the more informal check-ins. Adaptability is indispensable in the process. All principles of service learning still hold for international experiences, including linking community needs, students' learning objectives, and formal reflection of the experience. McKinnon and Fealy (2011) outline the core principles for developing global service learning programs in nursing, which "are based on the Seven Cs of Best Practice: Compassion, Curiosity, Courage, Collaboration, Creativity, Capacity building, and Competence" (p. 95).

Faculty interested in this type of experience for their students are encouraged to contact their office of international education (or equivalent), as it will provide logistical support. Many times it is the faculty themselves who have contacts in another country that are further developed for study abroad opportunities. As Bosworth and colleagues state, "it began with one professor of nursing ..." (2006, p. 34). An example of international service learning in Bangladesh is provided at the end of the chapter.

■ Potential Problems

Teaching in, and the facilitation of, a service learning course take time, so a major potential problem is lack of time. Time is required to form partnerships, prepare students, and involve partners in the design and implementation of the course. Another potential problem is the lack of preparation of the students (partnerships, reflection). The information needs to be in the course syllabus and class time needs to be devoted to describing service learning, explaining reflection, and the process of partnership. It is recommended that faculty teach only one service learning course at a time.

Lack of involvement of community partners in the design and implementation of the service learning projects can be a potential problem. As one of the components of service learning is reciprocity, involvement of community partners is mandatory. This can be remedied by clear and open communication. Regular contact with faculty is necessary so that issues can be dealt with early.

Another potential issue that has arisen is presenting service learning and the associated community-based participatory research work for promotion and tenure. There are now a number of resources available to faculty to support this work with communities and students. Nyden (2003) outlines some strategies that faculty can use, such as developing faculty networks, modifying tenure and promotion guidelines, and mentoring faculty and students. CCPH has developed a resource kit available on its website to provide health professional faculty with a set of tools to carefully plan and document their community-engaged scholarship and produce strong portfolios for promotion and tenure.

■ Conclusion

Service learning provides students the opportunity to develop transferable skills such as "the ability to synthesize information, creative problem solving, constructive teamwork, effective communication, well-reasoned decision making, and negotiation and compromise . . . and an increased sense of social responsibility" (Jacoby, 1996, p. 21). Service learning fits well with health professional education. Students need to get out of the classroom and become more involved in the community and with each other to make knowledge come alive. This strategy can provide students with insight into community conditions; community collaboration is lived, not just talked about in class.

Notes

One excellent resource on service learning is the Community-Campus Partnerships for Health (CCPH) website (http://www.ccph.info/). It contains a plethora of information, including discipline-specific sample syllabi and other resources that include service learning, to provide assistance to faculty who want to use this methodology. Additionally, the site contains sample partnership agreements, strategies for assessment (student, faculty, partner perspectives), and suggestions for how to institutionalize service learning on your campus and access to electronic discussion groups. The other important piece of this type of teaching scholarship, which is also available on the website, is how to incorporate this work into the reappointment/promotion/tenure process.

There is a National Service-Learning Clearinghouse (NSLC, 2013) website (http://www.servicelearning.org/), which has a range of information for elementary, high school, and tertiary education settings. It includes information on national and international conferences, e-mail discussion lists, service learning ideas and curricular examples, sample forms and templates, and technical assistance staff. This site has a link to the Corporation for National and Community Service (CNCS, 2013), which lists opportunities in a variety of organizations (http://www.nationalservice.gov/about). Access for the CNCS strategic plan is through this website, which has further information on service learning from kindergarten to graduate school.

Service learning is being used for international projects such as faculty-led study abroad courses. The International Service Learning (ISL) organization (http://www.islonline.org/about/) provides medical and educational teams of primarily student volunteers to provide services for the underserved populations of Central and South America, Mexico, and Africa. The goal of ISL is to partner student and professional teams from developed countries with service opportunities in developing countries. The International Partnership for Service Learning and Leadership (IPSL, 2009) is another organization that links academic programs and volunteer service, giving students a fully integrated study abroad experience. IPSL (http://www.ipsl.org/) promotes the theory and practice of service learning and development and promotion of service learning in institutions of higher education around the world. Faculty who want to incorporate service learning into study abroad options will need to consult with their own institutions' international offices.

TEACHING EXAMPLES:

Health Promotion Across the Life Span

The health promotion class is a junior nursing class and is now service learning based. The semester-long service learning project produces 30-second public service announcements (PSAs) to meet the course objectives of developing family education strategies, learning to give concise messages, and realizing that health education could be more than handing out pamphlets. Our community partner is the regional educational television network (RETN), the local producer and provider of media for learning and a public service organization. The production coordinator came to the class to teach the basics of developing and producing the PSAs. Groups of 4–6 students (78 students altogether, 14 groups) chose a health promotion issue for a particular age group and drafted a script and storyboard. This is approved by faculty and the RETN. Although this sounded simple, it actually took more time than we anticipated. Having both faculty and the RETN approve the scripts enabled students to incorporate their advice without stifling creativity. For example, one group who developed their PSA on toddler poisoning had the child actor carry the mock poison bottle rather than be seen drinking from the bottle. Once the scripts were approved, groups videotaped their PSAs with equipment borrowed from the university. It takes about an hour of videotape to edit down to a 30-second message. Editing was done by the RETN. The outcome was 14 health messages that are being shown throughout the state over the next several months. The PSAs are available at http://www.retn .org/programs/2010-health-promotion-across-lifespan. Reflection on the process was done through in-class writing assignments (unannounced), and outcomes indicated that the students learned about communication and the value (and difficulty!) of providing short messages. They found this a very enjoyable experience in which to learn about health education.

Public Health Nursing: Bangladesh

At the University of Vermont (UVM), following a grant to develop study abroad opportunities, a course was set up with partners in Bangladesh. This 3-week public health nursing immersion experience for senior undergraduate nursing students was organized in partnership with the International University of Business, Agriculture and Technology (IUBAT), College of Nursing. Nursing in Bangladesh is not a respected profession, with poor training and low pay (Berland, Richards, & Lund, 2010). The nursing program at IUBAT is working to change this and is among the first to teach nursing at international standards, in English and almost completely staffed by volunteers. The first cohort graduated in 2009 (Berland et al., 2010).

The majority of the Bangladeshi population is rural, and more than half live in poverty. It is the eighth most populated country in the world and third poorest. Between 1991 and 2003, the infant mortality rate dropped from 87 to 53 per 1,000 live births (in the United States, the rate is 7 per 1,000); the under-5 mortality rate was 76 per 1,000 live births in 2002 (United States, 8 per 1,000); and the maternal mortality ratio declined from 470 to 380 per 100,000 live births from 1991 to 2002 (United States, 14 per 100,000 in 2000) (World Health Organization, 2013). Although the rates have declined, infant and maternal mortality are still high.

To organize a study abroad course requires dedication and determination of the faculty member. Following course approval, students need to be recruited and a myriad of details need to be worked out. At UVM, the Office of International Education (OIE) assists with

(continued)

budget preparation, student applications, visas, flights, and risk management details. The UVM students meet about three times during the fall semester prior to departure to complete necessary paperwork, learn about Bangladesh and expectations for the course, and begin to come together as a team. IUBAT provides the on-the-ground logistics and contacts with a variety of facilities and transportation in country. It also enlists two to four students from its nursing program who are our interpreters and cultural brokers and travel with us during our time in Bangladesh.

The UVM students arrived in Dhaka (the capital of Bangladesh). The immersion experience began at the airport; small children dressed only in a pair of shorts came begging for food and money. Just in front of them was a fence lined with people at least 10 deep also holding out their hands. The noise and the smells of Dhaka poured over them. The bus trip from the airport to the hotel, while only a few miles, took almost an hour due to traffic that was crowded with buses, trucks, cars, rickshaws, tempos (a very small pickup truck-style motorized vehicle), and people. During our time in Bangladesh, we stayed in a rural village and in Dhaka, where we spent time in local hospitals. We traveled by train to the tea gardens, where the students learned about tea plantations and the people who work there. The students worked in small groups to complete community assessments and interview families to learn about health care in Bangladesh. Classes were held in the evening, and we discussed the events and sights of the day, connecting with the history, sociology, and health of Bangladesh. Students kept reflective journals throughout the experience and had some profound insights related to cultural competency, including the following statement:

> We went to Bangladesh with the intention of learning about the public health in a developing country. We discovered the common need for quality nursing care and access to resources and education. Visiting Bangladesh opened our eyes to the similarities of human health needs in that we all have common goals for our health. Our future nursing practice will be forever impacted by this experience.

During the first trip, the girls' high school in the rural village invited the nursing students to provide health education for their classes. This began with learning about schooling in Bangladesh, especially for girls. The following year, a photovoice project was completed to discover which nutrition and hygiene habits were already practiced by the families. Photovoice, a community-based participatory research method, is a photographic technique that enables people to record and reflect their community's strengths and issues, leading to discussion and policy considerations (Wang & Redwood-Jones, 2001, p. 560). With permission from the headmistress, five high school girls were given a digital camera to photograph their families' nutrition and hygiene habits. After training and discussion about the project, the girls returned with at least 50 photographs each. Using a portable photo printer and an interpreter, each girl told her story. Preliminary data analysis is providing indigenous beliefs, practices, and knowledge of food preparation and habits of these families. These stories will be the basis of a future nutrition program at the high school to be taught by the nursing students and IUB student interpreters.

Each trip is somewhat different, as what can be arranged may require timing changes, the desire to add to the experience, and the networking that happens on each trip. This type of international service learning requires a time commitment and a great deal of patience. While there are philosophical discussions about foreigners providing health care, what we do is support the college of nursing as our service learning work. It has a new nursing laboratory and few funds. Officials at the college are asked what they need, and we work to honor their request. For example, new nursing textbooks are collected from faculty to augment the library; maternity teaching models, IV arms, and CPR torsos have all been provided by our Sigma Theta Tau International Honor Society of Nursing, Kappa Tau Chapter; and smaller items such as glucometers, oximeters, and batteries have been collected. Students from both IUDAT and UVM stay in touch on Facebook following the experience. (Students from the first trip in 2008 still keep in touch with the Bangladeshi students!) The students learn from each other and all realize the importance of nursing. The best way we can help is to make their program successful so that Bangladesh grows its own strong nursing profession so Bangladeshi nurses can provide health care to the people of Bangladesh.

REFERENCES

Anders, R. L. (2001). A nursing study abroad opportunity. *Nursing and Health Care Perspectives, 22*(3), 118–121.

Ash, S. L., & Clayton, P. H. (2004). The articulated learning: An approach to guided reflection and assessment. *Innovative Higher Education, 29*(2), 137–154.

Bailey, P. A., Carpenter, D. R., & Harrington, P. (2002). Theoretical foundations of service-learning in nursing education. *Journal of Nursing Education, 41*(10), 433–452.

Bellack, J. P., & O'Neil, E. H. (2000). Recreating nursing practice for a new century: Recommendations of the Pew Health Professions Commission's final report. *Nursing and Health Care Perspectives, 21*(1), 14–21.

Bentley, R., & Ellison, K. J. (2007). Increasing cultural competence in nursing though international service-learning experiences. *Nurse Educator, 32*(5), 207–211.

Berland, A., Richards, J., & Lund, K. D. (2010). A Canada–Bangladesh partnership for nurse education: Case study. *International Nursing Review, 57,* 352–358.

Bosworth, T., Haloburdo, E., Hetrick, C., Patchett, K., Thompson, M. A., & Welch, M. (2006). International partnerships to promote quality care: Faculty groundwork, student projects, and outcomes. *Journal of Continuing Education in Nursing, 37*(1), 32–38.

Caffrey, R. A., Neander, W., Markle, D., & Stewart, B. (2005). Improving the cultural competence of nursing students: Results of integrating cultural content in the curriculum and an international immersion experience. *Journal of Nursing Education, 44*(5), 234–240.

Campus Compact. (2013a). Signatories. Retrieved from http://www.compact.org/resources-for-presidents/presidents-declaration-on-the-civic-responsibility-%20of-higher-education/signatories/

Campus Compact. (2013b). Who we are. Retrieved from http://www.compact.org/about/history-mission-vision/

Carter, J., & Dunn, B. (2002). A service-learning partnership for enhanced diabetes management. *Journal of Nursing Education, 41*(10), 450–452.

Cashman, S. B., Hale, J. F., Candib, L. M., Nimiroski, T. A., & Brookings, D. R. (2004). Applying service-learning through a community–academic partnership: Depression screening at a federally funded community health center. *Education for Health, 17*(3), 313–322.

Chabot, J. M., & Holben, D. H. (2003). Integrating service-learning into dietetics and nutrition education. *Topics in Clinical Nutrition, 18*(3), 177–184.

Chisholm, L. A. (2003). Partnerships for international learning. In B. Jacoby & Associates (Eds.), *Building partnerships for service-learning* (pp. 259–288). San Francisco, CA: Jossey-Bass.

Cohen, E., Johnson, S., Nelson, L., & Peterson, C. (1998). Service-learning as a pedagogy in nursing. In J. S. Norbeck, C. Connolly, & J. Koerner (Eds.), *Caring and community: Concepts and models for service-learning in nursing* (pp. 53–63). San Francisco, CA: American Association for Higher Education.

Community-Campus Partnerships for Health (CCPH). (2009). Promoting health equity and social justice (home page). Retrieved from http://ccph.info/CCPH

Community-Campus Partnerships for Health (CCPH). (2013). Service-learning: Definition. Retrieved from http://ccph.info/CCPH

Corporation for National and Community Service. (2013). About CNCS. http://www.nationalservice.gov/about

DeDonder, J., Adams-Wendling, L., & Pimple, C. (2011). A service-learning project facilitating leadership and management skills. *Journal of Nursing Education, 50*(7), 423–424.

Doyle, R. M. (2004). Applying new science leadership theory in planning an international nursing student practice experience in Nepal. *Journal of Nursing Education, 43*(9), 426–429.

Dunlap, R. K., Marver, D., Morrow, B. J., Green, B. R., & Elam, J. (2010). A community health service-learning roundtable: Nursing education partnership for community health improvement. *Journal of Nursing Education, 50*(1), 44–47.

Fuller, S. G., Alexander, J. W., & Hardeman, S. M. (2006). Sheriff's deputies and nursing students: Service-learning partnership. *Nurse Educator, 31*(1), 31–35.

Groh, C. J., Stallwood, L. G., & Daniels, J. J. (2011). Service-learning in nursing education: Its impact on leadership and social justice. *Nursing Education Perspectives, 32*(6), 400–405.

Hamel, P. C. (2001). Interdisciplinary perspectives, service learning, and advocacy: A nontraditional approach to geriatric rehabilitation. *Topics in Geriatric Rehabilitation, 17*(1), 53–70.

Harrison, L., & Malone, K. (2004). A study abroad experience in Guatemala: Learning first-hand about health, education, and social welfare in a low-resource country. *International Journal of Nursing Education Scholarship, 1*(1), Article 16.

Heffernan, K. (2001). *Fundamentals of service-learning course construction.* Providence, RI: Campus Compact.

Hoppes, S., Bender, D., & DeGrace, B. W. (2005). Service learning is a perfect fit for occupational and physical therapy education. *Journal of Allied Health, 34,* 47–50.

Hudson, C. E., Gaillard, S., & Duffy, N. (2011). Developing a community health clinical practicum service-learning model: An academic and VA medical center partnership. *Nurse Educator, 36*(1), 7–8.

Institute of Medicine (IOM). (2003). *Who will keep the public healthy? Educating public health professionals for the 21st century.* Washington, DC: Author.

International Partnership for Service-Learning and Leadership. (2009). International service-learning programs. Retrieved from http://www.ipsl.org/ http://www.ipsl.org/defaultIPSL.aspx

Jacoby, B. (1996). *Service-learning in higher education: Concepts and practices.* San Francisco, CA: Jossey-Bass.

Janke, R., Pesut, B., & Erbacker, L. (2011). Promoting information literacy through collaborative service learning in an undergraduate research course. *Nurse Education Today, 32,* 920–923.

Johanson, L. (2006). The implementation of a study abroad course for nursing. *Nurse Educator, 31*(3), 129–131.

Knowles, M. (1975). *Self-directed learning: A guide for learners and teachers.* New York, NY: Cambridge.

Koskinen, L., & Tossavainen, K. (2004). Study abroad as a process of learning intercultural competence in nursing. *International Journal of Nursing Practice, 10*(3), 11–120.

Kuiper, R. A. (2005). Self-regulated learning during a clinical preceptorship: The reflections of senior baccalaureate nursing students. *Nursing Education Perspectives, 26*(6), 351–356.

Lipson, J. G., & Desantis, L. A. (2007). Current approaches to integrating elements of cultural competence in nursing education. *Journal of Transcultural Nursing, 18*(1 suppl), 10S–20S.

Loewenson, K. M., & Hunt, R. J. (2011). Transforming attitudes of nursing students: Evaluating a service-learning experience. *Journal of Nursing Education, 50*(6), 345–349.

Mallette, S., Loury, S., Engelke, M. K., & Andrews, A. (2005). The integrative clinical preceptor model: A new method for teaching undergraduate community health nursing. *Nurse Educator, 30*(1), 21–26.

Maurana, C. A., Beck, B., & Newton, G. L. (1998). How principles of partnership are applied to the development of a community-campus partnership. *Partnership Perspectives, 1*(1), 47–53.

Mayne, L. & Glascoff, M. (2002). Service learning: Preparing a healthcare workforce for the next century. *Nurse Educator, 27*(4), 191–194.

McKinnon, T. H., & Fealy, G. (2011). Core principles for developing global service-learning programs in nursing. *Nursing Education Perspectives, 32*(2), 95–100.

National Service-Learning Clearinghouse (NSLC). (2013). America's most comprehensive service-learning resource. Retrieved from http://www.servicelearning.org/

Norbeck, J. S., Connolly, C., & Koerner, J. (1998). *Caring and community: Concepts and models for service-learning in nursing.* San Francisco, CA: American Association for Higher Education.

Nyden, P. (2003). Academic incentives for faculty participation in community-based participatory research. *Journal of General and Internal Medicine, 18*, 576–585.

O'Brien-Larivée, C. (2011). A service-learning experience to teach baccalaureate nursing students about health policy. *Journal of Nursing Education, 50*(6), 332–336.

Redman, R. W., & Clark, L. (2002). Service-learning as a model for integrating social justice in the nursing curriculum. *Journal of Nursing Education, 41*(10), 446–449.

Riedford, K. B. (2011). Bridging the gap between clinical experience and client access: Community engagement. *Journal of Nursing Education, 50*(6), 337–340.

Robinson, K., Sportsman, S., Eschiti, V. S., Bradshaw, P., & Bol, T. (2006). Preparing faculty and students for an international nursing education experience. *Journal of Continuing Education in Nursing, 37*(1), 21–29.

Ross, M. E. T. (2012). Linking classroom learning to the community through service learning. *Journal of Community Health Nursing, 29*, 53–60.

Rowthorn, V. (2012). Teaching health law: Health law service-learning trip, a how-to guide. *Journal of Law, Medicine & Ethics, 40*(2), 401–408.

Schneider, C. G., & Humphreys, D. (2005). Putting liberal education on the radar screen. *Chronicle of Higher Education.* Retrieved from http://chronicle.com/article/Putting-Liberal-Education-on/26781

Schoener, L., & Hopkins, M. L. (2004). Service learning: A tuberculosis screening clinic in an adult residential care facility. *Nurse Educator, 29*(6), 242–245.

Scott, S. B., Harrison, A. D., Baker, T., & Wills, J. D. (2005). Interdisciplinary community partnership for health professional students: A service-learning approach. *Journal of Allied Health, 34*(1), 31–35.

Seifer, S. D. (1998). Service-learning: Community–campus partnerships for health professions education. *Academic Medicine, 73*(3), 273–277.

Seifer, S. D., & Vaughn, R. L. (2002). Partners in caring and community: Service-learning in nursing education. *Journal of Nursing Education, 41*(10), 437–439.

Shinnamon, A., Gelmon, S. B., Holland, B. A. (1999). *Methods and strategies for assessing service-learning in the health professions.* San Francisco, CA: CCPH.

Tabi, M. M., & Mukherjee, S. (2003). Nursing in a global community: A study abroad program. *Journal of Transcultural Nursing, 14*(2), 134–138.

University of Vermont. (2013). Community-university partnerships & service learning. Retrieved from http://www.uvm.edu/partnerships/?Page=courses.php

University of Vermont, College of Medicine. (2013). Office of Primary Care and Area Health Education Centers. Retrieved from http://www.uvm.edu/medicine/ahec/

Walsh, L. V., & DeJoseph, J. (2003). "I saw it in a different light": International learning experiences in baccalaureate nursing education. *Journal of Nursing Education, 42*(6), 266–272.

Wang, C. C., & Redwood-Jones, Y. A. (2001). Photovoice ethics: Perspectives from Flint photovoice. *Health Education & Behavior, 28*(5), 560–572.

Warner, J. R. (2002). Cultural competence immersion experiences. Public health among the Navajo. *Nurse Educator, 27*(4), 187–190.

World Health Organization. (2013). Bangladesh country profile. Retrieved http://www.who.int/countries/bgd/en/

Worrell-Carlisle, P. (2005). Service-learning: A tool for developing cultural awareness. *Nurse Educator, 30*(5), 197–202.

CHAPTER 29

Study Abroad as a Strategy for Nursing Education

■ Julie Vosit-Steller ■

The American Association of Colleges of Nursing's *Essentials for of Baccalaureate Education* (AACN, 2008), the American Academy of Nursing Expert Panel of Global Health (Rosenkoetter & Nardi, 2007), and the International Council of Nurses (ICN, 2011) have called for nurses and nursing faculty to come together globally to educate nurses in greater numbers and in a forceful effort. Colleges and universities that educate nurses are encouraged to prepare and provide opportunities for students as global citizens and providers in global health programs (Leffers & Plotnik, 2011). As a result, nursing students have been offered national and international experiences for experiential learning to meet the criteria for service learning. It is worth exploring examples of U.S. university programs that model effective partnerships and prepare student groups prior to such immersion programs and the development of such programs to improve learning about being hosts to such partners. Study abroad opportunities are now considered mainstream in colleges of nursing and a means to immerse students and provide educators to train the culturally astute (Kostovich & Bermele, 2011). Due to globalization, immigration, and the fast-paced growth of ethnic diversity within the United States, the desire for nursing students to become culturally skillful, knowledgeable, and sensitive must be evaluated at the curricular level (Kostovich & Bermele, 2011).

The United States is experiencing the largest sustained immigration wave in its history, with an estimated 44.3 million documented and undocumented immigrants arriving each year from all parts of the world. At present, 15% of the U.S. population is composed of individuals who have emigrated both legally and illegally from Latin America. It is estimated that by 2050, the Latino population could number 102.6 million, or 24% of the U.S. population (Grieco, 2010). However, immigrants to the United States represent diverse populations from African, Asia, Europe, and the Pacific Islands (Min, 2006). The United States accepts more legal immigrants as permanent residents than any other country in the world (Lee & Rytina, 2008). Yet it is estimated that there are significant numbers of immigrants to the United States who have illegally entered the country (Associated Press, 2006).

Often these individuals are poor, do not speak English, and are leaving adversity and other family members in their own country.

■ Importance of Study Abroad Programs for Students' Education

As a result of globalization, nursing graduates are likely to care for individuals from diverse cultural and ethnic backgrounds and may find themselves in work settings outside the United States. Understanding the impact of culture and health and incorporating this understanding into the provision of evidenced-based and cost-effective patient care needs to be a component of clinical training. These concepts are the underpinning of the development of cultural sensitivity (Johns & Thompson, 2010). Research findings suggest that study abroad experiences contribute significantly to personal and intellectual development, as well as to global understanding of competently delivered nursing care (Johns & Thompson, 2010). The increase in immigration to the United States in recent years has resulted in dramatic changes in the cultural tapestry of American society. It has challenged our public and private institutions to respond to individuals and groups that are of different religions, cultural beliefs, and traditions. Among U.S. institutions, the healthcare system has been disproportionately impacted by immigration. Language, unfamiliar health beliefs and practices, and inability to pay for care are all challenges for healthcare institutions and healthcare providers. For many immigrants who come to the United States to work, their immigration is the result of seeking a better life and escaping poverty in their home country.

While there is an ongoing debate as to the ethics and cost of providing care to immigrants, especially those who have entered the United States illegally, there is no debate that immigration has changed the healthcare system. The U.S. healthcare system has historically been focused on providing health care for individuals of European descent and for African Americans. Increasingly, the healthcare system is responding to a global population, which is placing new demands on its organization. It has become critical that healthcare providers gain a broader perspective of health and treatment to adequately perform their roles. This challenge to gain a more multicultural perspective of health and traditions of health care is particularly essential among nurses, who represent the largest group of healthcare providers in the United States.

As described by Bennett and Holtz (2008), nursing as a profession is constantly striving to improve the delivery of health care to clients of all races, nationalities, and socioeconomic statuses. Patients from cultures other than that of the nurse often do not benefit from nursing care because of miscommunications, misunderstandings, and/or conflicts of values, beliefs, norms, and attitudes. True experts in care of the culturally diverse are nurses from the patients' countries of origin (Leffers & Plotnick, 2011). Because of the recent influx of international patients in the United States, comprehensive knowledge of the culture of the patient is imperative to adequately assess, plan, implement, and evaluate nursing care. In addition, understanding the patient's culture is likely to increase his or her satisfaction with the nursing care. Cultural competence is an ongoing process of seeking cultural awareness, cultural knowledge, cultural skill, and cultural encounters (Camphina-Bacote, 1994; Leininger, 1978; Purnell & Paulanka, 2003; Spector, 2004).

Hall, Stevens, and Meleis (1994) have shown that the future of successful transcultural nurse–patient communication depends on the nurses' abilities to meet the needs of an ever-growing diverse population. Madeline Leininger, the founder of transcultural nursing theory (1978, p. 11), stated, "Our American nursing care practices tend to rely upon unicultural values which are largely derived from our Anglo-American caring values and expectations." Maintaining an open attitude in examining one's own prejudices, attitudes, and stereotyped perceptions is essential before one can learn about people of other cultures. It is not the clients' responsibility to be understood, but the nurse's responsibility to understand and meet the clients' needs (Leininger, 1978). In our pluralistic society, nurses must develop an understanding about culture and its relevance to competent care. To provide this care, nurses must understand specific factors that influence individual health and illness behaviors. Life-changing educational experiences have been shared by both students and faculty when well-organized collaborations between international partners are developed and consistently followed (Johns & Thompson, 2010).

■ Overview of the Growth of Study Abroad Programs

It is the responsibility of universities to provide an education for students that will allow them to experience and compete in the global market, and it will be important for all students' education to help them become global citizens. For educators in the health disciplines, facilitating students in gaining a more global perspective, including cultural understanding of individuals from different health traditions, is an evolving component of their role as educators.

Carpenter and Garcia (2012) showed how a study abroad experience influenced the participants' awareness, sensitivity, knowledge, and skills related to culture of the people in a study in Guadalajara. This study was guided by the conceptualization of cultural competence as having the following four components: cultural awareness (affective dimension), cultural sensitivity (attitudinal dimension), cultural knowledge (cognitive dimension), and cultural skills (behavioral dimension). In choosing strategies for developing cultural competence that fit into otherwise full nursing programs and creating mechanisms to evaluate the results, nurse educators have been guided by the document, *Cultural Competency in Baccalaureate Nursing Education,* and its accompanying toolkit of resources (AACN, 2008). The toolkit in the study offers an extensive list of integrative classroom and clinical learning strategies, references, and Web resources to foster cultural competency (Carpenter & Garcia, 2012). The National League for Nursing toolkit on innovations in curriculum design (2011) also offers suggested strategies to enhance development of cultural competence. The Guadalajara experience described the use of some of the suggestions found in these toolkits—for example, offering an immersion experience, participating in community activities, arranging field trips, and encouraging students to keep a journal (Carpenter & Garcia, 2012). Again, study abroad is one way to broaden American nursing students' worldview, but nursing curricula are sequential and crowded with essential content and practice competencies; thus, nursing students rarely have the luxury of spending a semester abroad to experience another culture (Carpenter & Garcia, 2012). Depending on the location of the nursing program and available clinical experiences, students may be exposed to patients from diverse cultures, but such experiences are random. Although a recent search cited the existence of more than 220 study abroad programs for nursing students (Nursing Study Abroad, 2012), many nursing students are unaware of opportunities outside the prescribed curriculum.

Camphina-Bacote reminds us that effectively teaching cultural competence in nursing education "is a journey that reflects an ongoing transformational process" (2006, p. 244). We must keep working to address perceived barriers for ethnically diverse students; the challenges faced by students and faculty of color; gender and disability issues among nursing students; and cultural and linguistic issues in caring for culturally and ethnically diverse patients (Camphina-Bacote, 2003). Carpenter and Garcia (2012) demonstrated that a study abroad experience provided deeply personal learning opportunities resulting in enhanced awareness, sensitivity, knowledge, and skills important for addressing cultural differences in nursing practice.

Cultural competence is a relative term that suggests a level of understanding of another's culture expectations related to that culture. There are a variety of educational strategies that are used to introduce students to other cultures. Study abroad programs can be effective in exposing students and faculty members to individuals from other backgrounds than their own, providing a new level of understanding of these individuals' experiences, beliefs, and cultural traditions. The goal of such study abroad experiences is to expand the students' perspectives of the world, promote a new sensitivity to beliefs and traditions different from their own, and promote a sense of intellectual openness that supports ongoing learning that extends beyond the students' formal education (Bennett & Holtz, 2008).

Study abroad programs for university faculty members and students vary from short tourist-like visits, which can often give a quick and sometimes superficial glimpse of a country, with its language, culture, and various special attractions, to a long-term, more intense experience (an immersion experience) in which the participants live, work, and study within local populations. As described by Leininger and McFarland (2002), an "etic" experience involves only the view and belief of an observer, which may or may not be an accurate reflection of the genuine culture of a given people.

Study abroad education provides students with a distinct advantage upon graduation. In today's global economy, study abroad experiences are an enormous asset to a student's resume and academic experiences. An increasing number of healthcare corporations are looking for candidates who have the ability to communicate and work with people from various cultural backgrounds. This is especially true in the healthcare professions, where more and more healthcare industries are legally and competitively challenged to provide safe and culturally appropriate patient care. In addition, having a broader world perspective provides for greater depth of understanding of global health challenges, which gives nursing students greater opportunities to become better local citizens within their communities.

■ Common Goals of Study Abroad Programs

Study abroad embraces the notion of experiential learning leading to meaningful outcomes for all who participate. We must continue to develop and study innovative learning experiences throughout our nursing programs to ensure and enhance the development of cultural competence to provide better care to a diverse society. Common goals of such programs often include the following:

1. *Personal growth and experiential learning.* Students and faculty who return from a study abroad program often see it as an experience that matured them personally and intellectually. They praise being exposed to new ways of thinking and living, which encourages growth and independence. For many, going abroad to study is the first time they have really been away from home, from familiar surroundings of the United States, as well as from friends and family. This is seldom an easy experience, but it is worthwhile, often even life transforming. After immersing themselves in a new culture, mastering the challenges of learning in a new and different academic environment, and having the experience of being a foreigner, they often return home with increased self-confidence and pride in what they have achieved. Incorporation of service learning and time in a foreign classroom setting have been identified as primary aims toward personal growth for students (Kostovich & Bermele, 2012).

2. A *global perspective of the world.* Study abroad can broaden intellectual horizons and deepen knowledge and understanding of international, political, social, and economic issues. By having this experience, a person will learn how others view the United States and its world role. When living in a country where English is not the native language, or is spoken only by some, a person will learn the practical importance of learning another language and using it. Being immersed in an environment where communicating simple daily needs is a challenge can be an eye-opening experience for students, helping them move from the cognitive phase to the affective phase of well-known cultural curricular development models (Kostovich & Bermele, 2012).

3. *Career enhancement.* Study abroad also can enhance employment prospects, especially in the fields of health care, informatics, international affairs, and government service. Employers increasingly seek graduates who have studied abroad. They know that students who have successfully completed a study abroad program are likely to possess international knowledge and often

second-language skills. Such students are also likely to have other competencies that graduate and professional schools and employers value highly, such as cross-cultural communication skills, analytical skills, an understanding of and familiarity with local customs and cultural contexts, flexibility, resilience, and the ability to adapt to new circumstances and deal constructively with differences.

■ Study Abroad in Health Professions Versus Mission Trips

Study abroad in health professions within a university setting, such as a nursing elective course, provides a student with specific goals and objectives to achieve within an academic setting. The emphasis is intellectual, professional, and objective. Students must conduct themselves professionally and complete all necessary goals with activities within a certain time frame, and their professional performance and personal conduct are evaluated. Funding sources for the trip may differ. The entire course is evaluated by faculty teaching the course, by others within the university system, and by outside accrediting agencies. Mission trips may have similar goals, but they may also have a religious, political, or economic focus with other evaluation criteria. From an educational perspective, such trips may vary in purpose and philosophy. Pre- and post-trip planning can assist faculty in best preparation and expectation for abroad experiences.

■ Faculty and Student Experiential Learning in Eastern Europe: Brasov, Romania

Study abroad experiences, as a strategy to develop cultural sensitivity, are increasingly popular in nursing education. A collaborative relationship involved the forging of an intercollegiate relationship between two American colleges of nursing and a Romanian undergraduate program in nursing. The experience provided the faculty an opportunity to focus on development of cultural learning, and they also become proficient in organizing and coordinating trip logistics.

Through the study abroad experience, the student goals were identified to develop cultural sensitivity through immersion in two different cultural groups within the country—the Romanians at large and the palliative care/hospice nursing community. Additionally, the students' goals were to be able to meet the course clinical objectives at the graduate level for the family nurse practitioner program. Students' written reflections included descriptions of how the trip was life changing and altered their view of health care in a post-Communist system; their understanding of the relationship between health and poverty, and between chronic disease and death; and their awareness of their own cultural behavior norms that reflect materialism and spirituality.

Background

The need for palliative care for patients with malignant disease in southeast Europe is immense. In 2002, Romania had one practicing physician for every 580 people

(European Observatory of Health Care Systems, 2002). Deaths from cancer and other terminal illnesses number approximately 41,000 per annum in Romania, and in neighboring Serbia, cancer claims 20,000 lives annually. Cardiovascular disease and cancer account for 50% of deaths in Romanians who are under 64 years of age and 85% in those who are over 65 years (European Observatory of Health Care Systems, 2002). Lung and respiratory cancers are the most prevalent (World Health Organization, 2012); cancers of the lung, trachea, and bronchus account for 4% of deaths annually, followed by colon and rectal cancers, breast cancer, cervical cancer, and stomach cancer, which collectively claim 2% of lives annually. People suffering life-threatening or terminal illnesses such as advanced cancer are particularly vulnerable to poorly funded services. Many people do not seek health care because of fear. Education regarding prevention, early diagnosis, and treatment is lacking, and healthcare costs are assumed by individuals and their families. Surgery, chemotherapy, and radiation therapy are available only in Bucharest, Cluj, Oradea, and Tirgue Mures. Since diagnostic tests are very limited even in cities like Brasov, diagnosis takes more time and the patient bears the burden of lengthy hospital stays. As a result of these factors, individuals often present to their physician in very advanced stages of illness, when symptoms are severely affecting their level of functioning and quality of life. Consequently, Romanians who are diagnosed with a terminal illness are likely to be sent home from the hospital to perish, often without sufficient support or adequate pain relief. Ninety percent of Romanians die at home (World Health Organization, 2012). Romania's neighbors such as Serbia and Macedonia fare no better.

Creation of an Eastern European Nursing Collaboration

The creation of sustainable, international collaborations is congruent with the mission and values of nursing and the philosophy of nursing education. Establishing collaborative nursing education and practice programs ultimately improves clinical experiences and patient care. In 2003, a trans-Atlantic partnership was formed between a collaborative group called the New England Alliance (NEA) for Hospice of Hope and Hospice Casa Sperantei in Brasov, Romania (part of the Hospice of Hope organization). The NEA is an academic and collaborative relationship between the College of Nursing at the University of Rhode Island (URI) and the School of Nursing and Health Studies at Simmons College in Boston, Massachusetts. Hospice Casa Sperantei provides hospice and palliative care services to Brasov and the surrounding communities. Of note, the Romanian team considers hospice care to be part of the palliative care services.

The initial connection to the Romanian nurses was made through the American board of trustees of the hospice. The multinational nurses in the partnership sustain this collaboration to provide nursing education and professional development to foster evidence-based palliative care practice to nurses in Romania (Kirschling & Erickson, 2010). Eight members of the NEA have traveled to Romania 3 times; the visits provided clinical experiences for a total of 6 American nurse practitioner students. In 2009, the group also included a lymphedema therapist. Overall, these experiences influenced the participants' interest in interprofessional collaboration and continuing palliative care education. In June 2011, 12 members of the NEA traveled to Romania; 3 members were students, and 5 returned for a second or third experience.

The vehicles for collaborative education included clinical site visits at home, visits at the inpatient hospice, and continuing education programs with the Romanian nurses via on-site conferences. The collaboration was sustained following return of the visit by teleconferencing, research, and publications. The relationship has a dynamic vision to facilitate growth in the advancement of professional nursing in Romania, to foster transformational academic/service partnerships, and to a establish a mentorship model (Bleich, Hewlett, Miller, & Bender, 2004; Gerzevitz, Ferszt, Vosit-Steller, & Mitrea, 2009). The NEA's mission was inspired to build on the existing structure of Romanian nursing education and professionalism and to overcome cultural barriers to collaboration.

Establishing international collaborative relationships is both challenging and rewarding. In the process of strengthening relationships between the NEA and the hospice, members presented several teleconferences focused on improving the quality of life of terminally ill patients in Romania. The initial collaboration efforts in 2007 were somewhat limited in their effectiveness due to clinical challenges, cultural differences influencing learning styles, language difficulty, and a perceived mistrust that was described as a throwback to the previous oppressive Communist regime (Gerzevitz et al., 2009). The reported effects of the Communist regime consist of lack of self-esteem, lack of trust in people, and lack of support from the state infrastructure. Visiting the Romanian inpatient hospices, spending time face to face with the Romanian nurses and their patients, building trust, and encouraging and validating their nursing practice proved to be critical factors in forging this successful initiative (Gerzevitz et al., 2009).

In the beginning, cultural and language differences challenged the growth of the collaboration; however, a specific working relationship was established with a lead nurse who was fluent in English. Her commitment and enthusiasm aided the transition to a trusting relationship and rapport. In addition, translating nursing and academic resource material ahead of time allowed for non-English speakers to participate in the learning; this provided opportunity for involvement of the entire nursing team. The main factors that led to success were exchange of positive feedback and nurturing of the critical thinking of Romanian nurses. Appreciation of cultural differences, understanding of educational needs, advanced planning, good communication among the three site facilitators, and good technical support were essential to this fruitful educational endeavor.

In Romanian hospitals, clinical nursing practice does not change according to the new findings in the research field. Instead, every new generation inherits the archaic mode of delivering care; each nursing unit has its own way of doing things and therefore ignores the knowledge learned during basic nursing education (Mitrea, 2010). In general, face-to-face contact, as utilized by the NEA, provided opportunities to develop an understanding of cultural differences, to discuss expectations from educational approaches, and to begin to establish a relationship based on mutual respect (Memmott et al., 2010).

Another notable result of the collaboration was the creation of focus groups between the Romanian palliative care nurses and members of each hospital and/or specialty practice. These groups now meet regularly and have created pathways of communication for patients and families (Vosit-Steller, White, Barron, Gerzevitz, & Morse, 2010). The interdisciplinary collaboration among Romanian clinicians led to an increased trust across disciplines. A trusted relationship has replaced a competitive relationship that existed between separate clinical settings (Bleich et al., 2004).

The next phase of the NEA collaborative relationship with Hospice Casa Sperantei depends on communication, competence, and strategies (Bleich et al., 2004; Memmett et al., 2010). There is a need to sustain training resources, to acknowledge the need to translate any newly acquired techniques to their own practices, to expand education, and to transform support by reevaluating the role of collaboration on an annual basis. A current emphasis on developing nursing literature, obtaining skill for writing articles, and expanding support for palliative care training programs in remote countries affiliated with the Hospice of Hope are the current priorities of the NEA.

Collaboration is a dynamic process that benefits both the mentor and the mentee, particularly when both understand each other's needs. In our situation, the mentee is now an advisor, counselor, coach, guide, teacher, and friend whom others trust for valuable perspective. Our conversations with one another are uplifting and bring a sense of new possibilities to the relationship. Our Romanian colleagues go out of their way to set goals for themselves in the context of our collaboration and foster the development of their skills to reach these goals. The American team has gazed in silent wonder on our own professional growth following our many academic or face-to-visits; these moments are often unknown to our Romanian colleagues.

Mentorship has given each of us an opportunity to give back, to show our gratitude, and to reciprocate. These contributions provided the opportunity to prepare Romanian nurses for future leadership—a strength that is necessary in today's international nursing environment. We have all examined and validated what we have learned. We feel satisfied, proud, and rejuvenated as we see the benefits of our collaboration. The most powerful way to change the world, one person at a time, is to take the time to reach out to others, share wisdom, convey respect, and grow together.

The Nursing Practicum in Brasov, Romania, at Hospice Casa Sperantei

Objectives

The objectives of the nursing practicum program reflect the mission of the university and the community needs for college graduates, which is to possess global awareness and cultural sensitivity. More specifically, the objectives reflect the needs of nurses who will be working with Romanian patients in the community. The course objectives include the following:

1. Explore one's personal attitudes and beliefs about inpatients at the hospice in Brasov, Romania.
2. Examine the structure and function of healthcare delivery to patients at the hospices and patients receiving palliative care in Brasov and Bucharest.
3. Explore the main health issues of the local communities, including the Roma or gypsy community.
4. Actively participate in the healthcare delivery to patients enrolled in hospice and palliative care.
5. Improve Romanian language skills and communicate with patients, staff, and others in the community.
6. Explore the health beliefs and local Christian Orthodox cultural customs and practices of the Romanian community.

Setting up the Program

The initial process in developing the nursing experience in Brasov began with a visit to the area to determine the feasibility of establishing a 2-week intensive study abroad nursing course. Contact with the leaders of health care in the community was essential. The Simmons and URI professors contacted the Ministry of Health for the state of Romania. A discussion with the secretary and key healthcare community leaders of Hospice of Hope and Romania produced a dialogue regarding goals and expectations of the experience for students, the facilities and experiences available to students, the type of nursing faculty supervision expected for students working in the palliative care/hospice healthcare facilities, and potential benefits to the local healthcare system. When setting up a program such as this one, it is essential to establish a network of local people who will agree to coordinate student housing, transportation, Romanian language translation and courses at the hospice and with the nurses, student work experiences with the nurses in the field or at the hospice, and transportation for local cultural excursions and touring.

A leader within the NEA group coordinated the housing with a contact at the hospice. One meal daily was provided at the hospice. Breakfast and dinner were purchased with the group. Mealtimes were usually used as postconference time. The nurses knew which foods would be appealing and safe for American students to eat and communicated this to the American team. A coordinator from the hospice volunteered for local excursions. This person assisted with all transportation and agenda arrangements for weekend full-day cultural outings to nearby villages to see castles and shop at markets.

The NEA team visited Romania and practiced with nursing colleagues biannually in 2005–2011. The student nurses worked in both the inpatient and outpatient hospice settings in Brasov and went on home visits and discussed care planning and implementation. During meal times, the nurses discussed difficult clinical and social cases. Together, the group conducted education seminars to explore issues such as rituals at the time of death and terminal wound management. Quarterly teleconferences with the Romanian nurses have deepened the professional relationship. Topics include clinical case presentations and discussions of barriers to care. There has been visible growth within the international working group. Although the immersion to the Romanian culture was the initial introduction to their nursing practice, it has been the use of technology through teleconferencing and ongoing research that has sustained and fostered the foundation of trust over time in our relationship.

Nursing Student Experiences

Establishing international collaborative relationships is both challenging and rewarding. In the process of establishing a relationship between Romania and two colleges of nursing in the United States, two site visits were made by U.S. team members to Romania. Face-to-face contacts provided opportunities to develop an understanding of cultural differences, discuss expectations regarding educational approaches, and begin to establish a relationship based on mutual respect. During its 10-day visit, the team visited the inpatient hospice and the Princess Diana Education Center in Brasov. Team members also attended the Balkan Palliative Care Conference sponsored by Hospice of Hope, which forged other potential relationships with hospice professional staff working in outpatient hospices from Serbia, Moldova, Macedonia, and other Balkan countries.

One of the student experiences included a visit to a 60-year-old Romanian widow. She was a new patient to the hospice nurses. She was a practicing Christian Orthodox and received a modest pension from the government. Her medical history included cardiovascular disease. She was diagnosed with breast cancer the year of our visit and treated surgically with a unilateral mastectomy. She refused further treatment with chemotherapy or radiation. After several months, she presented with a fungating breast lesion. The major concern of the hospice nurses were related to the ineffective wound management, the pain management, and the patient's body image. These issues were addressed in postconference discussion and using suggestions from that post-conference, the nurses discussed those issues with the patient during a home visit the following day.

In Bucharest, the visiting American students and team members accompanied the hospice nurses on their home visits. In their journals and in postconference meetings, the students noted that meeting patients and hearing their stories was engaging and saddening. The lack of resources compared to the United States was striking. Patients, families, and hospice staff all had stories about the suffering that terminally ill patients face, the lack of services and supplies including medications for pain and symptom relief, lack of governmental financial support, and the need for further education in palliative care. The lack of hope in light of poverty, poor social services, and other effects of the post-Communist era had a profound impact on the U.S. team. However, the vision, commitment, and dedication of the Romanian hospice professional staff were inspiring. Selected comments from students follow.

"It gave me a better appreciation for the culture, the importance of family unity, and increased my language skills," said one. Another stated,

> I was impressed with what the nurses and doctors accomplished with so little supplies and materials. They were resourceful and careful. My experience in Brasov/Bucharest was very helpful to me with my nursing practice at home in the US. I am better able to relate and care for my end-of-life patients. This course was definitely a peak life experience for me. I have felt very drawn to the spirituality the people demonstrated, since I have worked at my hospital. This experience, being immersed in the culture, working with nurses, mothers and children, especially living in the Roma or gypsy communities, living with a family, was an opportunity to see inside a world that is rarely opened to outsiders or tourists. I am very grateful to have had this experience.

Another student made the following comment:

> I believe that I'm more knowledgeable about the Christian Orthodox culture, especially related to health care, as well as the language and medical care. With this knowledge I have been better equipped to plan and administer care that is individualized for the chronically ill pediatric population I come in contact with every day in my practice here in Boston. I consider this course to be the best I ever had. I learned so much besides nursing; I learned about politics, economics, post-communism society, the Romanian language, music and art, history, etc.

In both Romanian settings, it was clear that the patients were expertly cared for by nurses, doctors, and other professionals. Although the Romanian doctors and nurses have been well educated in palliative care, they seemed to have little confidence in their ability. This was surprising to the U.S. nurses given the excellent patient care that was provided by the Romanian nurses. The Romanian hospice team was willing to establish a collaborative relationship with the U.S. nurses and identified several areas where they felt they needed further education.

Despite the challenges posed by the inadequacies of the healthcare system, nursing care within the hospice network in Romania formally expanded during this time. The support of palliative care services and training of staff for the Romanian organization is largely the responsibility of the nursing staff at Hospice of Hope. The mission of the hospice includes raising awareness of the value of effective palliative care through education, advocacy, research, and promotion, and developing the provision of palliative care within the region through direct and indirect care. The core nursing team adapted the international End-of-Life Nursing Education Curriculum (ELNEC). The end-of-life nursing curriculum focuses on pain and symptom management, communication and culture, care at the time of death, and grief (Paice, Ferrell, Coyle, Coyne, & Callaway, 2008). Extensive support materials are used to provide supplemental resource materials to nurses who have financial constraints. Example protocols, policies, and education materials are offered.

The ELNEC program utilizes a train-the-trainer model, so it is realistic that one nurse could serve as the resource for an entire community. Training is a slow process, and access to health care at the end of life is difficult, particularly for patients who are living in poverty or cannot afford to pay for care. Continued education is offered by webcast and CD-ROM for professional development when technology is available. Sustaining palliative care initiatives has been possible by creating an infrastructure for coordination, information exchange, strategy, and advocacy at a national/regional level, yet facilitating empowerment, autonomy, and innovation for the nursing staff has been deficient.

Forging the Educational Initiative

The students and the faculty team discussed a number of alternatives for responding to the request from Romania. One student and two nursing faculty assumed the role of coordinators in their respective colleges of nursing and began to engage other interested faculty and clinicians, who met regularly to explore educational options. Teleconferencing was identified as the most cost-effective approach. However, Romania had no teleconferencing equipment. The administrators from Hospice Casa Sperantei began looking for a source of funding for the project, and a well-known philanthropic organization donated the equipment and oversaw the installation in the Princess Diana Educational Center in Brasov, Romania, and the mobile hospice in Bucharest. St. Elizabeth's Hospital in Boston was willing to donate time in its facility for the Simmons faculty to transmit to Romania. The URI instructional technology department was contacted, and a bridge was set up to facilitate the three sites transmitting simultaneously. The content and objectives of the first teleconference were identified based on the ELNEC.

Student Prerequisites and Preparation

Prerequisites for all student nurses included having completed at least the initial core graduate nursing courses with a clinical component, giving them skills in advanced health assessment. Most students were more advanced, with greater experiences in psychiatric, medical/surgical nursing and exposure to patients with complex chronic illness and patients who are actively dying. In addition, reading material assignments were given along with the student course syllabus so that students could prepare for their experiences ahead of time. Payment for the course included health insurance coverage during the students' stay in Romania. Insurance also included emergency air evacuation to the United States if needed. A list of vaccines required by the Centers for Disease Control and Prevention (CDC) was given. Students could obtain needed immunizations from the university's health clinic or another healthcare agency.

Recruitment of Students for the Trip

Faculty conducted informational sessions about the experience about 10 months prior to departure. Colorful and detailed flyers depicted photos of Brasov and a few very brief excerpts about the nursing elective course. Explanations regarding the costs, many available scholarships, and course elements were given. Some students were very creative in funding payments with a combination of scholarships, gifts from parents or other relatives, church donations, or extra overtime work in the hospitals. Students who really wanted to go found a way to achieve their goal.

Orientation

There were three mandatory student orientations. These were held 3 months prior to the trip, and within about 8 weeks before departure. During this orientation, students were given a written handout, and a group discussion addressed lodging, personal safety needs, documents, money, packing needs, special health challenges, housing, transportation, working in the field and in hospices, group dynamics and collaboration, culture shock and adjustments, cultural excursions, and, perhaps most important of all, cultural sensitivity and appropriate dress and behavior. Most of the students were excited about the experience and the direct patient care in the clinical settings. Some of the students were concerned about the language barriers and the need to present clinical expertise for the nurses in the field. Students were expected to be dressed professionally and prepared for drastic clinical situations, such as patients living in extreme poverty, patients with unclean wounds, and patients who were actively dying.

Donations of Supplies and Equipment

The Romanian nurses and the American faculty members noted that the hospice nurses did not have sufficient medical supplies and equipment for the patients being treated at home. These materials were assembled from a variety of sources. Some came from direct donations from physicians' private practices and some from local health departments or pharmacies within the greater Boston, Massachusetts, area. All donations were assembled, counted, and packed by faculty and students. A formal list, with types of supplies and quantities, was translated into Romanian for the customs office. The supplies were taken with the team into the country for an easier experience. Each student checked one box of supplies with his or her luggage, so that there were no additional fees for bringing the supplies into Romania. This experience taught the students in the beginning about sharing goods and thanking the health department ahead of time for supporting their medical experiences.

Educational Planning for the Visit

The Romanian hospice director provided the U.S. team with specific educational topics that they wanted addressed during their visit, including wound management, spiritual assessment, and end-of-life care. A carefully laid-out program for the visit included a day when individual U.S. team members were paired with the Romanian nurses to accompany them on home visits. They traveled throughout the surrounding countryside, into gypsy enclaves, high-rise apartments, and cottages. The U.S. nurses observed their Romanian counterparts provide perceptive, skillful, and compassionate palliative care. They were extremely creative and resourceful, particularly with the difficult constraints. Their practice was best practice despite their limited resources. The Romanian nurses seemed to lack confidence in their abilities and sought encouragement and validation from the U.S. nurses. At the end of the day, the U.S. nurses discussed their perceptions of the day and made plans for the following day's educational activities.

The site visit to Romania had proved to be the vehicle for developing a relationship based on mutual respect with the Romanian colleagues. Following this site visit, the Romanian team began to engage more actively in the teleconferencing format, demonstrating confidence and comfort with the U.S. team. The U.S. team continued to validate the quality of care they provided.

Teleconferencing

Teleconferencing is a very flexible and cost-effective teaching strategy. When well planned and delivered effectively, videoconferencing can be engaging and intellectually stimulating. Teleconferencing has been used successfully in medical education in a number of countries, including the United States. A geriatric team was able to model a patient-centered approach and provide for a patient and his physician without having to travel for consultation. In the United States, clinical supervision and education of 10 psycho-oncology staff was provided monthly through the use of videoconferencing. One-hour educational programs were followed by 1-hour discussions. Participants noted an increase in their knowledge, greater confidence in treating cancer pain, and increased effectiveness in management of psychosocial distress. After the study abroad immersion, attempts were again made for a more successful interchange in the teleconferencing format to sustain the collaborative relationship between the international nursing teams. Several topics were suggested by the Romanian team and addressed on a scheduled basis.

Several teleconferences have focused on improving the quality of life of terminally ill patients in Romania. The initial teleconferencing efforts were somewhat limited in their effectiveness due to technological challenges, cultural differences influencing learning styles, language difficulty, and a perceived element of mistrust, which was described as a throwback to the previous oppressive Communist regime. Visiting the Romanian hospices and spending time face to face with the Romanian nurses and their patients, building trust, and encouraging and validating their nursing practice proved to be a critical factor in forging this successful initiative. Electronic communication has presented opportunity to advance practice methods and provide validation for nursing actions. Appreciation of cultural differences and understanding of educational needs, advance planning, good communication among the three site facilitators, and good technical support have been essential in this fruitful, educational endeavor. Not surprisingly, there is little documentation of the excellent work of the Romanian nurses who serve dying patients in their country. Collaboration with these nurses confirms the value of their efforts made at the end of life to promote excellent clinical care and dignity.

Course Grade Requirements

The student work was graded according to the expectations and outcomes outlined in the course syllabi. Students were required to attend all pre- and post-practice conferences, as well as participate in the hands-on clinical work with the Romanian nurses. The course grading criteria followed the university or college criteria for undergraduate or graduate students—whatever applied to the individual student. The clinical participation was graded on a pass/fail basis. All students were asked to keep a journal in the format of critical reflective thinking. Their feelings, thoughts, responses, observations, and activities were recorded. Students were encouraged to write about their prior thoughts about Romania before they began the trip, and compare and contrast them to the actual experiences that they encountered; this is the premise of reflective journaling. The graduate students were required to write a major paper on an aspect of their experience that counted as 25% of their final course grade. They were also given an assignment to write a scholarly paper or participate in a group project (specific criteria were given) that addressed a health issue in Brasov, Romania. Both the journal summary paper and the scholarly course project/paper were due at the end of the following semester, giving the students ample time to collect information in Brasov (if they chose to do so) and complete the assignments well after they returned home. Students also assisted in collecting data for faculty research and presented it at conferences. In this manner, students would not be pressured to complete course assignments during their 2-week cultural experience.

Student Course Evaluations

Formative and summative evaluations usually provide valuable information about immersion experiences. Reported student observations during and after the visits can be helpful in shifting day-to-day priorities and course objectives to improve the experience for the future. Faculty may become aware of what students learn in the setting by offering course evaluations throughout the experience. Providing time within the conferences allows the students the opportunity to reflect and provide the evaluations while the memories are clear to them and they have designated time.

■ Guidelines for Setting up a For-Credit, Elective, Study Abroad Program for Student Nurses

The use of recommendations based on the collective wisdom of experienced nursing faculty who have participated in experiential learning can provide a rubric for successful study abroad courses. Whether the program is in the beginning stages of development or has been functioning for many years, working with diverse and international populations presents challenges for faculty and student learning. The following guidelines may provide a rubric for both structure, evaluation, and outcomes.

1. Create a proposal with the following:
   a. Goals and objectives of proposed program

    b. Location—distance, safety, costs, local interest and support for program, easy accessibility; collaborate with study abroad office

    c. Experiences for students and faculty—clinical experiences, participation in cultural activities, local language lessons

    d. Safety plan—political safety and stability, environmental safety (climate, local disease threats), health insurance and local health care available for participants, emergency evacuation plan

    e. Student prerequisites—nursing skills, language background, grade point average, orientation, disciplinary rules

    f. Number of faculty needed

    g. Number of students expected (interest survey given to students may give a more precise idea)

    h. Transportation—round trip to destination, as well as local transportation

    i. Estimated costs

2. Obtain support from the university's president, provost, dean, department chairs, and whoever else who may need to approve the endeavor. Obtain seed money to investigate the feasibility of the program and provide transportation, housing, and other costs needed to explore an area to make initial preparations for the proposed program. Gifts may also be required in some cultures to facilitate appointments for key people in the local proposed site.

3. Make a preparation visit to the proposed location.

    a. If possible, arrange all transportation and housing as you would expect to with students. Stay in a hotel or with a local family as you would expect students to experience to see how the experience would be for students. Always ask permission to take pictures to show the university administrators as well as prospective students.

    b. Keep a detailed record book of all costs encountered. This will help in designing a course with an accurate price to reflect real costs.

    c. Find a person who has experience and is willing to coordinate housing for students. This person will require a placement fee per student. Often the local university has such a person, or a secretary may be able to handle this. See if the university already has someone who assists foreign students with housing. Visit several homes or hotels for proposed housing and get specifics with prices.

    d. Obtain local language lessons. Find a local university or language school that is willing to give lessons to students at a reasonable price for 1 hour per day. This will help students to enhance their language and cultural background while they are at the proposed location.

    e. Meet with the minister of health (or equivalent person of high ranking in the community) to discuss the students' participation in caring for local patients within a healthcare setting (hospitals or clinics). Discuss specifically student roles, supervision by faculty, dress codes, hours of work, and length of stay, among other issues. If it is culturally appropriate, get a written contract.

Ask which types of supplies or equipment are needed for the purpose of donations in the future. After the meeting, send flowers and a thank you note to the person for giving his or her time and attention. Note: Students working within a different culture and language should not be giving medications because of the safety issue, which could be further threatened by a language barrier.

4. Meet with a tourist travel agency or find a specific person in the community who will agree to provide transportation and help with an agenda for visiting sites of interest. Take advantage of all local tourist attractions, emphasizing anything reflecting health care if available.

5. Recruit students.

   a. Prior to recruitment, make all decisions about transportation, tuition, housing, food, cultural sites, donations, health insurance, availability of scholarships, and other factors, and prepare a formal budget. Decide how much it will cost per student for the entire package.

   b. Create a brochure for the course/trip with detailed specifics of costs, inclusions, dates, course credits, prerequisites, and other information, and print flyers for a recruitment session. Several recruitment sessions may be necessary to contact all available students who may be interested in the program. Arrange a date, time, and location for the recruitments, and order food. If possible, bring photos or present a PowerPoint slide show of pictures of the area. Obtain a list of interested students with names and e-mail contacts, and provide a way for students to sign up for the course. If the university already has other study abroad programs in place, they may be extremely helpful in planning your program.

   c. Collect all fees prior to departure. Assemble supplies or equipment donations. Pack donations and send boxes with students to avoid mailing costs and possible theft of items.

   d. Create a mandatory orientation program prior to departure. Make sure that all students have all necessary passports, visas, and vaccinations. Supply food and invite all family or friends who are interested in the trip details. Review and give written handouts relating a typical day, dress and behavior codes, and health guidance including what to eat and which medications to bring. Include a list of what to pack, identifying the weight and number limitations for luggage. State where to meet at the airport and at what time. Emphasize the safety and health plan. Review rules and regulations. Pass out the course syllabus and review pre-trip readings available. A survey of student perceptions of the trip prior to leaving would make an interesting point of comparison to impressions after having had the experience. Encourage students to bring a small gift for their host family and nurse mentors at their location.

   e. Have students review and sign a code of behavior while studying in the location. Include the following:

      i. No alcohol or drug use is permitted.

      ii. Dress codes and rules for expected behavior with family, faculty, and all members of local community are to be written and enforced.

     iii. No leaving of the city under any circumstances without permission of faculty is permitted.

     iv. All students will stay all night with their host family, with no exceptions.

      v. Students will always follow the faculty's instructions and are subject to being sent home, incurring their own extra expenses, if they do not behave.

     vi. Students will fail the course if they do not behave as instructed by faculty.

6. Plan and document the experience while at the location.

   a. Plan an orientation with local health administration for tours and work assignments, to give donations of supplies, and offer to pay for snacks served. Bring a gift for key health administrator contacts.

   b. Keep a daily journal of visits, contacts, phone numbers and e-mail addresses, costs, problems to be solved, and daily agenda.

   c. Make student assignments with local agency administrators. Give students preferences when possible according to their previous experiences and language abilities.

   d. Make local community contacts on your own time. Meet the directors of all hospitals, clinics, housing, group excursions, and language centers. Bring small gifts or take them for coffee and pastries when meeting with them. Emphasize how much you appreciate the help that they are giving to you.

   e. Make friends in the local community with merchants, taxi drivers, restaurant owners, and other service providers, and if relationships are successful, bring students to them. Often you will receive a group discount on tickets, transportation, food, and other items with these relationships.

   f. Participate in all student activities. Take local language classes with students and assist with supervision in hospitals, in clinics, and on all cultural excursions. Find out about other activities in the community that may interest students.

■ Setting up for Success

The following is from many experiences in which faculty have learned something the hard way with no idea of what to expect, especially in the first few years. It is never possible to know ahead of time which problems may occur. Faculty as well as students need to be flexible and adaptable to new challenges.

1. Always write a code of behavior, emphasize it at recruitment, at orientation, and during the visit to the host country. Have students sign the behavior code.

2. Always have health insurance with evacuation coverage for all students and faculty. It is very reasonable. Do not rely on local healthcare facilities

for serious accidents or illnesses. For minor problems, they usually will be fine.

3. Make sure that all students stay in the local city at all times and spend the night with host families every night.

4. Review safety precautions for money (under-the-clothing money bags for traveling) and locking valuables such as passports, money, credit cards, and cameras with their host family.

5. Constantly remind students about what and where is safe to eat and drink, and be sure that they are always aware.

6. Always watch luggage and carry-ons at airports. Things may disappear very quickly, especially in developing countries, if they are valuable and unattended.

7. Be prepared to deal with culture shock. Language, customs, and in some locations tremendous, never-before-seen poverty can overwhelm faculty and students. Many poor people, including those begging in the streets, can be overwhelming. Giving away prepared sandwiches and fruit or bread can be a group activity that can help some of the overwhelming feelings of frustration.

8. Have students always travel in groups and always carry information with them regarding their host family homes and contact information for reaching faculty 24/7.

9. Always be available to students 24/7. This is not like the responsibility of a classroom on campus.

REFERENCES

American Association of Colleges of Nursing (AACN). (2008). The essentials of baccalaureate education for professional nursing practice. Retrieved from www.aacn.nche.edu/Education/essentials/htm

Associated Press. (2006). U.S. population hits 300 million. Retrieved from http://www.msnbc.msn.com/id/15298443/

Bennett, S., & Holtz, C. (2008). Building cultural competence: A nursing program in Oaxaca, Mexico. In C. Holtz (Ed.), *Global health care* (pp. 601–614). Sudbury, MA: Jones and Bartlett.

Bleich, M. R., Hewlett, P. O., Miller, K. L., & Bender, K. (2004). Beyond tradition: Synergizing intellectual and material capital to forge the new academic-service partnership. *Journal of Professional Nursing, 20*(5), 285–294. doi: 10.1016/j.profnurs.2004.07.007

Camphina-Bacote, J. (1994). *The process of cultural competence in health care: A culturally competent model of care* (2nd ed.). Wyoming, OH: Perfect Printing Press.

Camphina-Bacote, J. (2003). Cultural desire: The key to unlocking cultural competence. *Journal of Nursing Education, 42*(6), 239–240.

Camphina-Bacote, J. (2006). Cultural competence in nursing curricula: How are we doing 20 years later? *Journal of Nursing Education, 45*(7), 243–244.

Carpenter, L. J., & Garcia, A. A. (2012). Assessing outcomes of a study abroad course for nursing students. *Nursing Education Perspectives, 33*(2), 85–89. doi: http://dx.doi.org/10.5480/1536-5026-33.2.85

European Observatory of Health Care Systems (2002). Romaina HiT summary (2002). Retrieved from http://www.euro.who.int/en/who-we-are/partners/observatory/health-systems-in-transition-hit-series/hit-summaries/romania-hit-summary-2002

Gerzevitz, D., Ferszt, G. G., Vosit-Steller, J., & Mitrea, N. (2009). Cross-cultural consultation on palliative care: The use of teleconferencing. *Journal of Hospice & Palliative Nursing, 11*(4), 239–244.

Grieco, E. M. (2010). *Race and Hispanic origin of the foreign-born population in the United States: 2007.* Washington, DC: U. S. Census Bureau. Retrieved from http://www.census.gov/prod/2010pubs /acs-11.pdf

Hall, J. M., Stevens, P. E., & Meleis, A. I. (1994). Marginalization: A guiding concept for evaluating diversity in nursing knowledge development. *Advances in Nursing Science, 16*(4), 2–41.

International Council of Nurses (ICN). (2011). Disaster planning and relief. Retrieved from www.icn.ch /publications/disaster-planning-and relief/disaster-planning-and relief.html

Johns, A., & Thompson, C. (2010). Developing cultural sensitivity through study abroad. *Home Health Care Management & Practice, 22*(5), 344–348. doi: http://dx.doi.org/10.1177/1084822309353153

Kirschling, J. M., & Erickson, J. I. (2010). The STTI practice-academe innovative collaboration award: Honoring innovation, partnership, and excellence. *Journal of Nursing Scholarship, 42*(3), 286–294.

Kostovich, C. T., & Bermele, C. A. (2011). The top ten list: Lessons learned from teaching a study abroad course. *Nursing Education Perspectives, 32*(5), 308–312.

Lee, J., & Rytina, N. (2008). Naturalizations in the United States: 2008. Retrieved from http://www.dhs .gov/xlibrary/assets/statistics/publications/natz_fr_2012.pdf

Leffers, J., & Plotnick, J. (2011). *Volunteering at home and abroad: The essential guide for nurses.* Indianapolis, IN: Sigma Theta Tau International.

Leininger, M. (1978). *Transcultural nursing: Concepts, theories, and practices.* New York, NY: John Wiley & Sons.

Leininger, M., & McFarland, M. (2002). *Transcultural nursing: Concepts, theories, research, and practices* (3rd ed.). New York, NY: McGraw-Hill.

Memmett, R. J., Coverston, C. R., Heise, B. A., Williams, M., Maughan, E. D., Kohl, J., & Palmer, S. (2010). Practical considerations in establishing sustainable international nursing experiences. *Nursing Education Perspectives, 31*(5), 298–302.

Min, P. G. (2006). Asian immigration: History and contemporary trends. In P. G. Min (Ed.), *Asian Americans: Contemporary trends and issues* (2nd ed., pp. 7–31). Thousand Oaks, CA: Pine Forge Press/ Sage.

Mitrea, N. (2010). *Integration of palliative care training for the university level curriculum of nursing in Eastern Europe.* Unpublished dissertation, University of Transylvania, Brasov, Romania.

National League for Nursing. (2011). Faculty toolkit for innovation in curriculum design. Retrieved from www.nln.org/facultyprograms/facultyresources/Toolkit_Innovation_Curriculum_Design/index. htm

Nursing Study Abroad. (2012). GoAbroad.com. Retrieved from www.studyabroaddirectory.com/listings /cfm/deprogID/75

Paice, J. A., Ferrell, B. R., Coyle, N., Coyne, P., & Callaway, M. (2008). Global efforts to improve palliative care: The International End-of-Life Nursing Education Consortium training program. *Journal of Advanced Nursing, 61*(2), 173–180.

Purnell, L., & Paulanka, B. J. (Eds.). (2003). *Transcultural health care: A culturally competent approach.* Philadelphia, PA: F. A. Davis.

Rosenkoetter, M. M., & Nardi, D. A. (2007). American Academy of Nursing Expert Panel on Global Nursing and Health: White paper on global nursing and health. *Journal of Transcultural Nursing, 18*(4), 23–34, 305–315.

Spector, R. (2004). *Cultural diversity in health and illness* (6th ed.). Norwalk, CT: Appleton & Lange.

Vosit-Steller, J., White, P., Barron, A., Gerzevitz, D., & Morse, A. (2010). Enhancing end-of-life care with dignity: Characterizing hospice nursing in Romania. *International Journal of Palliative Nursing, 16*(9), 459–464.

World Health Organization. (2012). Mortality: Country fact sheet. Retrieved from http://www.who.int /countries/rou/en/

SECTION VI

Evaluation

The final section of this text presents a brief glimpse at a key aspect of any educational program evaluation. Whereas the importance of evaluation is often overlooked, it is an essential part of the teaching–learning process. Educators predominantly think of evaluation either in the form of testing and grading or in the form of clinical evaluation. Chapters in this section describe innovative approaches to evaluation that educators use. Program evaluation is also discussed to assist educators in updating and improving current programs and developing new ones. A thorough evaluation provides information for quality attainment.

CHAPTER 30

Program Evaluation

■ Astrid H. Wilson ■

Academic institutions and healthcare facilities are required to be account-able to their stakeholders and can no longer only be judged by reputation and resources. The public wants academic institutions and healthcare facilities to demonstrate measurable outcomes of their work. For example, in nursing, licensure pass rates are one outcome of a quality program and ensure students the ability to be employed. Likewise, the public has access to hospital mortality and morbidity rates and can make decisions whether to use those facilities with undesirable rates. Program evaluation can assure the public that academic institutions and healthcare facilities provide quality instruction and quality health care. This chapter defines program evaluation, provides benefits of the evaluation, discusses one accreditation model, and provides examples of evaluation research.

■ Definition

There are numerous definitions of program evaluation cited in the literature (Chen, 2005; Davidson, 2005; Fink, 2005; McNamara, 2006; Mertz, 2007). The common theme in the definitions is that of program evaluation being a process of collecting data to determine the effectiveness of a selected program and to make decisions. There is also an emphasis on systematic methods in collecting data to include process and outcome evaluations.

■ Purpose

Program evaluation may be comprehensive or directed at specific aspects of a program. There are many different types of evaluations and reasons to conduct program evaluation, such as effectiveness, accreditation, out-comes, impact, cost/benefit analysis, needs assessment, and research to provide empirical support. In addition, program evaluations can be used to demonstrate program effectiveness if the program has been funded and may be used to request additional funding. It is a valuable way to record the program's accomplishments. Most importantly, it is an opportunity to honestly consider ways to improve the implementation (process) and the effectiveness (outcome) of the program.

Data can be collected from an educational program to determine a program's worth and the success of its graduates (Bell, Pestka, & Forsyth, 2007). Inexpensive methods to collect information for a program evaluation include questionnaires, surveys, and checklists, which can be anonymous and provide a large amount of data. Interviews can elicit more information than questionnaires, surveys, and checklists and allow the interviewer to validate statements, but they take more time and are more costly due to the personnel needed. Focus groups, usually audiotaped, can yield rich narratives from groups of 4–12 participants; however, a skilled moderator is needed to lead each group. Transcribing and analyzing the tapes may be cost prohibitive. Case studies fully depicting participants' experiences can be used to showcase the program but are time consuming to develop.

■ Benefits

There are many benefits to conducting program evaluation—both to the members of the program and to outside stakeholders such as administrators, accreditation boards, and grant funders. The members of the program benefit by gaining self-understanding and self-accountability and provide a way to show the accomplishments of the program. Also, knowledge gained shows program strengths and identifies ineffective practices that can be helpful to program participants. In academic health-related programs and other programs, administrators such as deans, provosts, and presidents are keenly interested in the success of the university's programs that leads to credibility and visibility. The data collected in a program evaluation can be used for strategic planning and can substantiate requests for increased funding by providing evidence of effectiveness.

Accreditation Model

Accreditation for healthcare programs is usually developed through a nongovernmental accrediting agency set up through the board of directors of a specific national professional organization within a specialty profession such as medicine, nursing, physical therapy, nutrition, or other healthcare specialty. Each healthcare profession should have an accreditation process for educational programs that develop practitioners in their specialty. These educational programs are usually located within an institution of higher learning, although some healthcare agencies may provide programs in a specific profession, such as diploma nursing schools. There is a financial cost to the programs for the accreditation process and survey site visit.

The accreditation agency for the profession will develop standards, guidelines, and requirements that the program will need to meet to achieve accreditation for a undergraduate and graduate programs in a specific profession. Accreditation may be granted for a specific number of years, up to 10 years, depending on the accrediting agency's program. New programs receiving accreditation for the first time may have a shorter time frame, or if a program does not fully meet the criteria, the agency may require an earlier review.

An example of a comprehensive program evaluation in nursing is an accreditation review and site visit by peer evaluators. One such accrediting agency is the Commission on Collegiate Nursing Education (CCNE). The CCNE was developed by the American Association of Colleges of Nursing (AACN) to improve the existing accreditation process for baccalaureate and graduate nursing programs. The AACN developed a task force to explore the issue of developing an accrediting agency, and the CCNE program was developed and approved by the AACN membership in 1997 (CCNE, 2013). The CCNE was established as an autonomous agency contributing to the improvement of the public's health and does not report to the AACN, so that conflict of interest is not an issue. The program was developed to ensure the quality and integrity of baccalaureate, graduate, and residency programs in nursing and serves the public interest by assessing and identifying programs that engage in effective educational practices. The CCNE accreditation is a nongovernmental peer review process that operates in accordance with nationally recognized standards established for the practice of accreditation in the United States (CCNE, 2013).

An educational organization applies to the CCNE for initial accreditation of existing and new programs. Nursing programs with continuing accreditation are notified of the dates of an on-site visit and the process for reaccreditation about a year before the accreditation is due to expire. The accreditation process and site visit provide a nursing program the opportunity to conduct its own program evaluation using the CCNE's four standards and key elements of each standard. Standards I–III relate to program quality of its mission and governance, institutional commitment and resources, and curriculum and teaching–learning practices; Standard IV is focused on program effectiveness with aggregate student and faculty outcomes (CCNE, 2009).

The nursing program needs to develop a system to collect data related to the standards and prepare an analytical self-study report. Program faculty need to be actively involved in collecting data and developing the report. The university administration is also involved in collecting administrative and financial data relating to the program.

CCNE peer evaluators read the program's self-study report and visit the campus to validate what is contained in the report. During the visit to the institution, the site visitors meet with university and program administrators, faculty, students, and community agencies that employ graduates. At the end of the visit, they hold an open forum to discuss their preliminary findings of standards that appear to be met as well as noting areas that may need some improvement. The evaluators do not make recommendations about accreditation but rather prepare a report describing the results of their visit and send it to the CCNE, which in turn forwards the final report to the chief nurse administrator of the program. The chief nurse administrator has an opportunity to respond to the report in writing. This response may include additional data that were not available as the time of the site visit and what was done to respond to suggested areas for improvement. The program's self-study report, the evaluators' report and response, and third-party comments are forwarded to the CCNE

Accreditation Review Committee. That group reviews all materials and makes a confidential recommendation to the CCNE board of commissioners regarding accreditation. It is the board of commissioners that makes the final accreditation decisions.

Many aspects of a quality nursing program are addressed in the CCNE accreditation review process, such as mission, goals, student and faculty expectations and outcomes, student and faculty governance, institution support and resources, curriculum and teaching–learning practices, and program effectiveness based on aggregate data. Ongoing evaluation of these components of a nursing program assists in program improvement and effectiveness. For example, ongoing review of teaching–learning practices gives the program the opportunity to self-reflect on its teaching strategies and student learning in the classroom, clinical setting, and online instruction. Research studies to develop evidence for effective teaching strategies and student learning can enhance program effectiveness. Any empirical evidence developed by a program provides strong evidence for accreditation review.

■ Evaluation Research

Evaluation research provides empirical findings that can strengthen the value of selected programs and determine how they are working. Evaluation research can focus on the entire program or specific aspects of a program. There may be more than one part of the program being evaluated, such as the process or implementation, outcome, impact, or cost analysis (Polit & Beck, 2012). Different research methodologies can be used when conducting program evaluation, such as surveys, pretest-posttest designs, focus groups, and qualitative methods. Examples of the use of different methodologies in diverse program evaluations are provided.

Survey

Survey research is a common method used in social science research to collect data. The advantages of surveys include their flexibility, broad scope, and ability to focus on diverse topics (Polit & Beck, 2012). Surveys can be used to obtain data in personal interviews, questionnaires, and telephone interviews. Surveys have been used in evaluation research.

A program evaluation was conducted using questionnaires to determine nursing school instruction and students' perceived competence to emphatically communicate with patients (McMillan & Shannon, 2011). Six hundred nursing students from 14 nursing programs completed the questionnaire, *Nursing Student Empathic Communication Questionnaire,* using a five-point Likert scale. As the questionnaire was used for the first time, there was no prior reliability coefficients report; however, in this population, the Cronbach's alpha subscales ranged from 0.63 to 0.83. The results had implications for the program including practical steps to enhance classroom and clinical pedagogy such as providing situations that foster empathetic communication development, improving teaching methods, and providing evidence-based studies showing the relationship between empathetic communications in improving patient outcomes.

Another program evaluation study—focusing on a transplantation specialty pharmacy (TSP) program—utilized surveys (Hlubocky, Stuckey, Schuman, & Stevenson, 2012). The TSP program was instituted, and the purpose of the study was to determine the impact on patients' and healthcare providers' satisfaction, identified outcomes, and cost margin. In addition, data were collected related to medication adherence and hospital readmission within 90 days of the surgery. There was almost a 35% response rate ($n = 290$) from the surveys. The results were favorable for patients' and healthcare providers' satisfaction, continuity of care, and a substantial cost margin. These empirical findings support the use of the TSP program at this institution.

Pretest-Posttest Design

The pretest-posttest design involves the collection of data prior to an intervention and then again after the intervention. With this design, researchers can determine which changes occurred and see if any statistical significance was found in a quantitative study (Polit & Beck, 2012).

An evaluation study was conducted in a bachelor of nursing program in Australia to determine whether a structured learning program influenced student anxiety and efficacy (Watt, Murphy, Pascoe, Scanlon, & Gan, 2011). A pretest-posttest design was used to study three cohorts of students ($n = 118$) who completed questionnaires before and after participating in a structured learning program. There were statistically significant results in the scores on the posttest, with anxiety being decreased and efficacy being increased. This study supported implementing a structured learning program at this school.

Focus Groups

Focus groups are held to obtain perceptions about an area of interest. Their size may vary from 4 to 12 depending on the sensitivity of the discussion and the number of participants. This method enables a researcher to take advantage of the participants' discussion to collect more in-depth data (Doody, Slevin, & Taggart, 2013).

An evaluation study of a mentoring program designed to increase the diversity of the nursing workforce was conducted using focus groups. The purpose was to determine the effectiveness of a formal mentoring program entitled Preparing the Next Generation of Nurses Mentoring Program (Wilson, Sanner, & McAllister, 2010). The program paired at-risk nursing students (mentees) with a faculty mentor. Focus groups were conducted annually over a 3-year period separately among mentors and mentees. Themes flowed from the discussions that described faculty and student perceptions of the overall program and both groups' perceptions of a good mentor and mentee. The findings were helpful and in part refined the role of a faculty mentor and showed how to overcome some of the challenges, including scheduling conflicts.

Both surveys and focus groups were used in evaluating teams of interdisciplinary staff in an interprofessional education program (Bajnok, Puddester, MacDonald, Archibald, & Kuhl, 2012). The purpose was to determine whether interprofessional team development made a difference in team functioning, satisfaction, and improved patient well-being. The overall goals of the education project were met, including a positive reaction to the learning experience, an increased awareness of the roles and responsibilities of other healthcare providers, their ability to transfer their learning to the workplace, and greater collaboration in care decision making.

Case Studies

Case studies are in-depth descriptions of selected phenomena including an individual, group, or social unit. Data collection may relate to a present state or other factors related to the study of interest (Polit & Beck, 2012).

Researchers used a qualitative, cross-case analysis to describe evaluation systems related to comprehensive developmental school counseling (CDSC) programs in two states, Missouri and Utah (Martin & Carey, 2012).. Results of the study provided in-depth descriptions of the evaluation programs and the differences in each state's approach. Lessons learned included the importance of building the capacity of school counselors to evaluate their own programs with state leadership. The authors suggest one advantage for state leaders is that a systematic state evaluation program can be used to advocate for the necessity of school counseling in the educational system.

■ Conclusion

This chapter addressed program evaluation and its importance for maintaining high-quality nursing and other healthcare programs. The purposes and benefits of program evaluation were discussed and the term defined. The role of accreditation in identifying effective nursing programs was discussed using the standards and key elements of the CCNE. Examples of program evaluation research studies were presented, including the effect of a nursing school instruction program on students' perceived competence to emphatically communicate with patients, a structured nursing program to reduce student anxiety and increase efficacy, and a nursing mentoring program for at-risk nursing students. Additional studies presented were from other disciplines—an evaluation of a transplantation specialty pharmacy program, the effectiveness of interprofessional teams in the practice setting, and the evaluation capacity with state-level school counseling programs. Using data from program evaluations can be useful in better understanding a program, and it can provide insights into necessary changes for improvement. Also, research evaluations provide empirical data to support needed changes in specified programs.

REFERENCES

Bajnok, I., Puddester, D., MacDonald, C. J., Archibald, D., & Kuhl, D. (2012). Building positive relationships in healthcare: Evaluation of the teams of interprofessional staff interprofessional education program. *Contemporary Nurse*, 42(1), 77–89.

Bell, D. F., Pestka, E., & Forsyth, D. (2007). Outcome evaluation: Does continuing education make a difference? *Journal of Continuing Education*, 38(4), 186–190.

Chen, H. (2005). *Practical program evaluation: Assessing and improving planning, implementation, and effectiveness.* London, UK: Sage.

Commission on Collegiate Nursing Education (CCNE). (2009). Standards, procedures, and resources. Retrieved from http://www.aacn.nche.edu/ccne-accreditation/standards-procedures-resources/overview

Commission on Collegiate Nursing Education (CCNE). (2013). Mission, values, & history. Retrieved from http://www.aacn.nche.edu/ccne-accreditation/about/mission-values-history

Davidson, E. J. (2005). *Evaluation methodology basics: The nuts and bolts of sound evaluation.* Thousand Oaks, CA: Sage.

Doody, O., Slevin, E., & Taggart, L. (2013). Focus group interviews in nursing research: Part 1. *British Journal of Nursing, 22*(1), 16–19.

Fink, A. (2005). *Evaluation fundamentals: Insights into the outcomes, effectiveness, and quality of health programs.* London, UK: Sage.

Hlubocky, J. M., Stuckey, L. J., Schuman, A. D., & Stevenson, J. G. (2012). Evaluation of a transplantation specialty pharmacy program. *American Journal Health-Systems Pharmacists, 69,* 340–347. doi: 10.2146/ajhp110350

Martin, J., & Carey, J. C. (2012). Evaluation capacity within state-level school counseling programs: A cross-case analysis. *Professional School Counseling, 15*(3), 132–143.

McMillan, L. R., & Shannon, D. (2011). Program evaluation of nursing school instruction in measuring students' perceived competence to empathetically communicate with patients. *Nursing Education Perspectives, 32*(3), 150–154.

McNamara, C. (2006). *Field guide to nonprofit program design, marketing and evaluation.* Minneapolis, MN: Authenticity Consulting.

Mertz, A. J. (2007). *Why conduct a program evaluation? Five reasons why evaluation can help an out-of-school time program.* Publication #2007-31. Washington, DC: Child Trends.

Polit, D. F., & Beck, C. T. (2012). *Nursing research: Generating and assessing evidence for nursing practice* (9th ed.). Philadelphia, PA: Wolters Kluwer/Lippincott Williams & Wilkins.

Watt, E., Murphy, M., Pascoe, E., Scanlon, A., & Gan, S. (2011). An evaluation of a structured learning programme as a component of the clinical practicum in final year bachelor of nursing programme: A pre-post-test analysis. *Journal of Clinical Nursing, 20,* 2286–2293. doi: 10.1111/j.1365-2702.2010.0362

Wilson, A. H., Sanner, S., & McAllister, L. E. (2010). An evaluation study of a mentoring program to increase the diversity of the nursing workforce. *Journal of Cultural Diversity, 17*(4), 144–150.

CHAPTER 31

Evaluating a Program's Teaching Resources

■ Shanti Freundlich ■

The evaluation of teaching resources—the resources that exist to support an academic program—must be part of a holistic, systematic, and ongoing evaluation. In this context, program evaluation is "the process of weighing, interpreting, and subsequently making judgments about data collected from multiple components of education programming" (Menix, 2007, p. 204). To evaluate the resources available to support teaching and teachers in a professional health sciences program, the context, as well as the resources that faculty members have to draw on, must be examined. According to the National League for Nursing Accreditation Commission (2012), teaching resources include fiscal, physical, and learning resources. At a more granular level, they include the physical—buildings, classrooms, lab space; the technology—electronic databases and other information resources, the learning management platforms, simulation labs, and the staff available to support all of these resources; and the curriculum and professional development resources for the faculty, both as healthcare professionals and as teachers—teaching and learning centers, opportunities for professional growth, interprofessional opportunities, and the fiscal resources to support them all. As with any form of evaluation, the program should choose highly regarded and relevant standards as a measure against which to compare itself, and the perspective gained from evaluation should be incorporated into future changes to the program. Quite simply, if the results of an evaluation are not going be used as part of an ongoing evidence-based decision-making process, there is little value in evaluating a program's resources.

The accreditation standards for different health education programs all have different requirements, but there are enough commonalities between the resources needed that the context, resources, models, and future challenges discussed here will speak to a wide variety of programs.

■ Context

Nursing and other professional health sciences programs exist within a larger context that has changed dramatically in recent years, and this context affects the goals of nursing and other professional health sciences programs and shapes the resources they deem essential. There are recent and significant pieces of legislation affecting the work environment that newly graduated students enter—namely, the Patient Protection and Affordable Care Act (ACA) and the Health Information Technology for Economic and Clinical Health Act (HITECH). These are affecting the professional environment in which students have their clinical placements and where they will be working after graduation. The changes mandated by these laws are also affecting faculty members—they are adopting new systems and technologies in their places of work and into their teaching as they prepare students to enter this changed professional world.

The ACA addresses nursing education in multiple ways—addressing faculty shortages through raising funding caps, supporting faculty and student loans programs, including an emphasis on diversity, updating the Nurse Education, Practice and Retention grant program, and expanding the National Health Services Corps, among other grants and programs (Wakefield, 2010). It also affects educational programs indirectly; students need to be prepared for an increased number of patients as health care becomes more accessible and care models in hospitals and community health settings change.

Meanwhile, HITECH calls for the implementation of electronic health records (EHRs) and the achievement of their meaningful use—the use of EHRs to achieve health and efficiency goals (National Coordinator for Health Information Technology, 2013). For students to adhere to these health information technology standards, programs must train them to be proficient EHR users, to be comfortable integrating technology into practice, and to understand meaningful use standards so that they can help achieve those goals and improve quality of care.

Simultaneously, professional health education programs also exist within the context of academia: strategic plans; institutional mission and vision statements; accreditation standards; tenure concerns; faculty shortages; teaching versus research mentalities; high-stakes conversations about online education including blended courses, fully online programs, and MOOCs (massive open online courses); and ever-changing student demographics, dynamics, and expectations. Program evaluation must also examine how and if multiple learning styles are addressed, how they are reflected in student learning outcomes, and how programs support faculty members' continued professional development around teaching techniques.

Any one of the ACA-, HITECH-, or academia-related factors would have significant impact on the shape of a program and require fiscal, physical, and learning resources. However, programs are affected by all of them and so must allocate resources to address all of these factors. An evaluation is a chance to examine current levels of support and identify future goals in resource management.

■ Teaching Resources

To determine which resources are needed to support a curriculum, Schug (2012) recommends asking the following: "What resources (e.g. library, information technology) contribute to the curricular implementation? What features of the physical facilities were conductive to learning? What presented barriers/challenges?" (p. 303).

These fiscal, physical, and learning resources (National League for Nursing Accrediting Commission, 2012) that support faculty in their teaching are just one aspect of an academic program. Evaluating the resources that faculty use to create an environment that facilitates learning is separate from evaluating teaching (i.e., faculty output) or learning (i.e., what students take in). Resources can be categorized more specifically as:

- Physical resources—including the buildings, classrooms, lab spaces and the geographic location.
- The simulation/clinical resources necessary for students to gain hands-on experience and learn how to work with real patients, clinicians, and doctors under pressure.
- Technology resources—the electronic and print resources (via the library), learning management platforms, electronic health records, and the support to offer training and ensure functionality.
- Online learning resources—the specialized software and support necessary to ensure that students enrolled in blended or fully online courses receive the same level of attention and interaction as those enrolled in in-person courses.
- Curriculum/teaching resources—the materials and personnel usually found in cocurricular support centers that offer opportunities to refine teaching techniques, explore innovative teaching methods, and encourage the incorporation of new learning theories and styles.

Before it can be evaluated, a program must define and articulate its resources, map them to course and curricular goals, and describe at which level they currently exist.

▪ Theoretical Framework

At the program level, strategic mission statements and learning outcomes set the standards that a program aspires to meet. Based on these, resources can be evaluated to determine if they meet these standards. Once the program being evaluated has clear strategic goals, a theoretic framework on which to base the evaluation process can be chosen. Not every aspect of a program's resources should or can be evaluated at once, but Gard, Flannigan, and Cluskey (2004) recommend that any evaluation process start with the following four clear, practical questions:

1. What do we want to know?
2. Why do we want to know it?
3. What should we measure?
4. How should we measure it?

Once these questions have been answered, a more in-depth theoretical model can be chosen as a framework, or aspects of multiple frameworks can be combined into a customized model to best evaluate the program's resources. The literature is full of potential frameworks, and one should be chosen based on which aspect of the program is being evaluated; some focus on simulations (Jeffries, 2005), and others focus on online or distance education curricula (Avery, Cohen, & Walker, 2008), while many take a systematic approach (Gard, et al., 2004; Hamner & Bentley, 2003; Kalb, 2009; Matthiesen & Wilhelm, 2006).

Resources are one aspect of Kalb's (2009) three Cs model, which is designed as a comprehensive method to evaluate a program based on NLNAC accreditation standards. This model weaves together context, content, and conduct; maps them to the NLNAC standards; and from there maps them back to foundational documents including the 2003 *Nursing's Social Policy Statement*, the 2004 *Nursing: Scope and Standards of Practice*, and the 2001 *Code of Ethics for Nurses with Interpretive Statements*. Based on this model, resources are included in two of the three concepts—content and conduct. Resources both "promote the process of learning" and are the "technology to support learning" (Kalb, 2009, p. 179).

Meanwhile, Matthiesen and Wilhelm (2006) use a case study approach to argue that evaluation should not limit its scope solely to the curriculum, but rather should be an ongoing and systematic view of the program and the core components required by multiple accreditation bodies, licensure, and certification boards. Schug (2012) chooses to focus on just the curricular aspects of a program; however, she also acknowledges that they are components of a larger evaluation process. Her schema for curricular evaluation can be used to inventory and evaluate resources at a micro (i.e., course) level by asking which resources are available to support each aspect of a course and whether there is any room to improve said resource. Instead of simply asking if the following aspects are present in a course, Schug (2012) recommends evaluating which resources are available to faculty and students to best facilitate the creation, maintenance, use, or understanding of:

- Course objectives
- Curricular threads
- Course content
- Schedule
- Teaching and learning strategies
- Evaluation of student performance
- Textbooks/library holdings
- Student evaluations of the course
- Accrediting standards
- Liberal arts requirements

Evaluation is a "judgment process [that] compares evaluation data and purposes with correlated criteria to determine worth, value, or success or failure" (Menix, 2007, p. 203), and a theoretical framework serves as a scaffold for evaluation as a program articulates to itself what it wants to know and why, and what it wants to measure and how (Gard et al., 2004). As a program evaluates itself systematically, the findings of an in-depth examination of resources can help project its potential future directions.

■ Evaluation Process

One method to help jump-start the evaluation process is to consider the program through the eyes of a new faculty member or student. Determine the resources that are immediately available to them, those that are lacking, and which additional support for teaching/learning would ideally be present. This exercise can offer an outsider's perspective on the familiar and prompt a deep examination of program resources. This is a method that usability experts often use in academic libraries to evaluate a library's physical space from a student's perspective.

Much of the literature on program evaluation agrees that accreditation visits can be the catalyst for ongoing program evaluation (Gard et al., 2004; Hamner & Bentley, 2003; Jeffries, 2005; Suhayda & Miller, 2006), and a programmatic evaluation will often be led by a committee of invested faculty. This helps ensure that the process garners support and buy-in from the larger department, and programs that have developed evaluation models also recommend working with the existing academic calendar and accreditation schedules, rather than attempting to work independently from them. A comprehensive evaluation plan can combine theoretical elements from the systematic approach of Hamner & Bentley (2003) and the ongoing schedule of Gard and colleagues (2004). Hamner & Bentley's (2003) matrix includes space for the resource being evaluated, supporting documentation, the person responsible, the evaluation method, the evaluation standard, the committee findings, and the committee's recommendations for action. Gard and colleagues' (2004) schedule recommends planning the process in August, reviewing the existing documentation during the fall semester, focusing on the resources in the latter half of it, and collecting course evaluation data at the end. The fall semester can be used to focus on external accreditation; meanwhile, the spring semester can be used to write recommendations, and alumni feedback is collected throughout the year.

As a program initiates an evaluation process, it is essential to connect to the departmental, school, and institutional strategic planning processes so that the evaluation has a clear purpose and so that at the end of an evaluation cycle it is easy to report and connect the work of a single program to the vision of the larger institution. Hamner & Bentley (2003) also recommend clearly defining the program resources and elements that are being evaluated from the outset, so that it is a more manageable process. Once a framework has been articulated, a committee formed, and a schedule agreed upon, the information being gathered needs to be shared between committee members so that work is not duplicated. It may also benefit the evaluation committee to draw on documents their program has already created in response to other nationally recognized accreditation standards. To encourage faculty to participate in a program evaluation, it must be clear that the data collected are completely separate from individual faculty evaluations so that the committee can work from comprehensive data. These steps—gathering complete and comprehensive data, sharing information, and drawing on previous work—will make it more straightforward to reuse the findings and recommendations for other reports.

■ Evaluating Resources, Not Learning

The evaluation of student learning is core to all academic programs, and this discussion of teaching resources examines the context in which that learning occurs. Assessing how and what students are learning is an integral part of teaching, and assessment can be built into the essential aspects of each lesson, as well as the midterm and final exams that serve as comprehensive assessment measures.

Similar to evaluating resources, learning is more effectively measured if clear learning outcomes are set ahead of time, as outlined by Wiggins & McTighe's (2011) backward approach to curricular design. In their approach, course design starts with course outcomes, which learning outcomes connect back to, and which are tied directly to the program's mission, vision, and goals. Having a strategic scaffold in place means that faculty are under less pressure to develop all of those outcomes from scratch every time they teach, and if faculty lead the development of the program's learning outcomes as part of an ongoing process, no faculty members will feel too far removed from these goals in their own teaching.

Without a doubt, evaluating student learning is part of program evaluation, but when taking a holistic approach to evaluation, the measure of a program does not rest solely on students, but rather on all the elements that come together to create an environment that facilitates and encourages learning—one that is supported by teaching resources.

■ Future Challenges

A program that teaches evidence-based medicine must also draw on the same principles to inform its own teaching practices. Evaluating teaching resources is an integral part of a larger systematic program evaluation, and both the elements and process will benefit from being clearly defined from the outset. While evaluation examines the past and present, the findings and recommendations can inform future opportunities, even as events outside a program continue to evolve and shape expectations.

Nursing and professional health sciences programs are exploring interprofessional learning opportunities—in classrooms, clinical training settings, and community settings. As these interprofessional plans solidify, all the academic programs involved must ensure that they are held to the same evaluation standards as all of the other program elements. Interprofessional learning opportunities may also require different or additional teaching resources, so as these opportunities grow, faculty will need to look closely at their programs to ensure the resources are still meeting the program's needs.

As programs consider moving more teaching to blended or fully online formats, they must continue to evaluate resources, outcomes, and students against the same standard used for in-person programs. They will also have to determine which additional teaching resources must be provided to ensure faculty members are able to deliver the same high-quality teaching in a completely different format, which will offer new challenges as well as benefits.

■ Conclusion

Once a program evaluation becomes an ongoing process, the findings and recommendations for changes to teaching resources may seem overwhelming and challenging to implement. Rather than attempting to enact every recommendation simultaneously and at full scale, programs may consider running pilot projects and implementing incremental change. Scaling efforts also acknowledge that faculty and staff have limited amounts of time in which to participate in evaluation efforts and program reviews on top of their existing teaching, service, and clinicial responsibilities. An organization that is serious about creating an environment that uses the results of an evaluation for program improvement will encourage the implementation of the recommendations, even if it just starts at a small scale.

Evidence-based decisions are a driving force in health care and healthcare education today. Ensuring that the same evidence-based mind-set is also applied to the teaching resources that are being using to prepare the next generation of healthcare providers is a natural and essential step of the process.

REFERENCES

American Nurses Association. (2001). *Code of ethics for nurses with interpretive statements*. Washington, DC: Author.

American Nurses Association. (2003). *Nursing's social policy statement* (2nd ed.). Washington, DC: Author.

American Nurses Association. (2004). *Nursing: Scope and standards of practice*. Washington, DC: Author.

Avery, M. D., Cohen, B. A., & Walker, J. (2008). Evaluation of an online graduate nursing curriculum: Examining standards of quality. *International Journal of Nursing Education Scholarship, 5*(1).

Gard, C. L., Flannigan, P. N., & Cluskey, M. (2004). Program evaluation. An ongoing systematic process. *Nursing Education Perspectives, 25*(4), 176–179.

Hamner, J. B., & Bentley, R. W. (2003). A systematic evaluation plan that works. *Nurse Educator, 28*(4), 179–184.

Jeffries, P. R. (2005). A frame work for designing, implementing, and evaluating simulations used as teaching strategies in nursing. *Nursing Education Perspectives, 26*(2), 96–103.

Kalb, K. A. (2009). The three Cs model: The context, content, and conduct of nursing education. *Nursing Education Perspectives, 30*(3), 176–180.

Matthiesen, V., & Wilhelm, C. (2006). Quality outcomes and program evaluation in nursing education: An overview of the journey. *Quality Management in Healthcare, 15*(4), 279–284.

Menix, K. D. (2007). Evaluation of learning and program effectiveness. *Journal of Continuing Education in Nursing, 38*(5), 201.

National Coordinator for Health Information Technology. (2013). HealthIT: The official site for Health IT information. Retrieved from http://www.healthit.gov/

National League for Nursing Accrediting Commission. (2012). *NLNAC accreditation manual: Including the 2008 standards and criteria*. Atlanta, GA: Author.

Schug, V. (2012). Curriculum evaluation using National League for Nursing Accrediting Commission standards and criteria. *Nursing Education Perspectives, 33*(5), 302–305.

Suhayda, R., & Miller, J. M. (2006). Optimizing evaluation of nursing education programs. *Nurse Educator, 31*(5), 200–206.

Wakefield, M. K. (2010). Nurses and the affordable care act. *American Journal of Nursing, 110*(9), 11.

Wiggins, G., & McTighe, J. (2011). What is backward design? In W. Wiggins & J. McTighe (Eds.), *Understanding by design* (pp. 7–19). Retrieved from http://nhlrc.ucla.edu/events/startalkworkshop /readings/backward-design.pdf

CHAPTER 32

The Clinical Pathway: A Tool to Evaluate Clinical Learning

■ MARTHA J. BRADSHAW ■

The clinical pathway is a strategy that uses specific, essential evaluation criteria in unique clinical learning settings.

■ Definition and Purpose

The clinical pathway is an abbreviated form of clinical evaluation that provides a means for the instructor to evaluate student progress using specified criteria. Clinical pathways can be used to evaluate applied practice and clinical learning that occur in time-limited, less traditional care settings. Learning activities are directed toward the same clinical outcomes as would be expected in traditionally structured patient care settings. The emphasis is on application of principles in a new setting, rather than gaining experience via repeated opportunities in a familiar setting. As students apply principles, they recognize the development of individual practice-based judgment and decision making, and they begin to visualize themselves as professional healthcare providers. Faculty can determine how well the student uses guided thinking and clinical reasoning in unfamiliar settings, yet at the same time provides familiar and appropriate interventions.

■ Theoretical Foundations

Clinical pathways, also called critical pathways, are being used by nurses and other members of the healthcare team as a directed approach to goal-based outcomes; they are especially beneficial in quality improvement for cost-effectiveness (Broughton, 2011). Most nursing literature describes pathways for use in complex patient care situations, and use of pathways can have a positive influence on patient mortality (Panella, 2009). Consequently, if one thinks of clinical failure by a student as "mortality," then a pathway can be a valuable tool to avert student loss.

Pathways are also used for orientation of new nursing staff, quality improvement, evaluation and improvement of patient care interventions, and student-precepted experiences (Hunter & Segrott, 2010; Kersbergen & Hrbosky, 1996;

Kinsman & James, 2001). One of the advantages of a pathway is that it is a cost-effective means, in both time and money, by which the individual is directed to the goal(s) and progress is measured (Renholm, Leino-Kilpi, & Suominen, 2002). Pathways also enable all individuals involved to know exactly what the goals are, thus clarifying expectations and making energy expenditure more efficient (Kersbergen & Hrbosky). Clinical faculty are able to collaborate on student evaluations by examining how well the student meets outcome criteria from more than one perspective. This principle is similar to how integrated-care pathways are used in interdisciplinary clinical situations, in that student progress and achievement of outcomes is the focus (Atwal & Caldwell, 2002).

■ Conditions

In selected situations, student clinical learning activities are one-time experiences and may deviate from the more structured patient care experiences. In addition, many clinical experiences are short term because of decreases in hospitalization length and emphasis on wellness programs. Examples of these clinical experiences in nursing are community health fairs, outpatient surgery, and pediatric health screenings in day care settings. Whereas these unique clinical opportunities provide expanded observations and open up new areas of practice, one-time experiences do not always lend themselves to achievement of established clinical learning outcomes. If the learning outcomes are not readily identified, then the clinical instructor cannot easily evaluate clinical progress based on the experience. Therefore, instructors traditionally create one-time experiences as observation-only activities or as task-focused activities that may not represent a professional nursing approach. In doing so, many valuable learning opportunities may be lost to the students. Instructors also lose the opportunity to determine the extent to which students are able to adapt to unique settings, apply principles, and enact new roles. For these reasons, a clinical pathway should be developed for virtual learning experiences, such as with high-fidelity patient simulators. These behaviors, as part of clinical reasoning, are essential in evaluating patient safety. Tanicala, Scheffer, and Roberts (2011) address the need to effectively evaluate behaviors in students that have a bearing on patient safety and could make the difference between a passing and failing student.

Use of a clinical pathway for student experiences enables continued learning by students and maximizes the benefits of the one-time clinical opportunities. Just as the critical pathway is an abbreviated version of a patient's plan of care, so the student clinical pathway is an abbreviated version of the clinical evaluation tool. A major advantage of the pathway for both the student and course faculty is that it reduces the inconsistency or inadequacy of evaluation of one-time or isolated clinical learning opportunities. Variations in expectations and evaluation lead to variations in outcomes among students (Holaday & Buckley, 2008; Tanicala et al., 2011), and the pathway is a means to correct this problem.

At the time of the clinical experience, the student uses the pathway as a guide for fulfilling selected roles and completing specific responsibilities. Simultaneously, the student is aware of the criteria by which evaluation will take place. Therefore, use of clinical time and experience is maximized. The clinical pathway makes unique clinical experiences more purposeful, thus improving student clinical learning outcomes (Kinsman, 2004). Student clinical pathways are based on the same purposes as are patient- or staff-oriented pathways; they are goal directed, designed to be efficient, and effective in terms of time and energy. The components of the clinical pathway are derived directly from the clinical evaluation tool used by faculty in student evaluation.

▪ Types of Learners

Whereas the clinical pathway could be used with learners of all levels, it is best used with undergraduate students. The clinical pathway offers specific learning outcomes and can include recommended or structured activities that enable the student to meet these outcomes. Students in undergraduate clinical settings generally have more faculty supervision, which creates opportunity for direct observation and evaluation. The clinical pathway is designed for intended learning, even though students often acquire additional personal growth during the clinical experience.

The pathway also is quite suitable for students of all levels in brief clinical learning settings with a preceptor, such as a one-day event. The preceptor should not be expected to conduct an in-depth evaluation of the student, but preceptor feedback is exceedingly helpful in compiling comprehensive information on a student. Therefore, a succinct and purposeful tool can be easily completed and provide needed information. Preceptors also feel more empowered in their ability to make decisions about students and promote accountability for care (Kersbergen & Hrbosky, 1996).

▪ Resources

The basis for a clinical pathway is the learning outcomes for the course. These outcomes are based upon professional competencies (Oermann & Gaberson, 2006). Evaluation tools used by all clinical instructors are directed toward course outcomes and ultimately professional standards for practice. Instructors supervising students in selected experiences identify outcomes and expected behaviors from the evaluation tool. Based on anticipated clinical learning opportunities, the instructor develops a clinical pathway that guides the student in what will be accomplished during the experience and the activities or behaviors the instructor expects to observe in each learner.

▪ Using the Method

Implementation of an education-focused clinical pathway enables the faculty to develop student learning experiences that are directly related to the outcomes for the total clinical course. Two examples demonstrate how pathways are derived from the clinical evaluation tool and how components of the tool can be applied to more than one setting. Hearing and vision screening with school-age children can be conducted with nursing students at any level in the educational program. Such screenings have a place in a fundamentals course, in a course on nursing care of children, or in a community nursing course. A more sophisticated version of the screening (to include patient referral) can be developed for nurse practitioner students.

When students are assigned to a unique, one-time clinical experience, they may have some apprehension about being responsible for patient care in a new setting. Knowing that they have only one opportunity to demonstrate competence, students benefit from the direction that a pathway provides. In fact, many students like the opportunity to test themselves in the new setting. Time and opportunity do not permit the students to meet all criteria on the standard, comprehensive course evaluation tool. To maximize the learning experience, a sample pathway (see **Table 32-1**) was developed based on the following items from the course clinical evaluation tool:

■ Demonstrates preparation for assignment.
■ Performs nursing skills correctly.
■ Maintains professionalism.
■ Demonstrates professional inquiry activities.

As can be seen by the example in Table 32-1, other expectations are specified under the broad clinical outcomes. The pathway expectations are derived from the clinical evaluation tool and applied to the situation, such as communications with children or use of critical thinking. The expectations also indicate specific behaviors related to the clinical activity that must be demonstrated by the student, such as ability to complete vision screening.

Additional information that leaves no room for guesswork regarding preparation and professional behaviors is provided in the pathway for the student. Also, the standard for acceptable behavior (pass) is indicated as part of the directions, so that in the event a student demonstrates unacceptable behaviors, he or she has a clear understanding of how the final evaluation was determined (see **Exhibit 32-1**).

In developing the pathway, the focus is on outcomes (student learning), not process (tasks or activities). Therefore, the instructor may designate specified activities or behaviors that direct the student to the outcomes; not all behaviors must be seen to attain the goal. Furthermore, other, unanticipated activities related to the patient situation that enable the student to meet the outcomes may present themselves.

An evaluation sheet provides feedback to the student regarding the experience and serves as the evaluation measure and anecdotal record for the instructor. Information regarding clinical activities and evaluation is found in the clinical section of the course syllabus. In that section is the detailed information indicating that the one-time activity is a clinical day of equal importance to a day caring for a hospitalized

Table 32-1 Course Outcomes Applied to Clinical Pathways

Learning Outcomes of Clinical Pathways

1. Demonstrates professional behaviors and inquiry activities.

2. Demonstrates preparation and use of principles in screening techniques.

3. Assesses behaviors of patient and family/support in ambulatory surgery and provides appropriate nursing interventions.

4. Provides nursing interventions for a patient in the ambulatory surgery/operative unit.

Clinical Learning Outcomes of Course

1. Demonstrates professional behavior and accountability.

2. Demonstrates preparedness for assignment.

3. Provides a safe environment.

4. Complies with the regulations of the school of nursing and clinical agency.

5. Performs nursing skills or interventions appropriate to the patient's health.

6. Demonstrates safe administration of medications.

7. Establishes rapport and demonstrates good communication skills.

8. Demonstrates collaboration with other care disciplines.

9. Demonstrates patient and family teaching.

10. Demonstrates appropriate documentation.

11. Maintains confidentiality and respect for others.

12. Completes assignments on time.

13. Seeks assistance/guidance appropriately.

14. Adapts to changing or stressful situations.

15. Uses critical-thinking skills.

16. Demonstrates professional inquiry activities.

patient. Clinical instructors use the information from the pathway when formulating a final clinical evaluation report on each student.

Exhibit 32-2 is a clinical pathway developed for use with nursing students in an ambulatory surgery unit. In addition to typical nursing activities related to an operative experience, an emphasis of this experience includes patient and caregiver interaction, alleviation of anxiety, provision of information about the procedure, and presentation of postoperative teaching prior to discharge. The ambulatory surgery pathway also is constructed to indicate to the students what the expectations are for patient care. Prior to use of the pathway, students may be unsure of what they are permitted to do, and thus miss many learning opportunities.

Exhibit 32-1 Clinical Pathway: Hearing and Vision Screening

The clinical pathway identifies the specific nursing activities that will enable the student to meet the objectives for this one-time clinical experience. The student will be evaluated based on completion of items on this pathway. A student who fails this clinical pathway (i.e., fails to pass at least 7 of the 12 items on the clinical pathway) has failed the clinical day.

Objectives and Student Nursing Activities

1. Demonstrates preparation and use of principles in screening techniques:
   - Attends clinical experience promptly, appropriately attired, and with own supplies.
   - Establishes a positive working relationship with patient(s).
   - Initiates and completes screening in timely manner.
   - Correctly follows sequence of steps in screening assessment(s).
   - Shows familiarity with equipment, screening criteria, and documentation.
   - Individualizes assessments as needed based on unique attributes of each patient.
2. Demonstrates professional behaviors and inquiry activities:
   - Uses principles of therapeutic and professional communications when interacting with patient(s).
   - Shows appropriate level of independence and self-direction.
   - Demonstrates critical-thinking and problem-solving skills regarding screenings or patient interactions.
   - Documents or reports results of screening exam.
   - Seeks guidance or advice from instructor as needed.
   - Discusses screening results and/or patient responses with instructor and fellow students.

Student Preparation
   - Complete check-off on hearing and vision screening equipment in the skills lab. If needed, practice again before clinical experience.
   - You are permitted to bring your H&V booklet or some guidelines written on a card. This does not take the place of preparation and familiarity with the procedure. If you make too many references to the guidelines, your instructor will consider you unprepared. Bring these pathway sheets to give to your instructor.

Exhibit 32-2 Clinical Pathway: Ambulatory Surgery Experience

For this one-time clinical experience, the clinical pathway identifies the specific nursing care activities on which the student will be evaluated. Items on this pathway will enable the student to meet the objectives for the ambulatory surgery experience for NUR 3104 (shown). A student who fails the ambulatory surgery experience (i.e., receives a failing evaluation on two of the three sections of the clinical pathway) has failed a clinical day.

Objectives and Student Nursing Activities

1. Assesses behaviors of patient and family/support in ambulatory surgery and provides appropriate nursing interventions:
   ■ Introduces self to patient and family/support person; establishes a working relationship.
   ■ Identifies behaviors related to hospitalization and surgery; discusses conclusions regarding behaviors with instructor, giving specific examples.
   ■ Indicates how patient behaviors influence preoperative, surgical, and postoperative periods.
   ■ Gives specific examples of family/support coping abilities.
   ■ Makes conclusions and interventions that are correctly based on patient's developmental level.
2. Provides nursing interventions for a patient in the ambulatory surgery/ operative unit:
   ■ Demonstrates preparedness regarding knowledge of surgical procedure; discusses procedure and pertinent information with instructor.
   ■ Reviews patient's health history, lab, and other data as available on unit.
   ■ Teams with staff RN to provide care for patient.
   ■ Conducts assessments, including vital signs, in a timely manner, using correct technique.
   ■ Recognizes comfort and safety needs, specific for operative patients.
   ■ Provides interventions promptly.
   ■ Administers medications, based on the five rights and according to school of nursing guidelines.
   ■ Practices professional therapeutic communication skills in the areas of teaching, reassurance, and collaboration.
3. Demonstrates professional behaviors and inquiry activities:
   ■ Selects appropriate priorities for patient and family/support.
   ■ Conducts self in dignified, professional manner, including conversation and general appearance.

(continued)

Exhibit 32-2 (Continued)

- Shows organization and good use of time.
- Demonstrates initiative to be involved in patient care and to further own learning.
- Evaluates outcomes of patient's surgical experience; discusses patient responses and readiness for discharge/transfer with instructor.

Ambulatory Surgery Experience Clinical Pathway: Evaluation

Note: The student must receive a passing evaluation for at least two of the objectives to receive a passing grade for this clinical day.

1. Assess behaviors of patient and family/support in ambulatory surgery and provide appropriate nursing interventions.
   Pass/fail   Comments:

2. Provide nursing interventions for a patient in the ambulatory surgery/operative unit.
   Pass/fail   Comments:

3. Demonstrate professional behaviors and inquiry activities.
   Pass/fail   Comments:

_____   _____

Instructor   Date

Because the ambulatory surgery pathway is broader in scope, it uses both basic care items (same as in Table 32-1) and specific goals:

- Provides a safe environment.
- Establishes good rapport and maintains good communication.
- Recognizes skill and knowledge limitations and seeks assistance appropriately.
- Demonstrates safe administration of medications.
- Uses critical thinking in decision making and applying various problem-solving methods.

For this clinical experience, the student may be evaluated either by a different instructor or by a staff preceptor. Evaluation information is shared with the clinical instructor, added to other evaluation data, and used as part of the final course evaluation. One benefit of using the pathway in total course evaluation is that it provides the instructor with a glimpse at behavior patterns in a student, regardless of setting. In the event that the pathway does not provide beneficial evaluative feedback, the faculty must determine if the clinical experience and learning opportunities cannot be measured the way the pathway was constructed, or if the course evaluation tool needs to be revised to better reflect student learning outcomes (Kinsman, 2004).

■ Potential Problems

Any difficulties encountered in using the clinical pathway are related to the nature of this evaluation measure. It is intended to evaluate the student in a one-time experience, based on selected criteria.

Potential problems with this method include:

- Inability of the instructor to observe and evaluate all behaviors. The type of clinical activity and spontaneous events govern the student's participation in care and types of care provided.
- The new environment may have a negative effect on the students' behavior. Some students adapt more quickly than others to working in new settings. This is especially true of more experienced students and field-independent students who are able to sort out and select relevant information about the clinical setting. Students who are less able to adapt are therefore hampered in their performance and may appear to be weak in clinical judgment or nursing skills.
- It is easy to "rubber stamp" evaluation remarks. For the instructor who has 40 or 50 students progressing through the one-time experience, the evaluation remarks become repetitive and tiresome. Instructors must endeavor to make individual comments that are an accurate description of the student. Remarks that reflect abilities in other clinical settings will validate the student's total clinical evaluation.
- To some instructors, the clinical pathway may be seen as too behavioral. In some cases, this is the intent of the pathway: to evaluate psychomotor skills. An

immunization pathway is an example of psychomotor evaluation. The clinical pathway can be constructed in such a way as to provide opportunities for the student to use critical-thinking and problem-solving abilities in ways that the instructor can readily observe and evaluate. An example is priority setting and decision making related to immediate patient care needs. This is an advantage of the pathway in that it facilitates evaluation in spontaneous situations.

■ Conclusion

Clinical pathways are a means by which an instructor can objectively and effectively evaluate student learning and progress toward clinical outcomes. An advantage to use of pathways in one-time experiences is that the pathway serves as a criterion-based frame of reference for both the student and the instructor because the criteria are the same as for other clinical experiences in that course. The faculty member thus has an objective measure of student learning and performance, and the student always knows the measure on which he or she will be evaluated.

Clinical pathways are limited to brief experiences and are not designed to show professional growth and progress in learning over time. However, a pathway could be designed to appraise critical thinking and professional behaviors associated with spontaneous incidents, such as a problem patient. Nurse educators can use pathways as a creative means to address student performance in a variety of situations.

References

Atwal, A., & Caldwell, K. (2002). Do multidisciplinary integrated care pathways improve interprofessional collaboration? *Scandinavian Journal of Caring Sciences, 16*, 360–367.

Broughton, E. I. (2011). The "how" and "why" of cost-effectiveness analysis for care pathways. *International Journal of Care Pathways, 15*, 76–81.

Holaday, S. D., & Buckley K. M. (2008). A standardized clinical evaluation tool-kit: Improving nursing education and practice. *Annual Review of Nursing Education, 6*, 123–149.

Hunter, B., & Segrott, J. (2010). Using a clinical pathway to support normal birth: Impact on practitioner roles and working practices. *Birth: Issues in Perinatal Care, 37*, 227–236.

Kersbergen, A. L., & Hrbosky, P. E. (1996). Use of clinical map guides in precepted clinical experiences. *Nurse Educator, 21*(6), 19–22.

Kinsman, L. (2004). Clinical pathway compliance and quality improvement. *Nursing Standard, 18*, 33–35.

Kinsman, L., & James, E. L. (2001). Evidence-based practice needs evidence-based implementation. *Lippincott's Case Management, 5*, 208–219.

Oermann, M. H., & Gaberson, K. (2006). *Evaluation and testing in nursing education* (2nd ed.). New York, NY: Springer.

Panella, M. (2009). The impact of pathways: A significant decrease in mortality. *International Journal of Care Pathways, 13*, 57–61.

Renholm, M., Leino-Kilpi, H., & Suominen, T. (2002). Critical pathways: A systematic review. *Journal of Nursing Administration, 32*, 196–202.

Tanicala, M., L., Scheffer, B., K., & Roberts, M. S. (2011). Defining pass/fail. Nursing student clinical behaviors phase I: Moving toward a culture of safety. *Nursing Education Perspectives, 32*, 155–161. doi: 10.5480/1536-5026-32.3.155

Index

Note: Page numbers followed by *b*, *f*, or *t* indicate material in boxes, figures, or tables, respectively.